AF668981

THE SANKARA NETHRALAYA

Atlas of OPHTHALMIC ULTRASOUND AND ULTRASOUND BIOMICROSCOPY

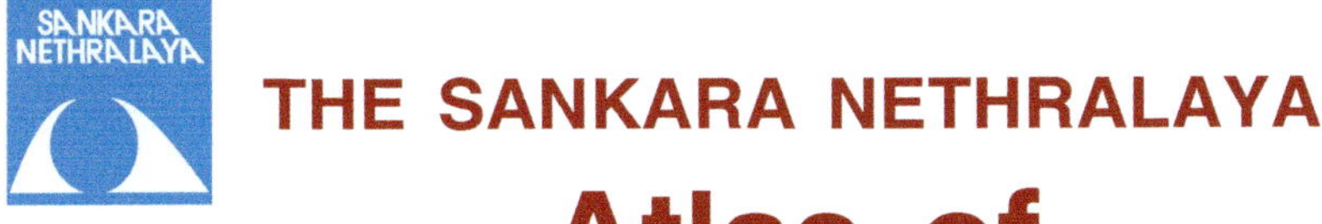

THE SANKARA NETHRALAYA

Atlas of OPHTHALMIC ULTRASOUND AND ULTRASOUND BIOMICROSCOPY

SECOND EDITION

Muna Bhende
Senior Consultant
Vitreoretinal Service

Harshali Kamat
Fellow, Vitreoretinal Surgery

Tandava Krishna
Fellow, Vitreoretinal Surgery

B Shantha
Deputy Director and
Senior Consultant, Glaucoma Service

Parveen Sen
Senior Consultant
Vitreoretinal Service

Vikas Khetan
Consultant, Vitreoretinal Service

Suchitra Pradeep
Consultant, Uvea Service

Sankara Nethralaya
18, College Road
Chennai, Tamil Nadu, India

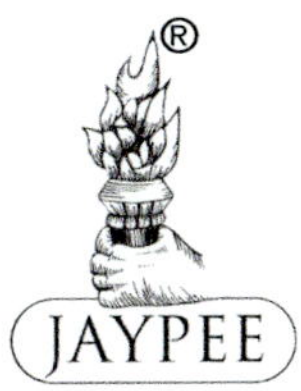

JAYPEE BROTHERS MEDICAL PUBLISHERS (P) LTD

New Delhi • Panama City • London • Philadelphia

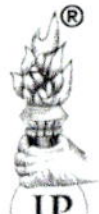

Jaypee Brothers Medical Publishers (P) Ltd

Headquarters

Jaypee Brothers Medical Publishers (P) Ltd
4838/24, Ansari Road, Daryaganj
New Delhi 110 002, India
Phone: +91-11-43574357
Fax: +91-11-43574314
Email: jaypee@jaypeebrothers.com

Overseas Offices

J.P. Medical Ltd
83 Victoria Street, London
SW1H 0HW (UK)
Phone: +44-2031708910
Fax: +02-03-0086180
Email: info@jpmedpub.com

Jaypee-Highlights Medical Publishers Inc.
City of Knowledge, Bld. 237, Clayton
Panama City, Panama
Phone: + 507-301-0496
Fax: + 507-301-0499
Email: cservice@jphmedical.com

Jaypee Medical Inc.
The Bourse
111 South Independence Mall East
Suite 835, Philadelphia, PA 19106, USA
Phone: + 267-519-9789
Email: joe.rusko@jaypeebrothers.com

Jaypee Brothers Medical Publishers (P) Ltd
17/1-B Babar Road, Block-B, Shaymali
Mohammadpur, Dhaka-1207
Bangladesh
Mobile: +08801912003485
Email: jaypeedhaka@gmail.com

Jaypee Brothers Medical Publishers (P) Ltd
Shorakhute, Kathmandu
Nepal
Phone: +00977-9841528578
Email: jaypee.nepal@gmail.com

Website: www.jaypeebrothers.com
Website: www.jaypeedigital.com

Inquiries for bulk sales may be solicited at: jaypee@jaypeebrothers.com

The Sankara Nethralaya Atlas of Ophthalmic Ultrasound and Ultrasound Biomicroscopy

First Edition: 2006

Second Edition: **2013**

ISBN 978-93-5090-535-7

Printed at Replika Press Pvt. Ltd.

Foreword to the First Edition

Although ophthalmic ultrasound is now widely accepted as an important tool for the diagnosis and management of many ocular and orbital disorders, most academic centers do not have formal training programs to teach the skills necessary for performing precise and accurate ultrasound examinations. Unless an individual can spend several months or more at one of the few centers in the world that have an expert echographer, most ophthalmic ultrasound is self taught by attending lectures, reading articles, and studying one of the few textbooks available in this field. A welcome addition to the collection of teaching materials currently available for ophthalmic ultrasound is *The Sankara Nethralaya Atlas of Ophthalmic Ultrasound.*

This group, consisting of mainly vitreoretinal surgeons who are also experienced echographers, has put together a concise, yet comprehensive text that is extremely well illustrated and very readable. Excellent examples of almost every ocular and orbital disorder, one might expect to encounter in the clinical practice of ophthalmic echography, are represented in this atlas. The reader's understanding of the ultrasound illustrations is enhanced with color fundus photographs and external photos, as well as CT scans and MRI scans of the orbit. One of the text's outstanding features is the use of "nuggets" in most of the chapters; charts which provide pearls of information that are important for the differentiation and diagnosis of particular conditions.

The authors are to be congratulated for carefully assembling this wealth of information in such a practical and straightforward manner. It demonstrates their thoughtful insight into the field of ophthalmic ultrasound as well as their skills as educators. This atlas will undoubtedly be an invaluable resource for new practitioners and will be of great interest to those already familiar with ultrasound of the eye and orbit.

Ronald L Green MD
Professor
Doheny Eye Institute
Department of Ophthalmology
University of Southern California Keck School of Medicine
Los Angeles, California
USA

Preface to the Second Edition

The first edition of *The Sankara Nethralaya Atlas of Ophthalmic Ultrasound* was intended to be both a teaching and practical reference tool for the ophthalmologist. Though more sophisticated imaging techniques in certain areas of ophthalmology have evolved over the past years, ultrasonography is still a useful tool that can be done in a clinic by the ophthalmologist. While updating some of the chapters of the first edition with more images and examples of representative cases, we have retained the original outline and pattern.

In this second edition *The Sankara Nethralaya Atlas of Ophthalmic Ultrasound and Ultrasound Biomicroscopy,* we have now included an entirely new section on ultrasound biomicroscopy that has widened the scope of this atlas to include anterior segment imaging as well. With text being kept to a minimum, the salient clinical and ultrasound features have been described with practical tips for technique, interpretation, and implications on management. Where possible, we have provided corresponding color photographs, pathology images as well as other diagnostic reports, such as CT and MRI. The combined experience of ophthalmologists from almost all the ophthalmic subspecialties has resulted in a large collection of cases both common and rare, where ultrasound imaging has been a valuable diagnostic aid.

We hope that this new, revised edition will prove to be useful to students, practising ophthalmologists, and radiologists who perform ophthalmic ultrasound.

Muna Bhende

Preface to the First Edition

Ultrasonography is an important investigative tool in ophthalmology, in particular for vitreous surgery, oncology, and orbital diseases. The ultrasonography department at Sankara Nethralaya consists of ophthalmologists, most of whom are trained vitreoretinal surgeons. The department performs about 40 procedures every day and has been doing so far almost two decades. This atlas is a compilation of the numerous classic and unusual cases that have been seen here, along with a brief outline of the salient clinical and ultrasound features. The nuggets at the end of the chapters are intended to serve as a quick reference in difficult situations. We are honored that an authority on the subject, Prof Ronald L Green, who has coauthored a classic textbook on Ophthalmic Ultrasound, has written the foreword for this atlas. This atlas is meant as both a basic text as well as a reference tool for both students of ophthalmology and practising ophthalmologists.

Muna Bhende

Acknowledgments

As we have continued most of the material from the first edition, we acknowledge the original contributors once again as without their help the foundation would have needed to be re-laid. Our mentor and chief Dr SS Badrinath continues to guide and inspire us in our endeavors. Dr Lingam Gopal and Dr Tarun Sharma, both stalwarts in vitreoretinal surgery, have provided encouragement, wise counsel and guidance through every stage of the preparation of the atlas.

The vitreoretinal department both consultants and fellows, has contributed in a huge way toward the material in this atlas.

The incorporation of the new section on ultrasound biomicroscopy has meant active involvement of more subspecialities notably glaucoma, uvea oncology, and optometry.

As always, we rely heavily on our support staff from photography, biomedical engineering, IT, and medical records as well as our secretarial staff. Their contribution to the creation of this atlas is invaluable.

To our patients—many of whom patiently underwent repeat evaluations in order to obtain the best images for the atlas—your contribution will go a long way in making this atlas a purposeful one.

Thanks to Shri Jitendar P Vij (Group Chairman), Mr Ankit Vij (Managing Director), Mr Tarun Duneja (Director - Publishing), Ms Sunita Katla (Publishing Manager), Ms Chetna Malhotra Vohra (Sr Manager, Business Development), Mr DC Gupta (Sr Editor), Ms Seema Dogra (Cover Designer), Mr Jayanandan (Bengaluru Branch), Ms Samina Khan (PA to Director), Mr Rajesh Sharma (Production Coordinator), Sandeep Tomar (Graphic Designer), and Arvind Kumar (DTP Operator) of M/s Jaypee Brothers Medical Publishers (P) Ltd, New Delhi, India who made this atlas a reality.

The list of individuals acknowledged below is by no means exhaustive and the authors apologize, if they have left out anyone inadvertently.

VR Consultants

Dr Pramod Bhende
Dr Dhanashree Ratra
Dr Pratik Ranjan Sen
Dr Ekta Rishi
Dr Pukhraj Rishi
Dr Chetan Rao
Dr Kasinathan
Dr Pradeep S
Dr Vinata Rajendran
Dr G Suganeswari
Dr Aditya Verma
Dr Kumar Saurabh
Dr Rupak Roy
Dr Sudipta Das

Uvea Department

Dr J Biswas
Dr Mamta Agarwal
Dr Partho Prathim Majumder

Glaucoma Department

Dr L Vijaya
Dr Aditya Neog
Dr Manish Pandey

VR Fellows

Dr Aditi Gupta
Dr Lakshmi Kunyal
Dr Bindu Appukuttan
Dr Shruti Thiagarajah
Dr Gaurav Mathur
Dr Mohd Kazi

Optometry

Ms Yamuna Devi L
Ms Shenbagam N
Ms Archana Babu

Neuroophthalmology

Dr Vijay Ananth

Oculoplasty

Dr Bipasha Mukherjee

Radiology

Dr Veena Noronha

Ocular Pathology

Dr Krishnakumar
Ms Vanitha

Secretarial Staff

Ms Anuradha
Ms Bindu
Ms Kalaivani

Photography department

Mr Krishna MS
Mr K Chidambaram
Mr CS Hariharan
Mr T Ravishankar
Mr M Thilak
Mr Shankar K

Biomedical Engineering

Mr P Krishnamurthy
Mr P Vinoth Kumar

Medical Records and IT teams

Contents

SECTION 6: Congenital Anomalies and Disorders of the Pediatric age Group

SECTION 7: Surgical Considerations

SECTION 8: Orbital Lesions

SECTION 9: Optic Nerve Disorders

SECTION 10: Ultrasound Biomicroscopy

Section 1

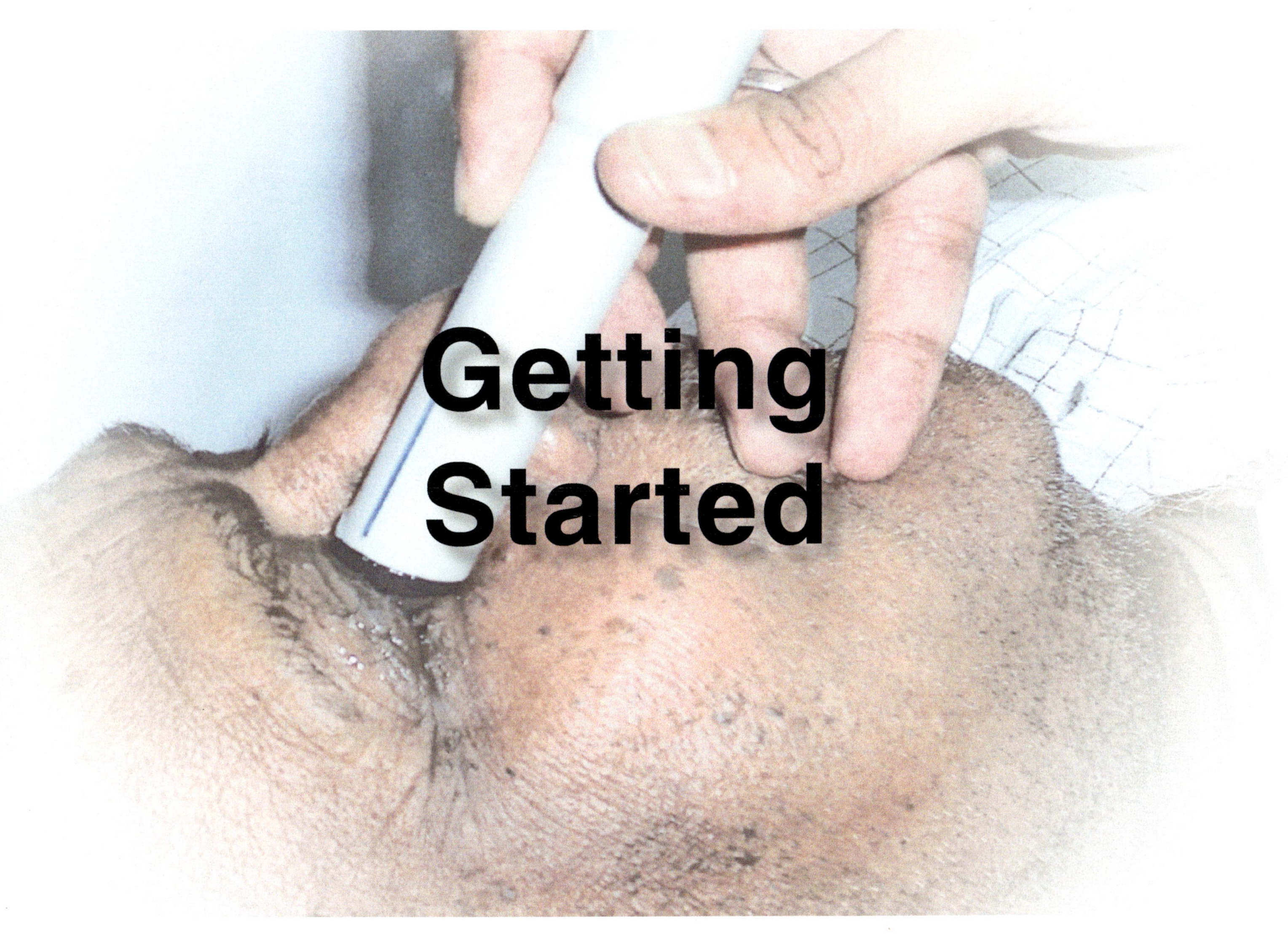

Getting Started

1 Principles of Ophthalmic Ultrasound

The acoustic spectrum extends from the audible range of 10–20,000 Hz to the vibrational states of matter with frequencies of $>10^{12}$ Hz. While abdominal ultrasound uses frequencies of 1–2 MHz, ophthalmic ultrasound incorporates frequencies of 8 MHz and above to produce images of the eye and orbit. These structures are more easily accessible from the surface, which permits the use of a higher frequency probe. Frequencies of 8–12 MHz comprise conventional ophthalmic ultrasound, while high frequency systems utilize a 20 MHz probe. Probe frequencies of 35–100 MHz comprise ultrasound biomicroscopy.

The physical principles are similar for all ultrasound systems and require an understanding of a few terms:

- *Pulse echo system:* The basic unit which includes a piezoelectric transducer to generate the ultrasonic wave, a receiver which processes the returning waves and a display screen
- *Acoustic impedance:* The difference between the strength of the returning echoes from tissue boundaries with abrupt changes in acoustic properties. These surfaces are also known as acoustic interfaces. The greater the difference between the acoustic impedance of adjacent structures, the stronger is the returning echo
- *Angle of incidence:* This refers to the angle of the sound beam relative to the area of interest. The more perpendicular the beam, the stronger is the returning echo
- *Resolution:* The ability to distinguish between adjacent echoes, both axial and lateral. This is enhanced by the use of a focused sound beam
- *Amplification:* This is an important part of the signal processing that occurs before the returning sound beam is displayed on the monitor. Three types of amplification are commonly used:
    1. *Linear:* Limited range of echo densities, but can show minor differences within this range
    2. *Logarithmic:* Wider range of echo densities, but does not show very minor differences between echo intensity
    3. *S curve:* A method that tries to combine the benefits of both the above to enable better tissue differentiation
- *Gain:* This is the procedure of increasing or decreasing the amplitude of echoes that are displayed on the screen
- *Time gain compensation (TGC):* The technique used to enhance the returning echoes from deeper structures by reducing those from the structures closer to the surface. This is typically utilized in studying the orbit
- *Display of signals:* The ultrasound signal that is received can be displayed in 3 ways: A mode, B mode or a combination of the above. Other modifications include the three-dimensional ultrasound which uses a rotating transducer rather than the oscillating one used in the conventional ultrasound system and a combination of color Doppler with the B scan

- *A scan:* One-dimensional time—**A**mplitude display in which the echoes, represented by spikes from the baseline, are spaced depending on their distance from each other and the probe. The amplification is linear in the A scan used for axial biometry, logarithmic when combined with the B scan and S-shaped in the standardized A scan for tissue differentiation
- *B scan:* Two-dimensional **B**rightness display where the strength of the returning echo is displayed as a dot on the screen, the brightness being directly proportional to the echo strength

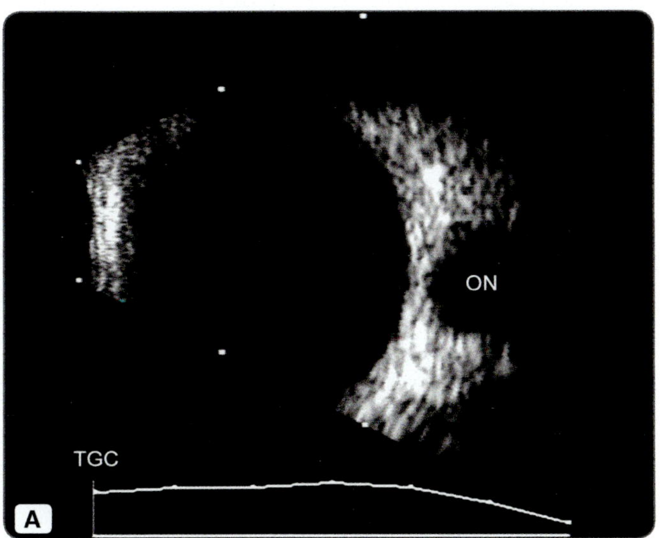

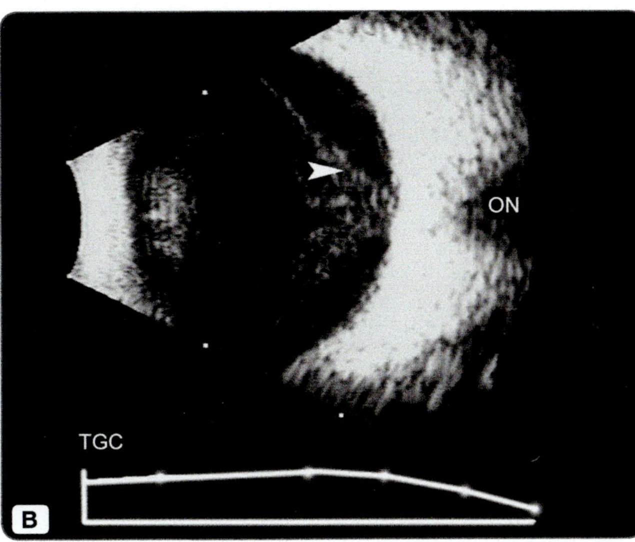

Figures 1.1A and B: B scan images of an eye with vitreous hemorrhage. Note the clear vitreous cavity when the scanning is done at a lower gain. Figure B shows that at higher gain there are significant intragel echoes (arrowhead) and an incomplete posterior vitreous detachment (PVD).

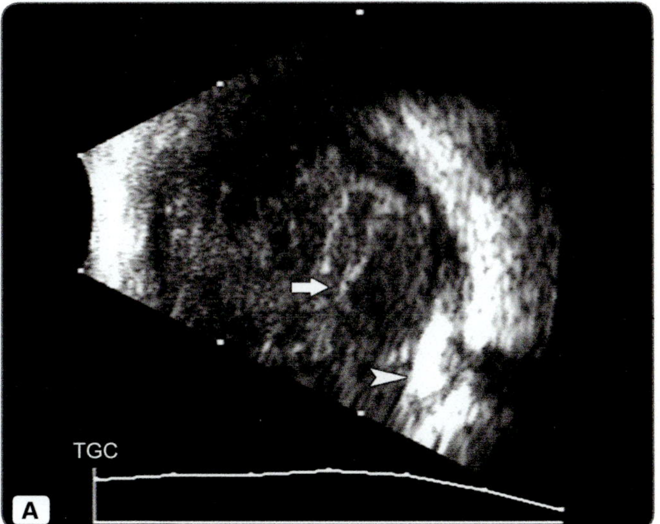

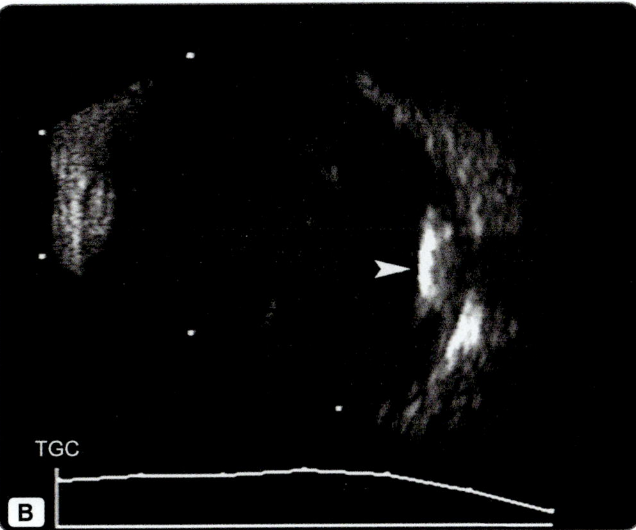

Figures 1.2A and B: B scan images of an eye with vitreous hemorrhage (arrow) and a retained IOFB (arrowhead). This set of images demonstrates the usefulness of reducing the gain to better delineate the IOFB (arrowhead) as seen in Figure B.

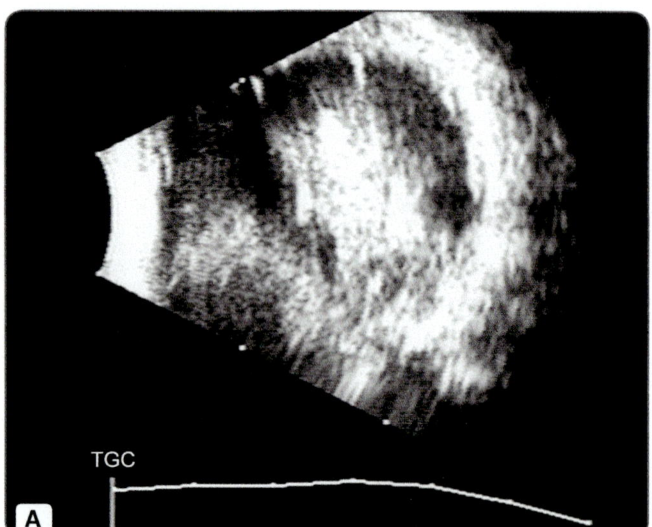

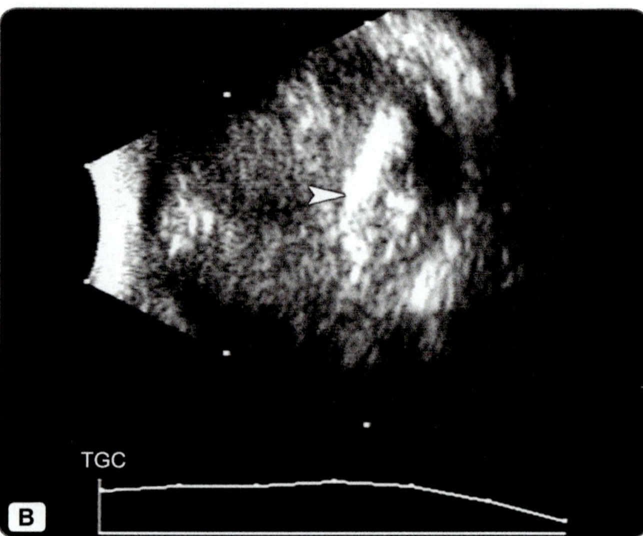

Figures 1.3A and B: B scan images of an eye with retinoblastoma. Note the high reflective nature of the tumor. Clumps of very high reflectivity are seen within the mass that are suggestive of calcification. By reducing the gain in Figure B, the calcification (arrowhead) and shadowing is seen much better.

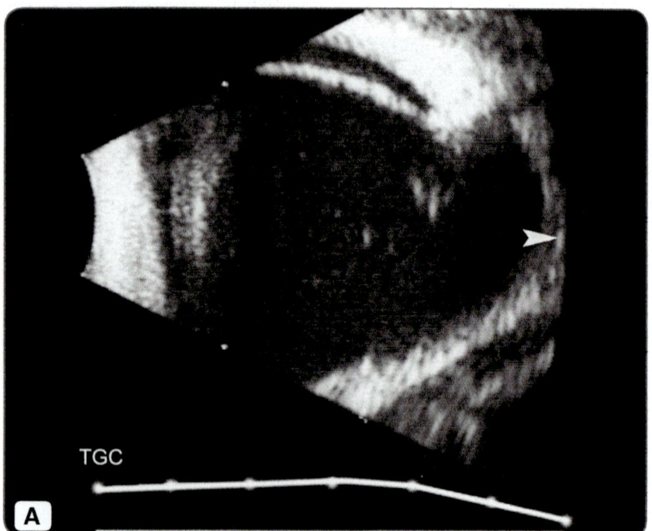

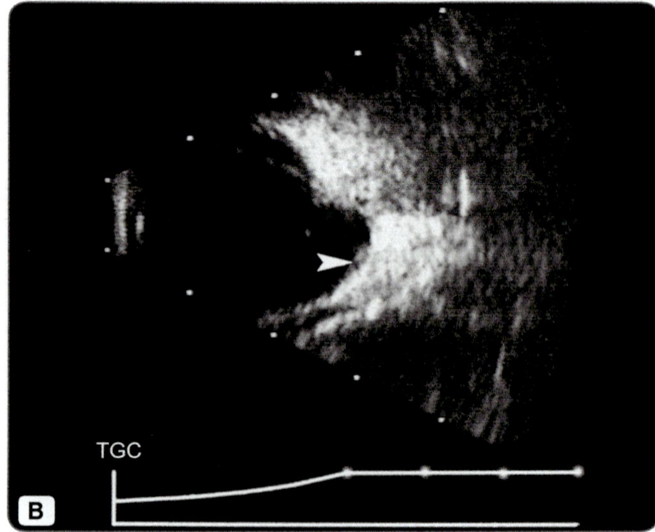

Figures 1.4A and B: B scan images of an eye with a large choroidal coloboma. Note that at the depth setting of 3 cm, the posterior ectatic area of the coloboma (arrowhead) is not well seen (Fig. A). In Figure B, the depth has been increased to better study the posterior globe contour. Note also the TGC scales at the bottom of the images. In Figure A, the TGC setting is raised to image the vitreous echoes. Figure B shows how, by dampening the TGC anteriorly, one is able to enhance the returning echoes from the orbit.

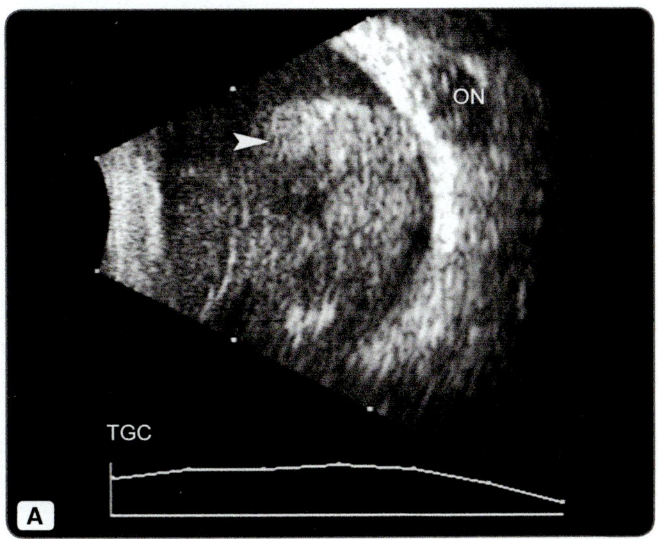

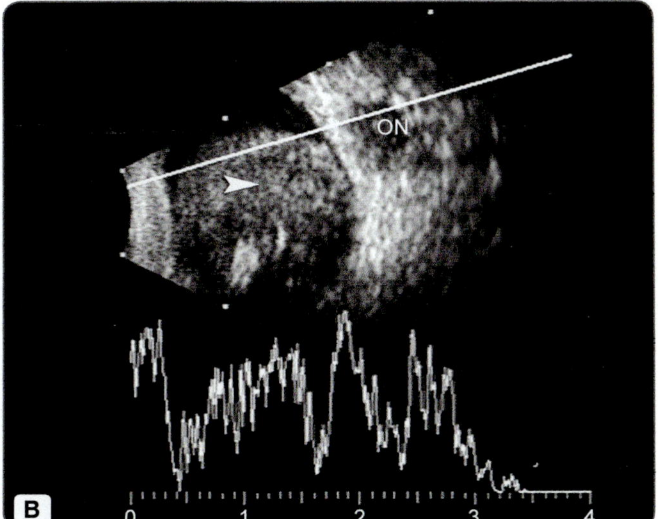

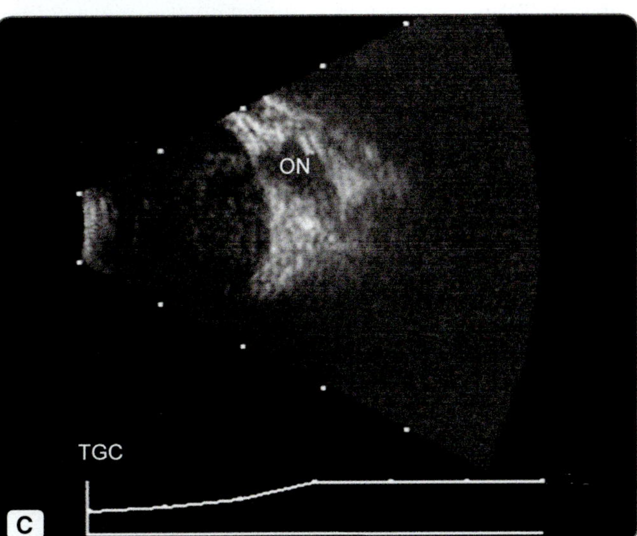

Figures 1.5A to C: These images are of an eye with retinoblastoma and optic nerve involvement. Figure A shows the large exophytic tumor with calcification (arrowhead). Figure B includes an A vector as well as a deeper probe penetration to better visualize the optic nerve(ON). Note that the TGC setting is such that the tumor as well as the enlarged optic nerve shadow is seen. In Figure C, the depth penetration has been further increased, and with a change in the TGC settings, the vitreous echoes have been dampened so as to get an excellent view of the thickened optic nerve.

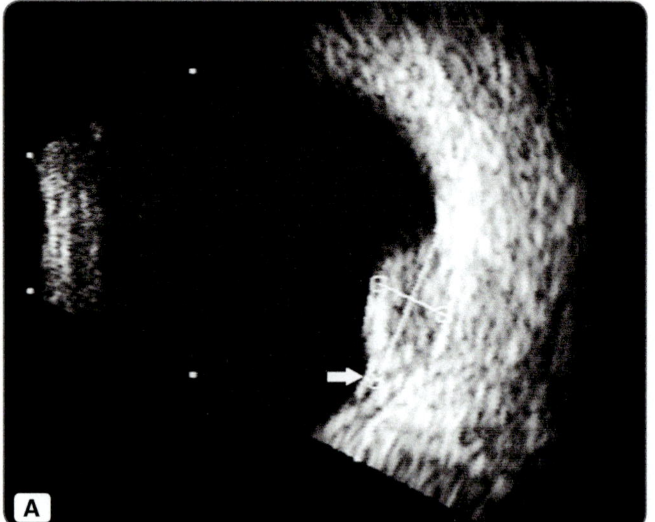

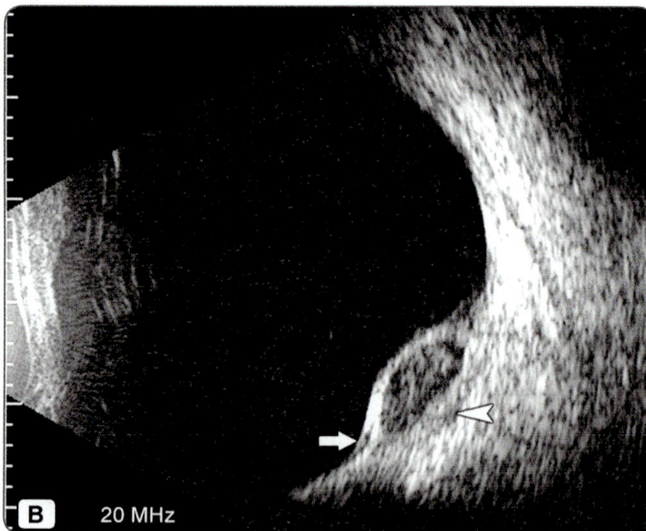

Figures 1.6A and B: B scan images of similar sized choroidal melanomas. Figure A is an image taken with a 10 MHz probe, whereas Figure B is a 20 MHz image. Note the improved resolution with the 20 MHz probe where the shallow retinal detachment (arrow) is well seen as well as the small extrascleral nodule (arrowhead) *(Figure B courtesy Dr Vincenzina Mazzeo, Italy).*

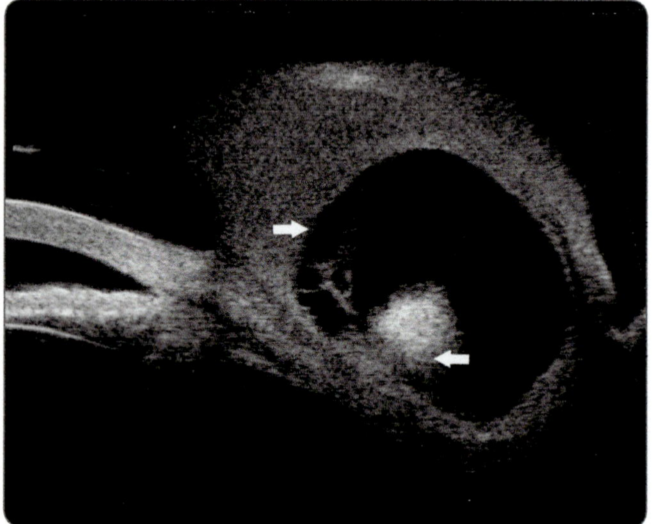

Figures 1.7: Ultrasound biomicroscopy with a 35 MHZ probe shows that anteriorly located structures till the pars plana can be imaged better than with the 10 or 12 MHz probe. In this case, a subconjunctival cysticercus cyst.

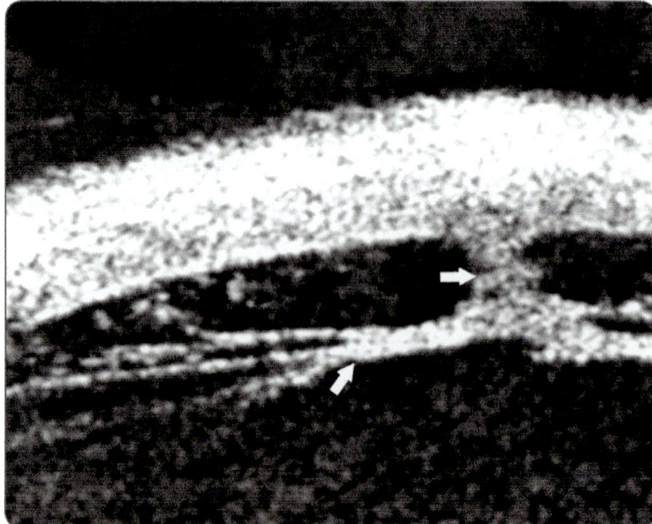

Figure 1.8: An ultrasound biomicroscopy image of proliferation from the sclerotomy site (arrows) using a 50 MHz probe. This image is of still higher resolution; however, note the corresponding decrease in depth penetration.

2 Technique of Evaluation and the Normal Ultrasound

Ultrasound evaluation of the eye and orbit is performed in the supine or sitting position. The probe is placed directly over the conjunctiva or cornea or placed over closed lids. The former has the advantage of reducing the sound attenuation caused by the lids; however, it requires sterilization of the probe between procedures. The latter technique is more frequently followed and is more advisable in cases where there is suspicion of a breach in the ocular surface. A coupling solution is used to provide standoff and avoid attenuation caused by air.

The ideal sequence of events during an ultrasound evaluation would be:

- History including symptoms, findings of previous ultrasound or other imaging techniques performed and details of previous treatment including surgery. Details of clinical findings, provisional diagnosis and information required from the ultrasound are essential.
- Clinical examination especially in cases with a clear media.
- B scan evaluation of the eye. This gives details of any abnormality seen including its topography. Being a two-dimensional evaluation, the structures are better appreciated than on A scan evaluation alone.
- A scan examination with the vector passing through the area of interest. This would provide further details regarding the reflectivity of the lesion.
- Evaluation of the optic nerve and orbit. This is of particular importance in cases of trauma, inflammations and intraocular tumors.
- Use of calipers to measure the size of the mass lesion if any, as well as measurements of intraocular structures if required.
- In case of suspected orbital pathology, evaluation of the eye first, followed by the orbit is essential. It is also important to examine the opposite orbit for comparison.
- In cases of congenital or developmental glaucomas, axial length measurement is recommended.

OCULAR SCANS

Probe Positions

- Transverse: Gives the lateral extent of a lesion
- Longitudinal: Gives the anteroposterior extent of the lesion
- Axial: Demonstrates the lesion in relation to the lens and the optic nerve

ORBITAL SCANS

Probe Placement

- Transocular: Best for demonstrating lesions of the mid and posterior orbit
- Paraocular: Demonstration of lesions of the lids and anterior orbit.

Extraocular muscles are best evaluated both by transverse and longitudinal scans. The widest part of the muscle is chosen while measuring the thickness, and rather than the individual thickness, it is the comparison with the same muscle of the other eye that is of significance as is the relative change in appearance and thickness on follow-up.

NUGGETS

The vitreous cavity is normally echolucent, and abnormal findings are usually high reflective hence easily detected.

The orbital echoes are high reflective due to the presence of orbital fat. Abnormalities that are low reflective are more easily picked up.

Due to the variable echoes within the orbit, it is essential that the opposite orbit be examined before any pathology is diagnosed.

NORMAL APPEARANCE OF OCULAR AND ORBITAL STRUCTURES

The first few millimeters comprising the cornea, anterior chamber and anterior lens capsule are not easily visualized without adequate standoff or an immersion technique.

Lens

The entire lens can be seen with the standoff technique or an immersion scan. It is seen as an oval high reflective structure with intralesional echoes varying from none to highly reflective depending on the amount of cataract.

Vitreous

This is acoustically clear but can show low reflective echoes depending on the amount of syneresis. A senile posterior vitreous detachment can be seen in the elderly as a smooth, mobile low reflective membrane having no posterior pole attachments. Similar findings can be seen in high myopia.

Retina, Choroid and Sclera

All three are seen as a single high reflective structure. The layers are seen distinctly only in pathological conditions such as retinal detachment, choroidal effusion, scleritis, etc.

Optic Nerve

This is seen as a wedge-shaped acoustic void in the retrobulbar region on an axial scan. This view, however, gives limited information. The vertical transverse approach at low gain settings is the ideal view for imaging the optic nerve.

Extraocular Muscles

These are seen as echolucent to low reflective fusiform structures within the orbit, extending posteriorly from their tendinous insertions towards the orbital apex. The superior rectus-LPS complex is the thickest and the inferior rectus is the thinnest of the muscles. The inferior oblique is usually not imaged except in pathological conditions.

Axial Length

This is best assessed with the A scan. It is approximately 17 mm at birth and reaches the full length of approximately 23 mm by the age of 10 years.

Description of a Lesion

- Location in relation to the easily demonstrable landmarks, e.g. optic disc or lens in an intraocular lesion; optic nerve, globe and extraocular muscles in an orbital lesion
- Extent—both anteroposterior and lateral
- Dimensions—in case of tumors and other solid lesions
- Shape and configuration—whether point like, membrane like or a mass

- Internal reflectivity—whether echolucent, low, moderate or highly reflective. The sclera is considered as 100% reflective and the reflectivity of other structures is compared with that of the sclera.
- Structure—whether solid or cystic, regular or irregular
- Degree of sound attenuation, if any
- Mobility—includes active movements, such as internal vascularity within a mass, movement of a live intravitreal cysticercus; and after-movements such as that seen with a complete posterior vitreous detachment

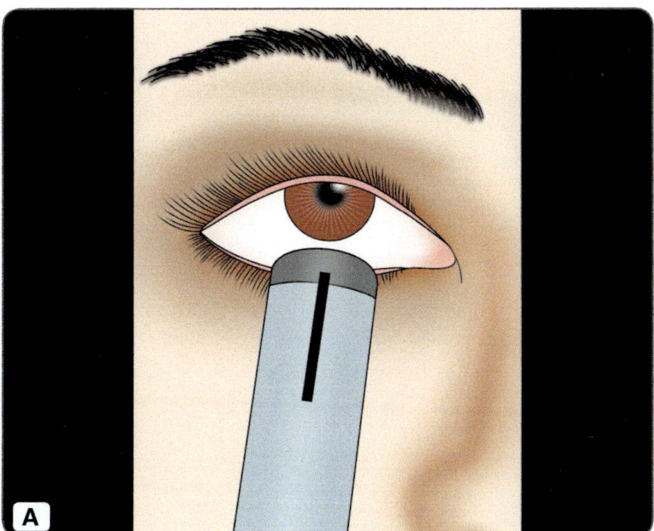

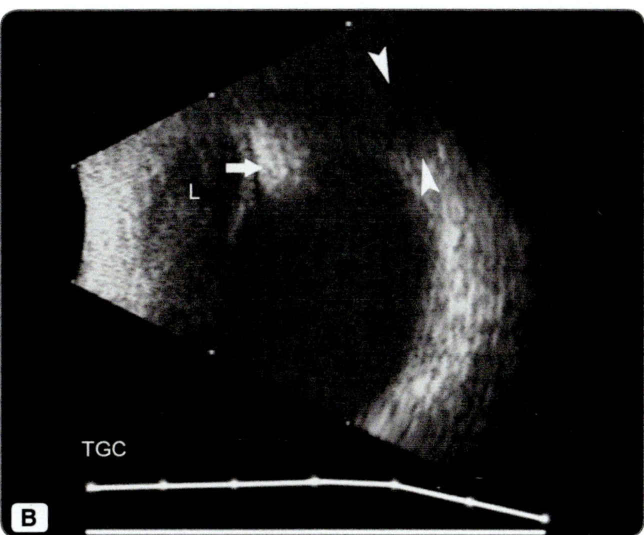

Figures 2.1A and B: Schematic and ultrasound image using the horizontal transverse technique of examination. This is able to demonstrate a foreign body located just behind the lens in the temporal periphery (arrow); arrowhead shows area of orbital shadowing. Note the indicator on the probe showing that the temporal quadrant is uppermost in the image.

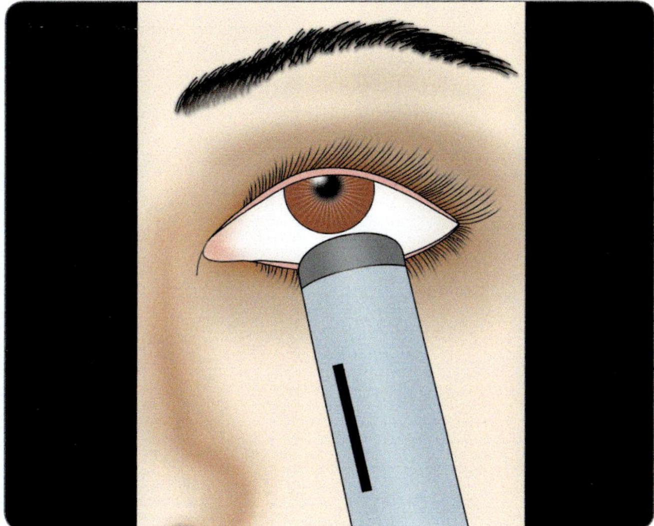

Figure 2.1C: Schematic showing the probe indicator placed nasally during transverse scanning.

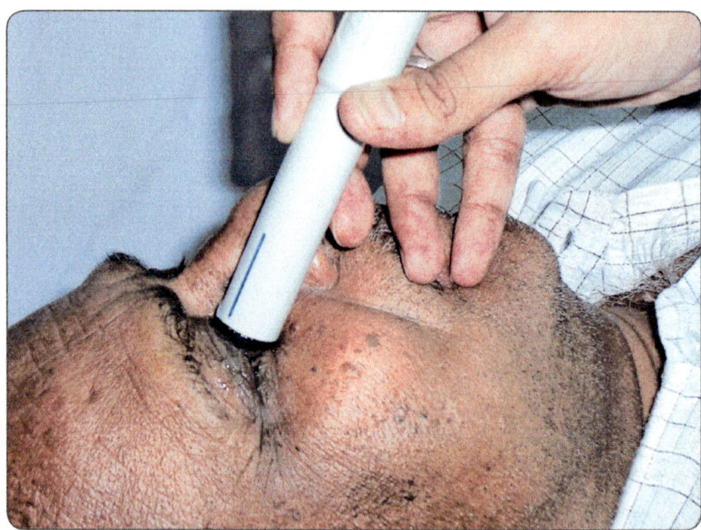

Figure 2.2A: Photograph showing the longitudinal scan technique. Here the probe is placed inferior to the limbus, scanning the upper half of the eyeball.

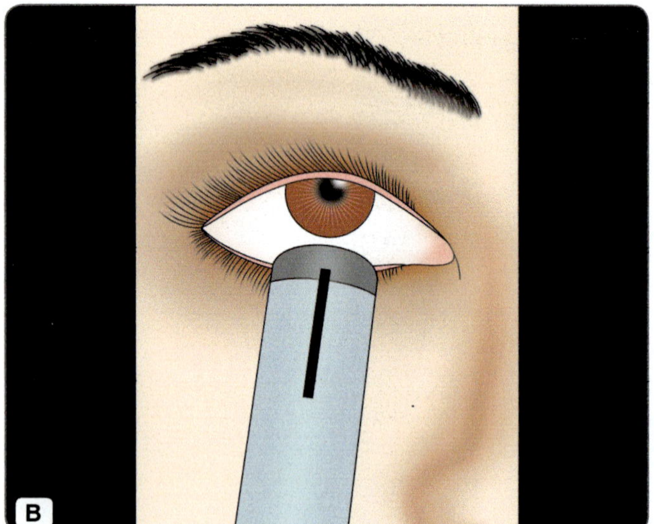

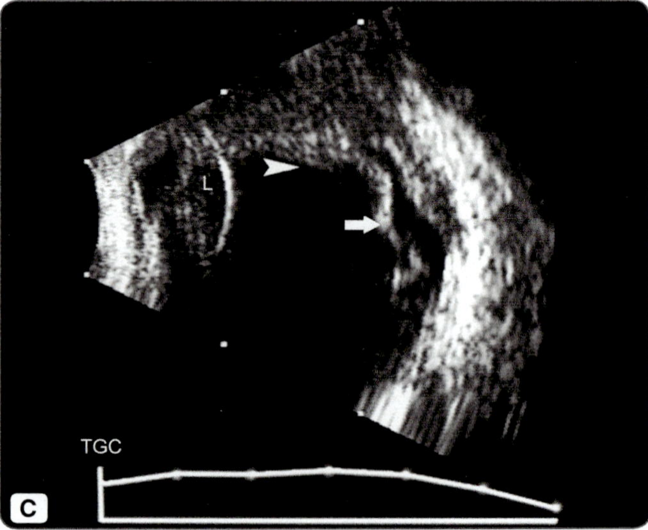

Figures 2.2B and C: The schematic shows the location of probe placement over the open lids. Figure C is a longitudinal scan showing a ciliochoroidal mass lesion (arrowhead) in the upper half with a secondary retinal detachment (arrow). Note the optic nerve shadow in the lower part of the image.

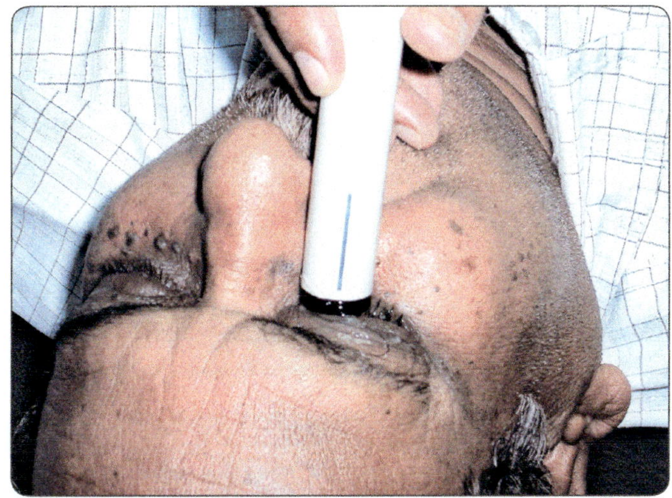

Figure 2.3A: Technique of performing the axial scan. The photograph shows the probe centered vertically above the closed eyelids.

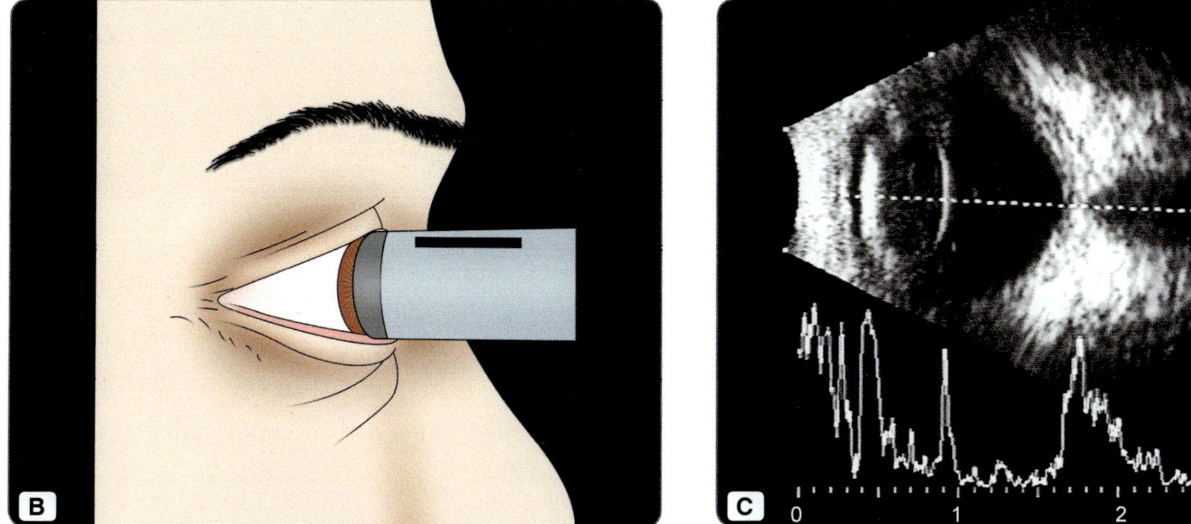

Figures 2.3B and C: The schematic shows the placement over the cornea. The ultrasound image shows the vertical axial image of an eye. Here the cornea, lens and optic nerve shadow are well aligned in the center of the image.

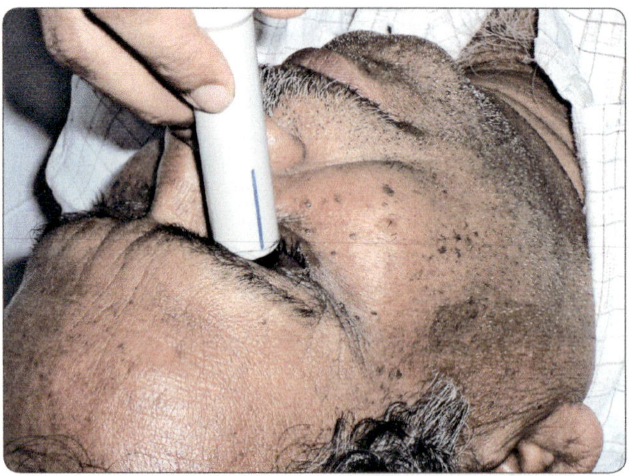

Figure 2.3D: Photograph showing the transverse axial technique.

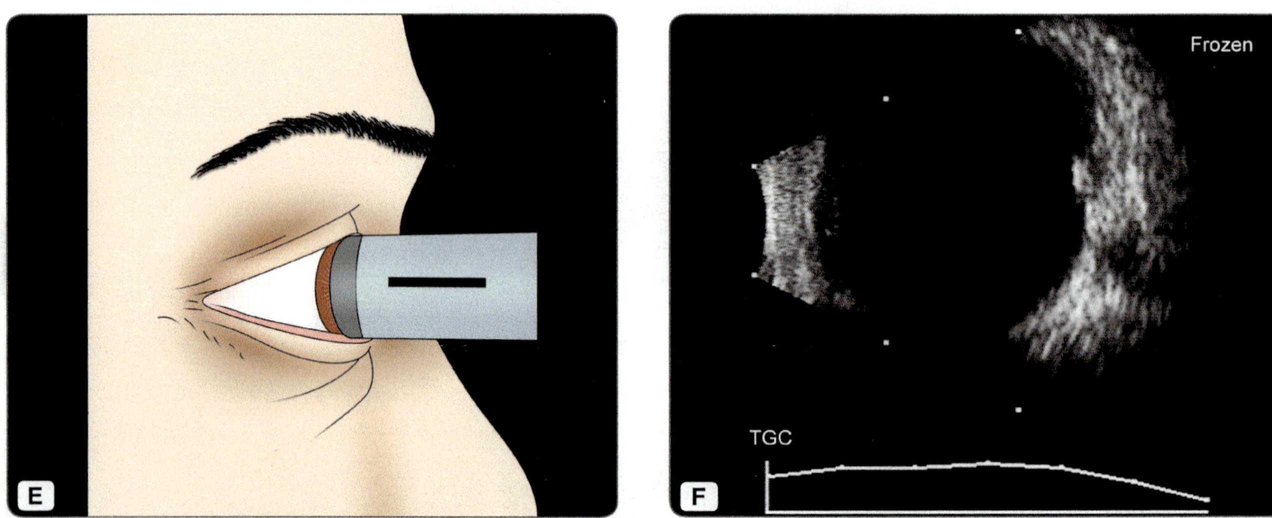

Figures 2.3E and F: The schematic shows this over the open lids. The ultrasound image shows an elevation temporal to the optic disc in the region of the macula.

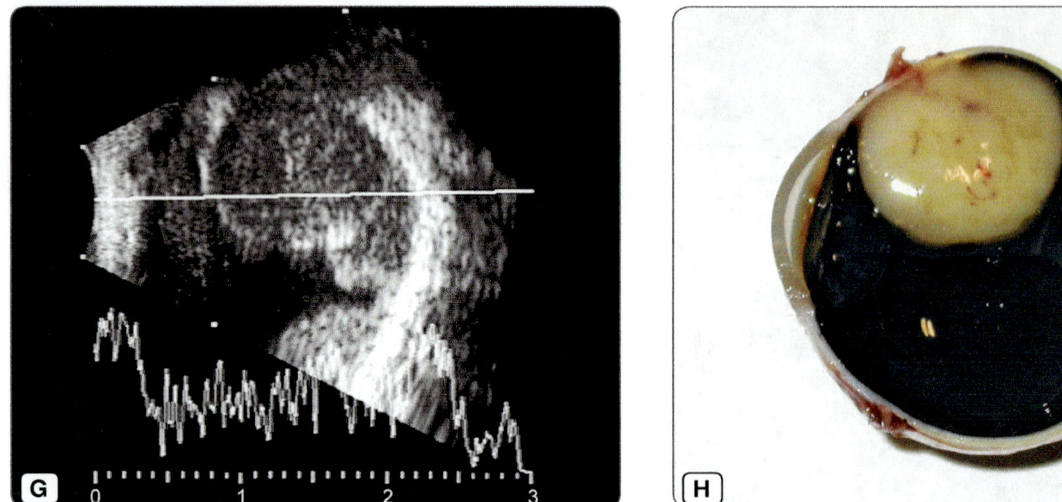

Figures 2.3G and H: The gross photograph of the sectioned globe after enucleation shows a mass lesion in the temporal quadrant. Axial B scan with vector A shows a choroidal mass in the temporal quadrant with a secondary retinal detachment.

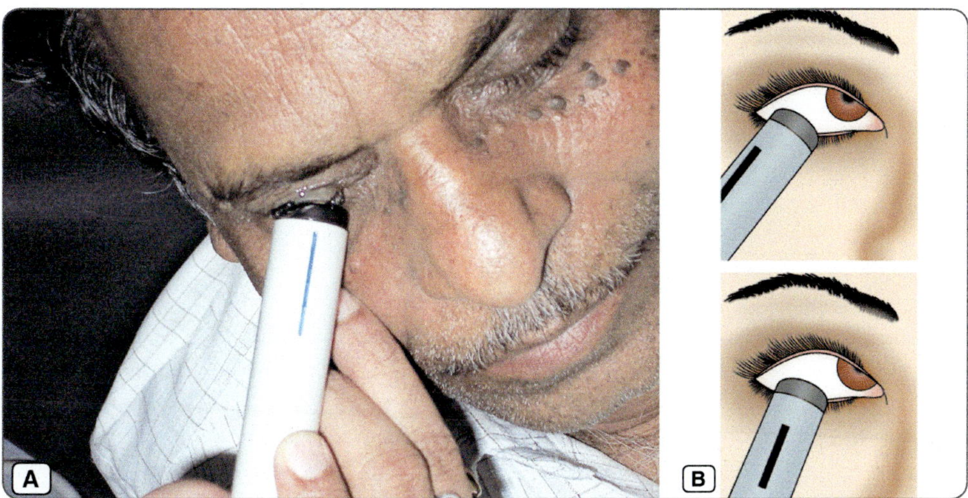

Figures 2.4A and B: Photograph and schematic showing the oblique probe placement to examine lesions that are not directly in the horizontal or vertical plane.

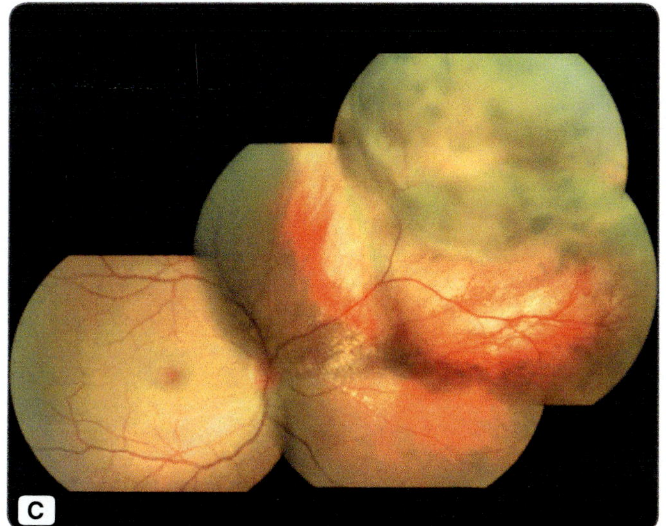

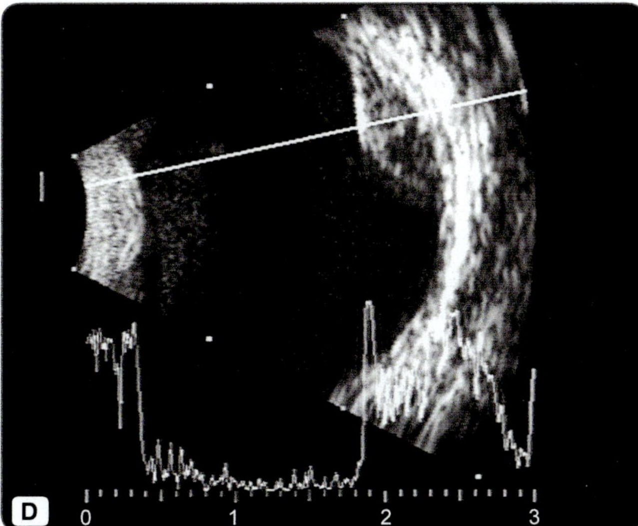

Figures 2.4C and D: The clinical photograph shows a pigmented choroidal tumor in the superonasal quadrant. The obliquely placed probe picks up the lesion which is demonstrated in the upper half of the image. The absence of the optic nerve shadow indicates that the scan is not axial.

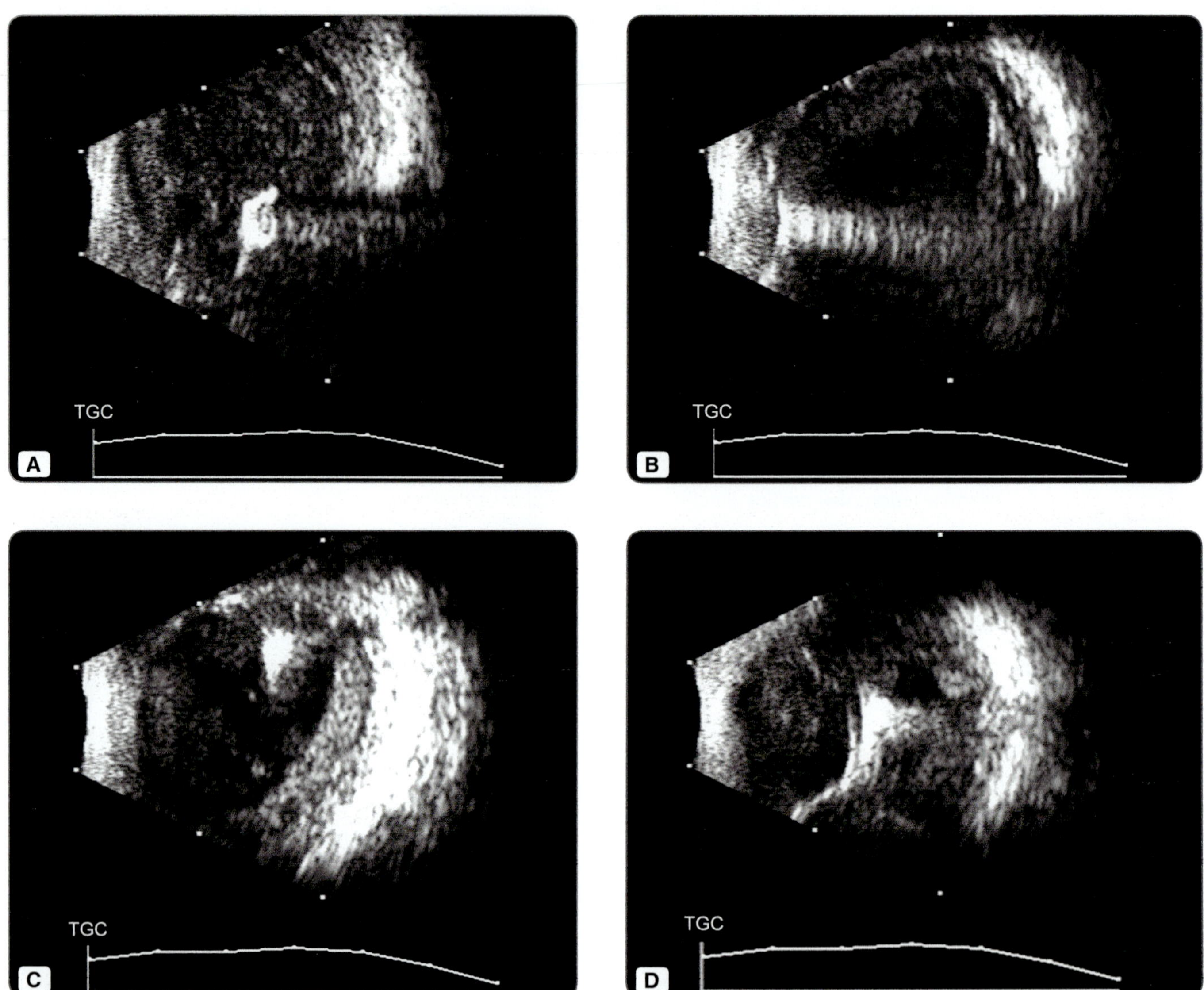

Figures 2.5A to D: A series of B scan images of an eye with history of penetrating trauma. Note the apparent multiple intraocular foreign bodies each one seen with a different probe position. Figure D is one position where a continuity between echoes is established, confirming the presence of a single large IOFB, in this case, a broken spring. This emphasizes the importance of scanning in various positions to obtain an accurate impression.

3 Imaging Artifacts

Artifacts are defined as reflections or echoes that appear on the image but do not correspond in location or intensity to an actual interface in the eye being studied.

Production of artifacts depends on the following factors:

- Differences in acoustic impedance of the structures being studied by decreasing or increasing the speed of sound
- Angle of incidence of the sound wave on the object
- Shape of the object
- Path through which the sound has to travel before reaching the object of interest.

Types of artifacts commonly encountered in ophthalmic ultrasound:

- **Reverberation artifacts**—occur when sound waves are reflected between two highly reflective surfaces. This causes an artificial delay in the return of the signal, which repositions the interface further from the probe than it actually is. The most common cause of this type of artifact is insufficient coupling gel between the eye and the probe, when an air bubble can be trapped between the two (external reverberation). Other structures that can cause such artifacts are IOLs and air gun pellets (internal reverberations). One can avoid this type of artifact by manipulating the probe to vary the distance between the probe and interface or change the angle of the probe relative to the interface of interest. The artifact will either disappear or change position to lie on the side of the object of interest away from the probe.
- **"Ring-down" or "comet tail artifact"**—occurs with small highly reflective objects such as air bubbles or metal. This occurs due to the vibrations of the object that are caused by the ultrasound wave. These vibrations cause a change in the return time of the reflected sound resulting in very high intensity reverberations adjacent to the object. These echoes rapidly trail off causing the comet tail effect. The reverberations are equidistant and generally decrease in strength with increasing distance from the probe.
- **Shadowing** is blockage of sound wave transmission by a highly reflective interface. This appears as a hypointense area behind a bright echo. It can be caused by calcium, glass, bone, air, metal or gas.
- **Angle of incidence artifact**—is produced when the probe is oriented perpendicular to the surface of a very smooth and highly reflective interface. This can cause the mistaken impression of an IOFB or calcium, e.g. a sound beam perpendicular to the macula can sometimes show up a highly reflective linear echo that is mistaken for a scar.

- **Refractive artifacts**—occur when the emitted sound beam traverses the edge of the lens, especially in an axial scan. This causes a difference in the perceived posterior globe contour, the peripheral retina appearing elevated relative to the central area. Sometimes, shadowing may also be caused behind the elevated area. This artifact can be avoided by redirecting the probe away from the lens edge. Tumor like elevations at the posterior pole caused by refraction of sound through the margins of the lens are called Baum's bumps. These can be avoided by taking a scan plane through an area outside the limbus. To be doubly sure, whenever a mass is seen at the posterior pole, scans should pass through different planes to rule out this refraction artifact.
- **Enhancement**—Increase in reflectivity posterior to a weakly attenuating lesion, e.g. serous orbital cyst.

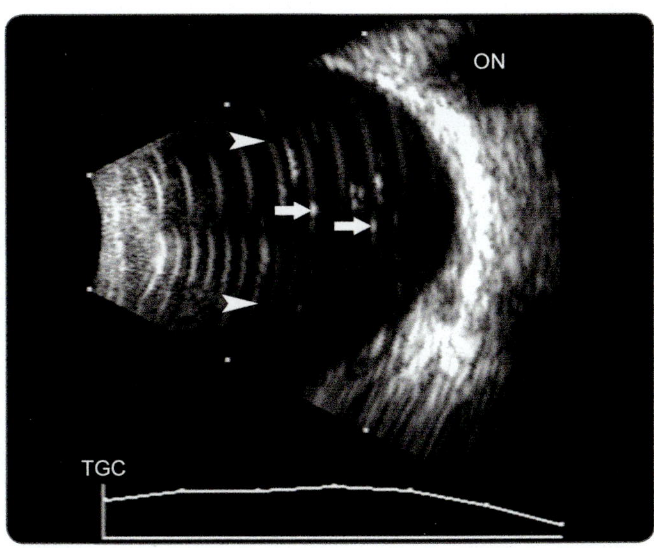

Figure 3.1: Reverberation artifact. This is caused by bubbles of silicone oil in the anterior chamber (arrowheads showing the reverberations). Tiny emulsified droplets are seen as high reflective dot echoes (arrows). ON = optic nerve.

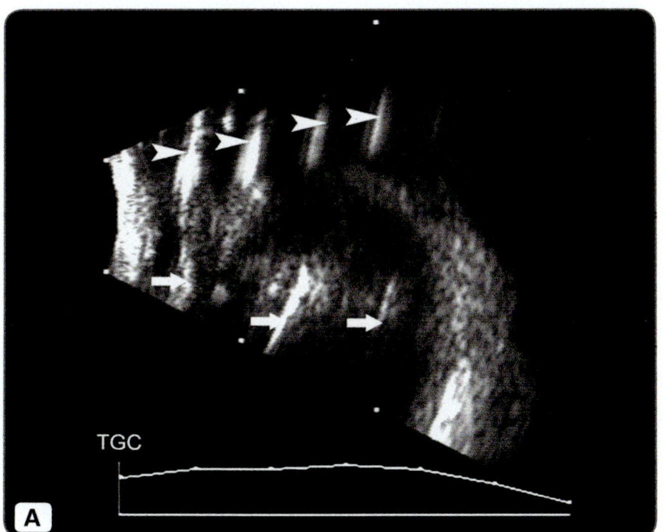

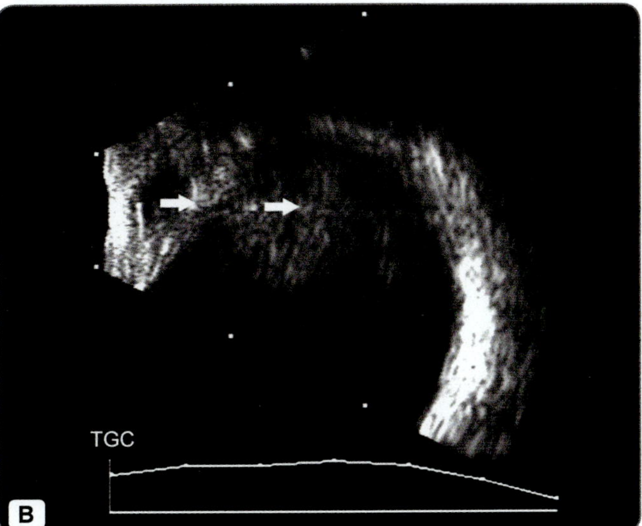

Figures 3.2A and B: Artifact due to insufficient coupling between the probe and the eye. This is a pseudophakic eye in a young child with posterior capsule opacification. The trapped air bubble between the probe and the eye causes reverberations (arrowheads) that may mimic an IOFB and hinder proper evaluation of the posterior segment. The IOL reverberations are also seen (arrows). Figure B shows that by increasing the amount of gel, the artifact disappears. This artifact is commonly encountered when the probe is placed just below the superior orbital rim to examine the upper orbit.

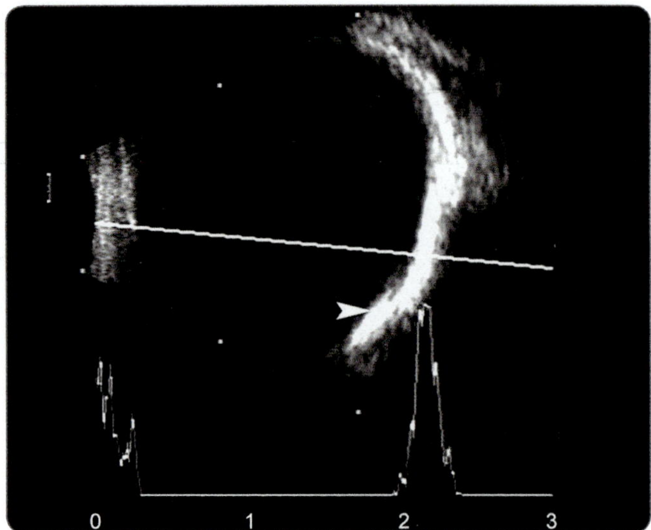

Figure 3.3: Shadowing caused by a plaque of calcification (arrowhead) on the posterior globe wall in a case of choroidal osteoma.

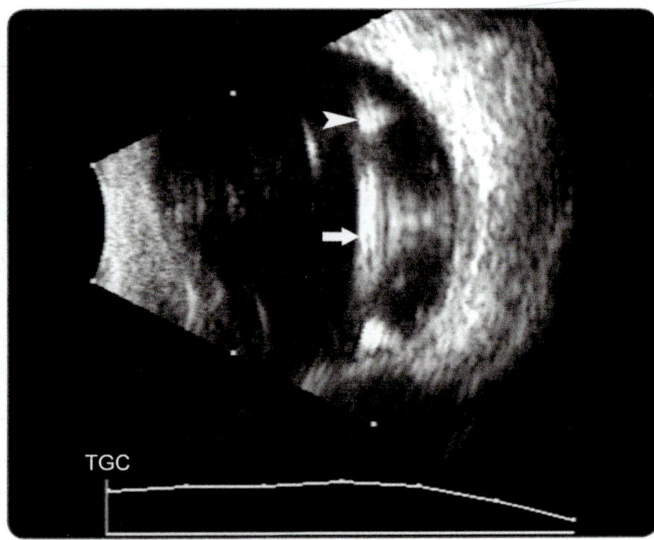

Figure 3.4: Reverberations caused by the optic (arrow) and haptic (arrowhead) of a posteriorly dislocated IOL.

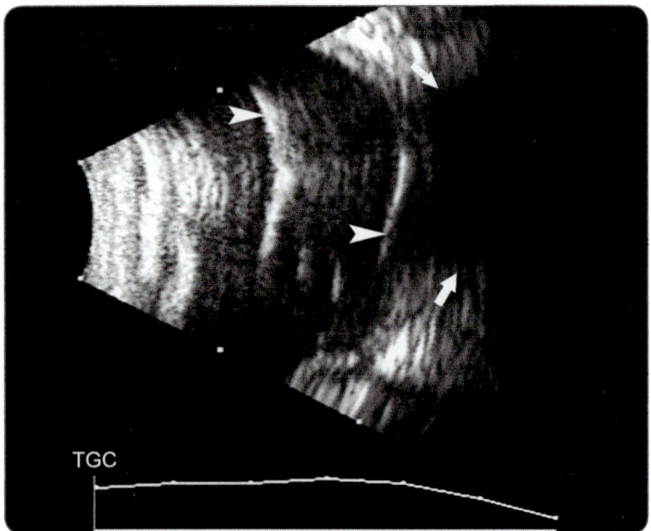

Figure 3.5: Both reverberation (arrowheads) and shadowing (arrow) artifacts can be caused by large air bubbles as is seen in this case.

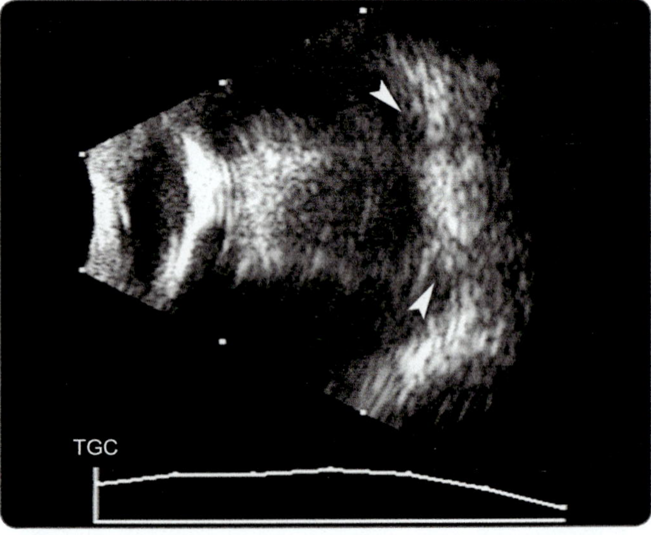

Figure 3.6: Refraction artifact. Note the difference in perceived globe contour (arrowheads) when the ultrasound beam traverses the edge of the IOL.

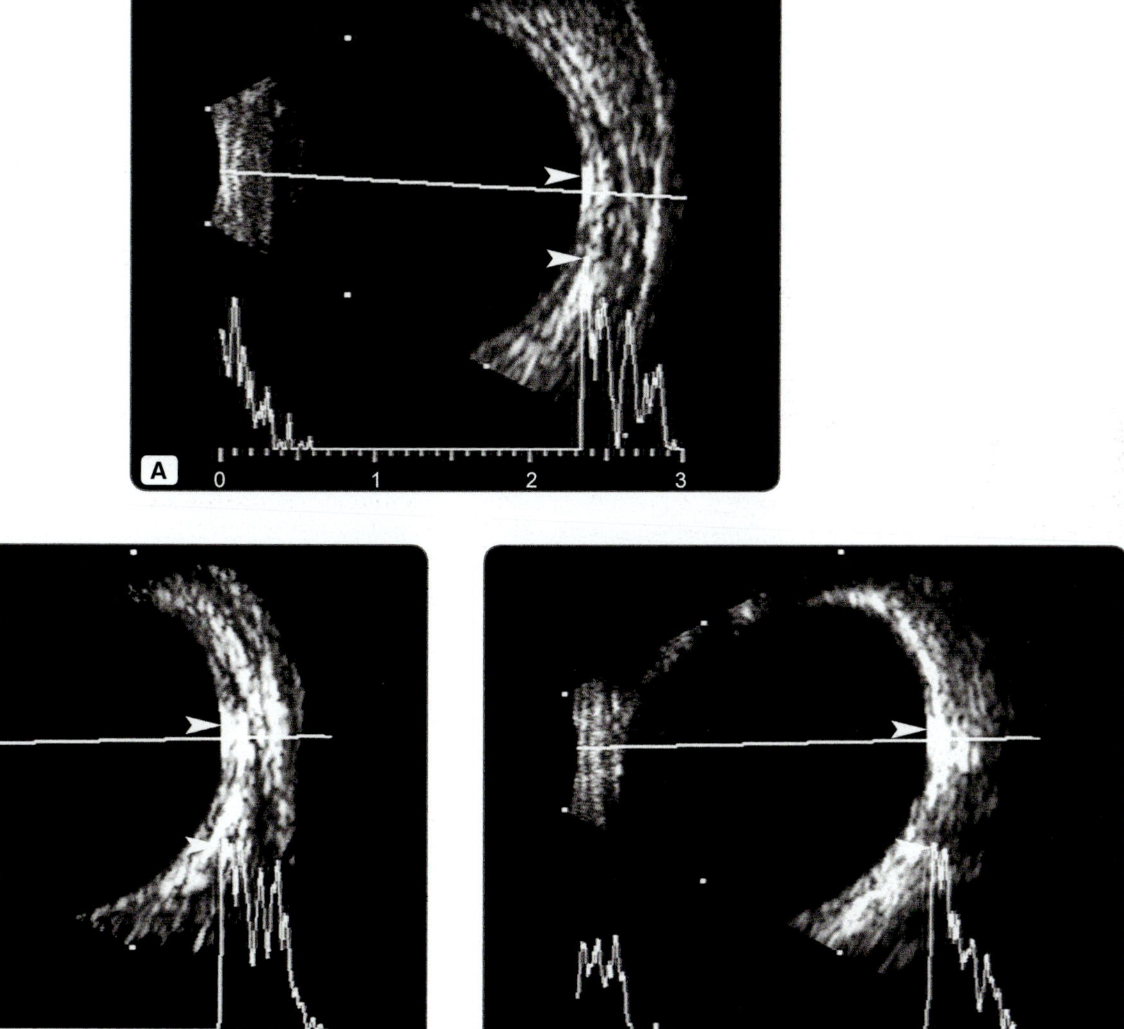

Figures 3.7A to C: Angle of incidence artifact. B scan with vector A of an eye with a pigmented flat lesion in the right eye. The Figure A shows a high reflective flat lesion on the globe wall with high reflectivity. Note that the probe and vector pass perpendicular to this area. Figures B and C are images of the opposite eye showing the same high reflective area which changes position with change of gaze, confirming that this is an artifact.

Section 2

Vitreoretinal Diseases

4 Vitreous Hemorrhage

CLINICAL FEATURES

- Vitreous hemorrhage is a common cause of reduced vision and occurs due to proliferative vascular retinopathies, trauma, disorders of coagulation, retinal breaks, polypoidal choroidal vasculopathy and tumors.
- Long-standing vitreous hemorrhage, hemorrhage in a one-eyed patient, bilateral vitreous hemorrhage and that associated with a retinal detachment and secondary glaucoma are indications for vitreous surgery.
- Ultrasonography is useful as a diagnostic, prognostic and follow-up tool.
- It helps to determine the source of vitreous hemorrhage and associated pathology.

ULTRASONOGRAPHY

- Fresh vitreous hemorrhage is echolucent or very low reflective. These dot-like echoes on B scan may need higher gain settings for detection. A similar finding is seen in hemorrhage in a vitrectomized eye where the blood is dispersed and freely mobile.
- In old or long standing vitreous hemorrhage, the dot-like echoes organize to form membranes of varying reflectivity across their extent. These are most dense inferiorly as a result of gravity.
- Vitreous hemorrhage may or may not be associated with a posterior vitreous detachment (PVD).

POSTERIOR VITREOUS DETACHMENT

- May be a physiological or pathological phenomenon.
- Can be complete or partial.
- Seen as a freely mobile membranous echo with variable attachments to the optic nerve head or retina. These could be focal or broad, single or multiple. This is in contrast to a rhegmatogenous retinal detachment where the attachment is to the optic disc, unless it is a peripheral or localised detachment.
- The reflectivity of the membrane would depend on the etiology, e.g. an age related PVD is mobile and low reflective whereas a blood lined PVD is moderate to high reflective.
- The mobility of the PVD is more than that of a retinal detachment; this helps in differentiation between the two.
- Multiple low reflective dot echoes posterior to a PVD are suggestive of subhyaloid hemorrhage. As subhyaloid hemorrhage remains fluid, it can be seen as a layering of echoes with a straight surface, seen to move with position of the head. This is sometimes referred to as posterior hyphema.

- The vitreoretinal adhesions may be associated with a tractional retinal detachment or a retinal tear where the PVD is seen attached to the flap.
- Splitting of the posterior cortical vitreous or vitreoschisis is described in diabetic retinopathy and other vascular retinopathies such as Eales' disease, the detection of which helps the surgeon to look for a second membrane during vitreous surgery.

MIMICKING CONDITIONS

- Asteroid hyalosis may mimic vitreous hemorrhage on ultrasound, however the echoes are discrete, very highly reflective and an echolucent gap is seen between the echoes and the posterior globe wall
- Vitreous echoes due to inflammation and infection are similar to those due to hemorrhage. However, other features of inflammation such as retinochoroidal thickening, exudative retinal detachment, optic disc elevation or Tenon's space widening may be seen
- Distinguishing a PVD from an RD may not be always easy. An RD is usually uniformly high reflective and of even thickness. Tilting the probe in different directions may reveal uneven thickness and reflectivity of the membrane indicating a PVD.

NUGGETS

Increase the gain to visualize vitreous echoes in a patient suspected to have a fresh vitreous hemorrhage.

Look carefully for a retinal tear in a patient with sudden onset vitreous hemorrhage with no obvious etiology.

In an elderly patient with massive vitreous hemorrhage and no PVD - look for a mound at the macula, to suggest bleeding from polypoidal choroidal vasculopathy. Also look for drusen in the fellow eye.

Rarely malignant tumors such as melanomas can cause massive vitreous hemorrhage - so look carefully for a mass in a patient with vitreous hemorrhage of uncertain etiology.

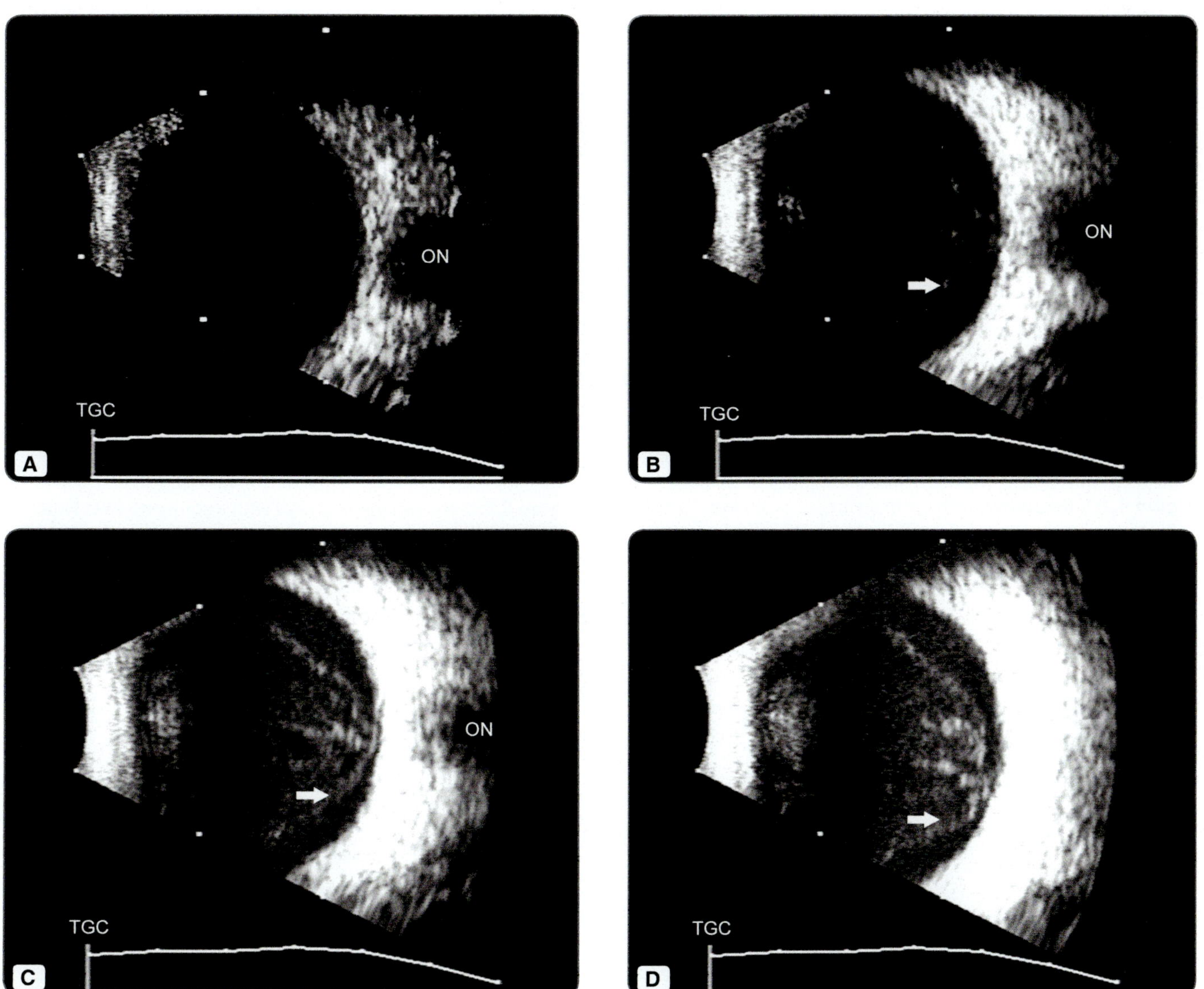

Figures 4.1A to D: B scan images at gradually increasing gain showing relatively fresh vitreous hemorrhage. Note that at lower gain the vitreous cavity appears echolucent, and as the gain is increased, low reflective dot-like echoes are seen, along with a low reflective membrane (arrow) attached to the optic disc. This is indicative of an incomplete PVD. (Optic nerve = ON).

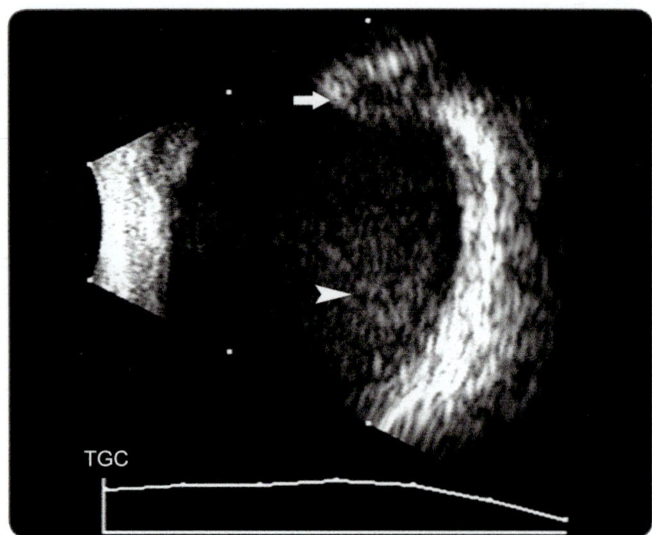

Figure 4.2: Vitreous hemorrhage in a vitrectomised eye. The low reflective echoes are evenly distributed in the vitreous cavity indicative of dispersed hemorrhage (arrowhead). Note the globe indentation caused by an encircling band (arrow).

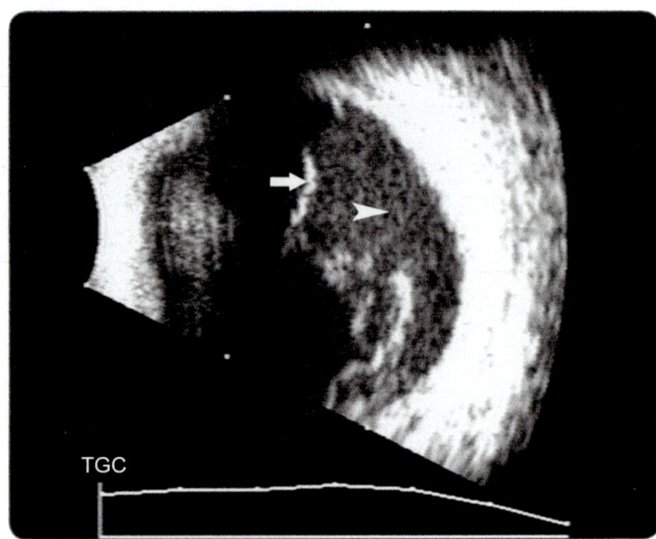

Figure 4.3: B scan image of an eye with a complete PVD. Note the echolucent intragel space. There is an irregular shaped membrane with no posterior pole attachments indicating a complete PVD (arrow). Plenty of low reflective echoes are seen behind the membrane, due to subhyaloid hemorrhage (arrowhead).

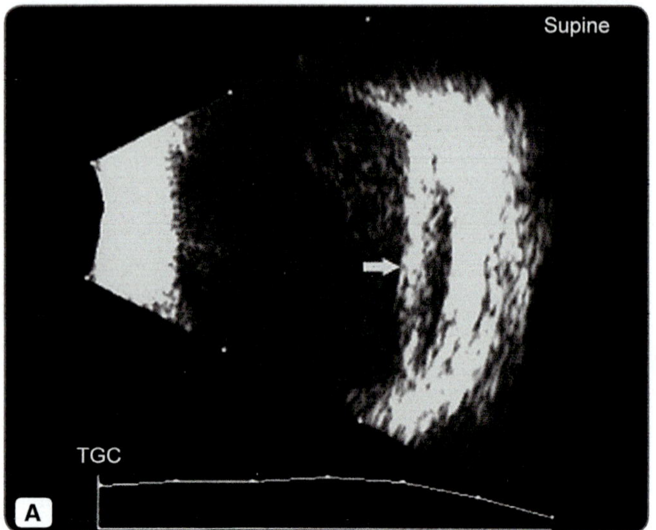

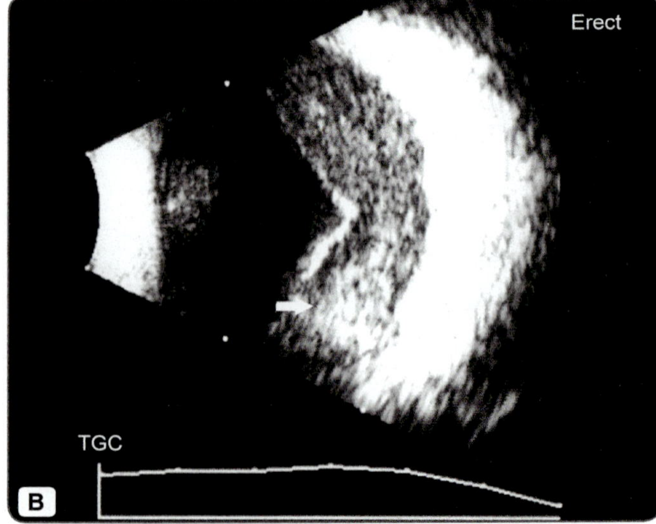

Figures 4.4A and B: Posterior hyphema in an eye with complete PVD. Note the configuration of layered subhyaloid echoes (arrow) with the patient in supine position. With erect position these echoes disperse downwards.

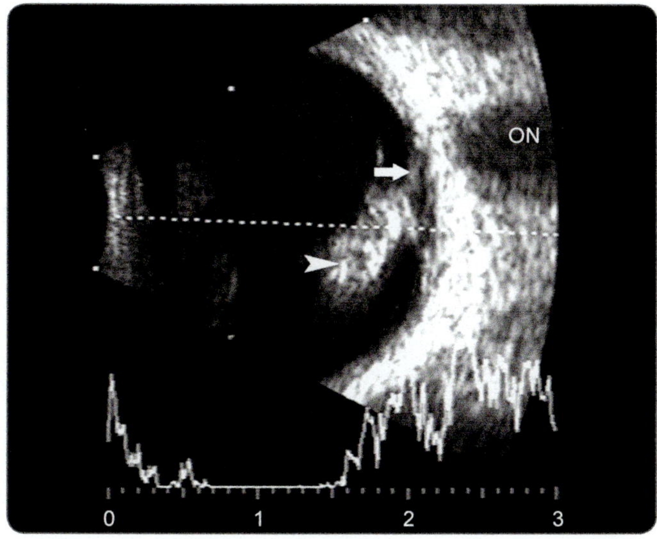

Figure 4.5: B scan image showing a clump of high reflective echoes extending into the vitreous cavity from the optic disc. It is attached to a tented membrane in the peripapillary area. This is indicative of fibrovascular proliferation (arrowhead) at the disc causing a peripapillary tractional retinal detachment (arrow).

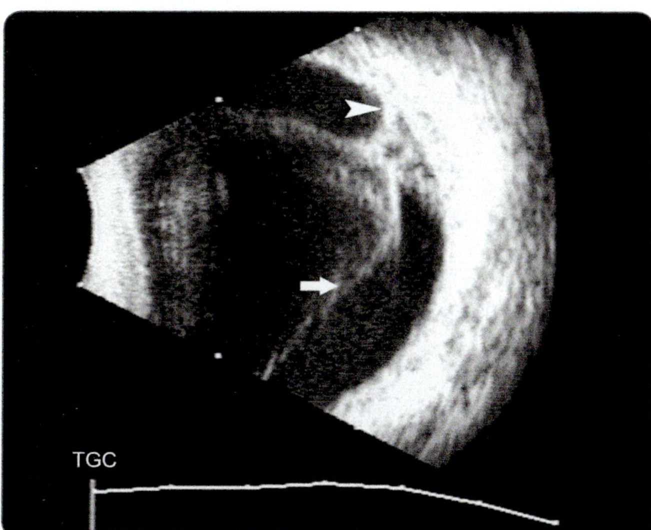

Figure 4.6: B scan image showing low reflective intragel echoes in the mid-vitreous cavity. There is a moderate to high reflective membrane (arrow) attached to a tented membrane at the posterior globe wall. The picture suggests an incomplete PVD with focal tractional retinal detachment (arrowhead).

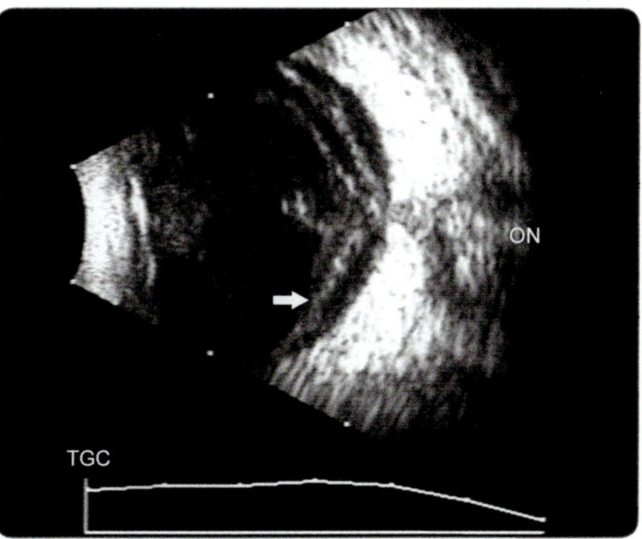

Figure 4.7: Double membrane configuration that can be seen in eyes with vitreoschisis. Note two membranes of similar reflectivity attached to the optic nerve. The membranes merge in the lower part (arrow), one of the clues for diagnosis of vitreoschisis.

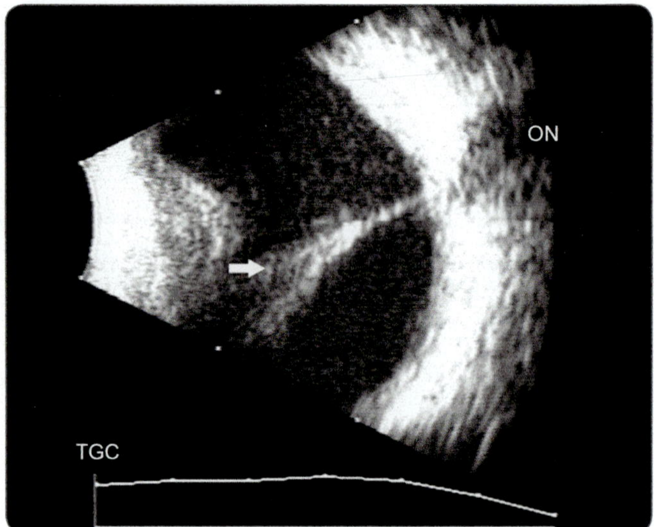

Figure 4.8: B scan image of an eye following penetrating trauma. Note the high reflective taut membrane (arrow) extending to the optic disc. Both ends of the anterior part appear to originate from below the lens, suggesting possible vitreous incarceration in an anterior wound and a hemorrhagic vitreous track extending posteriorly.

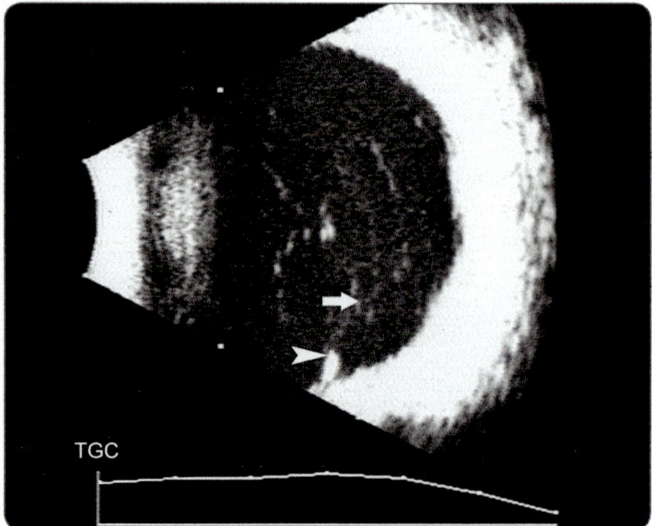

Figure 4.9: B scan image showing a complete PVD. The edge of the vitreous (arrow) is seen lifting up the flap of a retinal tear (arrowhead) in the inferior part of the image.

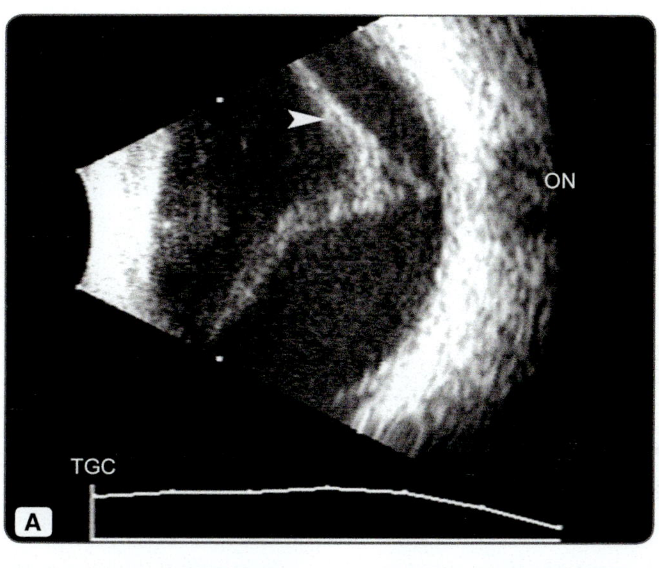

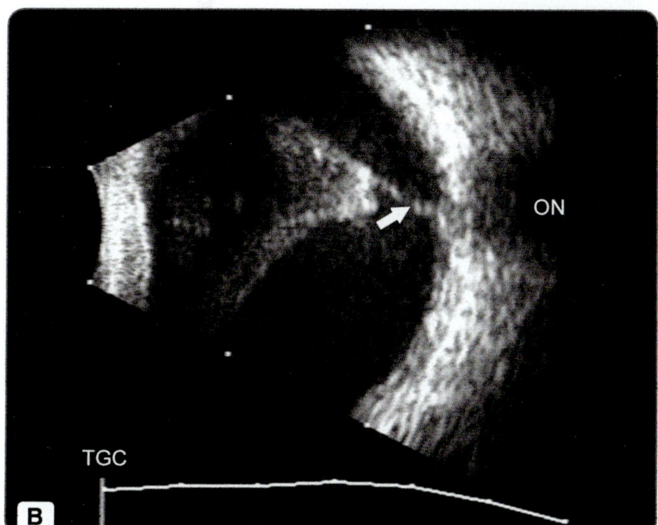

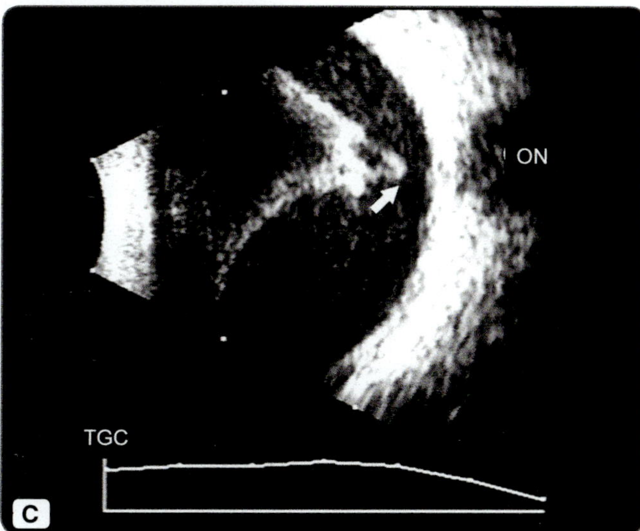

Figures 4.10A to C: B scan images showing a high reflective funnel shaped membrane (arrowhead) attached to the optic disc, which appears as a total RD. However, with a minimal tilt of the probe, it is seen that there is a variable thickness in the membrane and only a small strand (arrow) inserts at the disc, confirming that it is a PVD and not an RD.

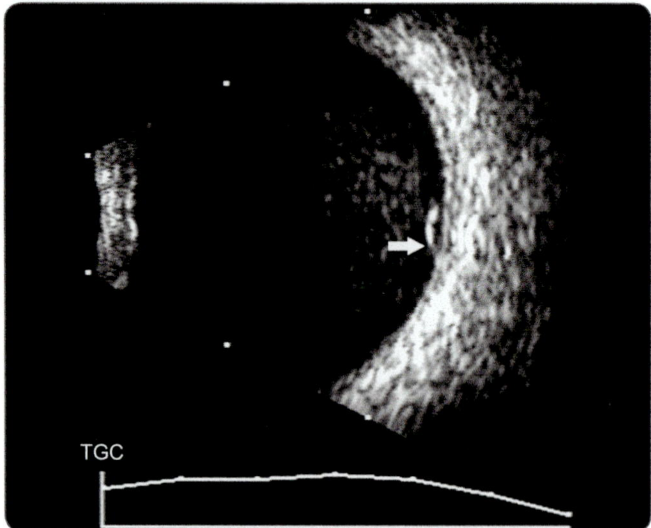

Figure 4.11: B scan image through the macula in a case of vitreous hemorrhage in a healthy adult. The vitreous cavity shows dot-like echoes suggestive of hemorrhage. The macular area shows a small dome-shaped elevation (arrow) with very low to absent internal echoes, suggestive of a hemorrhagic pigment epithelial detachment due to polypoidal choroidal vasculopathy.

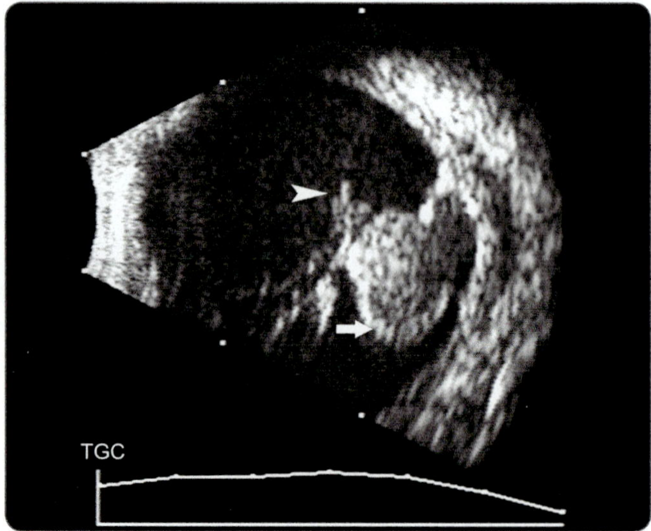

Figure 4.12: B scan image of an eye with massive vitreous hemorrhage (arrowhead). Note the mushroom shaped choroidal mass lesion (arrow) indicating that the hemorrhage is due to bleeding from a choroidal melanoma.

5 Retinal Breaks and Detachment

CLINICAL FEATURES

- Significant cause of visual morbidity.
- Can be either rhegmatogenous, tractional, combined traction-rhegmatogenous or exudative.
- Ultrasound is indicated to diagnose a retinal detachment (RD) in opaque media, to look for other associated findings in clear media, and to diagnose macular involvement in tractional detachments.

ULTRASONOGRAPHY

Rhegmatogenous Retinal Detachment

- Thin, continuous, membrane on the B scan separated from and located anterior to the echoes from the globe wall.
- A highly elevated, totally detached retina appears as convex bullae extending far into the vitreous from attachment points at the nasal and temporal ora serrata and at the optic nerve.
- The space posterior to the elevated retina is sonolucent. In longstanding detachments, the subretinal space may show echoes of varying reflectivity. High reflective echoes suggestive of subretinal hemorrhage can be seen in cases of traumatic RD.
- Retinal echoes on A-scan have high amplitude—100% of the scleral spike. The reflectivity remains equal along the entire extent of the membrane as long as the probe is perpendicular to it.
- Cyst formation can occur in a long-standing detachment and is seen as a thickened and convoluted echo pattern continuous with the retina. It may contain hemorrhage in which case echoes are seen within the cyst.
- Restricted after movements are seen in retinal detachment compared to a highly mobile posterior vitreous detachment. The mobility of the retina can vary depending on the duration of RD, the presence of PVR and associated retinal incarceration.
- In cases of PVR, the retina loses its mobility and assumes a triangular or funnel shaped configuration which can range from open to tightly closed.

Retinal Breaks

- Can be seen at the edge of the detached vitreous in cases of attached retina as high reflective elevations from the retinal surface with a free edge.
- Giant retinal tears are seen as convoluted membranes often with unusual configuration. There is often a free end which is very mobile.
- Retinal breaks in conditions such as acute retinal necrosis can be seen as large areas of discontinuity within the relatively stiff detached retina.

Tractional Retinal Detachment

- Typically seen as a concave membrane with a varying extent of vitreous adhesion. It may be either focal or broad depending upon the extent of vitreoretinal adhesion.
- Tractional retinal detachment (TRD) often occurs in vascular retinopathies such as diabetic retinopathy, vascular occlusions, trauma, endophthalmitis or uveitis in which there is vitreous membrane formation.
- In diabetic retinopathy TRD is found most commonly around the optic disc and along the vascular arcades. Traction may present as mild elevation of retina, a shallow or highly elevated detachment or as a complete funnel shaped detachment.
- Vascular retinopathies such as Eale's disease commonly have proliferative changes in the midperiphery, hence the TRD may be at or even anterior to the equator.
- Equatorial (peripheral) traction secondary to anterior hyaloidal fibrovascular proliferation typically occurs after vitrectomy for proliferative diabetic retinopathy in phakic patients and is characterized by a ring-like tented configuration of the peripheral detached retina.

Exudative Retinal Detachment

- Typical features on ultrasound include the presence of smooth bullae, and shifting fluid. The latter can be diagnosed by having the patient sit up or change head position which changes the configuration of the RD.
- Often, the detachment may be confined to the macula in inflammatory or infective conditions.
- In exudative retinal detachment caused by extensive panretinal photocoagulation, the detachment may be in the periphery, or seen as isolated pockets of elevated retina. In addition, one may find a shallow peripheral choroidal detachment.
- Presence of retinochoroidal thickening would indicate an inflammatory etiology such as scleritis, VKH or sympathetic ophthalmia.
- It is necessary to look for a tumor mass or granuloma if no break or inflammatory signs are noted.

NUGGETS

Low reflective retinal detachments may be seen in long standing cases, endophthalmitis or retinal disruption.

The presence of shifting fluid does not rule out a rhegmatogenous retinal detachment.

In the presence of dense subretinal echoes such as in Coats' disease, the retina may not be clearly seen. The cavity of the funnel is identified as an echolucent area extending to the optic disc.

If a concave membrane shows a convex configuration on follow up, it is indicative of development of a rhegmatogenous element.

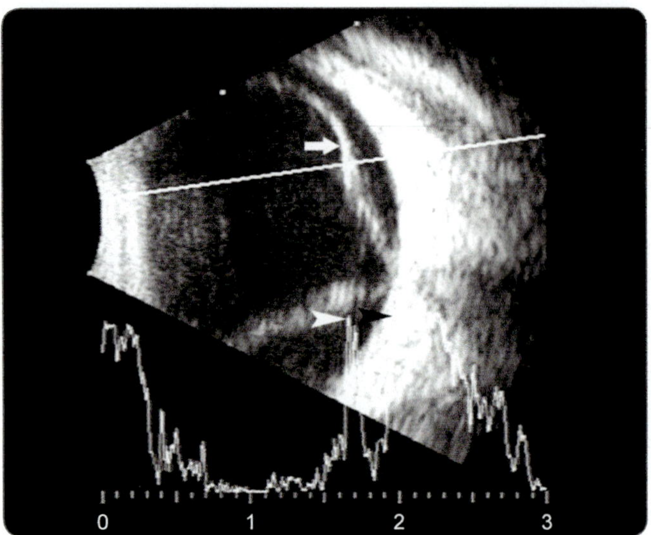

Figure 5.1: B scan with vector A scan showing a high reflective smooth membrane attached to the optic disc (arrow). The configuration is convex and the echoes are uniformly bright. The A scan passing through the membrane (white arrowhead) shows 100% reflectivity compared to the scleral echo (black arrowhead). The features are typical of a retinal detachment.

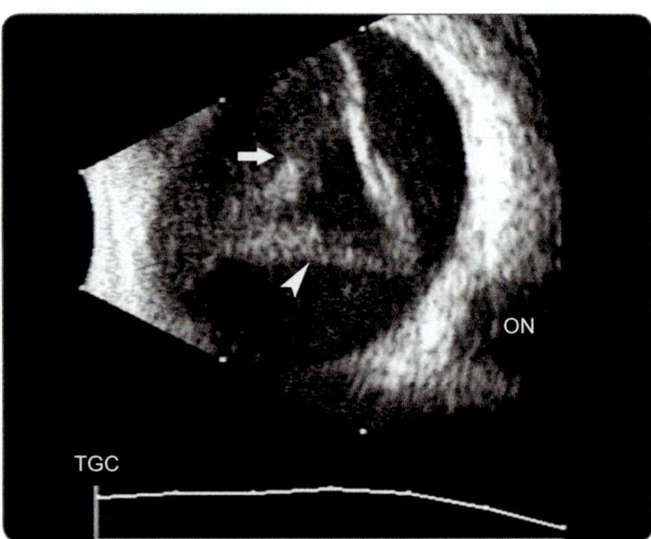

Figure 5.2: The B scan image shows a funnel-shaped or triangular membrane (arrowhead) attached to the optic disc (ON). The membrane looks taut and there is a second membrane bridging it (arrow). The features are suggestive of PVR with an open funnel configuration.

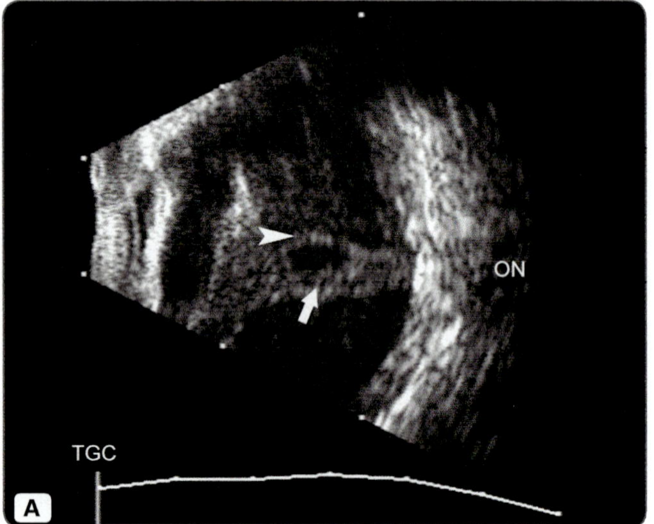

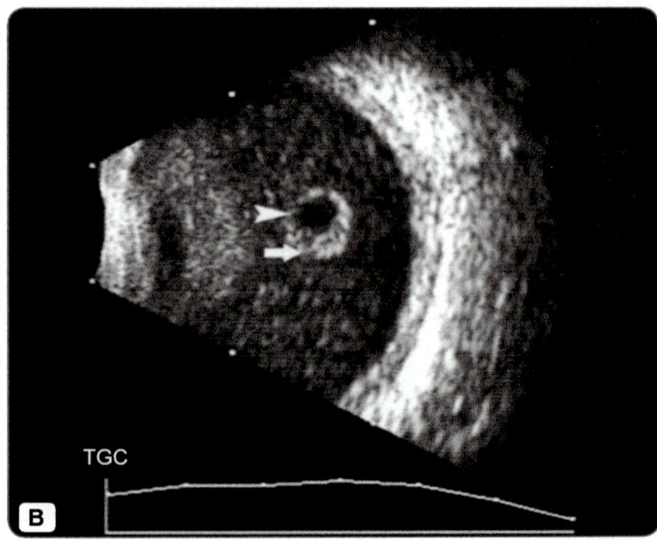

Figures 5.3A and B: Axial and transverse B scans of an eye with long-standing RD and retinal cyst formation (arrowhead). Extensive subretinal echoes are seen. The transverse scan shows the cyst in cross section. The closed funnel without an obvious lumen is seen at the lower border of the cyst (arrow). ON = Optic nerve

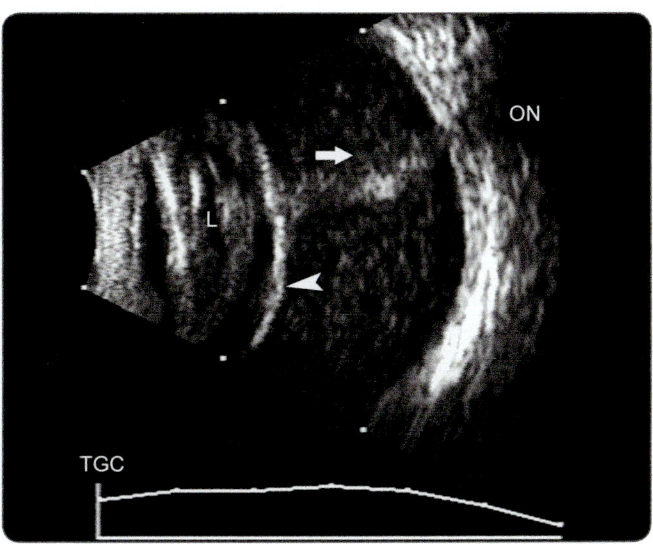

Figure 5.4: B scan image of an eye with a long-standing retinal detachment. Note the retrolental membrane (arrowhead) and the closed funnel appearance of the retina (arrow). The subretinal space is filled with low reflective echoes, again signifying the long duration of the detachment. (L- lens, ON - optic nerve)

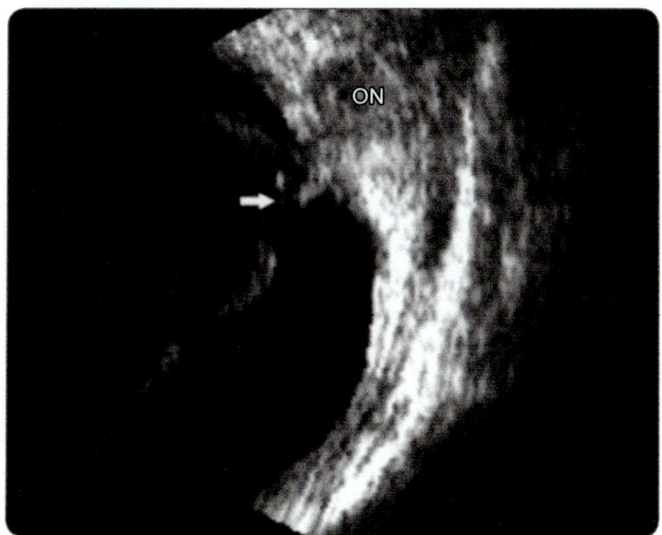

Figure 5.5: A magnified B scan image of an eye with retinal detachment. There is an area of discontinuity in the retina just below its insertion into the optic disc (ON). There is also a high reflective echo above this membrane indicating an operculated break (arrow).

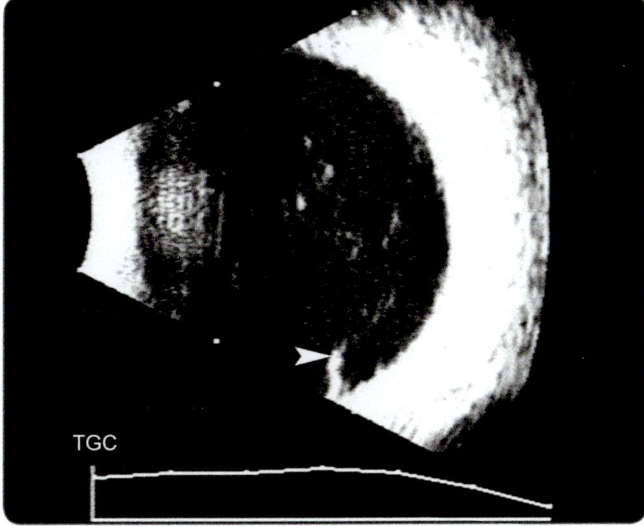

Figure 5.6: This B scan image shows a retinal break in attached retina in an eye with vitreous hemorrhage and a complete PVD. It is seen as a linear high reflective membrane like echo (arrowhead) with one end attached to the globe wall and the other attached to the edge of the posterior vitreous detachment.

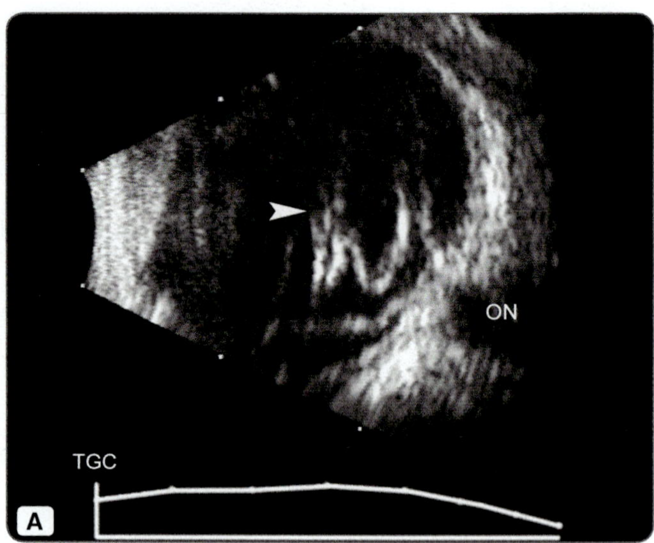

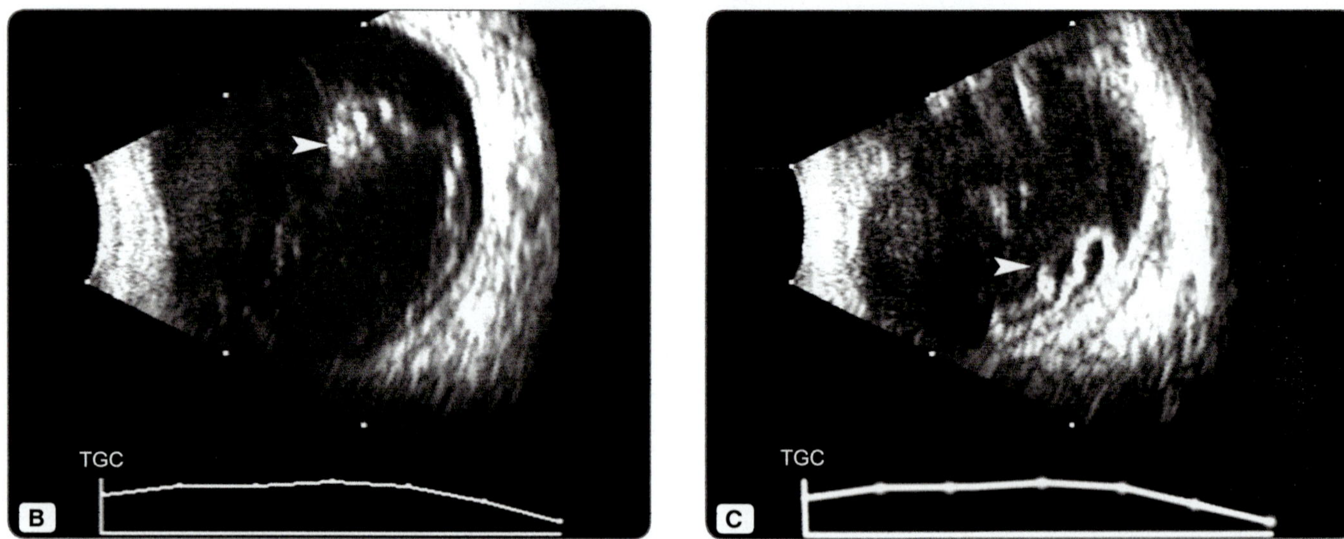

Figures 5.7A to C: B scan images of an eye with a giant retinal tear. Note the convoluted membrane with no attachment to the superior periphery. The vitreous is seen attached to the free end (arrowhead). The membrane is also folded upon itself indicating the large free edge that is highly mobile.

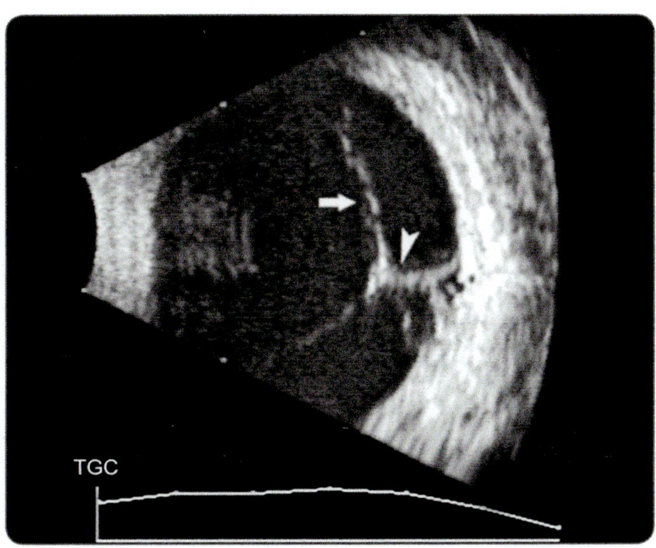

Figure 5.8: B scan image of an eye with an incomplete PVD causing a focal tractional retinal detachment. The detachment is triangular in shape (arrowhead) with the apex attached to the partly detached posterior hyaloid (arrow).

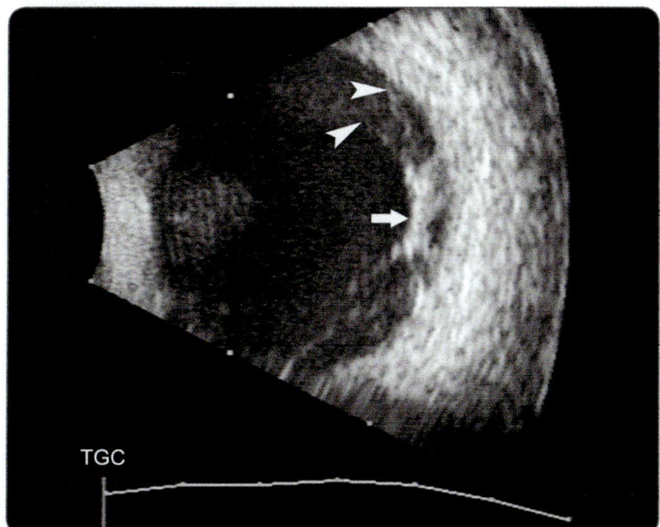

Figure 5.9: B scan image of a broad attachment of the posterior vitreous causing a shallow but more extensive TRD (arrow). The other features seen are the presence of subhyaloid echoes signifying hemorrhage and the splitting of the posterior hyaloid into two layers (arrowheads).

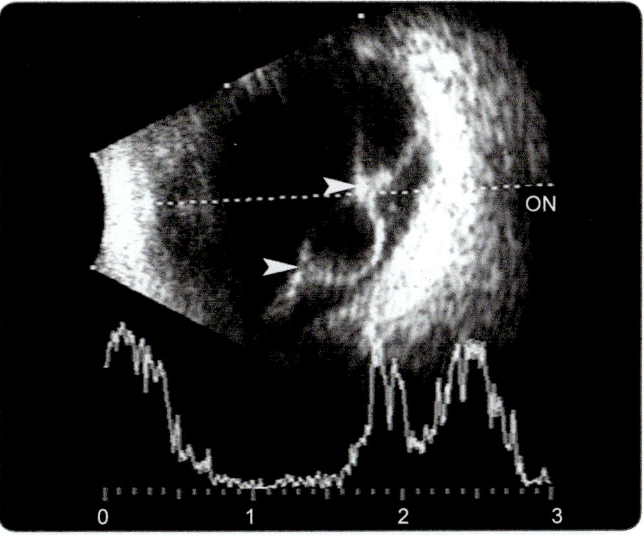

Figure 5.10: B scan image showing two areas of focal attachment (arrowheads) causing a hammock-like configuration of the TRD.

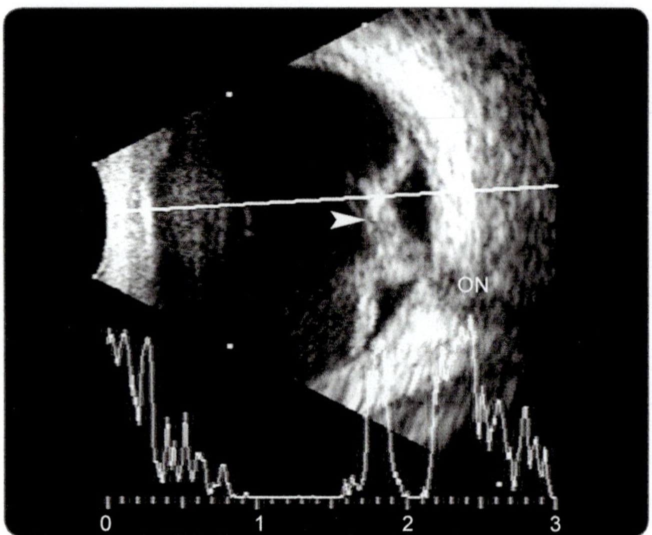

Figure 5.11: A B scan image showing a broad vitreoretinal adhesion causing a posterior pole detachment. Note the convex configuration of the detachment (arrowhead) indicating a possible rhegmatogenous element.

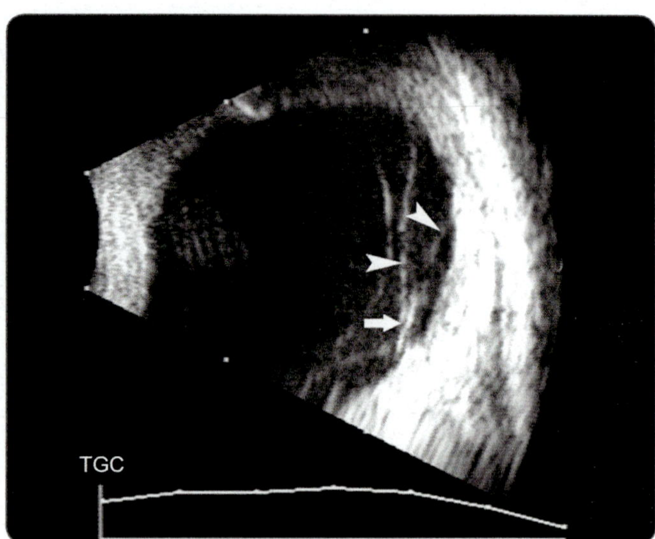

Figure 5.12: Multiple membranes attached to the optic disc of similar reflectivity. Note the splitting of the layers (arrowheads) which is described as vitreoschisis. The third membrane (arrow) can easily be mistaken for a TRD except for its medium reflectivity and direct continuity with the second membrane.

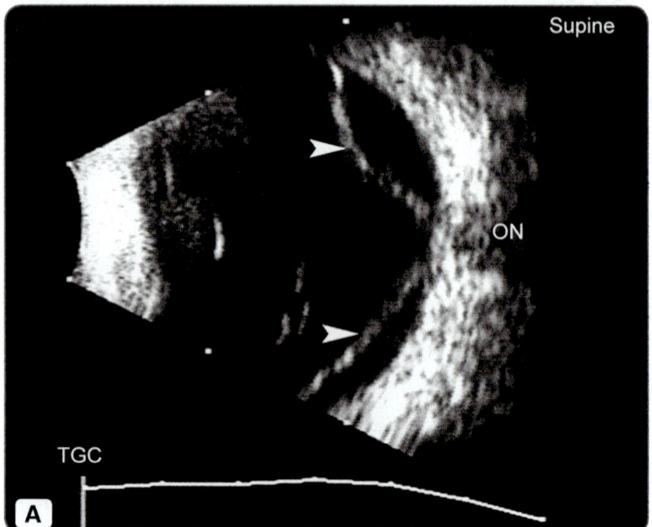

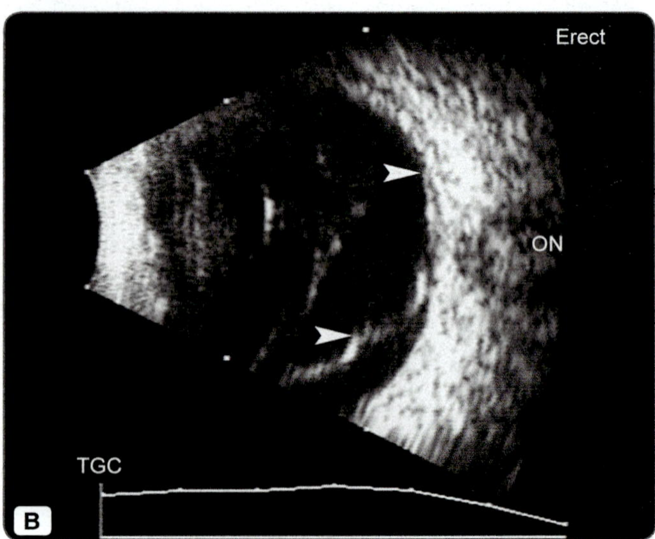

Figures 5.13A and B: Two B scan images demonstrating shifting fluid in an eye with an exudative retinal detachment. The first image in supine position shows a total retinal detachment (arrowheads) with equal elevation of the retina above and below the optic disc. The second, taken in erect position shows that the fluid has shifted inferiorly, and the superior retina appears attached.

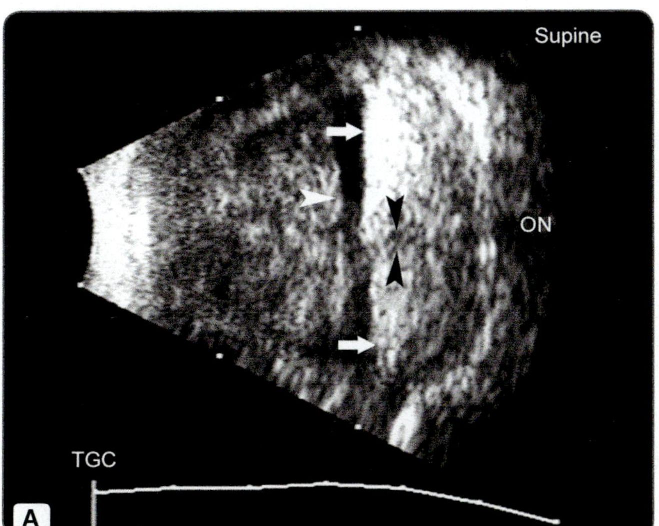

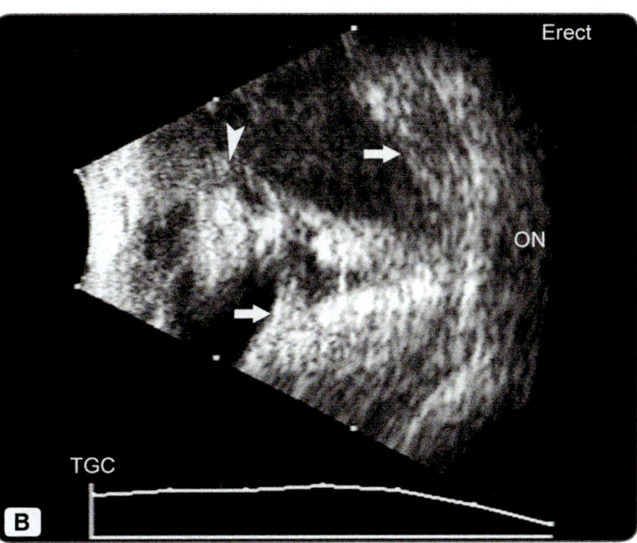

Figures 5.14A and B: Mobile subretinal blood (arrows) in an eye with a closed funnel retinal detachment (white arrowhead). Note the straight line configuration of high reflective subretinal echoes which change position with erect posture. The closed funnel of the retinal detachment is seen in contrast to the high reflective subretinal echoes as a low reflective band (black arrowheads) inserting into the optic disc (ON).

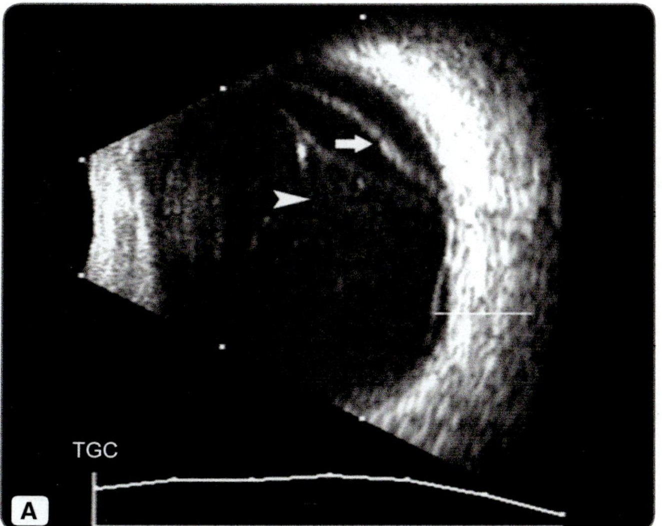

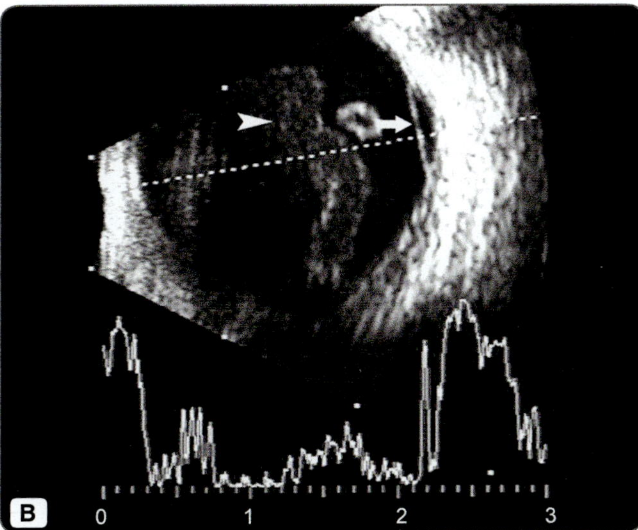

Figures 5.15A and B: B scan images of an eye with acute retinal necrosis and retinal detachment. Note the intragel echoes (arrowhead) signifying vitreous inflammation. There is a complete PVD. There is a retinal detachment seen, more extensive superiorly. Small areas of discontinuity within the membrane (arrow) are suggestive of necrotic retinal breaks. The RD in this situation is rhegmatogenous rather than exudative or tractional.

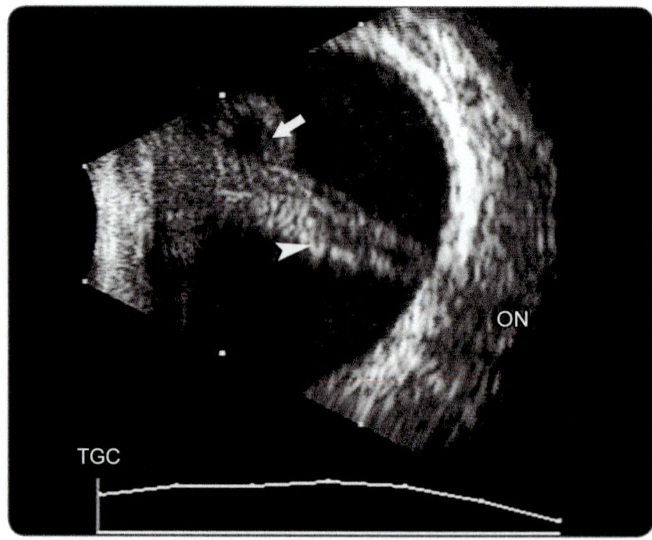

Figure 5.16: In this B scan image, there is a double membrane inserting into the optic disc (ON) with a closed configuration suggestive of RD with severe PVR (arrowhead). Note the retinal cyst (arrow) which indicates a long-standing detachment.

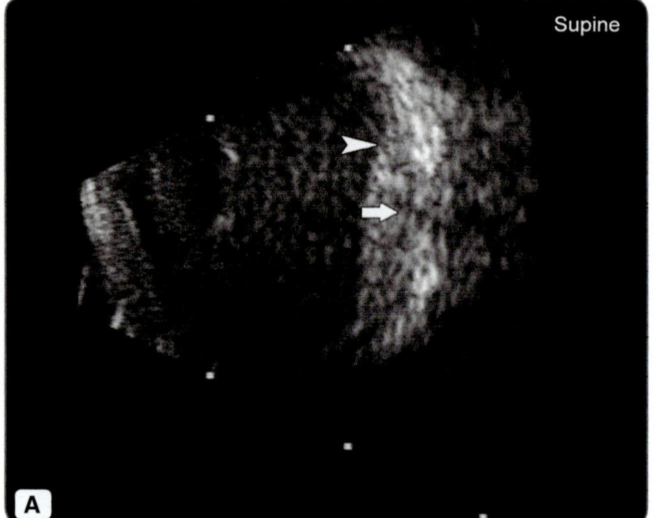

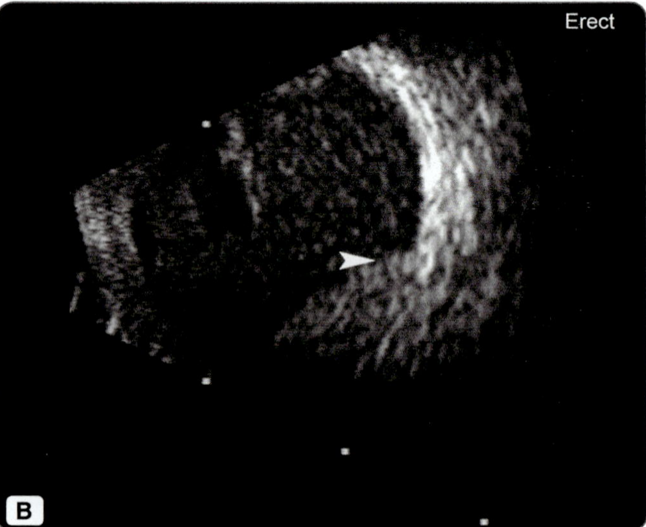

Figures 5.17A and B: Dual mode B scan showing the shift in the subretinal hemorrhage with a change in head position from supine to erect. This helps to differentiate hemorrhage from a membrane which will not move with change in position. Note that due to the subretinal echoes, the funnel of the detachment is only seen as a faint echolucent line in Figure A (arrow) and not visible in Figure B.

6 Choroidal Detachment

CLINICAL FEATURES

- Choroidal detachment can occur spontaneously or as a sequel to hypotony, trauma, a surgical procedure or even photocoagulation
- Clinically, it appears as single or multiple, dome shaped elevations with a smooth surface
- Choroidal detachments are either serous or hemorrhagic
- Ultrasonography is useful in diagnosing and differentiating the type and extent of choroidal detachment, and for follow-up.

ULTRASONOGRAPHY

- Smooth, thick, dome shaped membrane in the periphery with little or no after movement, which usually does not extend beyond equator as it is limited by the vortex vein exit
- The A scan shows a typical double peak or M-shaped spike signifying echoes from the choroid and the retina. The space behind the membrane is echolucent in case of serous choroidal detachment
- The suprachoroidal space shows multiple dot-like moderate to high reflective echoes in case of hemorrhagic choroidal detachment. Clumps of high reflective echoes signify clotted blood and relatively low reflective ones signify lysed or liquid blood. This is important in planning the timing of suprachoroidal drainage
- Massive hemorrhagic choroidal detachments may extend upto the posterior pole
- Shallow peripheral detachments may be flat or concave instead of dome shaped
- Ultrasound in unexplained hypotony may reveal a shallow peripheral choroidal detachment with disc elevation and possibly a shallow posterior pole retinal detachment
- In an eye with rhegmatogenous RD that develops a choroidal detachment, a progressive decrease in the height of retinal detachment may be seen with the development of a secondary choroidal detachment. In contrast, in an eye with choroidal detachment that develops an exudative or secondary RD, there may be an increase in the retinal detachment along with the height of the choroidal detachment.

NUGGETS

Serial ultrasound examinations are useful in monitoring the resolution of choroidal detachment and clot lysis of suprachoroidal blood.

A cord like moderate to high reflective echo stretched between the sclera and choroidal dome at the equator in case of bullous serous choroidal detachment represents a vortex vein.

Serous choroidal detachments do not insert on the optic nerve head even when they are massive (kissing choroidal detachment)

Nanophthalmos should be suspected in an eye with reduced axial length and choroidal detachment.

Hemorrhagic choroidal detachments can occur spontaneously in eyes with PEHCR (Peripheral Exudative Hemorrhagic Chorioretinopathy) as well as in patients with chronic renal failure who are on anticoagulants.

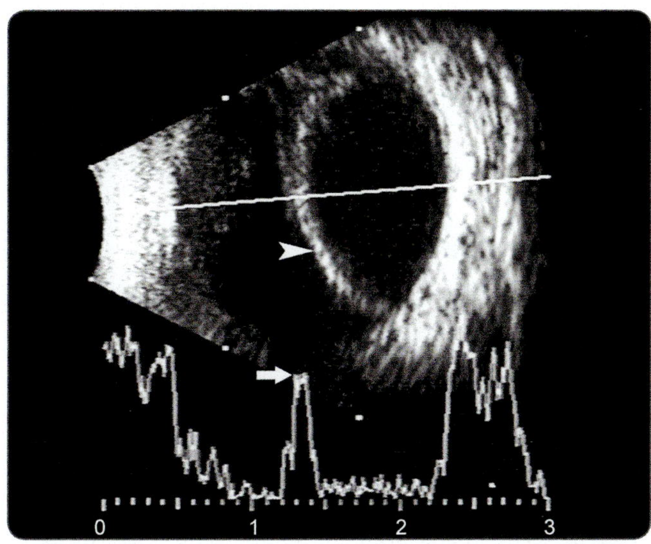

Figure 6.1: B scan with vector A scan showing a high reflective dome-shaped membrane (arrowhead). The membrane echo shows a characteristic 'M' spike (arrow) on the A scan which is of 100% reflectivity. There are no echoes behind the membrane confirming that it is a serous choroidal detachment.

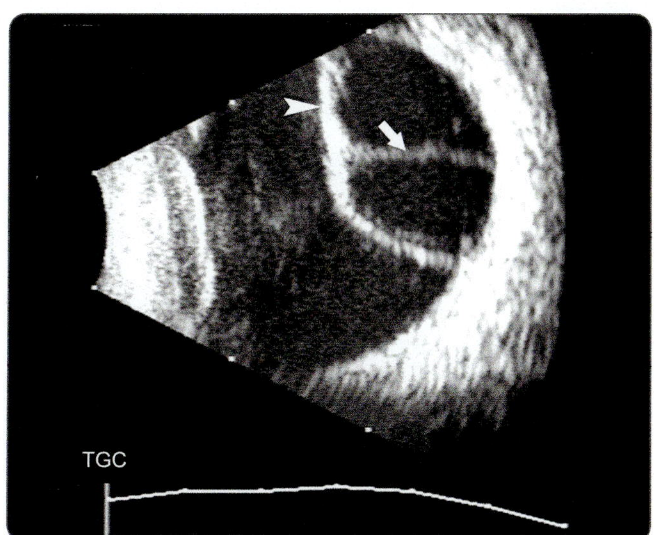

Figure 6.2: B scan image showing a dome-shaped membrane (arrowhead) suggestive of a choroidal detachment. Note the linear cord-like band running across the membrane (arrow) – such bands are believed to be vortex veins, one rarely sees more than one in a quadrant.

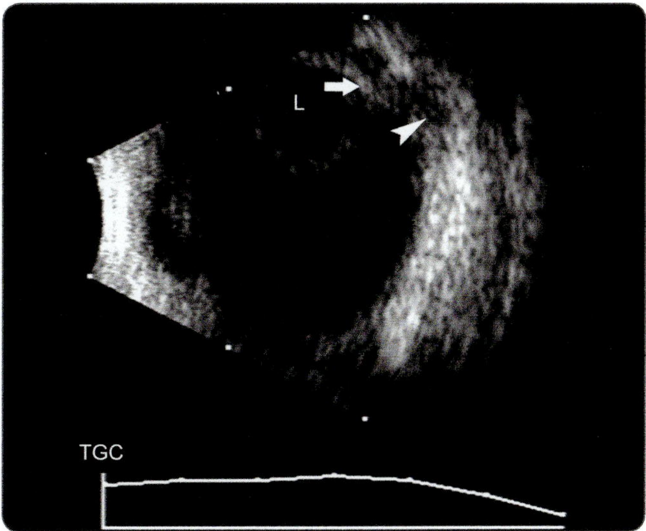

Figure 6.3: This obliquely viewed B scan image shows a ciliary body detachment (arrowhead) causing shallowing of the anterior chamber. The lens (L) is seen as a globular structure behind the iris (arrow).

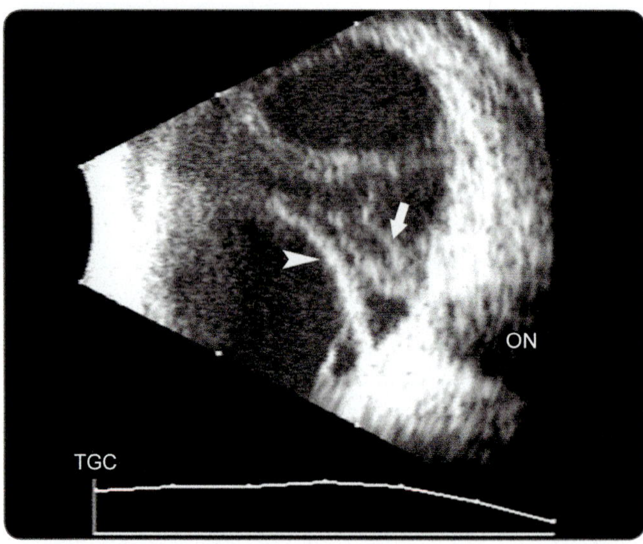

Figure 6.4: Serous choroidal detachment can be secondary to a rhegmatogenous retinal detachment. The B scan image shows a funnel-shaped membrane (arrow) inserting into the optic nerve indicative of a retinal detachment. There is also a large serous choroidal detachment (arrowhead). Note that this does not extend till the optic disc.

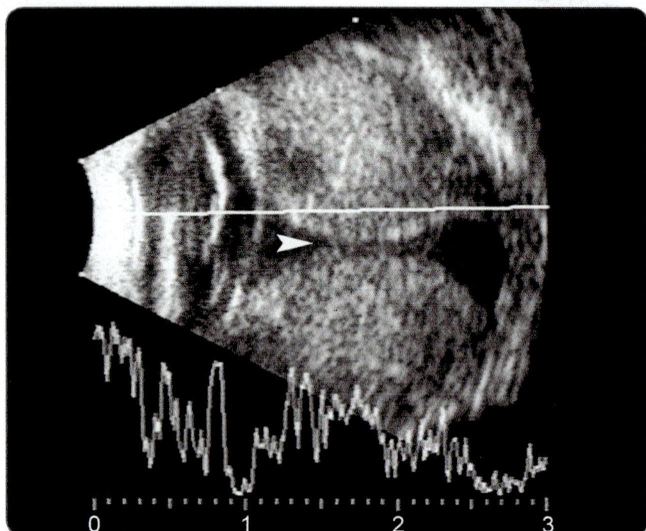

Figure 6.6: B scan with vector A scan showing a dome-shaped high reflective membrane with moderate to high reflective echoes between the membrane and the globe wall. The membrane extends almost till the lens with the two mounds touching each other (arrowhead). This is a hemorrhagic choroidal detachment and is most often seen as an intraoperative catastrophe or due to trauma.

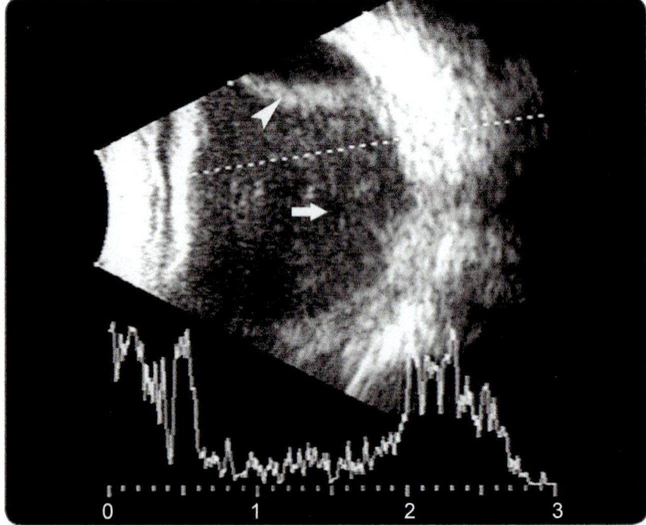

Figure 6.5: B scan image in an eye with chronic endophthalmitis and hypotony. The vitreous cavity is filled with low reflective dot-like echoes (arrow). There is a peripheral shallow serous choroidal detachment (arrowhead). Note the choroidal thickening at the posterior pole. This can occur in hypotony and is of high reflectivity on the A scan.

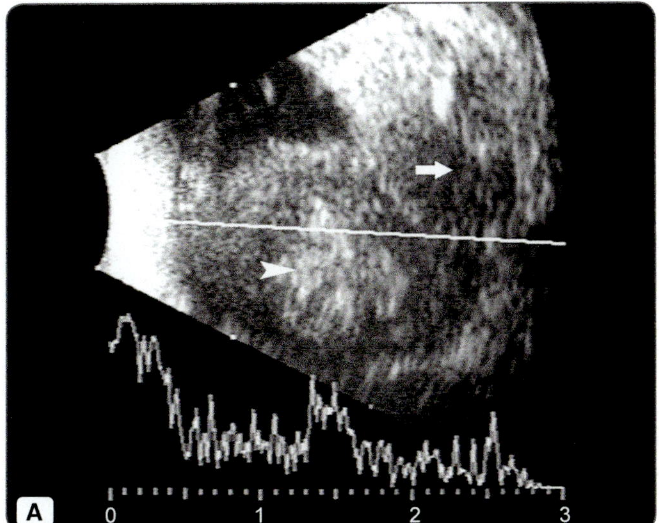

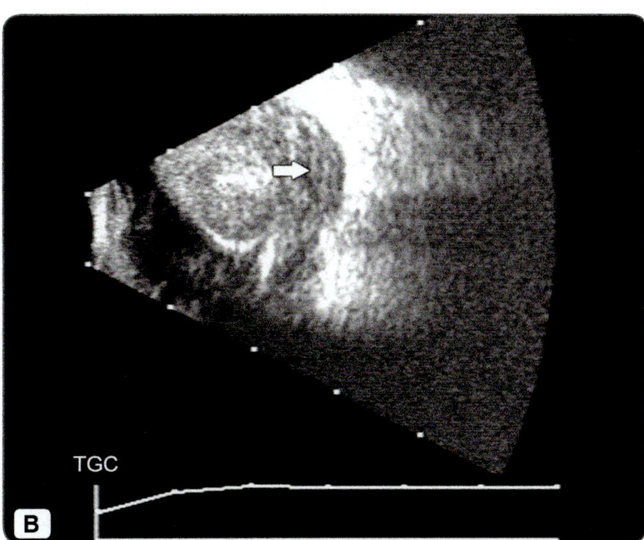

Figures 6.7A and B: B scan images of a patient with an intraoperative non-expulsive suprachoroidal hemorrhage during cataract surgery. The lens echoes are not seen. There are two elevated dome shaped membranes touching each other- "kissing choroidal detachments." The suprachoroidal echoes are variable. The very high reflective echoes suggest clotted blood (arrowhead) and the lower reflective echoes (arrow) suggest lysis of the clot.

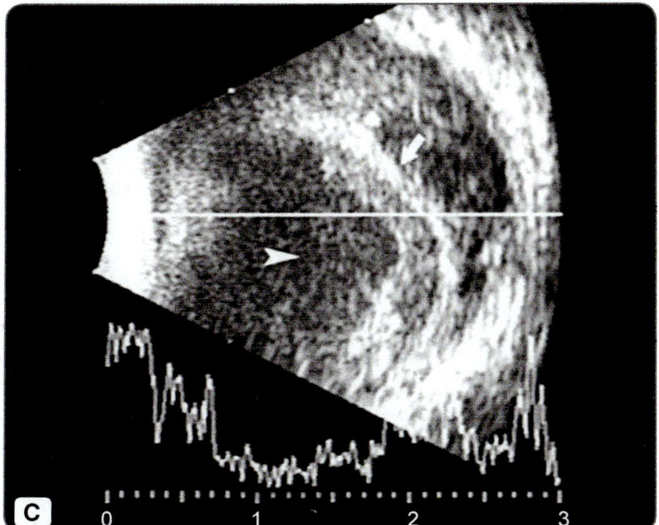

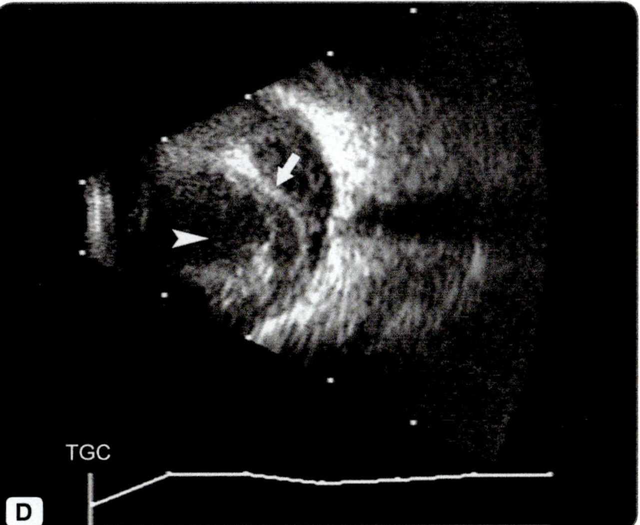

Figures 6.7C and D: B scan images taken a few days later show the change in size of the choroidal detachment. The upper membrane now has a relatively concave configuration (arrow) – this is not seen in serous choroidal detachments. More significantly there is a large area of low reflectivity in the suprachoroidal space indicative of significant clot lysis (arrowhead). This indicates that surgical evacuation of the blood could be considered.

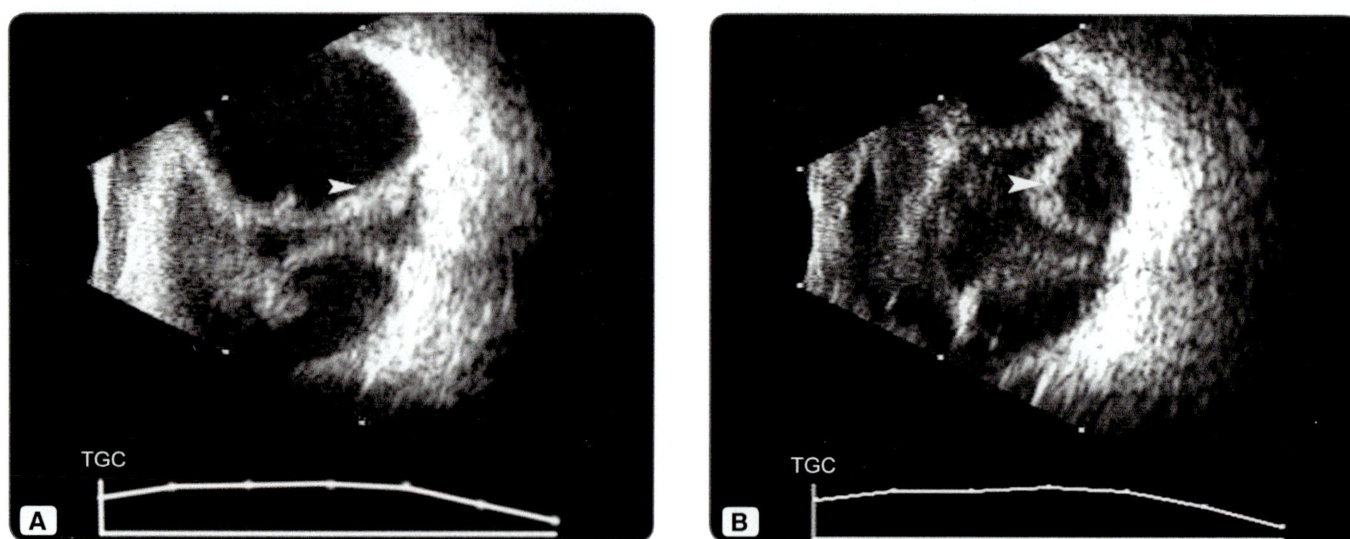

Figures 6.8A and B: B scan images of an eye with vitreous hemorrhage and serous choroidal detachment (arrowhead). Note the scalloped appearance of the 360 degrees choroidal detachment when the scan is performed obliquely as in Figure B.

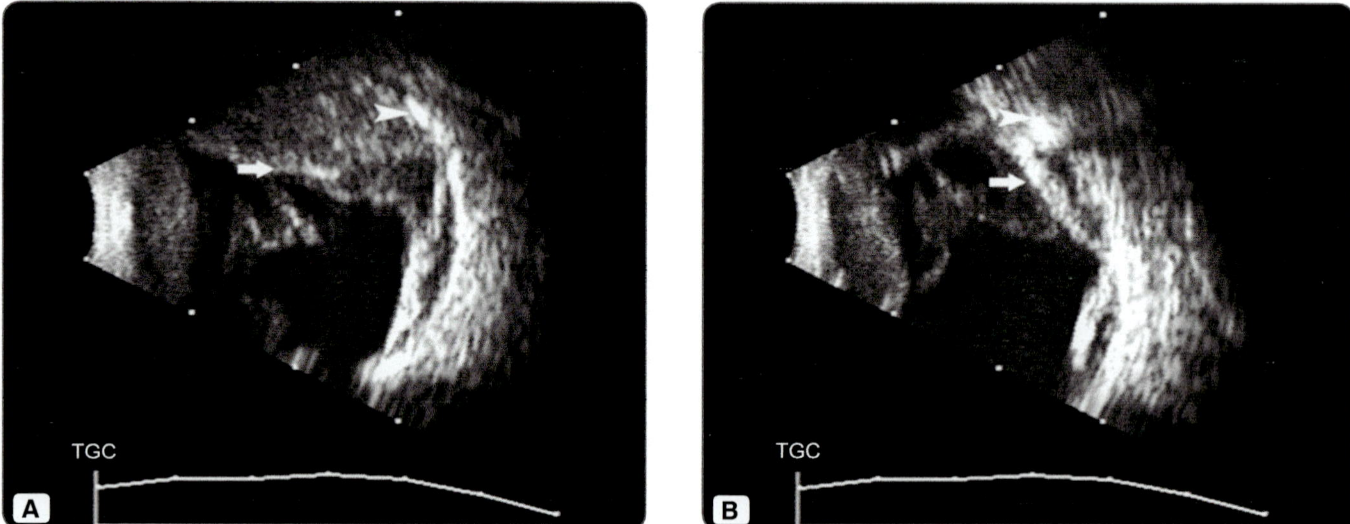

Figures 6.9A and B: B scan images taken at a 2 week interval of an eye with vitreous hemorrhage and suprachoroidal hemorrhage (arrow) following trauma. The patient had undergone scleral buckling previously (arrowhead indicates the band). Note the change in configuration of the detachment from convex to concave as the hemorrhage resolves.

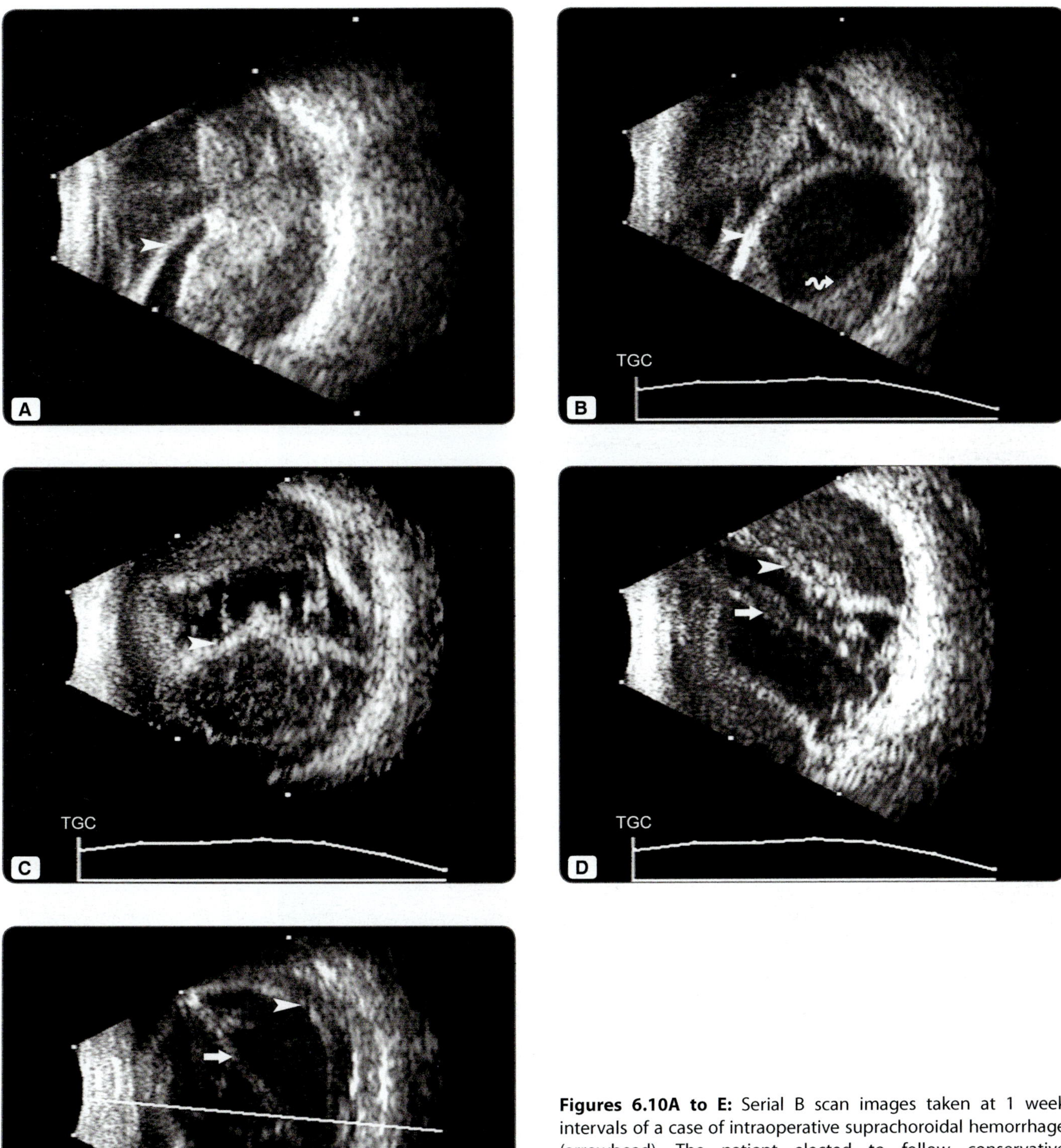

Figures 6.10A to E: Serial B scan images taken at 1 week intervals of a case of intraoperative suprachoroidal hemorrhage (arrowhead). The patient elected to follow conservative management. The images show progressive liquefaction of the hemorrhage with passage of time as well as a change in contour from convex to concave. The curved arrow shows layering of the blood in the suprachoroidal space. In the last 2 images also note the vitreous band (arrow) caused by the compressive effect of the massive choroidal detachment. This remains stretched across the vitreous cavity into the limbal wound, after the choroidal detachment has subsided.

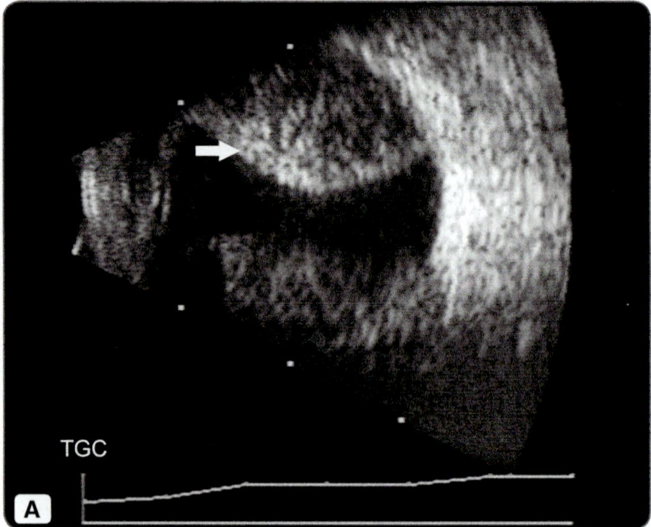

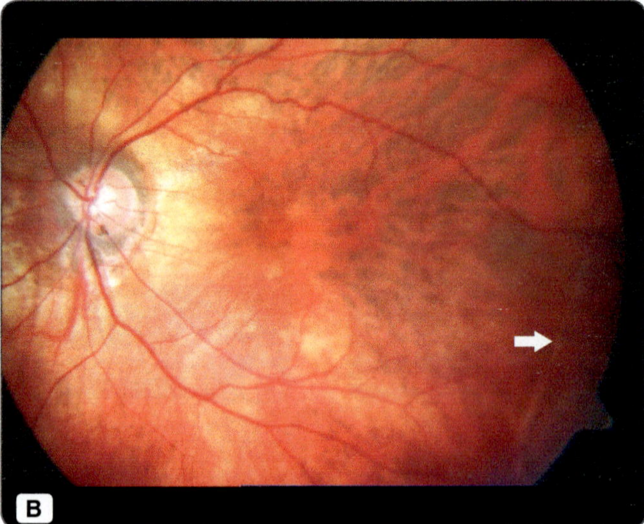

Figures 6.11A and B: Postoperative ultrasound of a 56-year-old high myope who developed choroidal detachment during cataract surgery. Note the choroidal mounds with high reflective suprachoroidal echoes suggestive of hemorrhage. The color photograph shows the fundus after successful surgery for drainage of the suprachoroidal blood and vitrectomy for breakthrough hemorrhage (arrow in Figure A). The arrow points to a demarcation line indicative of resolving choroidal detachment.

7 Subretinal Hemorrhage

CLINICAL FEATURES

- Commonly occurs as a feature of advanced macular degeneration (AMD) or idiopathic polypoidal choroidal vasculopathy
- Can present as a massive lumpy mass with variable degrees of pigmentation
- Vitreous hemorrhage can occur due to breakthrough of the hemorrhage into the vitreous cavity
- In cases of massive hemorrhage, the visual prognosis is very poor
- Can also occur following trauma, and rarely bleeding from a large, choroidal melanoma
- Ultrasound is indicated as a diagnostic as well as follow-up investigation. It is often used to differentiate between dark hemorrhage and a melanoma.

ULTRASONOGRAPHY

- Bumpy lobulated surface with indistinct margins. Presents as a thickening of the retinochoroidal layer
- Commonly located in the macula but can be present anywhere in the fundus
- Occasionally may be quite extensive
- Internal reflectivity is typically variable due to the presence of clotted and lysed blood as well as fibrous tissue
- Secondary retinal detachment over the lesion may be noted
- Plaque-like areas similar to calcification may be seen
- Overlying vitreous hemorrhage can occur due to break through from the subretinal space
- Tendency for change in contour and reduction in height over a period of time. The reduction may be due to the development of breakthrough vitreous hemorrhage as well as to the actual resolution of the subretinal hemorrhage itself.
- The retinal status of the fellow eye can give a clue to the origin of the vitreous hemorrhage, e.g. features of AMD or PCV

NUGGETS

Choroidal melanomas are also a common differential diagnosis, but here the features of uniform low reflectivity, choroidal excavation and acoustic hollowing can help differentiate between the two.

Choroidal metastases may show similar features, however the internal reflectivity is uniform and the retinal detachment is likely to be more extensive.

Not all cases of subretinal hemorrhage show a decrease in height over time. Some may rapidly increase, more so if the patient is on anticoagulants.

Bullous hemorrhagic retinal detachments can occur spontaneously in polypoidal choroidal vasculopathy.

Features of AMD or PCV in the fellow eye can give a clue to the cause of hemorrhage.

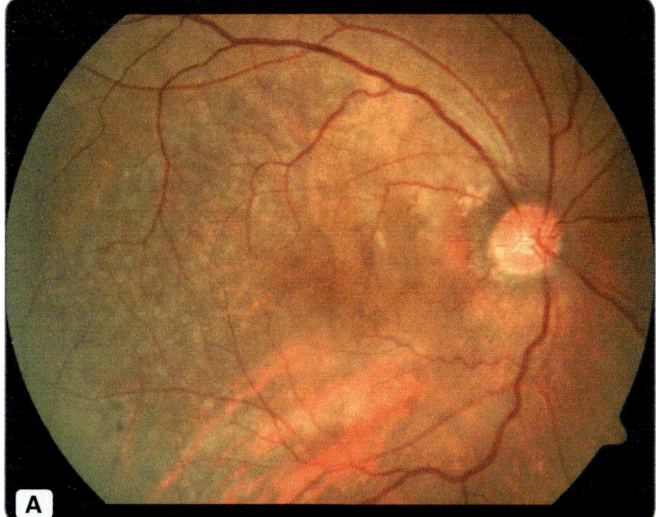

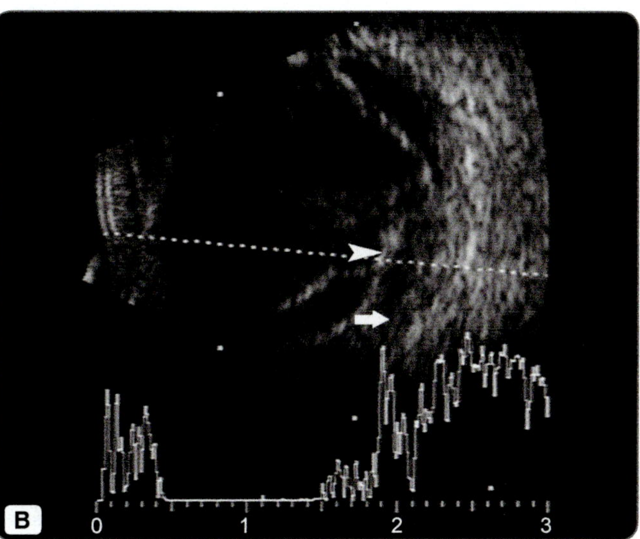

Figures 7.5A and B: A 55-year-old lady presented with decreased vision in the left eye for 1 month after intravitreal bevacizumab. Clinical examination revealed features of AMD in the right eye (Fig. A) and vitreous hemorrhage in the left. B scan image (Fig. B) revealed intragel echoes and a PVD attached over an area of sub retinal elevation suggestive of subretinal hemorrhage with breakthrough bleed. During vitrectomy she was noted to have a large sub macular hemorrhage which scarred down in the postoperative period leaving a best corrected vision of counting fingers close to face.

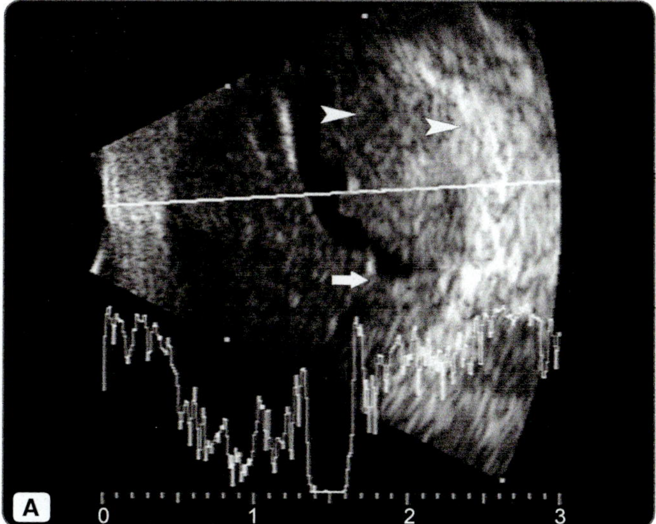

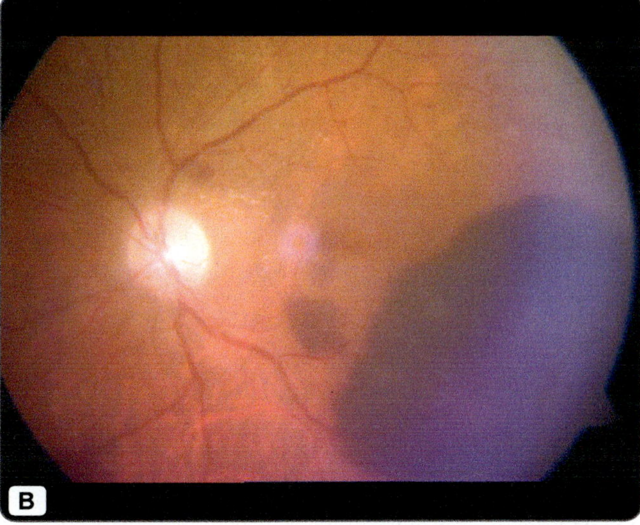

Figures 7.6A and B: B scan image of a patient with bilateral dense cataracts and poor view of the retina. Right eye shows moderately reflective intragel echoes and large subretinal mounds with a lobular surface. Note the vitreous echoes attached to an area on the surface of the mound indicating the site of breakthough hemorrhage. (Fundus of the left eye after cataract surgery showing a large subretinal bleed just inferotemporal to the fovea).

8 Asteroid Hyalosis

CLINICAL FEATURES

- Asteroid hyalosis is a degenerative condition of the vitreous of unknown etiology in which calcium soaps accumulate on vitreous fibrils in the eye
- It is characterized by shiny discrete objects suspended in the vitreous disturbing a clear view of the retina
- In most instances it is an asymptomatic condition, but occasionally the patient may complain of floaters or reduced vision
- Thirty to seventy percent of patients with asteroid hyalosis have diabetes mellitus
- Fundus fluorescein angiography can give surprisingly good information although ophthalmoscopic visualization may be inadequate. However, very dense asteroids may require that ultrasound be performed to assess the posterior segment.

ULTRASONOGRAPHY

- The vitreous cavity shows a varying number of discrete mobile point like bright echoes on the B scan with a high spike on the A scan vector
- There is classically a clear space between the particles and the posterior globe wall, and this can mimic a posterior vitreous detachment
- In a patient with associated vitreous hemorrhage, clumps of low to moderate reflective echoes may be interspersed and it may be difficult to distinguish between the two.

NUGGETS

Falsely short axial length measurements may be obtained using automated biometry in patients with asteroid hyalosis, leading to significant error in intraocular lens power calculations. This occurs due to abnormal automatic placement of the retinal gate on one of the vitreous spikes, resulting in the error. The problem can be avoided by performing a manual biometry to confirm the reading especially when asteroid hyalosis has been noted either clinically or on B scan ultrasound.

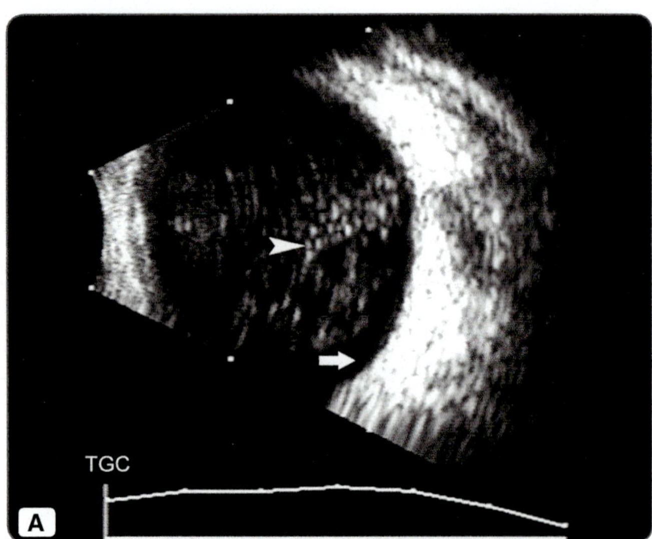

Figure 8.1A: B scan image showing multiple discrete point like echoes (arrowhead) in the vitreous cavity. Note the relative echolucent space between the echoes and the posterior globe wall (arrow). There is no separation of the posterior hyaloid.

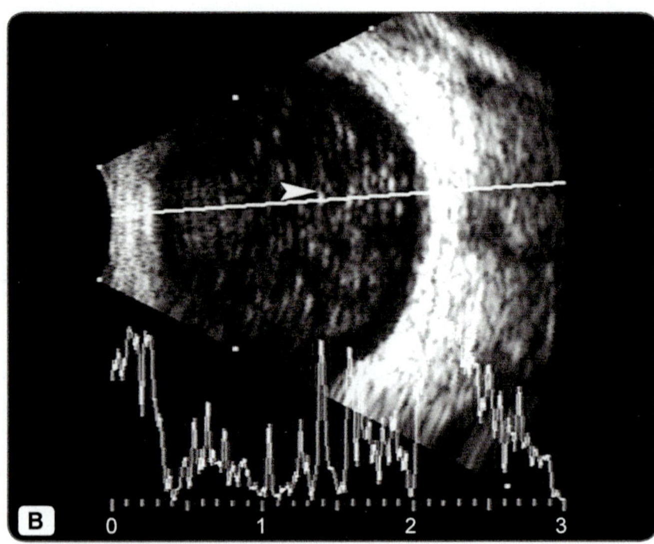

Figure 8.1B: The A scan vector shows 100% reflectivity of the echoes.

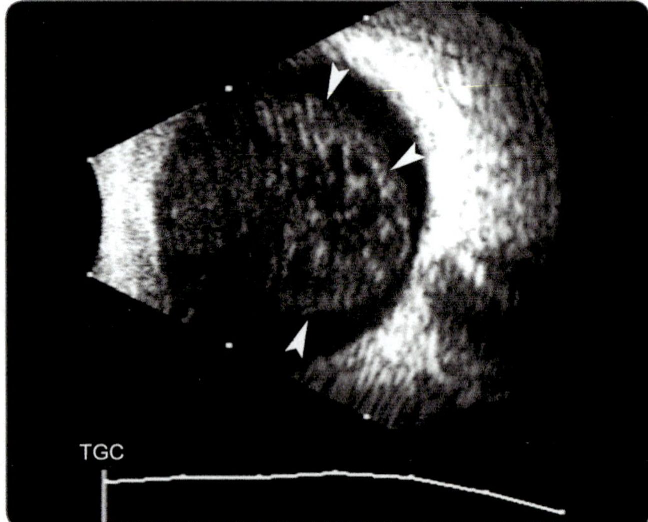

Figure 8.2: B scan image of a patient with asteroid hyalosis and posterior vitreous detachment. Note the smooth posterior contour (arrowheads) separating the asteroid particles in the gel vitreous from the retrohyaloid space.

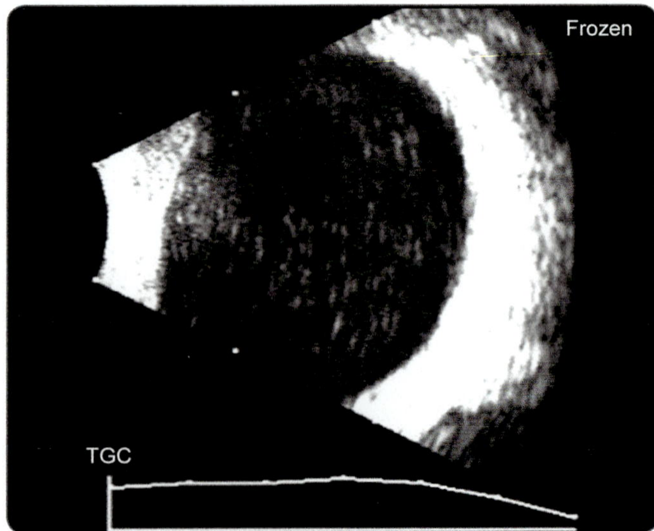

Figure 8.3: B scan image showing relatively few asteroid particles in the vitreous cavity.

Section 3

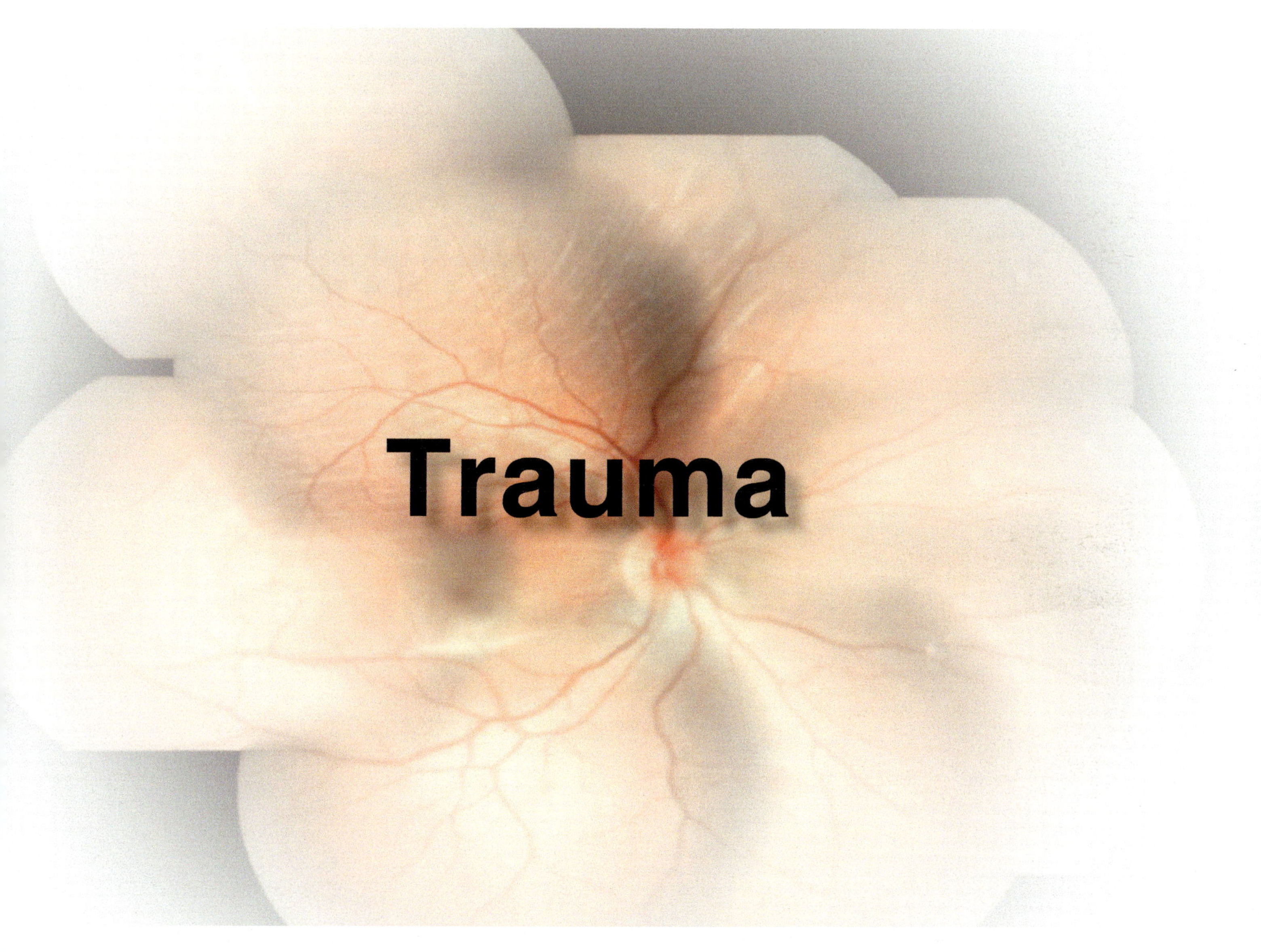

Trauma

9 Intraocular Foreign Body

CLINICAL FEATURES

- Most cases with intraocular foreign body (IOFB) are due to workplace related injuries, the commonest being metal on metal hammering.
- Can lead to secondary changes in the eye such as cataract, hemorrhage, infection, retinal tears and detachment, and retinal degeneration such as siderosis (in case of iron containing IOFB).
- Ultrasound is indicated for the following purposes:
  Detection of an IOFB—its location, number, size and possible nature
  Detection of associated ocular damage
  Documentation for medicolegal purposes.

ULTRASONOGRAPHY

Typical Features

- Echodense signal with shadowing
- Persistence of the signal at lower gain
- The foreign body may be quite small and linear, and may be missed if the probe is not perpendicular to the flat side of the foreign body.

Specific Features

- Metal and stone being prominent reflectors of ultrasound, produce higher amplitude echoes than any normal structure except bone. Stone foreign bodies are usually larger and more irregular in shape. Knowing the circumstances of injury can also help distinguish between the two
- Wood and vegetable matter reflect only intermediate amplitude echoes and may be quite difficult to distinguish. In case of a long-standing injury and retained IOFB, degradation of the organic matter may make the IOFB undetectable
- Glass has specific echographic characteristics. It is only when the sound beam strikes the long, smooth surface of a glass sliver with perpendicular incidence, that it is likely to be picked up by ultrasound
- Spherical IOFBs produce very strong reverberations due to their regular structure

- Air has special characteristics. An air bubble may mimic a foreign body because of the comparatively higher speed of sound through air compared to vitreous. The change in impedance at the interface between the bubble and the surrounding media is very high and produces a very strong echo.

NUGGETS

Irregular shaped IOFBs may mimic multiple foreign bodies, this is particularly seen in large glass pieces with multiple reflecting surfaces, IOLs and certain airgun bullets.

In case of a long-standing IOFB, due to disintegration, the reflectivity may not be as high as expected. In such cases, the presence of siderotic changes may lead one to suspect and look for an IOFB more diligently.

Due to the decrease in speed of sound in blood compared to aqueous or vitreous, one may miss a small IOFB in the presence of dense vitreous hemorrhage. Here sound may not reflect well off the surface of an object surrounded by blood.

Multiple IOFBs may be seen in blast injuries, spectacle damage and road traffic accidents.

Areas where an IOFB may not be easily picked up are the anterior chamber, lens, ciliary sulcus and pars plana. Standoff, immersion scans or high frequency ultrasound can be used if in doubt.

The B scan tends to overestimate the size of the IOFB.

In certain case where the echographic characteristics may be atypical, a CT scan along with ultrasound may help confirm the findings.

Remember not to ask for an MRI confirmation if you suspect a magnetic or metallic foreign body!

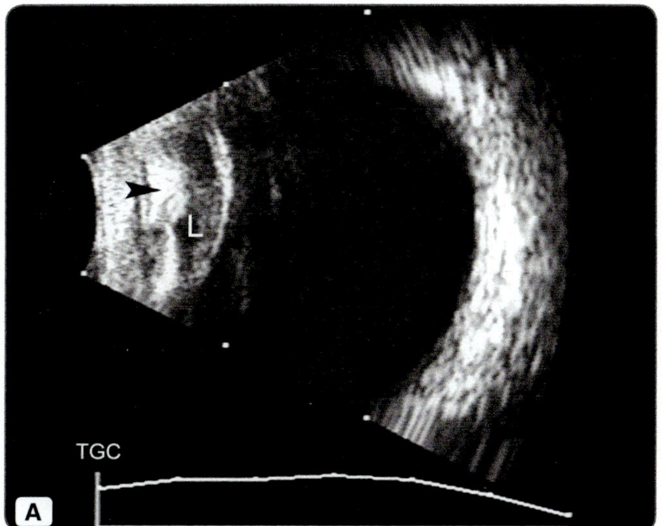

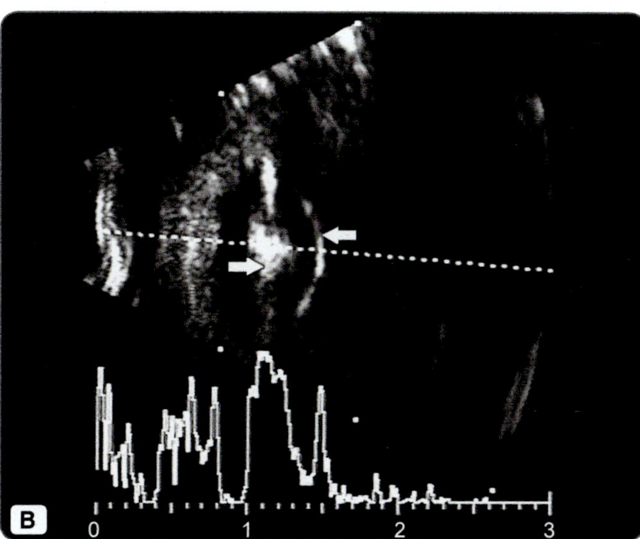

Figures 9.1A and B: B scan image of two eyes with penetrating injury, traumatic cataract with an intact posterior capsule, and an apparently normal posterior segment on ultrasound. There is a linear high reflective structure within the lens (L), causing a small amount of reverberation, indicating an intralenticular foreign body (arrowhead). In Figure B, using the standoff technique, the IOFB is seen much better (arrow). The thin arrow shows the intact posterior capsule of the lens.

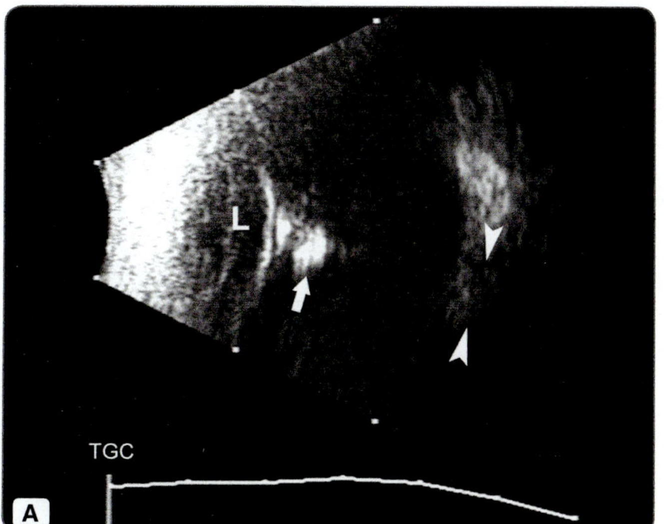

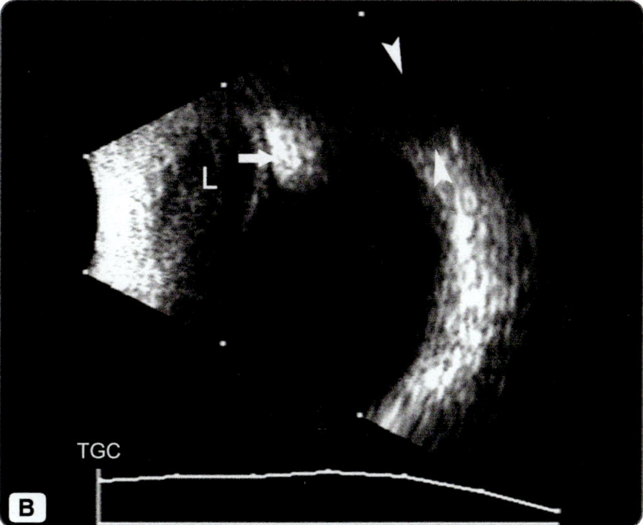

Figures 9.2A and B: B scan images of an IOFB (arrow) located just behind the lens (L). The IOFB is irregular in shape, of high reflectivity and causes orbital shadowing (arrowheads). Though it is fairly large, such an IOFB can be missed on regular ultrasound due to its very anterior location.

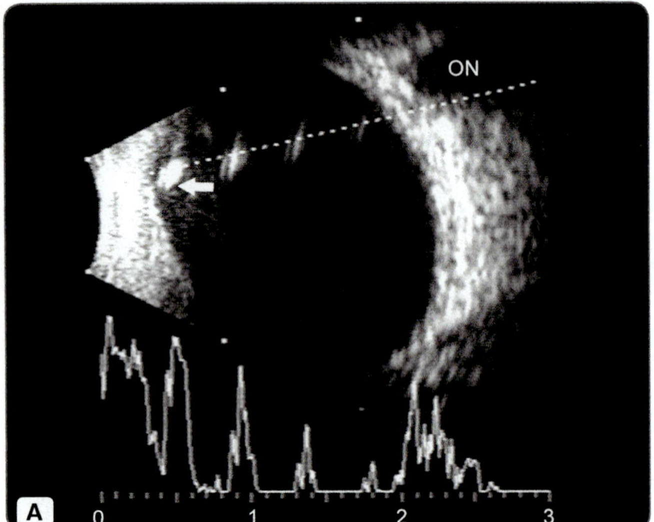

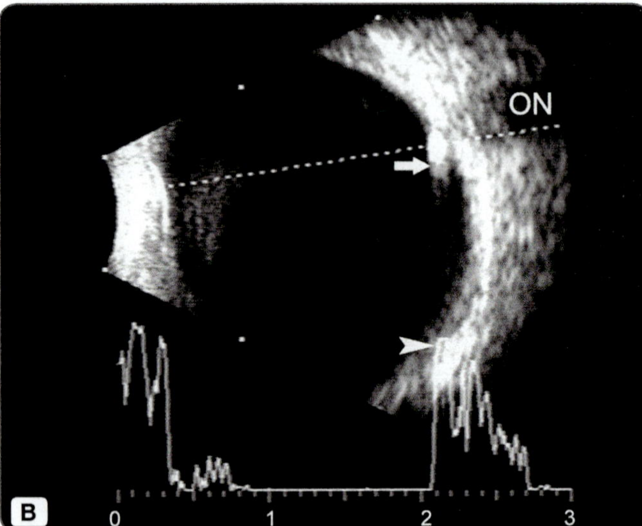

Figures 9.3A and B: B scan with vector A scan showing obliquely placed reverberations (arrow) from an anteriorly located foreign body. The A scan spikes are at regular intervals and of gradually decreasing reflectivity. Figure B is a B scan with vector A scan of the same eye showing a second foreign body (arrow) located on the optic disc. This is of 100% reflectivity (arrowhead). Shadowing is not obvious as it is located on the optic disc. Such multiple foreign bodies usually are spectacle glass pieces or fragments from a blast injury.

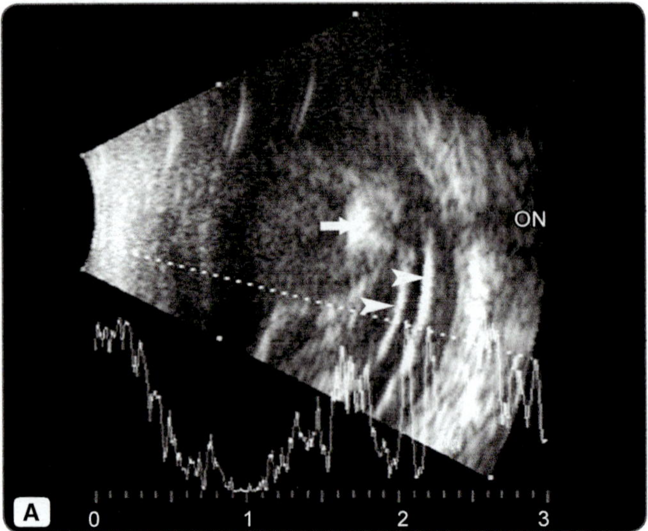

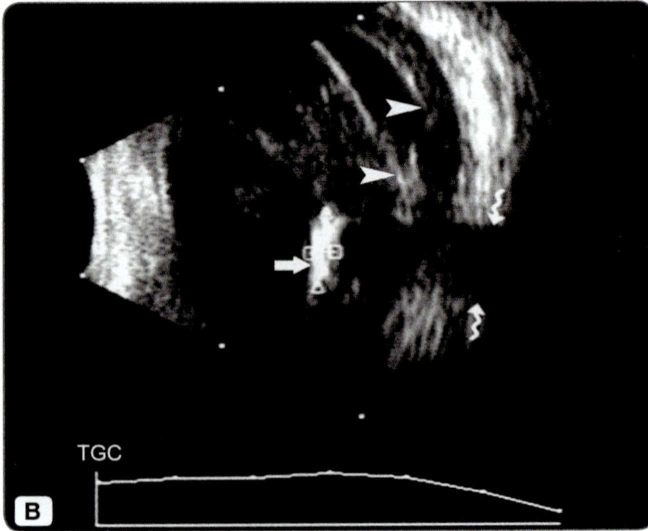

Figures 9.4A and B: B scan with vector A scan demonstrating the presence of an IOFB (arrow) in the vitreous cavity with dense vitreous hemorrhage and multiple high reflective membranes (arrows). Note that the image at high gain does not demonstrate the IOFB clearly. In the second image, taken at low gain, the IOFB is well seen, and features such as 100% reflectivity and orbital shadowing (curved arrows) are clearly made out.

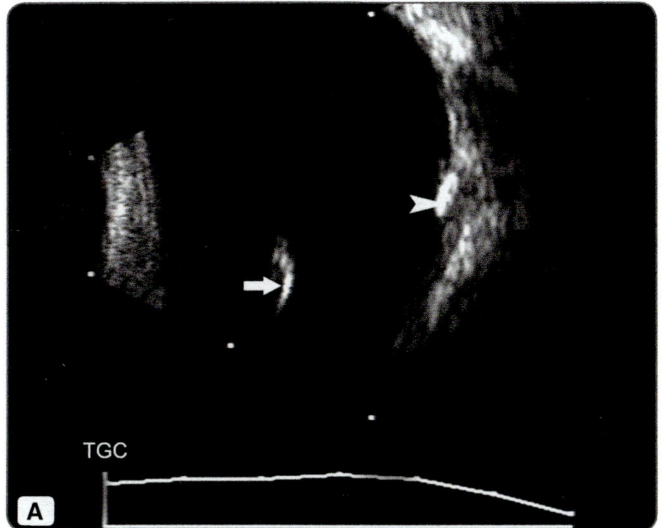

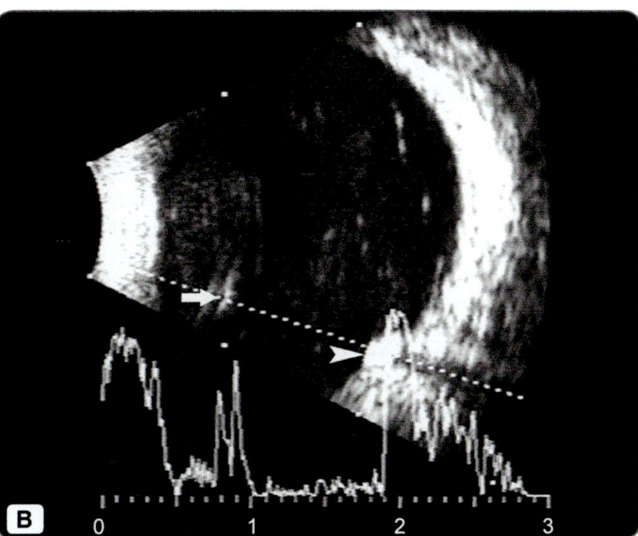

Figures 9.5A and B: B scan image showing two high reflective lesions, one in the vitreous cavity (arrow), and a second on the retinal surface (arrowhead). The intravitreal foreign body is of lower reflectivity, and the second, of very high reflectivity. The former was from an old injury and the latter from a recent one. The vector A scan is seen passing through both lesions showing their relative reflectivity.

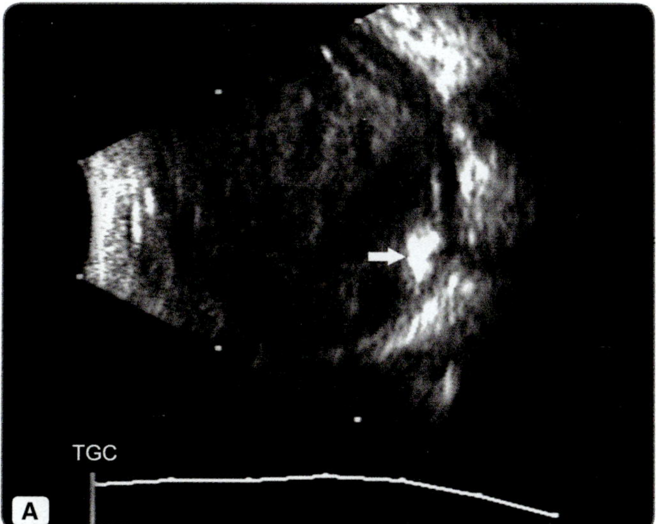

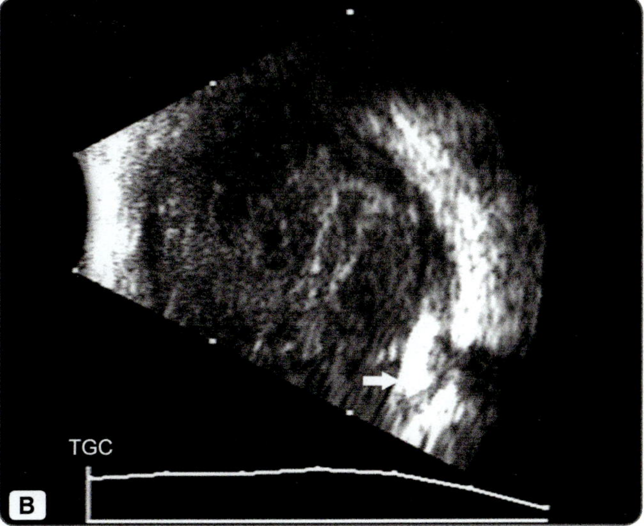

Figures 9.6A and B: These images show the importance of placing the probe perpendicular to the longest axis of the IOFB to best demonstrate its characteristics. The first image shows a relatively smaller and irregular IOFB (arrow) on the retinal surface, but the second, done with a minimal change in probe position demonstrates a larger size and high reflectivity with dense orbital shadowing.

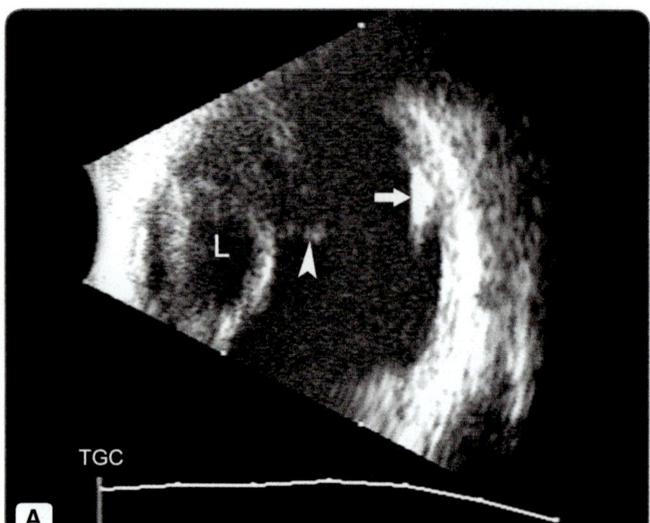

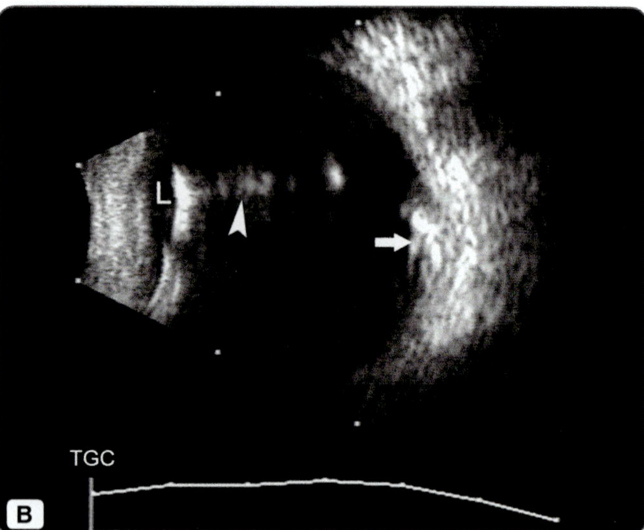

Figures 9.7A and B: These B scan images show a vitreous track (arrowhead) from the posterior surface of the lens (L) and an IOFB lying on the retinal surface (arrow). Such tracks are helpful in locating a possible IOFB. In the first image, the IOFB lies along the track, but in the second it is seen at a lower level.

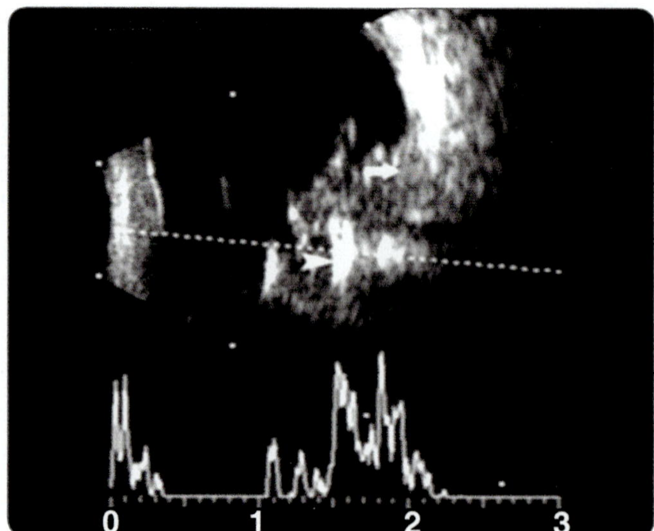

Figure 9.8: B scan images with vector A scan showing a large clump of variably reflecting echoes at the posterior globe wall. The globe wall is not clearly seen indicating a possible scleral rupture with incarceration of ocular contents (arrow). Within this area are seen linear high reflective echoes with orbital shadowing, suggestive of an IOFB (arrowhead), possibly with multiple reflective surfaces. The IOFB is seen partly within the eye and partly within the ocular coats.

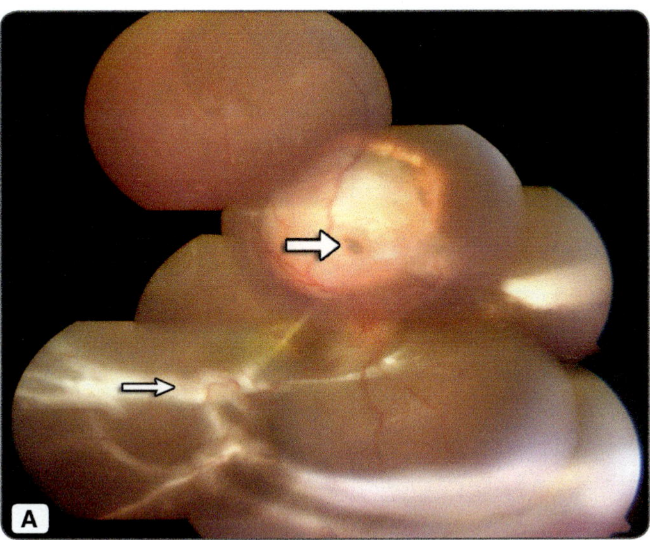

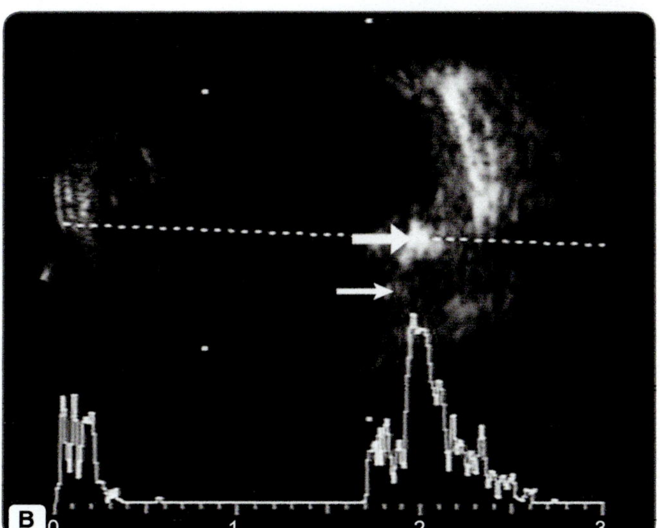

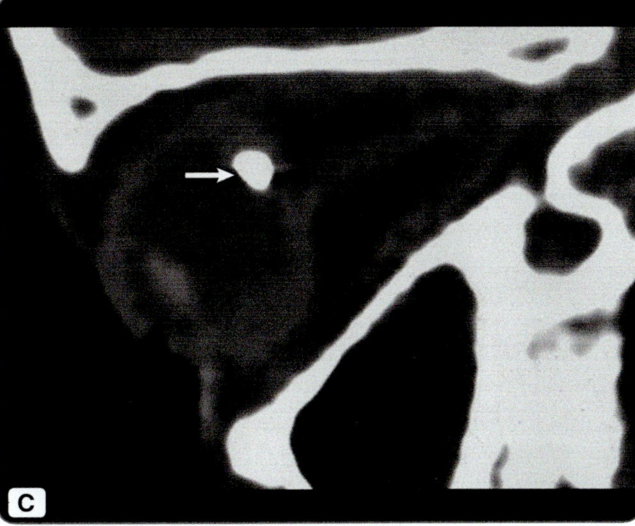

Figures 9.9A to C: Fundus photography of a young girl with a long-standing retinal detachment following trauma. Note the subretinal bands (arrow) and a granuloma above the disc with a small pigmented spot (broad arrow). Ultrasound B scan with vector A shows a moderately reflective subretinal mass in the area of the granuloma. Within this is a very high reflective clump of echoes indicative of a foreign body. The CT scan confirms the presence of a foreign body within the mass (arrow).

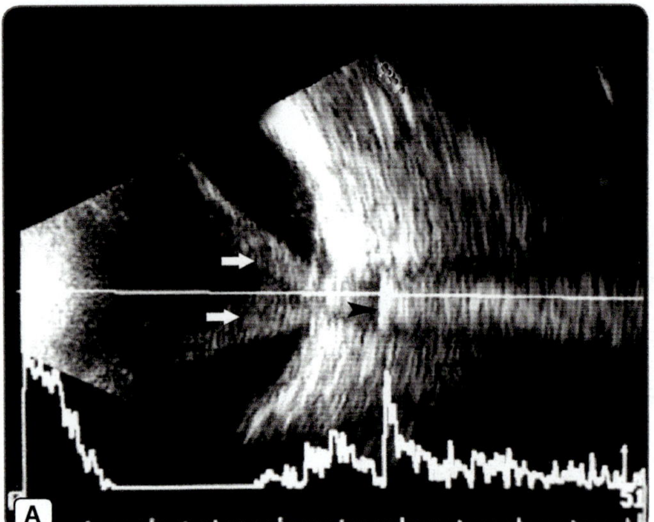

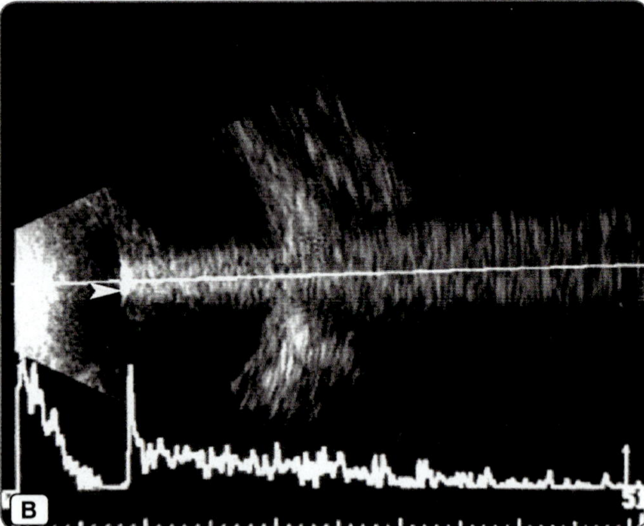

Figures 9.10A and B: B scan with vector A scan following injury with an air gun. In figure A, note the high reflective vitreous membranes attaching at the optic disc and an IOFB within the optic nerve (black arrowhead). The high reflectivity with strong reverberations indicates a spherical object. The fellow eye shows a similar IOFB within the anterior vitreous cavity (white arrowhead).

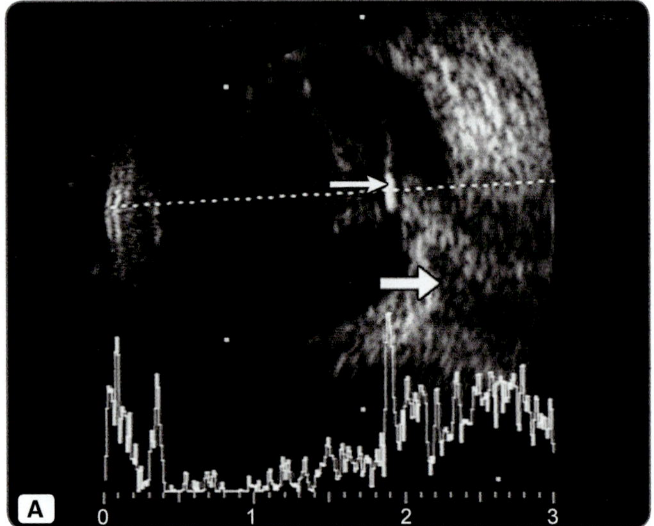

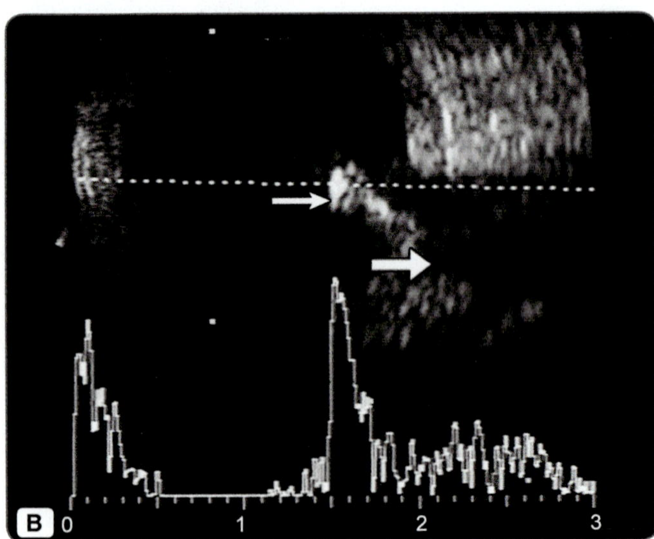

Figures 9.11A and B: Ultrasound B scan images of an eye with IOFB partly embedded in the optic nerve. Note the high reflective echo on the surface of a large clump emanating from the optic nerve. The widened distorted optic nerve shadow is seen in the second figure (broad arrow).

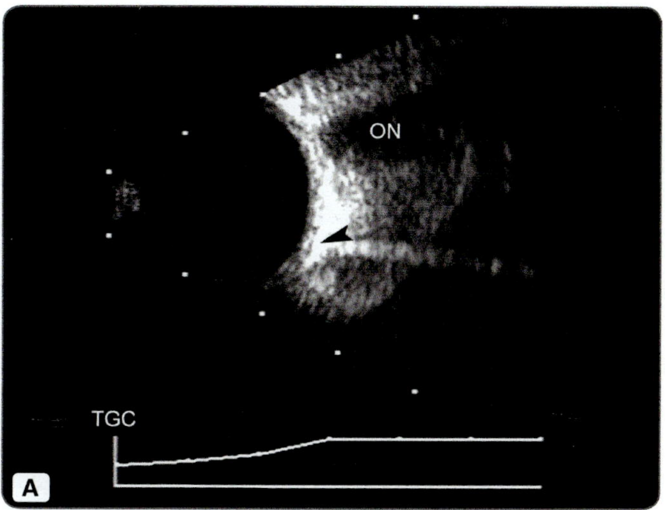

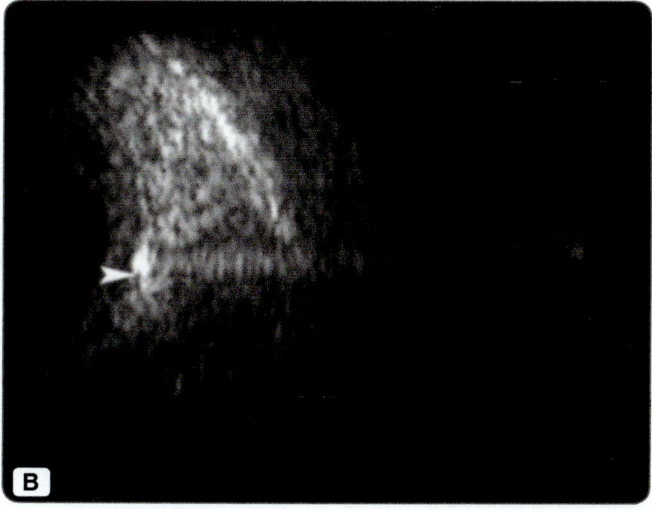

Figures 9.12A and B: B scan images of a case of orbital foreign body lying just external to the ocular coats. In this case the foreign body is seen as a high reflective area (arrowhead) just adjacent to the globe wall, causing strong reverberation echoes (Optic nerve = ON).

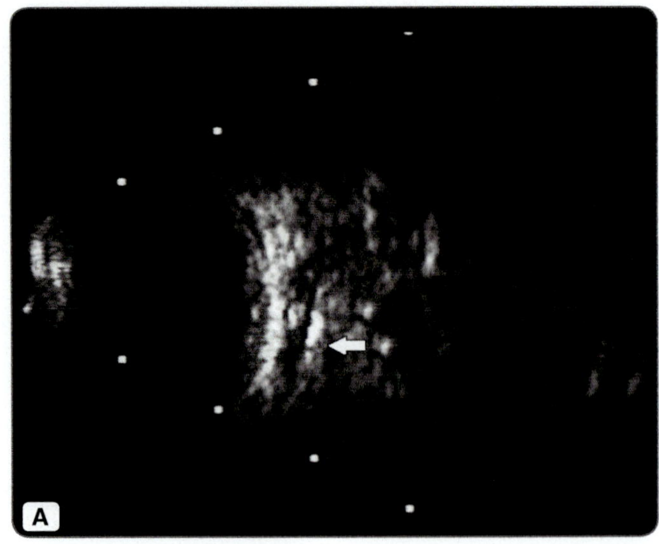

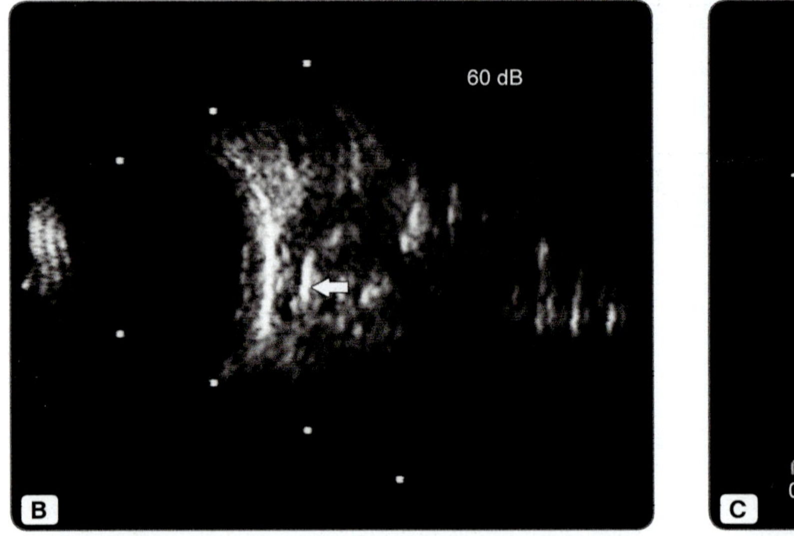

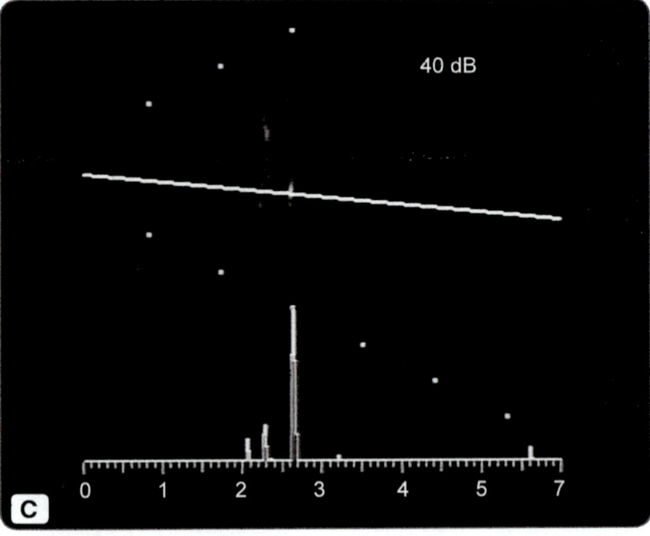

Figures 9.13A to C: Ultrasound B scan images of the orbit showing an orbital foreign body (arrow). The anterior echoes have been dampened to view the orbit better. The high reflective echoes within the orbit make detection of an orbital foreign body difficult. In Figure C, the gain has been reduced to dampen all echoes. Note the solitary high reflective echo arising from the orbital foreign body.

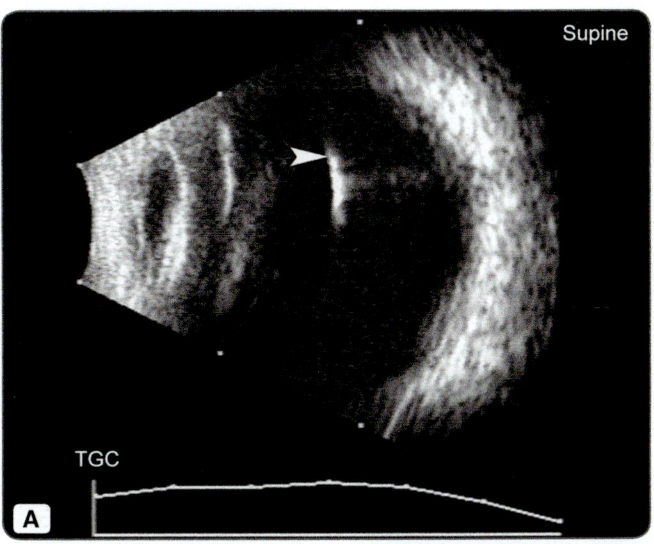

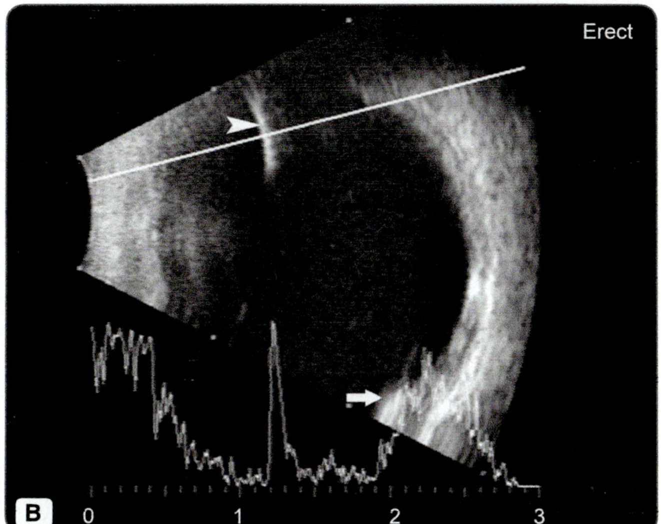

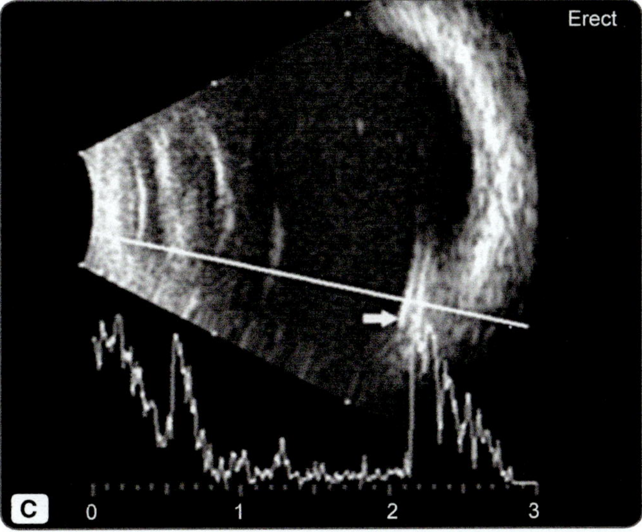

Figures 9.14A to C: B scan with vector A scan images showing the differing behavior of air and IOFB. In the supine position a linear echo of high reflectivity showing a comet tail artifact (arrowhead) is seen in the mid vitreous. With the patient looking down (Fig. B), this echo tends to move to the superior part, indicating that it is an air bubble. Note the high reflective echo on the retinal surface inferiorly (arrow), indicative of an IOFB. The third image, again with the head position changed, shows that the air bubble is no longer visible, but the IOFB has remained stationary on the retinal surface.

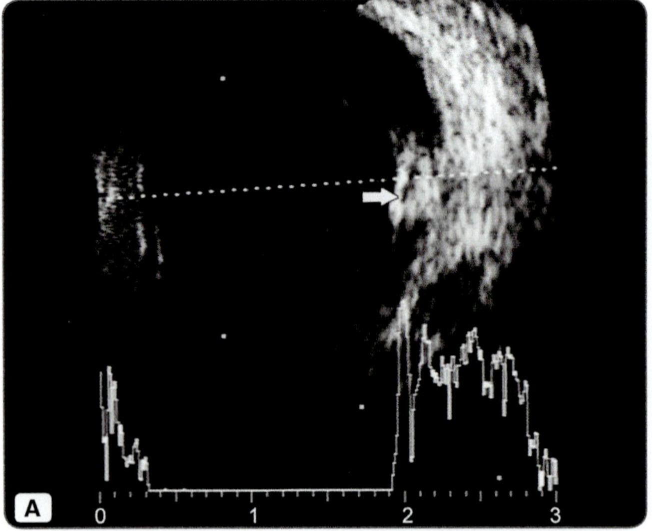

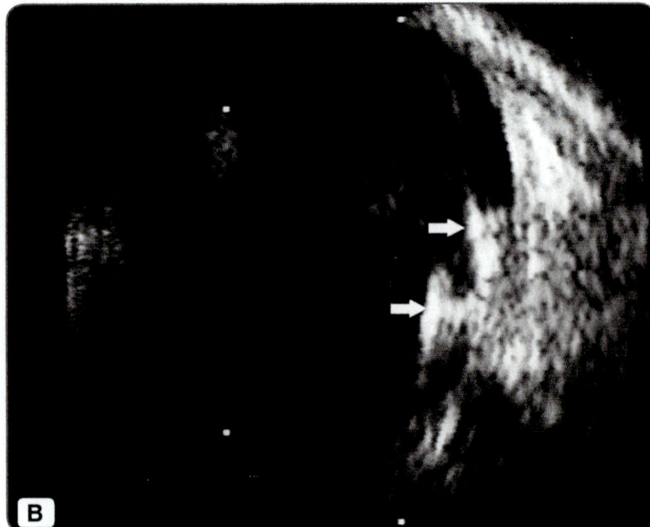

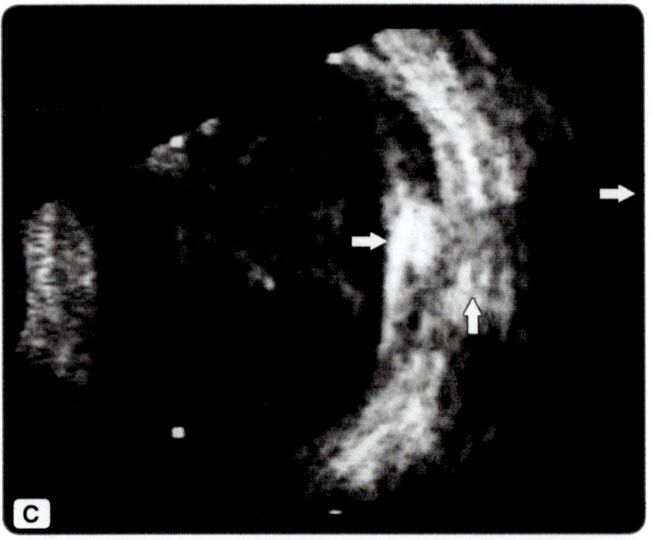

Figures 9.15A to C: Ultrasound B scans with vector A in an eye with multiple glass foreign bodies. Note that the first image shows a clump of high reflectivity. In the second and third images by adjusting the position of the probe so that it is perpendicular to the long axis of the foreign body, the reverberations are more prominent, causing shadowing just above the optic nerve shadow (arrow). It is also seen that there are two foreign bodies.

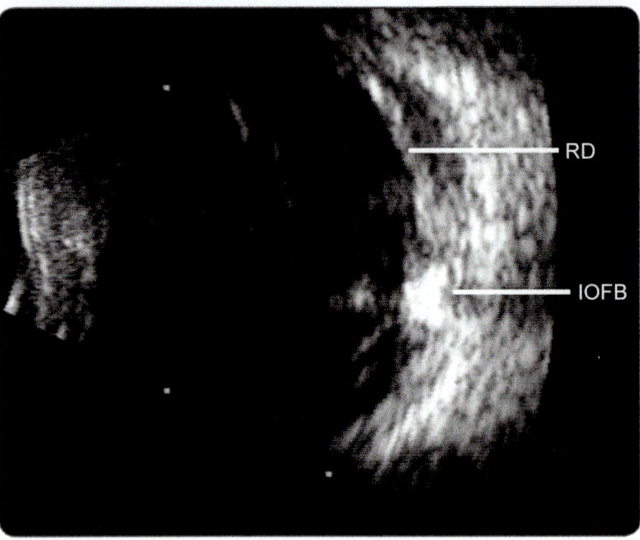

Figure 9.16: B scan images of a high reflective IOFB partly embedded in the ocular coats with vitreous incarceration and an RD.

10 Trauma

INDICATIONS FOR ULTRASOUND

- To assess internal ocular damage/anatomy following trauma in eyes with opaque media.
- To detect and localize intraocular foreign bodies.
- To detect posterior vitreous detachment.
- To detect retinal tears and detachments.
- To detect a posterior scleral rupture.

Advantages

- Easy access.
- Real time images.
- Greater resolution of intraocular soft tissue (0.1 to 0.01 mm) than MRI or CT scan.
- Useful in serial follow-up of eyes with hemorrhagic choroidal detachment.

Difficulties and Disadvantages

- The normal anatomy of the eye may be grossly disturbed. This may be due to abnormal displacement of normal ocular structures or introduction of abnormal structures into the eye. This, along with abnormalities in the media, such as blood or air, may cause misleading signals, which require careful interpretation.
- Hypotony can also cause distortion of structures and difficulty in interpretation is expected.
- There is a possibility of adding to the trauma if the procedure is not performed gently.
- Less sensitive in orbital trauma due to the normally variable echographic patterns of the orbit, and the inability for the conventional ultrasound beam to penetrate the deep orbit.

Specific Conditions where Ultrasound is Useful

- Hyphema
- Traumatic cataract
- Vitreous hemorrhage, follow-up for spontaneous PVD, RD.

- Traumatic endophthalmitis
- Detection and localization of intraocular foreign bodies.
- Differentiation between serous and hemorrhagic choroidal detachments and follow-up for clot lysis.
- Suspected posterior exit wounds with associated incarceration of intraocular contents.

LENS CHANGES

- The normal clear lens is low reflective. This feature is lost when the lens is damaged either by blunt or penetrating injury.
- The lens may be subluxated or dislocated, either anteriorly or posteriorly, or even expelled out of the globe.
- In case of penetrating, or sometimes even after blunt trauma, a posterior capsule rupture may be seen. The lenticular contents may be disturbed within the capsule, in which case the lens appears very high reflective due to hydration of the cortex. In other situations, the lens matter may prolapse into the vitreous where it can get admixed with vitreous and blood.
- Small posterior capsule ruptures may be missed by ultrasound.
- In penetrating injuries, one may even see an intralenticular foreign body.

NUGGETS

Use immersion or standoff techniques with the regular ultrasound probe to image the anterior segment or the lens. A higher frequency probe such as the 20 MHz probe is ideal to study the posterior capsule.

It is recommended to suspect, and carefully look for, an intralenticular foreign body if there is a positive history, presence of cataract and an intact posterior capsule on ultrasound.

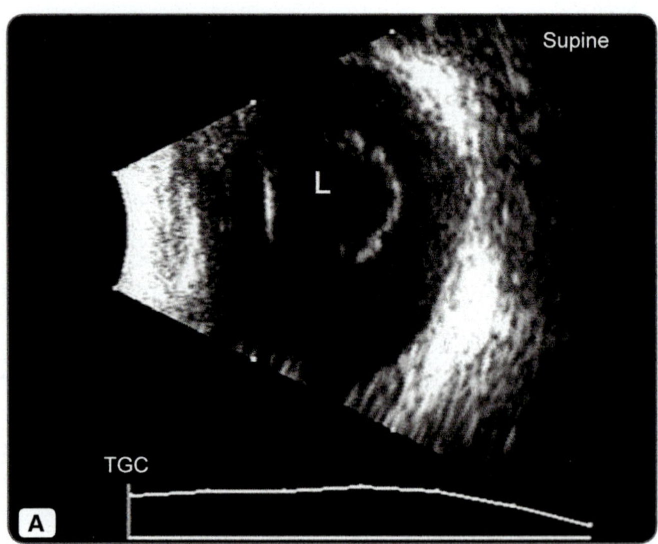

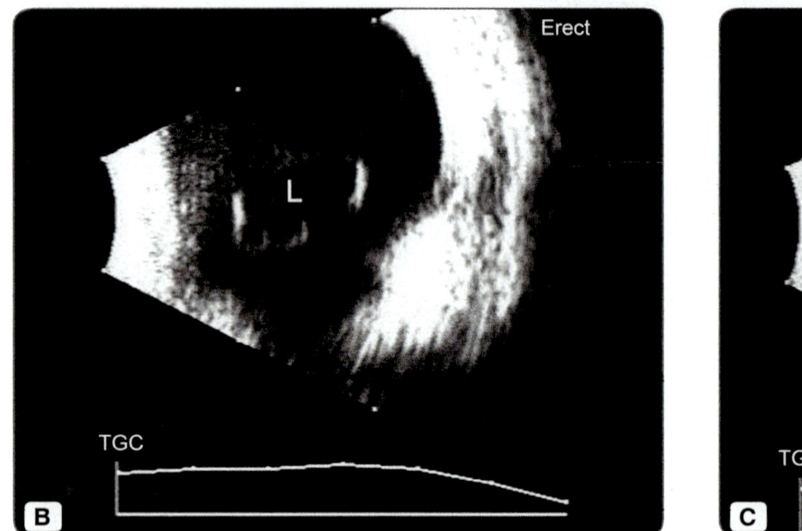

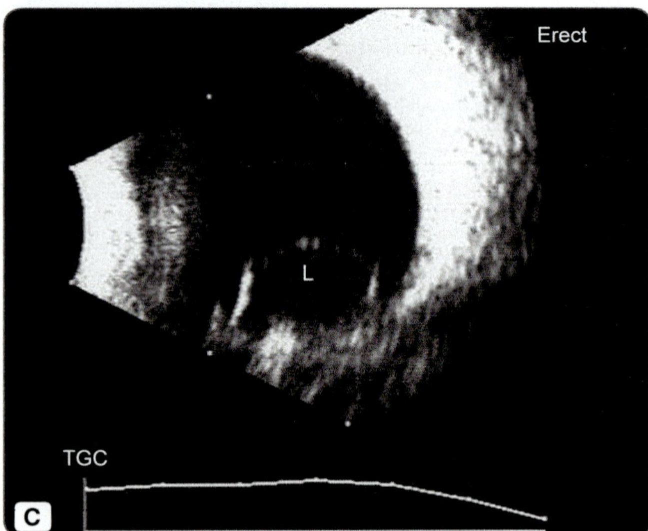

Figures 10.1A to C: B scan images showing a mobile dislocated lens in the vitreous cavity following blunt trauma. The clear lens is seen as a biconvex structure with no internal echoes (L). It is seen to move downwards as the position is changed from supine to erect.

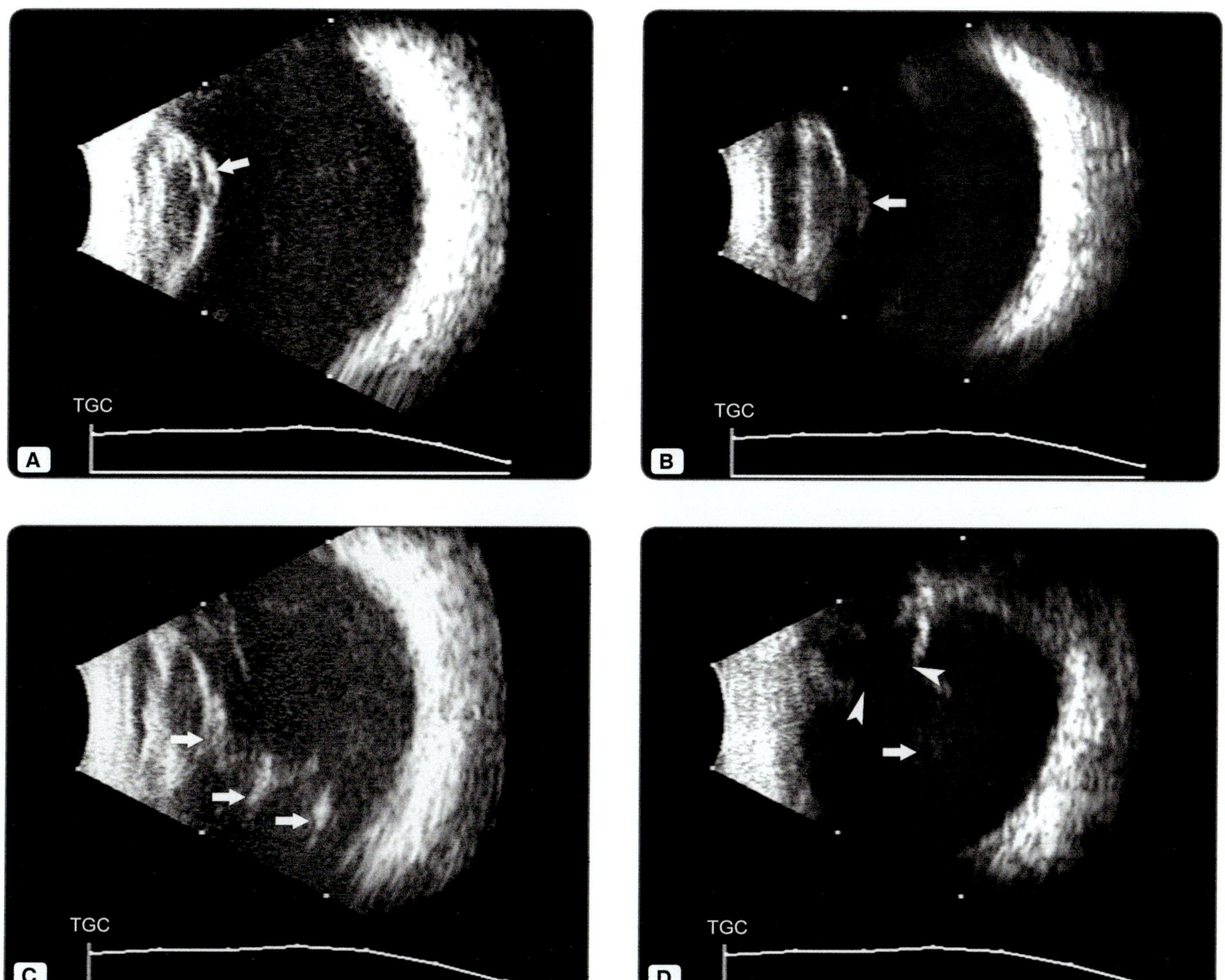

Figures 10.2A to D: B scan images showing varying degrees of posterior capsule rupture following penetrating injury. Figure A shows a posterior capsule dehiscence (arrow) but no prolapse of lens matter. Figure B shows a small amount of prolapsed lens matter in the anterior vitreous just behind the lens (arrow). Figure C shows a posterior capsular dehiscence with lens matter in the vitreous following the track of injury (arrows). Figure D shows a very large posterior capsule rupture (arrowheads) with low reflective vitreous echoes (arrow).

VITREOUS CHANGES

- These include hemorrhage, inflammation, infection, incarceration and membrane formation.
- It is important to look for a PVD and note its extent in order to plan the timing of surgery in a traumatized eye. In an eye with vitreous hemorrhage, the PVD may be lined by blood and hence appear highly reflective, not unlike a retinal detachment. However, the reflectivity may not be uniform and tends to be higher inferiorly because of the tendency for blood to settle with gravity.
- The blood may organize into membranes and these may converge towards an area of vitreous incarceration at the site of a scleral rupture .
- Vitreous tracks may be seen extending from the point of penetration to the posterior ocular structures and may lead to an area of rupture or incarceration diagonally opposite to the site of injury.

NUGGETS

A vitreous track extending from a posterior capsular rupture into the vitreous can alert one to the presence of a posterior segment IOFB

Similarly an area of posterior vitreous incarceration along with a scleral rupture could indicate a possible orbital foreign body. However, incarceration without evidence of scleral rupture or an IOFB at the site could also signify an impact site with the IOFB most often located inferiorly in the pars plana region.

The presence of intraocular air in a patient with endophthalmitis in the absence of an open globe or recent surgical intervention is suggestive of clostridial or bacillus infection.

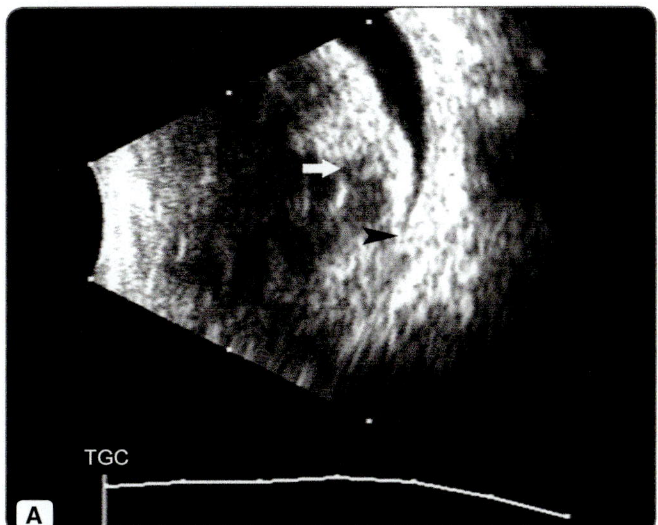

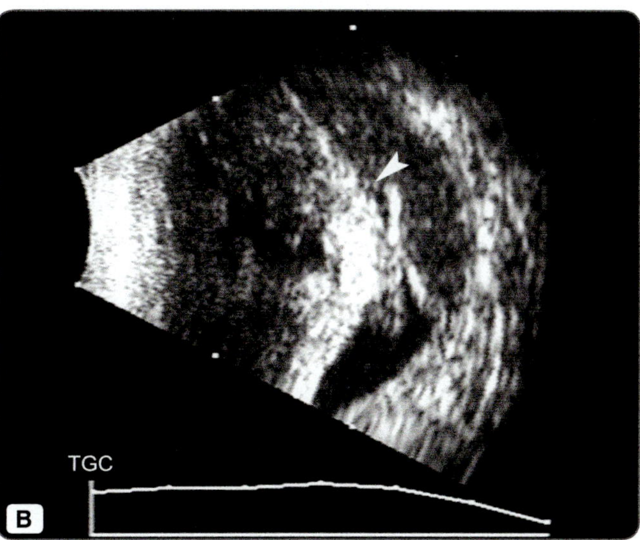

Figures 10.3A and B: B scan images of an eye with dense vitreous hemorrhage following blunt injury. The intragel echoes are fairly high indicating organized blood (arrow). There is a PVD posteriorly. In the periphery, the vitreous is densely adherent to an area of scleral rupture (black arrowhead). Figure B shows that there is also a mound of subretinal hemorrhage (arrowhead) that has broken into the vitreous cavity.

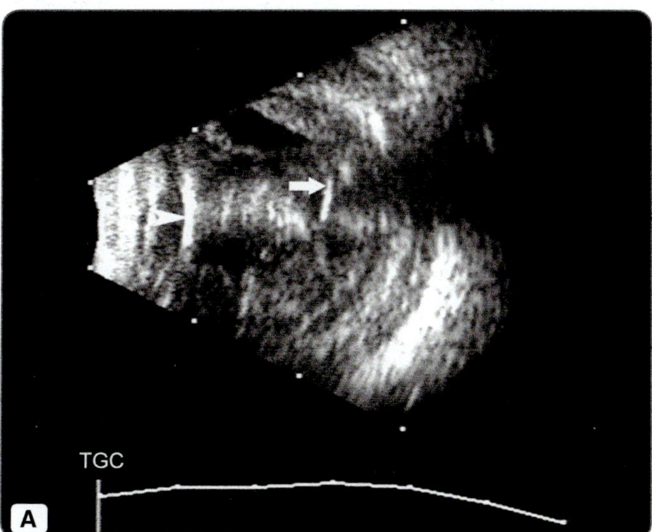

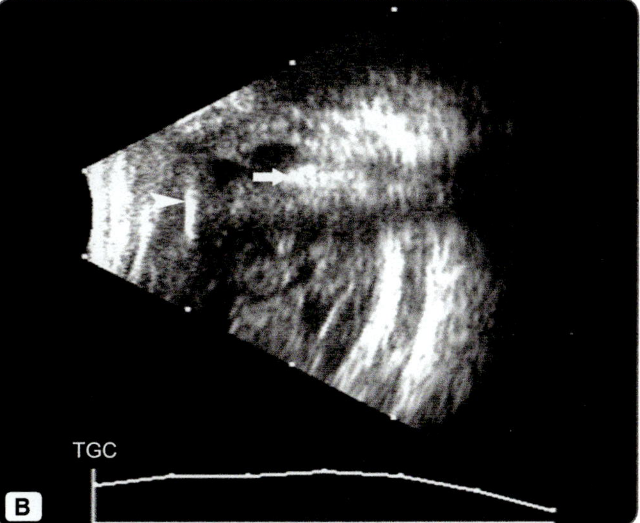

Figures 10.4A and B: Transverse and longitudinal B scan images of a young boy with traumatic panophthalmitis following a broom-stick injury. Note the intragel echoes suggestive of vitreous inflammation. There is gross choroidal thickening as well as Tenon's widening. Two linear high reflective echoes are seen, one just behind the lens capsule (arrowhead), with significant reverberations, suggestive of intraocular air. The second echo (arrow), more obliquely placed, causes shadowing in one of the views. This echo represents a broken end of the broomstick within the vitreous cavity.

RETINAL CHANGES

- Retinal breaks can occur as a consequence of both blunt and penetrating injury. They can occur at the periphery with the edge of the PVD attached to the apex. Dialysis and giant tears can also occur. Often the tear is seen diagonally opposite an area of vitreous incarceration. An associated PVD may not be present in cases, such as recent trauma, in a young patient and in the case of a retinal dialysis
- Giant tears have an unusual configuration and often appear as highly convoluted membranes with no peripheral attachments
- Retinal detachments due to penetrating trauma may have very restricted movements due to incarceration of intraocular contents at the wound site. Retinal insertions may be atypical in cases of severe penetrating trauma and may be confusing to interpret
- Subretinal hemorrhage is common and is seen as an area of thickening of the retinochoroidal layer that is of variable reflectivity depending on the stage of clot lysis. It is also often seen at the site of incarceration or an area of scleral rupture.

NUGGETS

The retina may not be as highly reflective as normal if there is associated endophthalmitis or retinal disruption, and also in very long-standing detachments.

The presence of subretinal hemorrhage at the posterior pole signifies a poor prognosis.

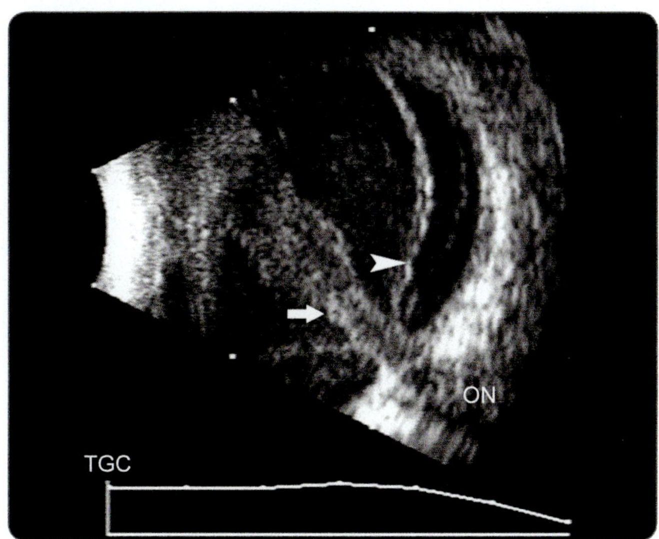

Figure 10.5: B scan image of an eye following penetrating injury. Note the thick, highly reflective vitreous stalk (arrow) extending along the track of penetration upto the optic disc area (ON). The second membrane of equally high reflectivity is a retinal detachment (arrowhead). It is often difficult to distinguish between the two in cases of trauma.

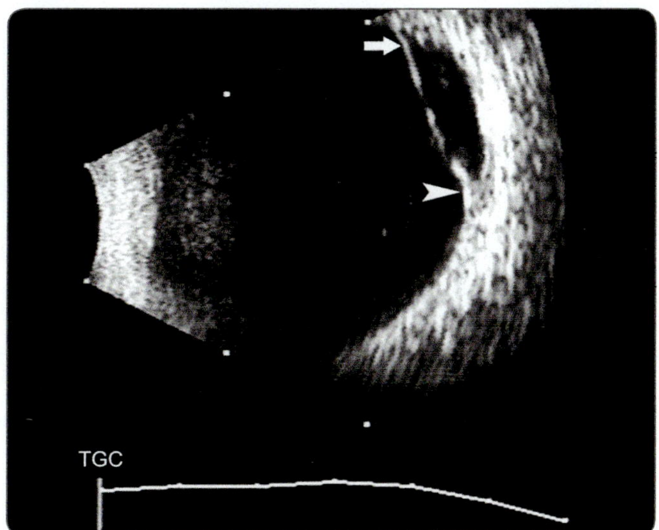

Figure 10.6: B scan image of an eye many years after penetrating injury with a hypodermic needle. Note the thin highly reflective membrane (arrow) extending along the track of the needle. The membrane is thicker near the globe wall (arrowhead) where an area of fibrous proliferation was seen clinically.

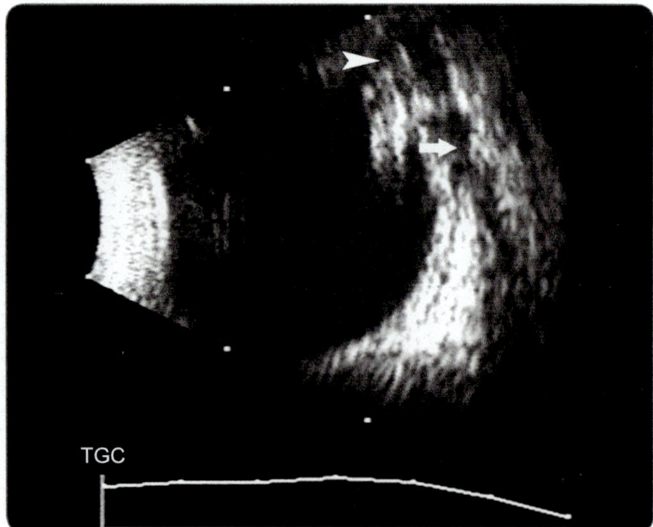

Figure 10.7: B scan image of an eye with accidental globe penetration during squint surgery on the medial rectus muscle. The vitreous cavity shows high reflective echoes clumped at the site of rupture indicative of incarcerated vitreous with hemorrhage (arrowhead). There is scleral echolucency at the site of penetration. The medial rectus insertion is not seen; instead the muscle insertion is folded upon itself and trapped within the scleral fibers (arrow).

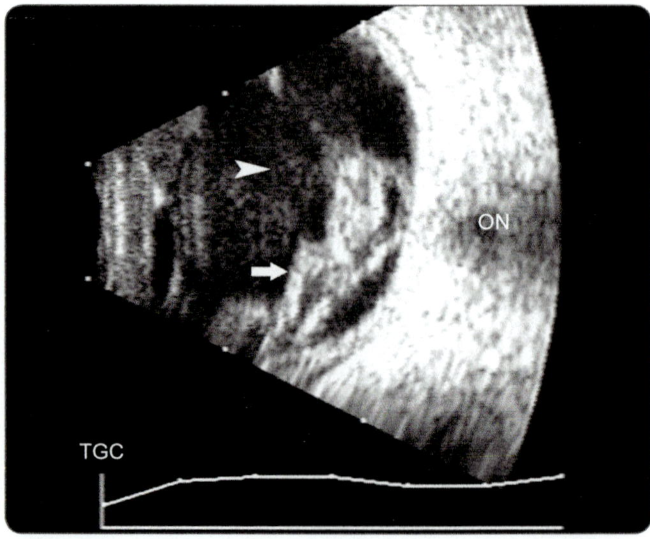

Figure 10.8: B scan image of an eye following severe blunt trauma. The lens echoes are not seen. The vitreous shows low reflective echoes suggestive of hemorrhage (arrowhead). There is a convoluted membrane attached to the optic disc (ON). The superior part of the membrane has no peripheral attachment and appears to be folded down over the inferior part (arrow). This picture is suggestive of a retinal detachment due to a giant retinal tear, which has folded upon itself.

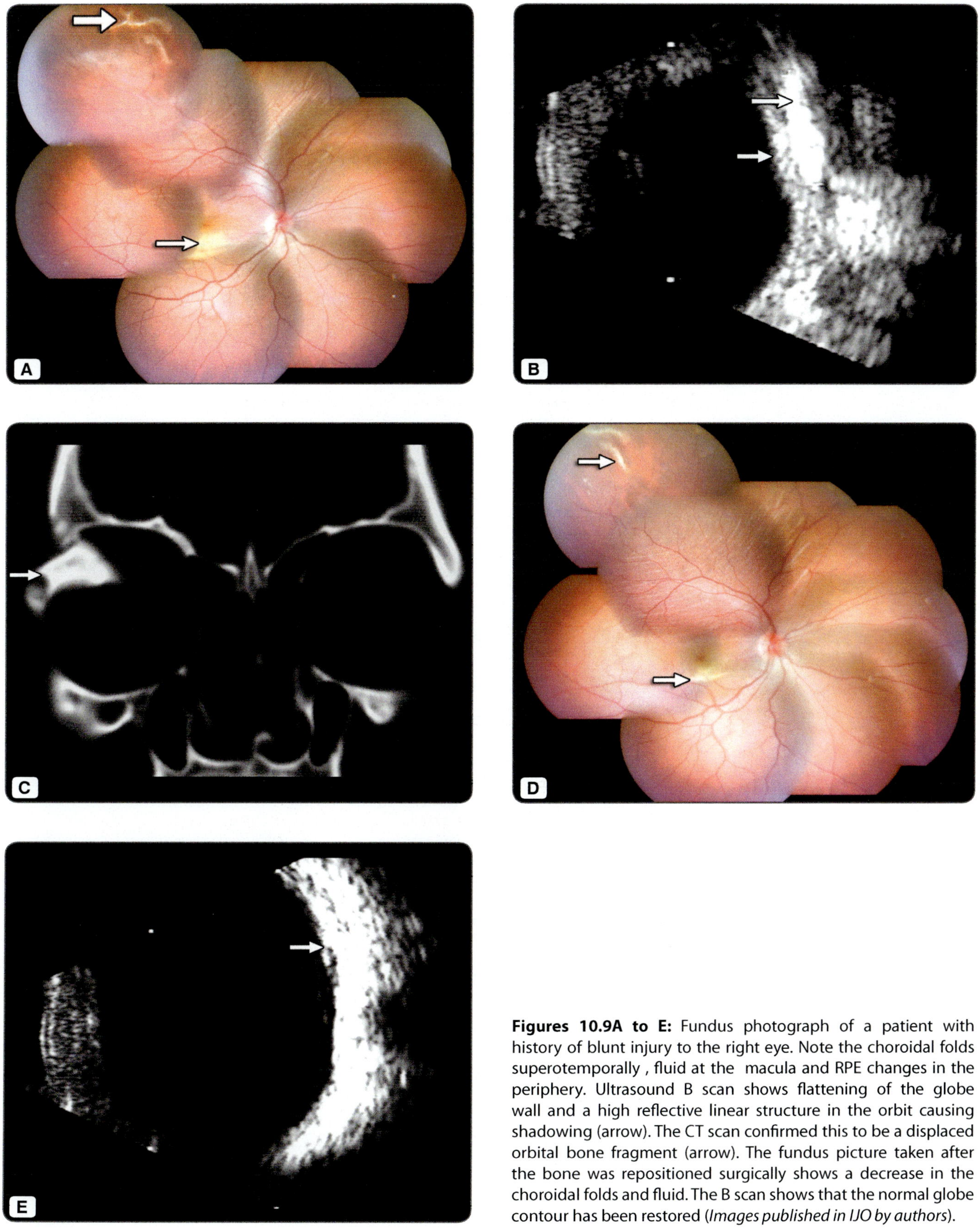

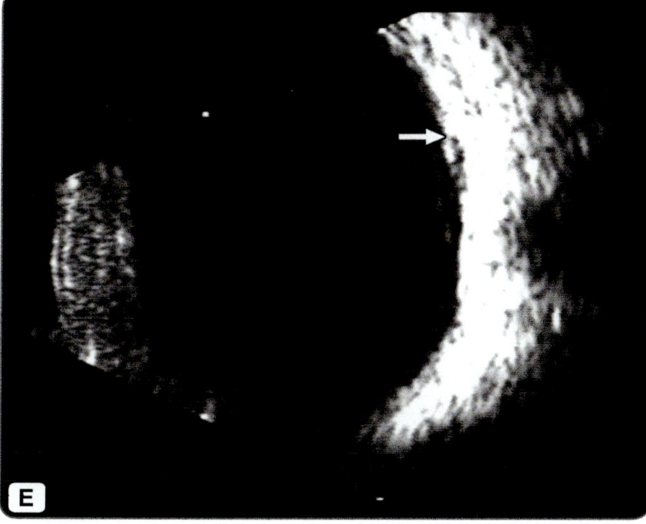

Figures 10.9A to E: Fundus photograph of a patient with history of blunt injury to the right eye. Note the choroidal folds superotemporally , fluid at the macula and RPE changes in the periphery. Ultrasound B scan shows flattening of the globe wall and a high reflective linear structure in the orbit causing shadowing (arrow). The CT scan confirmed this to be a displaced orbital bone fragment (arrow). The fundus picture taken after the bone was repositioned surgically shows a decrease in the choroidal folds and fluid. The B scan shows that the normal globe contour has been restored (*Images published in IJO by authors*).

SCLERAL RUPTURE

- Can occur either in penetrating or severe blunt trauma.
- Presents as chemosis, subconjunctival and/or vitreous hemorrhage and hypotony.
- Ultrasound features at the site of rupture include an area of irregular scleral echolucency, often with incarceration of vitreous and retina. In addition, Tenon's widening due to edema or hemorrhage may be seen.
- Other features include choroidal detachments and scleral folds due to hypotony.

SCLERAL FOLDS

- They can be seen in eyes with severe hypotony
- Appear as dome shaped elevations of the globe wall with intense orbital shadowing. They can mimic IOFBs, or calcification
- Resolve with restoration of intraocular pressure (IOP).

NUGGETS

Scleral ruptures adjacent to the optic nerve can be seen in optic nerve avulsion.

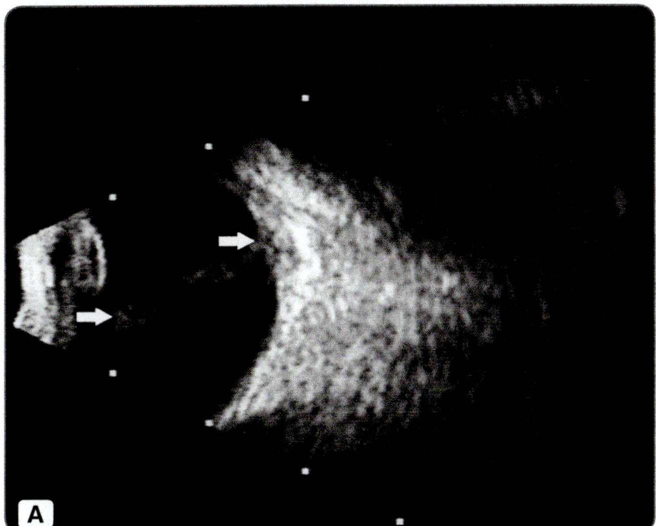

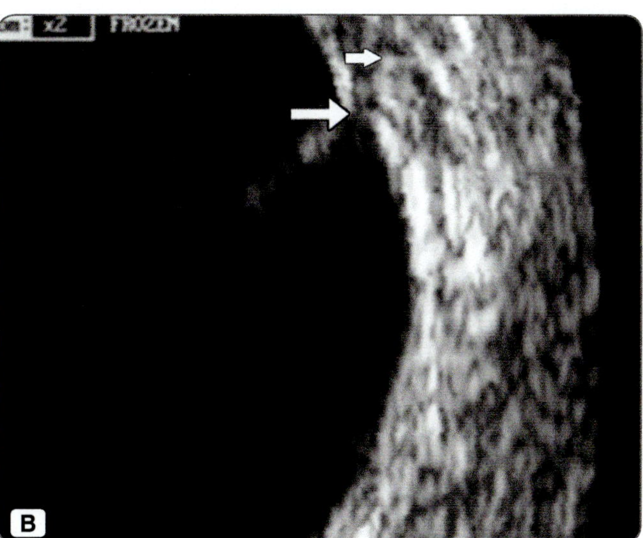

Figures 10.10A and B: Ultrasound images of a young boy who presented with poor vision following penetrating injury with a nail. Figure A shows the track of vitreous extending from the entry point to the posterior globe wall. Figure B is an enlarged image of the point of posterior perforation showing an area of scleral discontinuity and echolucency.

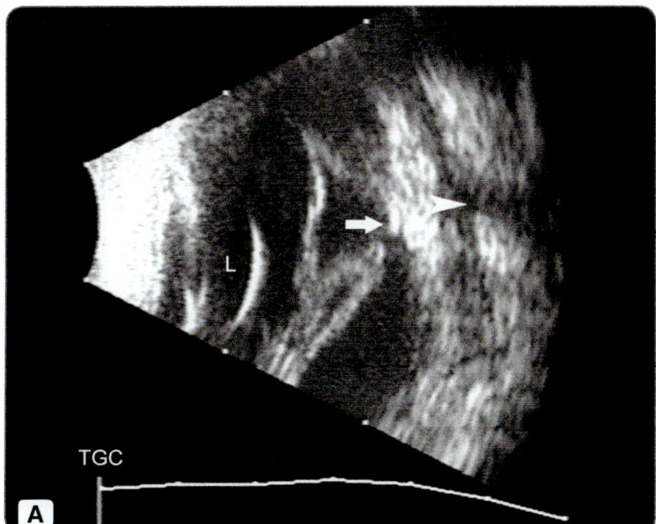

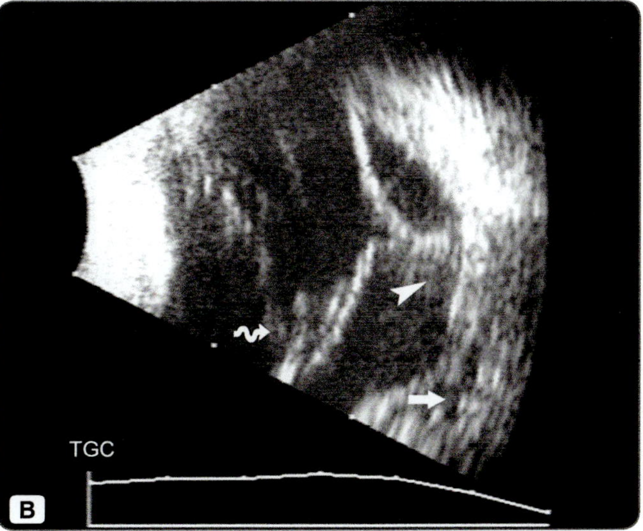

Figures 10.11A and B: B scan images of an eye following severe penetrating trauma in a road traffic accident. Note the smaller size of the globe. There are multiple vitreous membranes (arrow) incarcerated in a scleral rupture (arrowhead). Irregular choroidal thickening is also seen at this site indicating the presence of choroidal hemorrhage. The nature of the membranes is not clearly made out in Figure A. By changing the probe position, the retinal detachment is made out clearly in Figure B (arrow). The vitreous membrane is seen pulling up the retina (curved arrow).

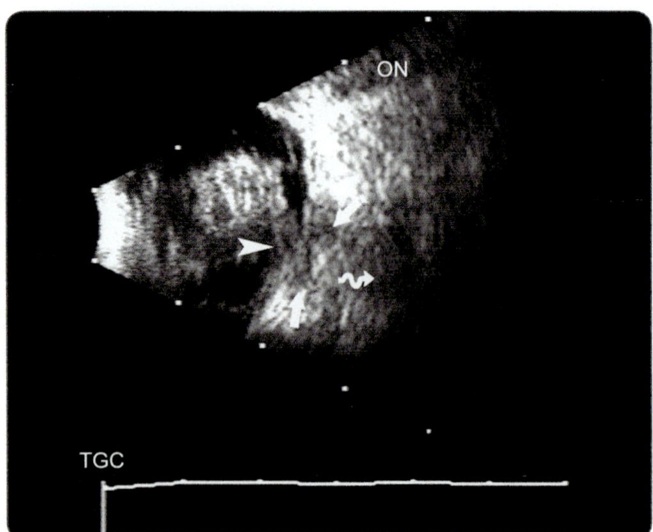

Figure 10.12: B scan image of an eye with dense vitreous hemorrhage along with choroidal hemorrhage and scleral rupture. Note the incarceration of ocular contents (arrowhead) in the area of irregular scleral rupture (arrows). The increased depth penetration of the beam in this image helps to get a better perspective. There is also an area of orbital hemorrhage (curved arrow). (Optic nerve = ON)

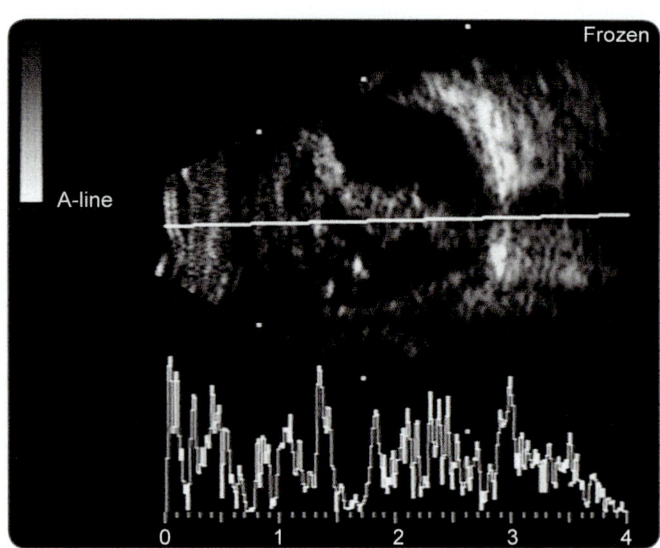

Figure 10.13: Ultrasound B scan with vector A image of a patient who sustained a bull horn injury. Note the vitreous membranes of high reflectivity and irregular contour (broad arrow). The thin arrow points to an area of suspected incarceration of intraocular contents. The long arrow shows echolucency in the surrounding orbital tissues which is suspicious of a globe rupture and wall discontinuity.

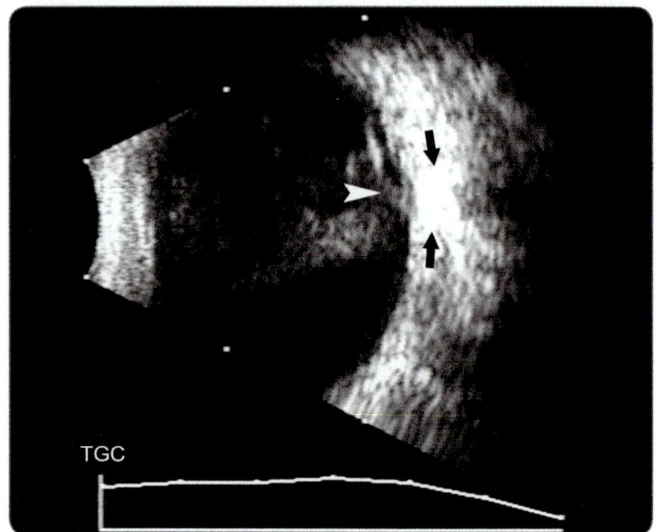

Figure 10.14: B scan image showing vitreous incarceration (arrowhead) into a scleral wound with an orbital foreign body just outside the coats (black arrows). Orbital foreign bodies are less easily visualized because of the high reflectivity of the surrounding orbital tissues.

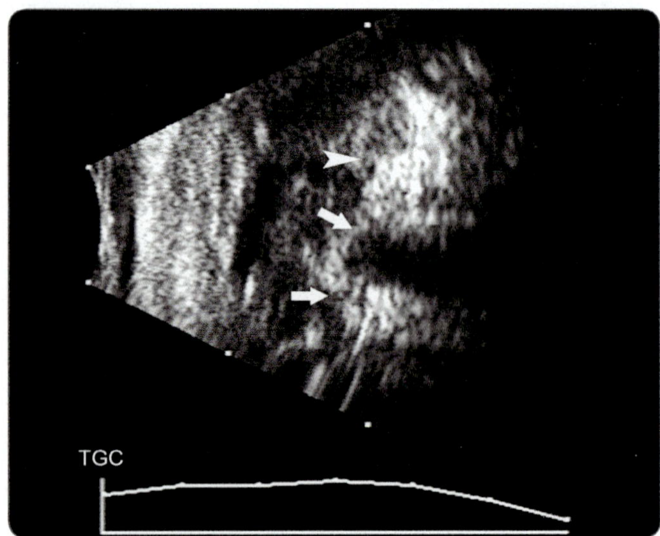

Figure 10.15: Scleral fold in a ruptured globe seen as a high reflective dome shaped structure (arrows) with orbital shadowing. Note the gross thickening of the retinochoroidal layer (arrowhead) and the intragel echoes suggestive of hemorrhage.

Section 4

Infections and Inflammations

11 Endophthalmitis

CLINICAL FEATURES

- Endophthalmitis is a potentially catastrophic intraocular inflammation with or without infection occurring as a complication of intraocular surgery, trauma, systemic infection or uveitis.
- Pain, redness and decreased vision are the most common presenting symptoms.
- Corneal haze, hypopyon and fibrinous reaction may be seen in the anterior segment.
- Fundal view may be hazy or absent.
- Ultrasonography is indicated to determine the presence of inflammation in the vitreous cavity and diagnose associated findings. Serial ultrasound evaluations are indicated to assess the response to conservative treatment and surgical intervention.

ULTRASONOGRAPHY

Common Findings

- Low reflective vitreous echoes—dot-like or cobweb-shaped membranes are suggestive of vitreous inflammation. In more severe cases, thick high reflective membrane like echoes may be seen.
- Presence of thicker echoes anteriorly suggests an anterior locus of infection.
- Posterior vitreous detachment (PVD) may or may not be present initially. As PVD develops in an eye with endophthalmitis, a tractional retinal detachment (TRD) like configuration may be seen. This is due to the thickened inflamed posterior hyaloid which is adherent to the retina. A close watch is to be kept for development of rhegmatogenous RD.

Associated Findings

- Exudative or tractional retinal detachment, choroidal detachment, retinochoroidal thickening and optic nerve head elevation may be seen. In presence of choroidal detachment or thickening, a 6 mm infusion cannula should be planned during vitrectomy
- Intraocular foreign body may be present in case of post-traumatic endophthalmitis.
- Presence of a peripheral granuloma with a tractional radial retinal fold could indicate toxocara infection.

Features Indicative of Poor Prognosis

- Choroidal detachment—may be serous in case of hypotony or may show echoes in the suprachoroidal space signifying direct infection. The latter carries a very poor prognosis
- Presence of thick vitreous membranes, retinal detachment and marked retinochoroidal thickening.
- Panophthalmitis—associated with scleral thickening, T sign and orbital inflammation.

NUGGETS

Always look for nuclear fragments in the vitreous cavity in eyes with severe postoperative inflammation, posterior capsule rent and inadequate surgery details.

The vitreous cavity may not show many echoes or may even appear relatively echolucent in cases where the vitreous cavity is full of pus.

Intraocular lens (IOL) reverberations may mask the echoes in the vitreous cavity. In this situation, by tilting the probe, one can bypass the reverberations to image the vitreous clearly.

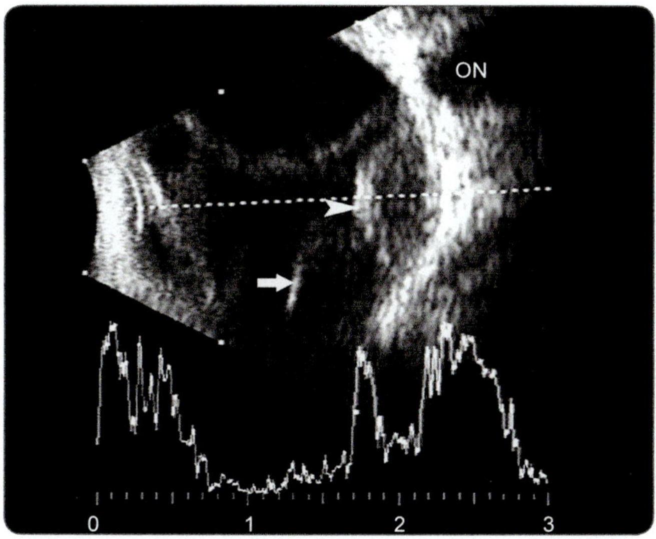

Figure 11.1: B scan with vector A scan of an eye with endophthalmitis. Note the low reflective membrane like echoes (arrow) inserting into the optic disc (ON). There is a dome-shaped lesion at the posterior pole with low internal reflectivity indicating a subretinal abscess formation (arrowhead).

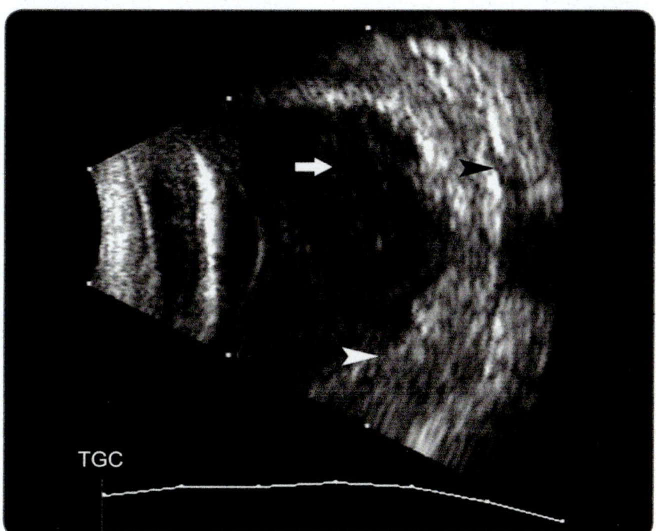

Figure 11.2: B scan image of an eye with severe postoperative endophthalmitis and orbital cellulitis. Note the cobweb-like echoes in the vitreous cavity (arrow). There is significant thickening of the retinochoroidal layer (white arrowhead) along with widening of Tenon's space (black arrowhead).

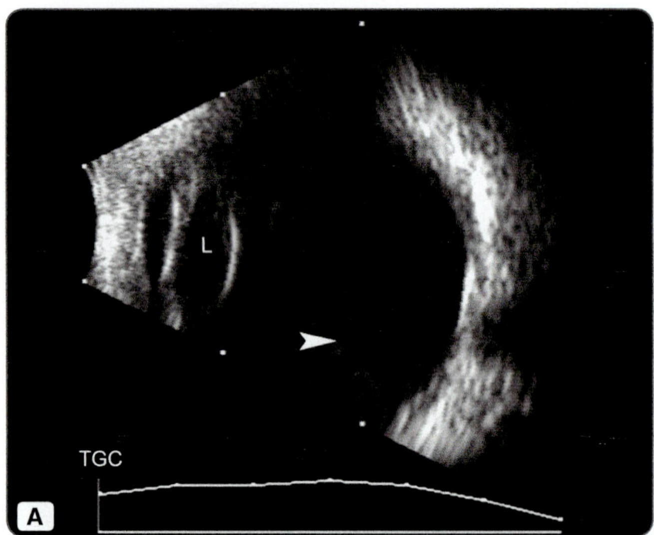

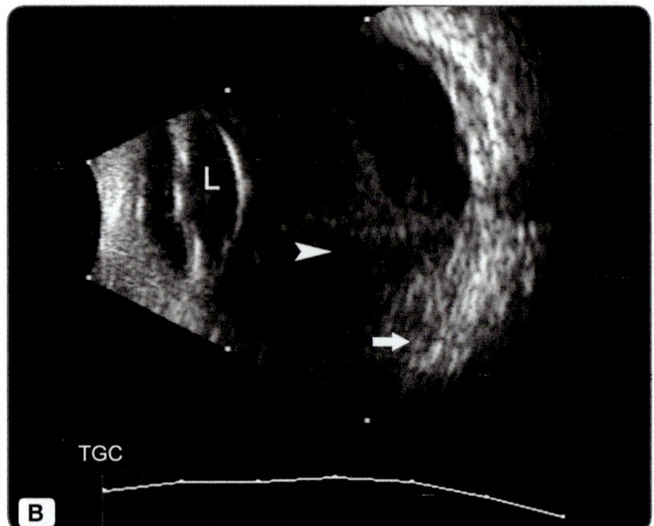

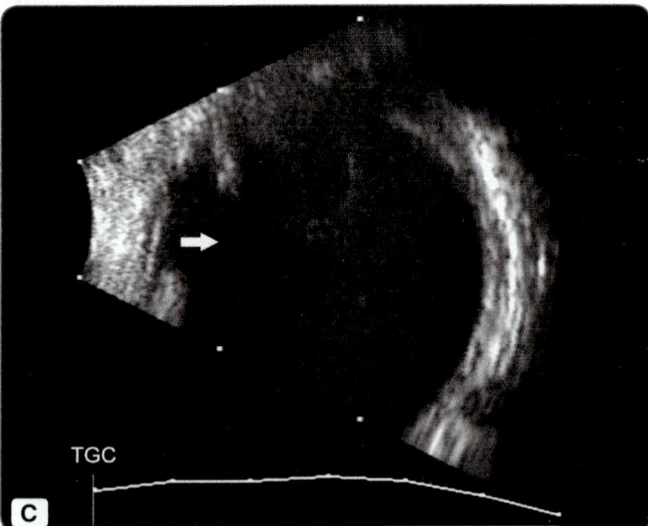

Figures 11.3A to C: B scan images of an eye with endogenous endophthalmitis (L = lens). The first images show relatively few intragel echoes (arrowhead). Figure B shows the increase in the echoes on follow-up with conservative management. At this point, retinochoroidal thickening is also seen (arrow). Figure C shows the clearing of echoes in the vitreous following lensectomy and vitrectomy. Note the absence of lens echoes (arrow).

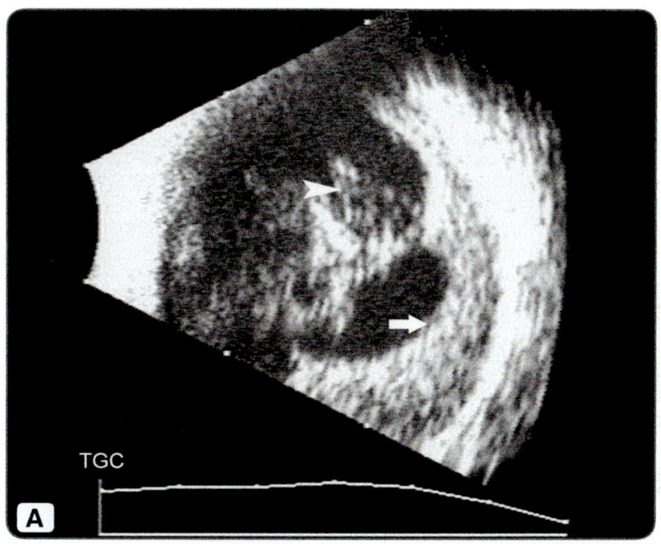

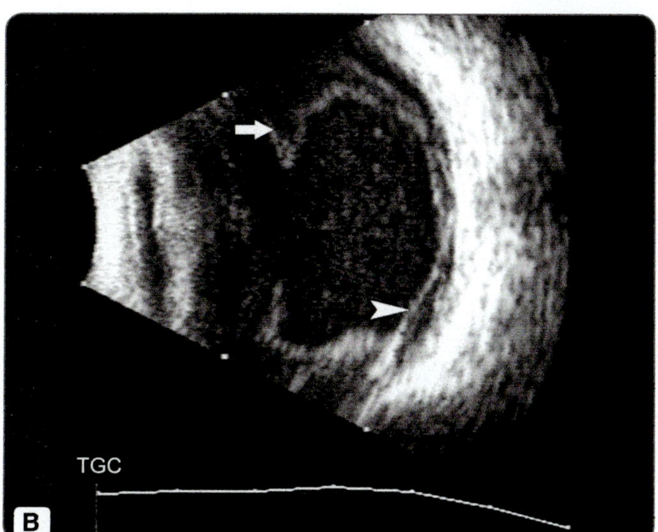

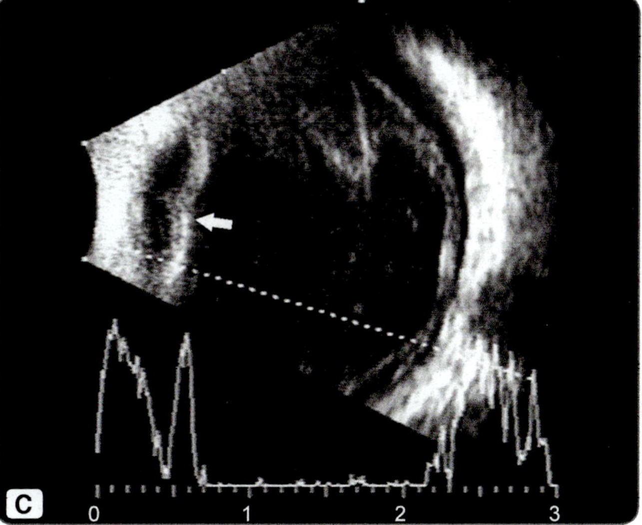

Figures 11.4A to C: B scan images pre- and post-vitrectomy in a case of endophthalmitis. The preoperative image shows plenty of intragel echoes (arrowhead) along with a thick layer of echoes along the globe wall (arrow). The postoperative images (Fig. B) show residual posterior hyaloid (arrowhead) and residual peripheral gel (arrow). Figure B shows a few echoes in the vitreous cavity, which are absent on the subsequent visit, signifying a good response to therapy. The high reflective membrane in the lens plane (arrow in Figure C) is a postoperative inflammatory membrane that preclude visualization of the posterior segment.

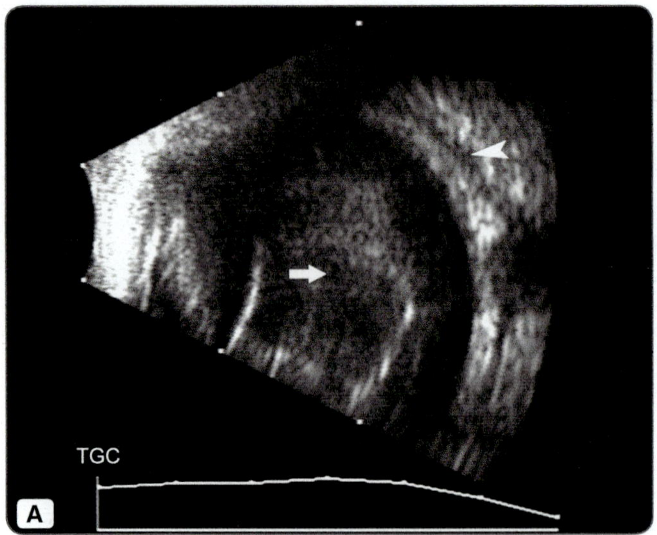

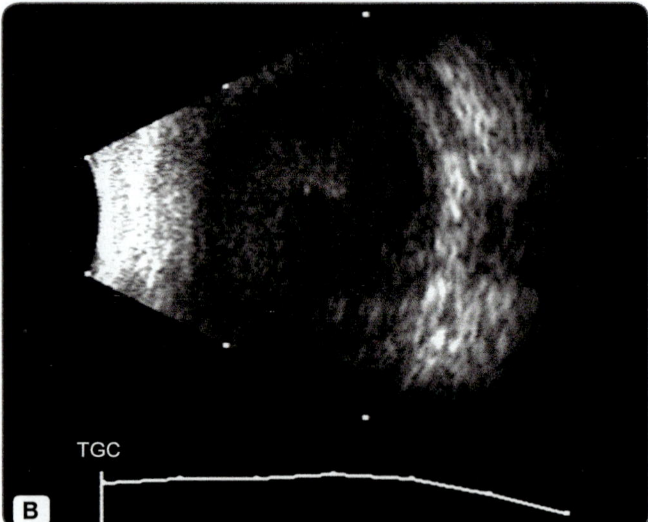

Figures 11.5A and B: B scan images of an eye with significant vitreous echoes (arrow) and orbital inflammation (arrowhead showing the T sign) at presentation. Figure B shows the relatively clear vitreous cavity with resolution of the Tenon's widening with vitrectomy and intravitreal antibiotics.

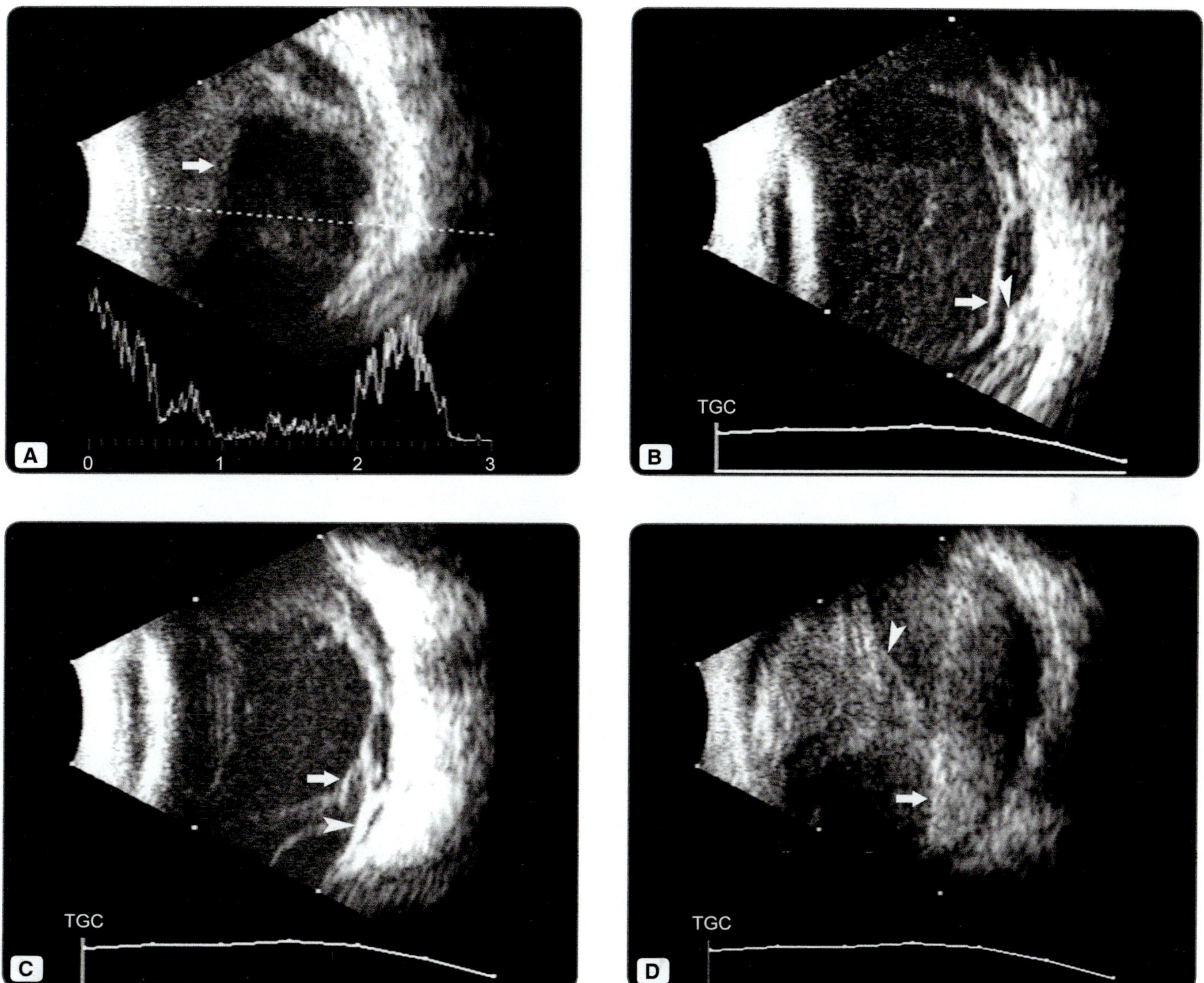

Figures 11.6A to D: B scan images of traumatic fungal endophthalmitis. The image at presentation shows a significant amount of intragel echoes in the vitreous cavity (arrow in Figure A). There is no PVD. The post vitrectomy images (Figs B and C) show development of PVD (arrow) with a shallow tractional detachment (arrowhead) due to inflammatory adhesions between the retina and vitreous. Figure D is the B scan image after one month showing a total retinal detachment (arrowhead) with closed funnel and densely layered subretinal echoes (arrow).

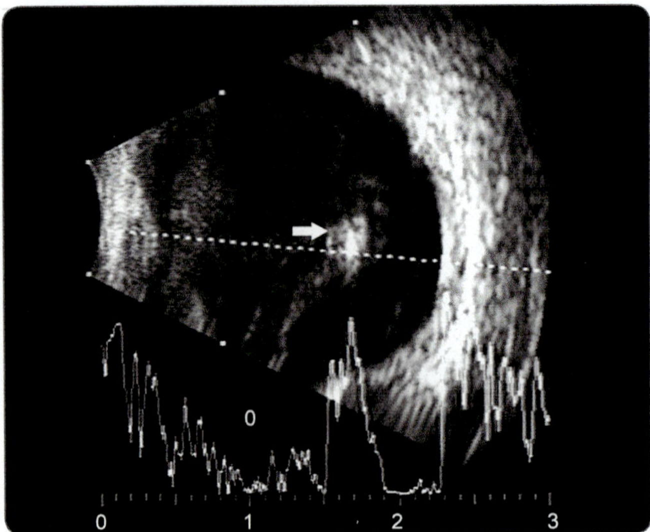

Figure 11.7: B scan with vector A scan showing vitreous echoes in an eye with severe postoperative inflammation following an apparently uneventful cataract surgery. The mid vitreous cavity shows a clump of high reflective echoes suggestive of dropped lens fragments (arrow) during surgery.

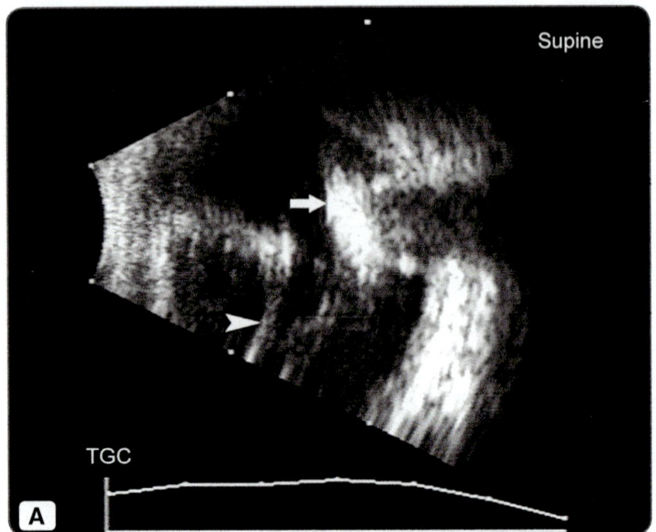

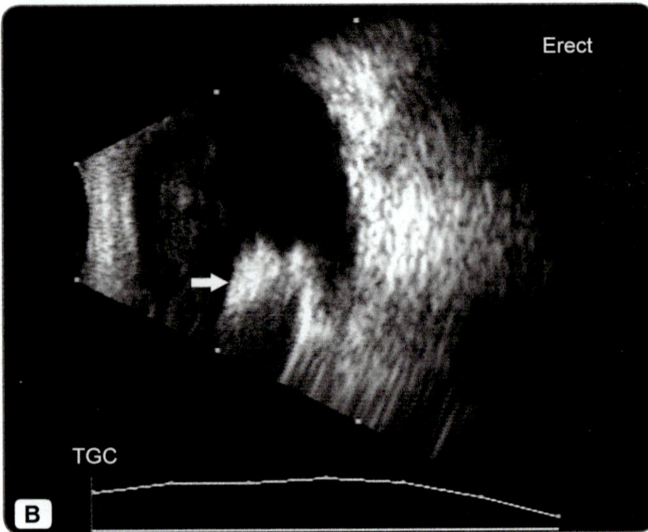

Figures 11.8A and B: B scan images of an eye with clinically diagnosed postoperative endophthalmitis. The anterior and mid vitreous cavity show moderate to high reflective echoes and a complete PVD (arrowhead). The posterior vitreous shows a very high reflective lesion causing orbital shadowing (arrow). This is suggestive of a hard nucleus. This is further confirmed by the inferior movement of the lesion with a change from supine to erect posture (Fig. B).

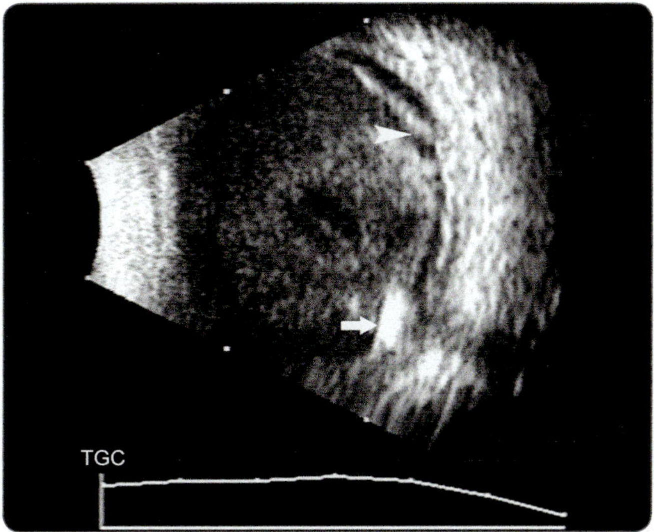

Figure 11.9: B scan with vector A scan of an eye with endophthalmitis following a workplace related injury. The vitreous cavity is full of low reflective intragel echoes. There is a very shallow membrane partly separated from the posterior globe wall suggestive of an incomplete PVD (arrowhead). In addition, there is a highly reflective structure on the globe wall causing orbital shadowing indicative of a retained IOFB (arrow).

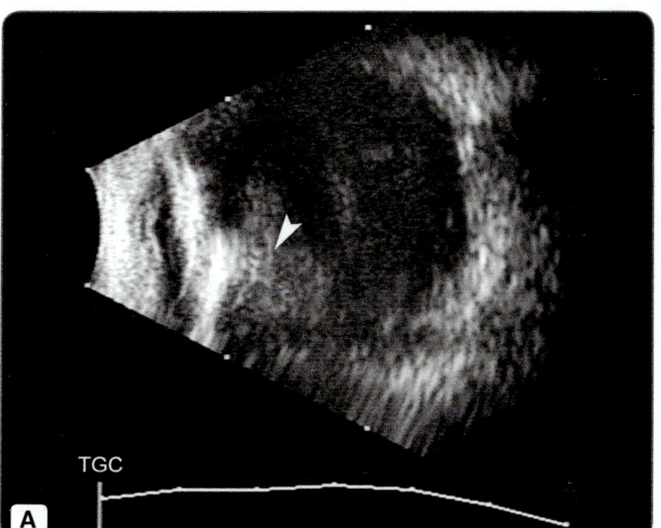

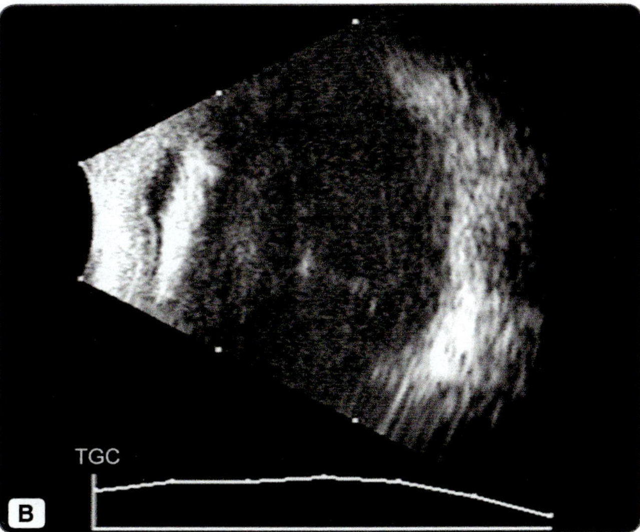

Figures 11.10A and B: B scan images of a case of pseudophakic endophthalmitis. In Figure A, the reverberations of the IOL (arrowhead) do not permit an accurate assessment of the vitreous echoes. By bypassing the IOL as in Figure B, one is able to study the vitreous cavity accurately.

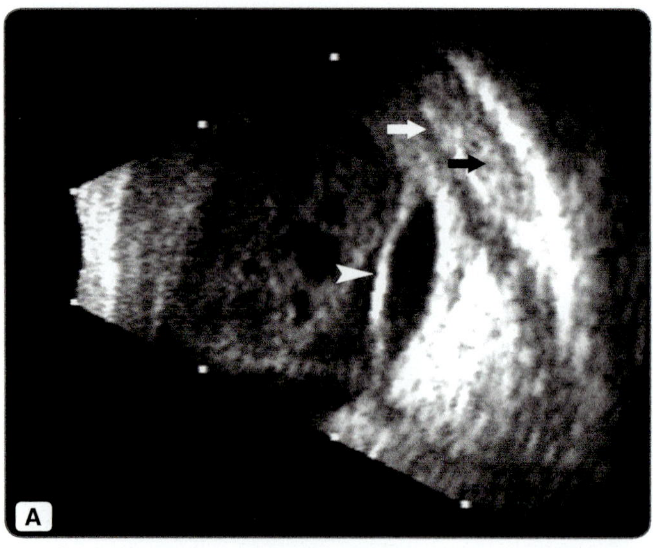

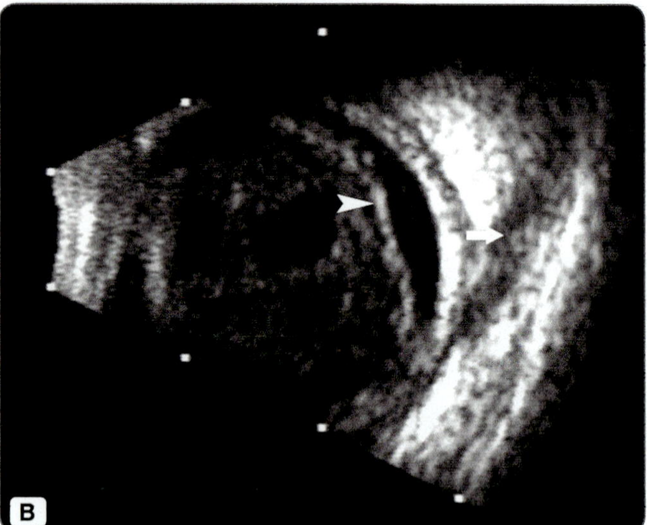

Figures 11.11A and B: B scan images of a child with panophthalmitis following penetrating injury with a wooden stick. He denied light perception on presentation.The images show extensive vitreous echoes with a total retinal detachment (arrowhead). There is Tenons widening as well. Note the thickened insertion of the superior (Fig. A) and lateral (Fig. B) recti (white arrows). There is also an area of low reflectivity in the anterior orbit suggestive of orbital cellulitis (black arrow).

12 Vogt-Koyanagi-Harada Syndrome

CLINICAL FEATURES

- Idiopathic bilateral panuveitis causing exudative retinal detachment associated with neurological, auditory and dermatological manifestations
- Ocular features include granulomatous uveitis, exudative retinal detachment, sunset glow fundus and chorioretinal atrophy
- Treatment includes high dose of systemic steroids and immunosuppressives.

ULTRASONOGRAPHY

Classical Features

- Diffuse, low to medium reflective thickening of the choroid at the posterior pole.
- Serous retinal detachment, located inferiorly or at the posterior pole.
- Mild vitreous opacities with no posterior vitreous detachment.
- Thickening of the sclera and/or episclera posteriorly.
- Optic disc elevation.
- Resolution of the findings with systemic corticosteroids or immunosuppressives.

Unusual Feature

- Annular choroidal detachment without serous retinal detachment.

MIMICKING CONDITIONS

- Choroidal thickening with serous retinal detachment is also seen in scleritis. However, in this condition the reflectivity of the choroid is high and the Tenon's widening is prominent
- Increased choroidal thickness along with an exudative retinal detachment is also seen in uveal effusion syndrome. Here the reflectivity is high and one may also get shallow peripheral annular choroidal detachments. The axial length in these eyes may be reduced and the scleral thickness is more than normal

- Shifting of subretinal fluid along with thickening of the choroid can also occur in eyes with a long-standing rhegmatogenous retinal detachment. However, the choroidal reflectivity is high in these cases
- Cases of multifocal CSR may present with bilateral bullous retinal detachments. Here, the vitreous is usually echolucent and choroidal thickness is normal.

NUGGETS

In eyes with the VKH syndrome, resolution of the retinal detachment occurs first and then the choroidal thickness reduces with successful therapy.

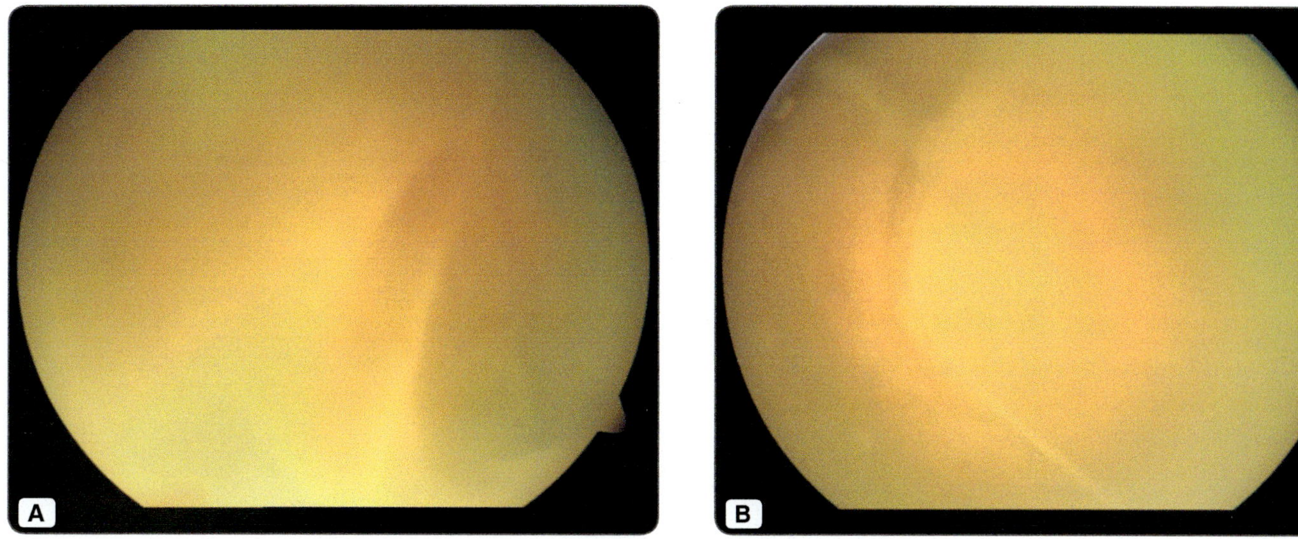

Figures 12.1A and B: Color photographs of bilateral exudative retinal detachments in a young lady with the retina touching the posterior lens surface. Note the poor picture quality due to the vitreous haze and massive detachment.

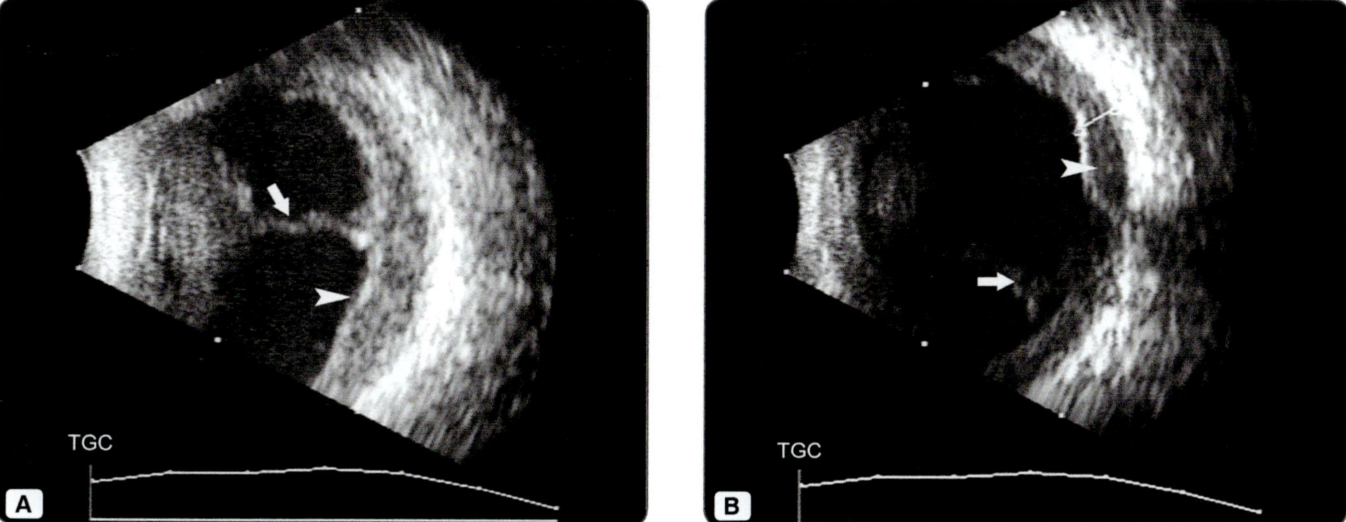

Figures 12.2A and B: B scan ultrasound images of the right and left eye showing the bullous retinal detachment extending anteriorly. The two large bullae are seen touching each other (arrow). The choroid is thickened in an irregular manner (arrowhead) and the internal reflectivity is uniform and low suggesting an infiltrative process. Figure B is the B scan image of the left eye showing a similar pattern of choroidal thickening (arrowhead). The retinal detachment appears indistinct and low reflective (arrow) due to the oblique placement of the probe in relation to the retina.

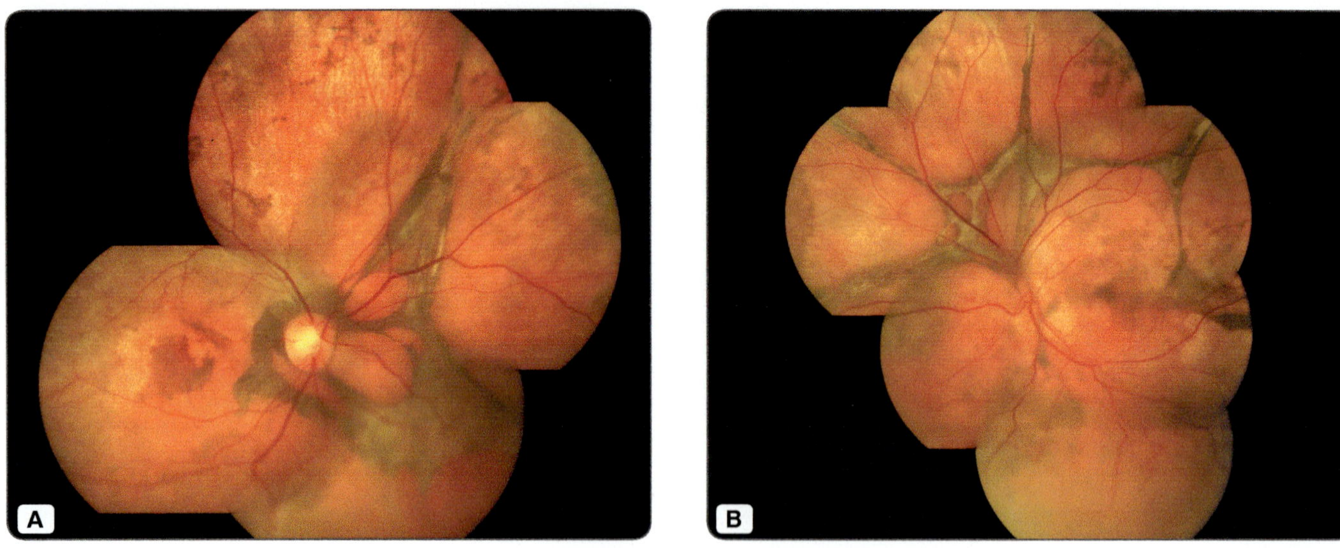

Figures 12.3A and B: Color photographs of the same patient 2 weeks after starting high dose corticosteroid therapy showing good resolution of the retinal detachment. Subretinal fibrotic bands are seen.

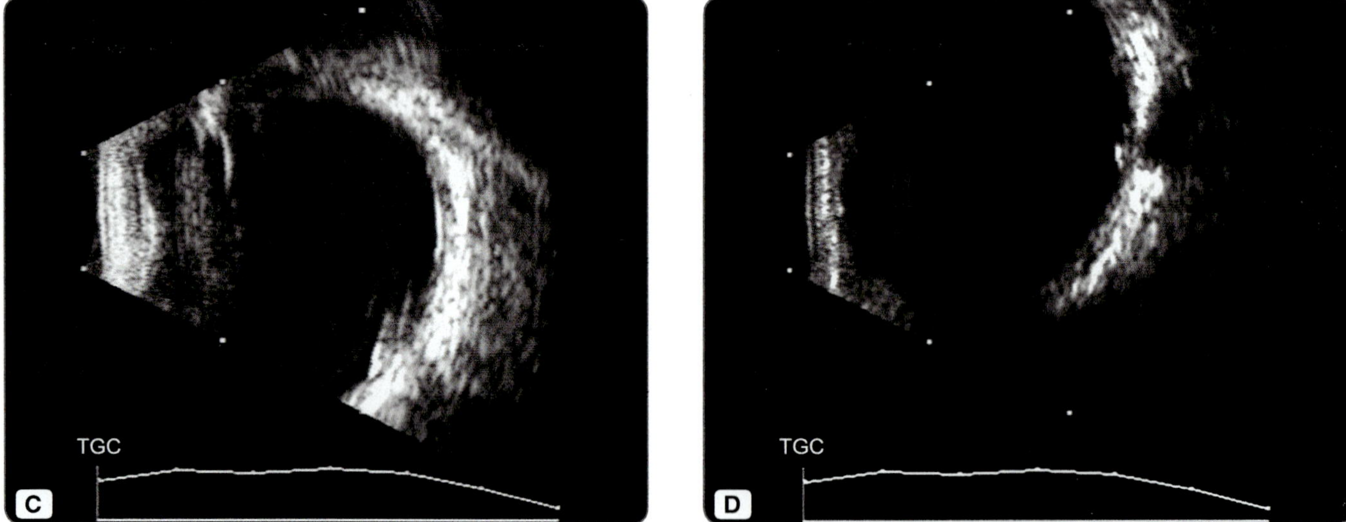

Figures 12.3C and D: B scan images after treatment showing a decrease in choroidal thickness and resolution of the detachment.

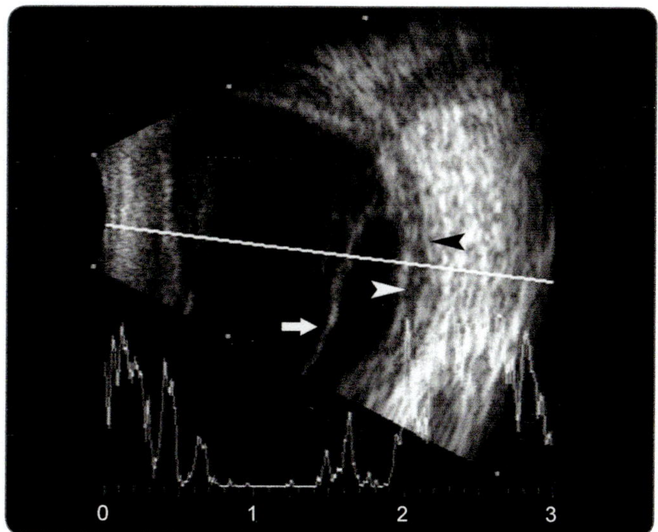

Figure 12.4: B scan with vector A scan of a patient with VKH syndrome. There is a bullous retinal detachment (arrow). The choroid is thickened and irregular (white arrowhead). The internal reflectivity is homogeneous and low. Distinguishing the sclera as a separate layer (black arrowhead) is easy if there is choroidal thickening as seen in this image.

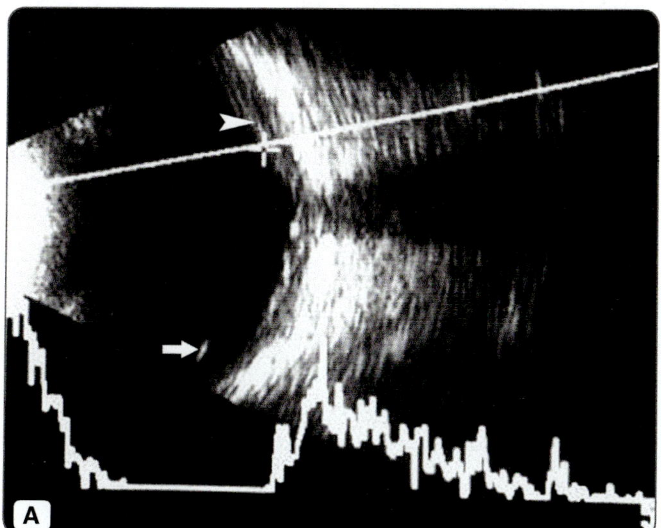

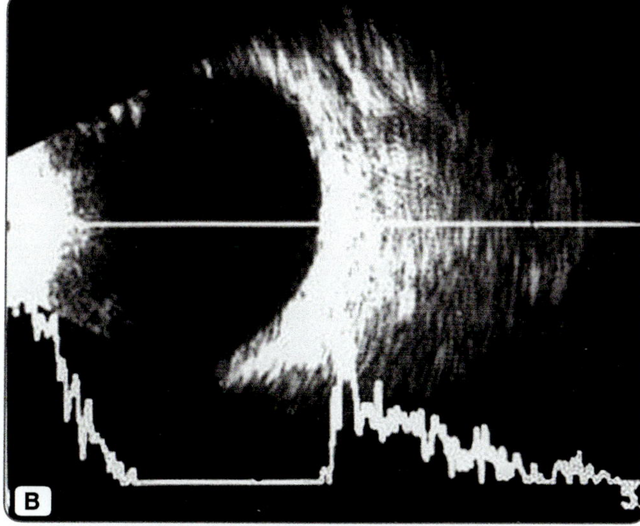

Figures 12.5A and B: B scan with vector A scan showing a shallow retinal detachment (arrow) and low reflective choroidal thickening (arrowhead). The right image is of the same case 3 months after corticosteroid therapy showing resolution of the retinal detachment and decrease in choroidal thickness.

13 Scleritis and Subretinal Abscess

CLINICAL FEATURES

- Inflammatory disease of sclera either anterior or posterior.
- Can be idiopathic, infective or secondary to collagen vascular disease like rheumatoid arthritis.
- Posterior scleritis may mimic other diseases, most importantly amelanotic melanoma.
- Ultrasound is indicated as a diagnostic aid and also to monitor response to treatment.

ULTRASOUND

- Diffuse or localized high reflective scleral thickening.
- Associated with swelling of underlying Tenon's and episclera causing an echolucent area. When peripapillary in location this causes a 'T' sign.
- Exudative retinal and choroidal detachment, optic nerve edema and nerve sheath edema may be seen.
- Severe scleritis may extend along the muscle sheaths causing thickening of the tendon and belly. This is most often seen in cases of panophthalmitis.
- The giant nodular form may mimic a choroidal tumor.

NUGGETS

T sign is indicative of posterior scleritis. However, it can also be seen in case of large intraocular tumors and temporarily after local treatment (e.g. cryo, brachytherapy) of small choroidal tumors.

Nodular form can be differentiated from choroidal melanoma by absence of sound attenuation and choroidal excavation.

Infectious scleritis is more likely to cause severe inflammatory changes and abscess formation both in the sclera and orbital soft tissue.

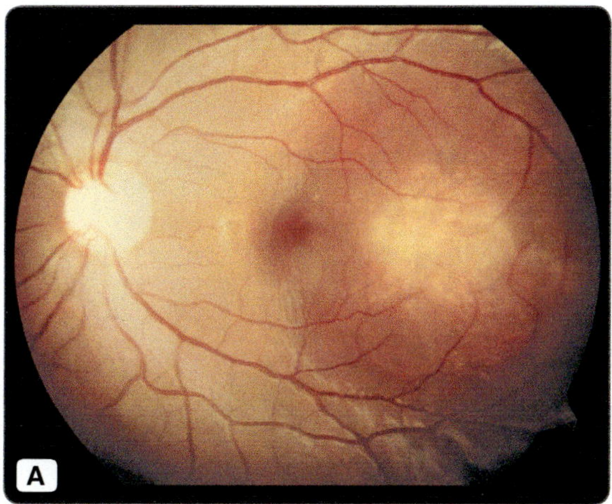

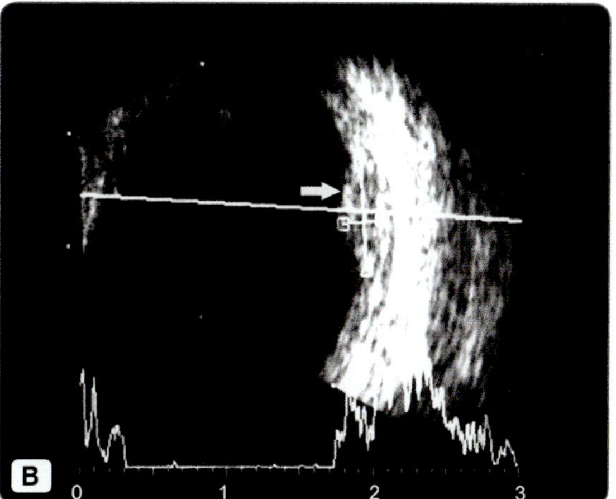

Figures 13.1A and B: Color photograph and B scan image of a case of posterior scleritis. The color photograph shows a mass lesion at the posterior pole. The B scan image shows a localized thickening of the choroid (arrow) with an area of Tenon's widening at the base.

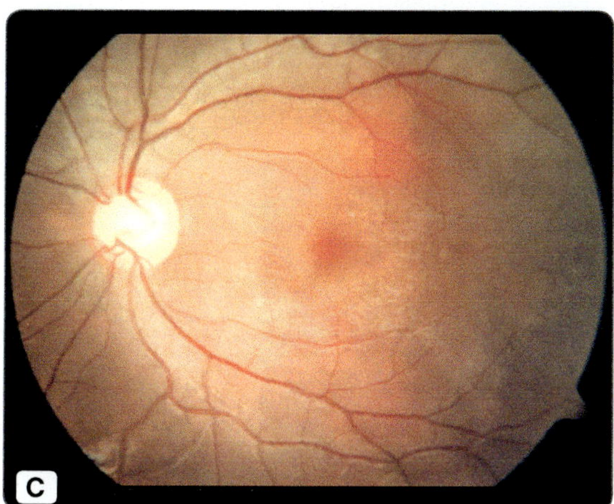

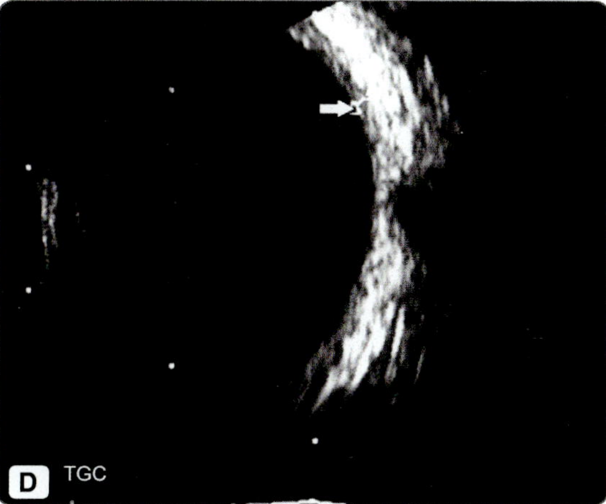

Figures 13.1C and D: Color photograph and B scan image of the same eye after corticosteroid treatment showing resolution of the mass and normal appearance of the choroid (arrow).

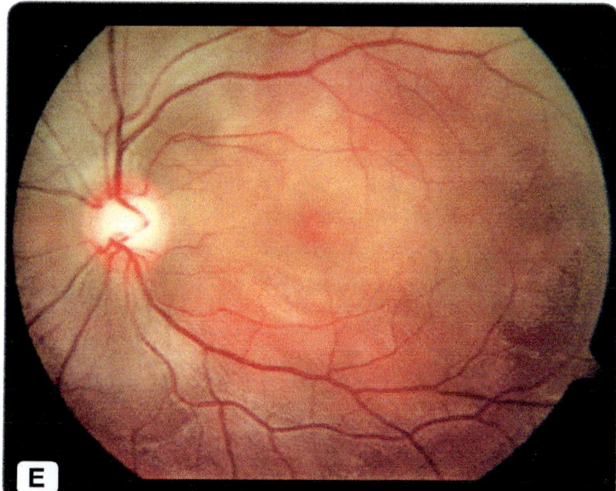

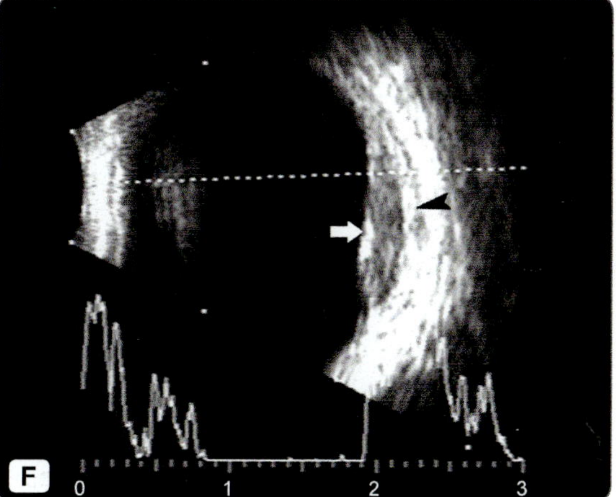

Figures 13.1E and F: Color photograph and B scan image of the patient one year later with a recurrence of scleritis. The choroid is thickened and high reflective (arrow) with Tenon's widening at the base (arrowhead). A localized secondary retinal detachment is seen inferior to the lesion.

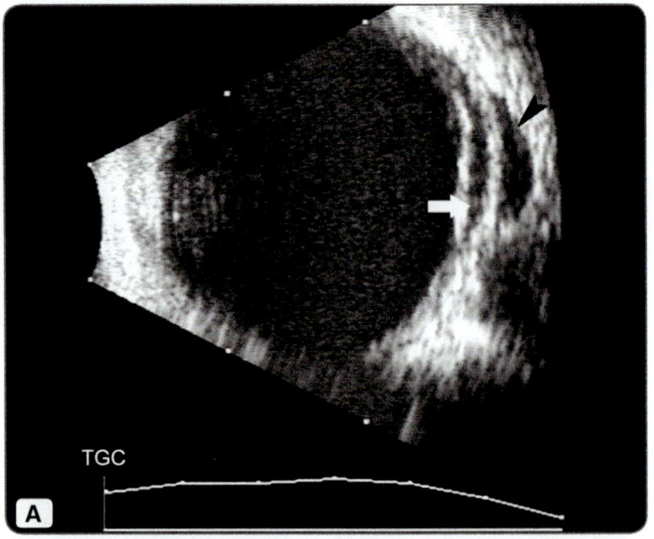

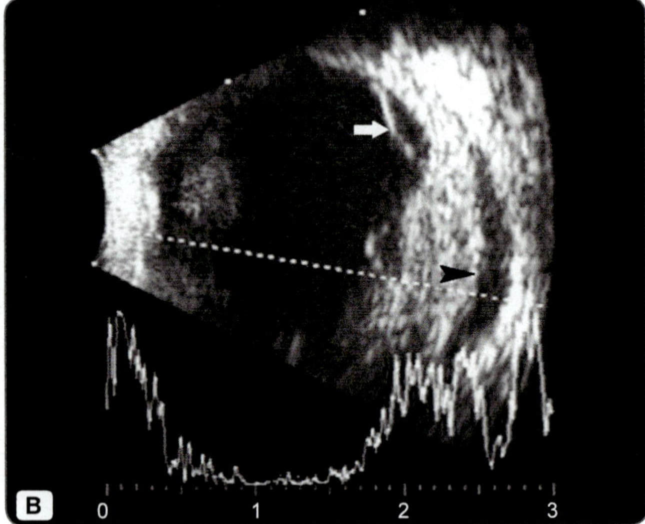

Figures 13.2A and B: B scan images showing choroidal thickening with prominent Tenon's widening in two cases of scleritis. Figure A shows choroidal thickening (arrow) with Tenon's widening (arrowhead). Figure B shows significant scleral edema (arrowhead) along with a secondary retinal detachment (arrow) in addition to the other findings.

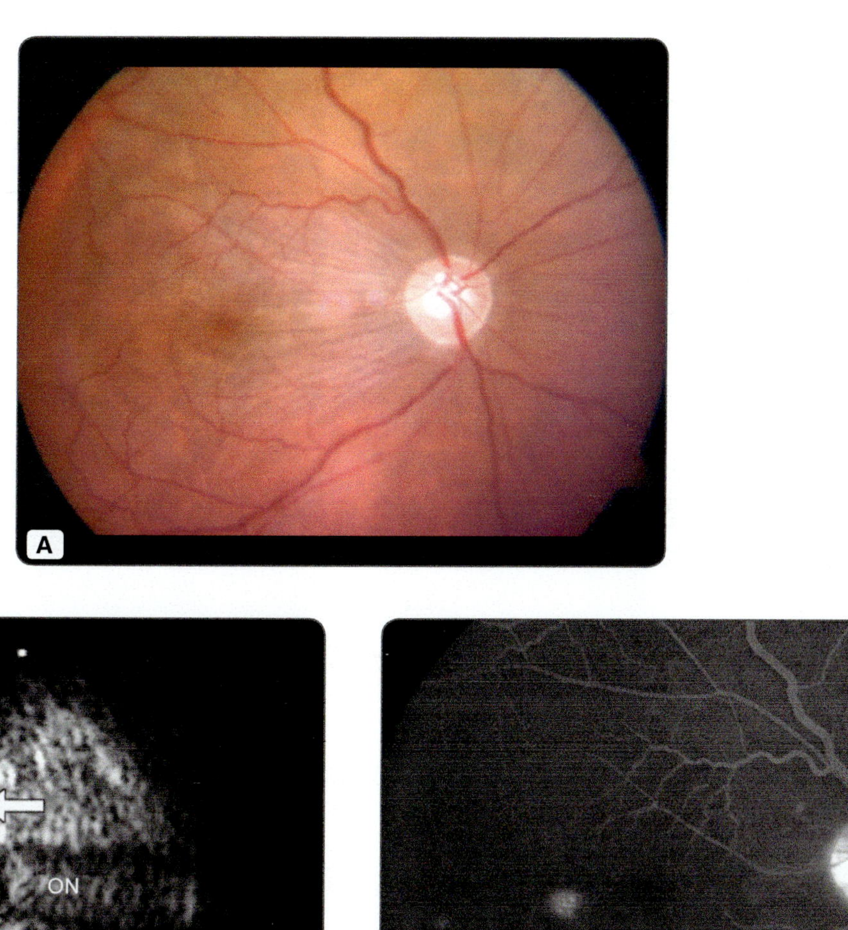

Figures 13.3A to C: Fundus photograph, ultrasound image and fluorescein angiography late phase images of a female with painful loss of vision in the right eye. Note the choroidal folds at the posterior pole. Ultrasound B scan shows choroidal thickening at the posterior pole (thin arrows) including the peripapillary area and Tenon's widening continuous with the optic nerve shadow (broad arrows). The FFA shows late staining of the optic disc and an area of mottled fluorescence in the area of a small pigment epithelial detachment.

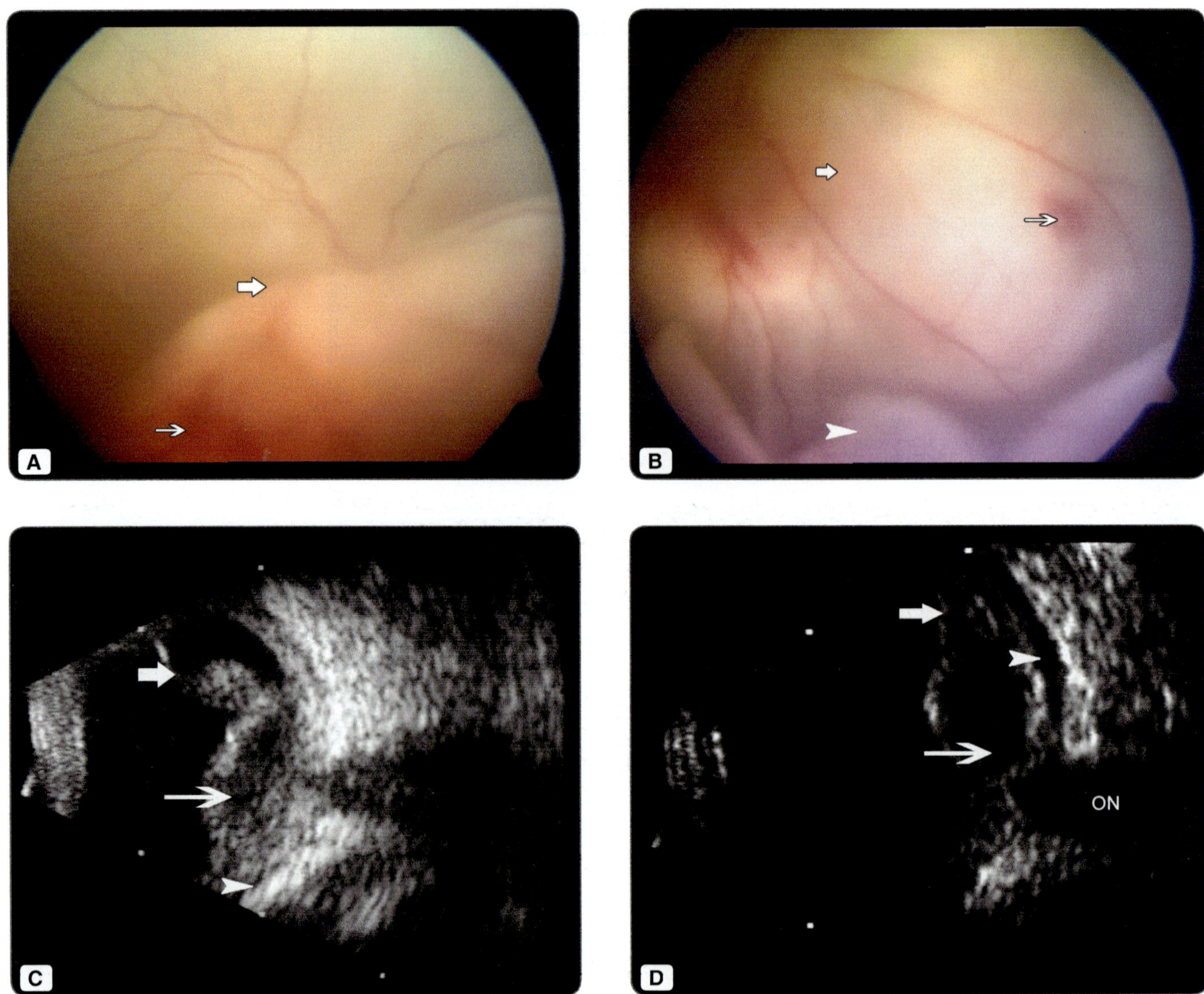

Figures 13.4A to D: Clinical and ultrasound images of an eye with subretinal abscess. The fundus photographs show a large subretinal mass (broad arrow) obscuring view of the optic disc. There are hemorrhages on the surface (thin arrow) and an associated bullous RD (arrow head). B scan ultrasound shows the retinal detachment (broad arrow), subretinal mass with an area of echolucency within it (thin arrow) and Tenon's widening (arrow head).

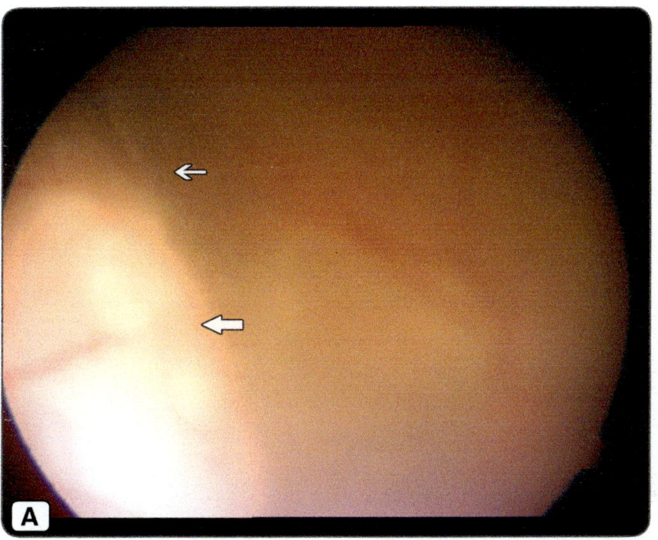

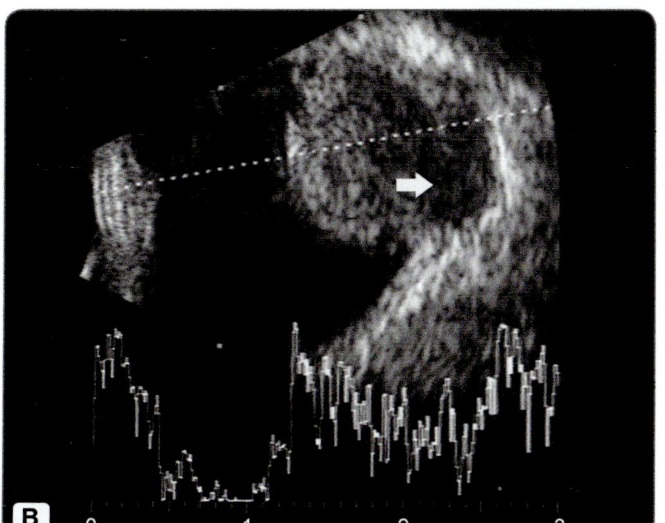

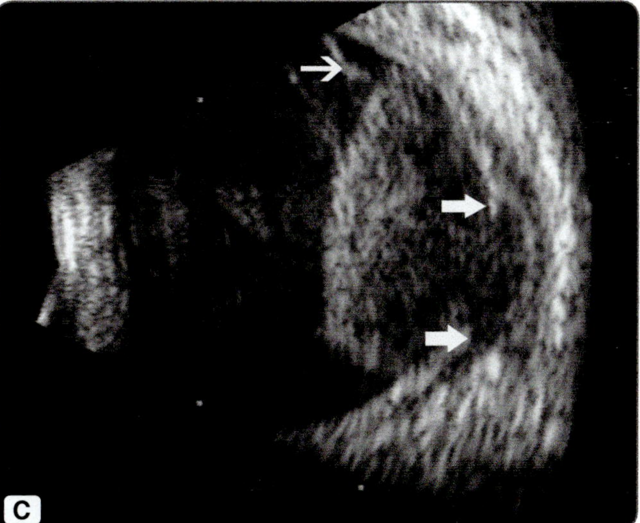

Figures 13.5A to C: Fundus photograph and ultrasound images of a 10-year-old girl with loss of vision in the right eye. Note the vitritis and yellowish mass at the posterior pole. B scan ultrasound with vector A shows a large retinochoroidal mass with moderate-to-high reflective intralesional echoes, secondary retinal detachment (arrow) and extrascleral extension (broad arrows). The vitritis is seen as low reflective intragel echoes.

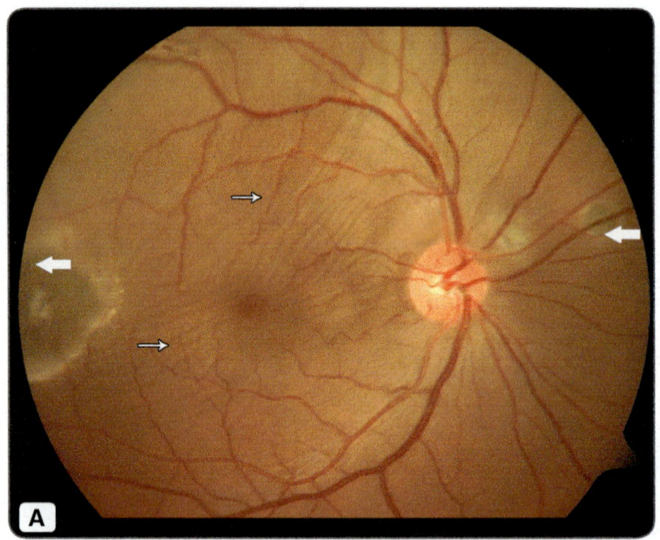

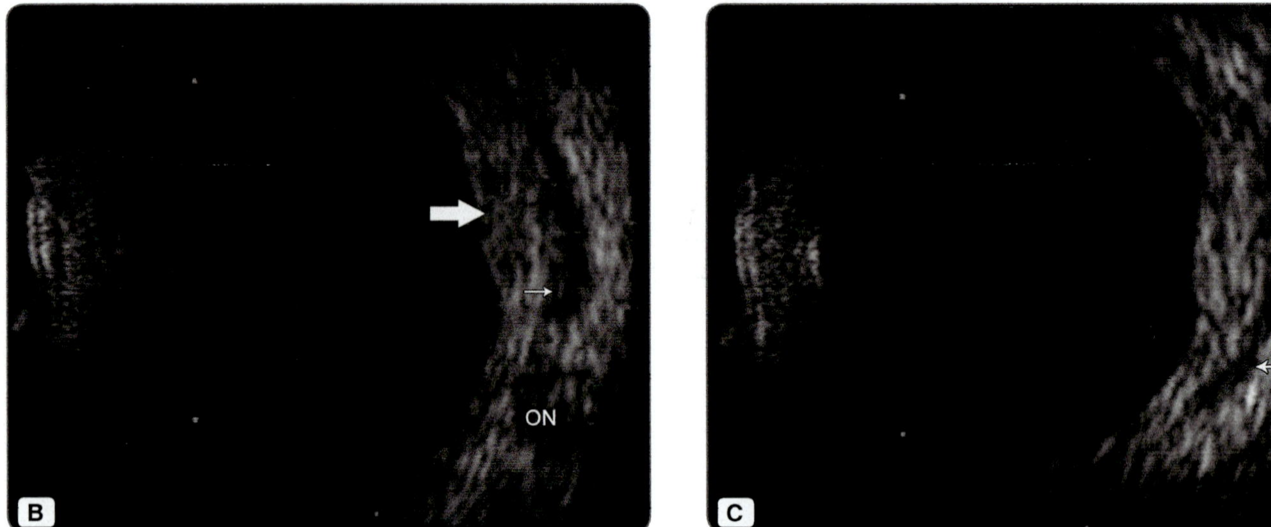

Figures 13.6A to C: Ultrasound and fundus images of a middle-aged man treated with posterior subtenons steroid for choroiditis and complained of pain and drop of vision following the same. Note the choroidal folds (arrows) at the posterior pole along with patches of healed choroiditis. Ultrasound images show an area of choroidal thickening (broad arrow) and Tenon's widening (thin arrows). The circumferential scan (Fig. C) shows the Tenon's widening very clearly.

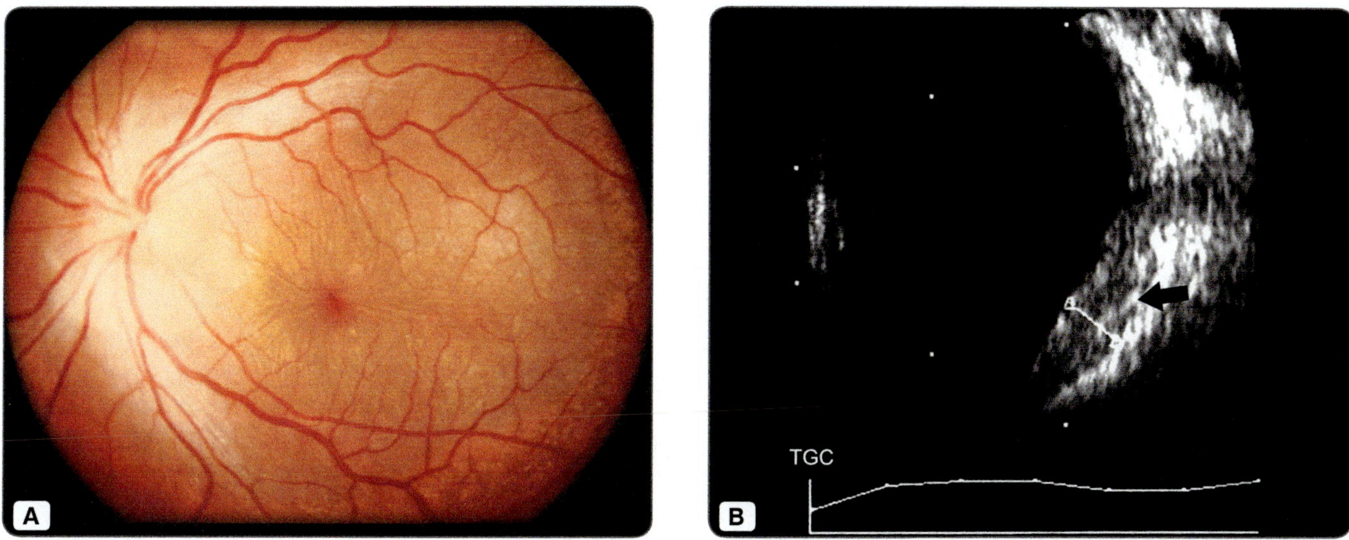

Figures 13.7A and B: Color photograph and B scan image of an eye with posterior scleritis and disc edema. Note the localized area of retinochoroidal thickening along with scleral edema (arrow). There is optic disc elevation as well.

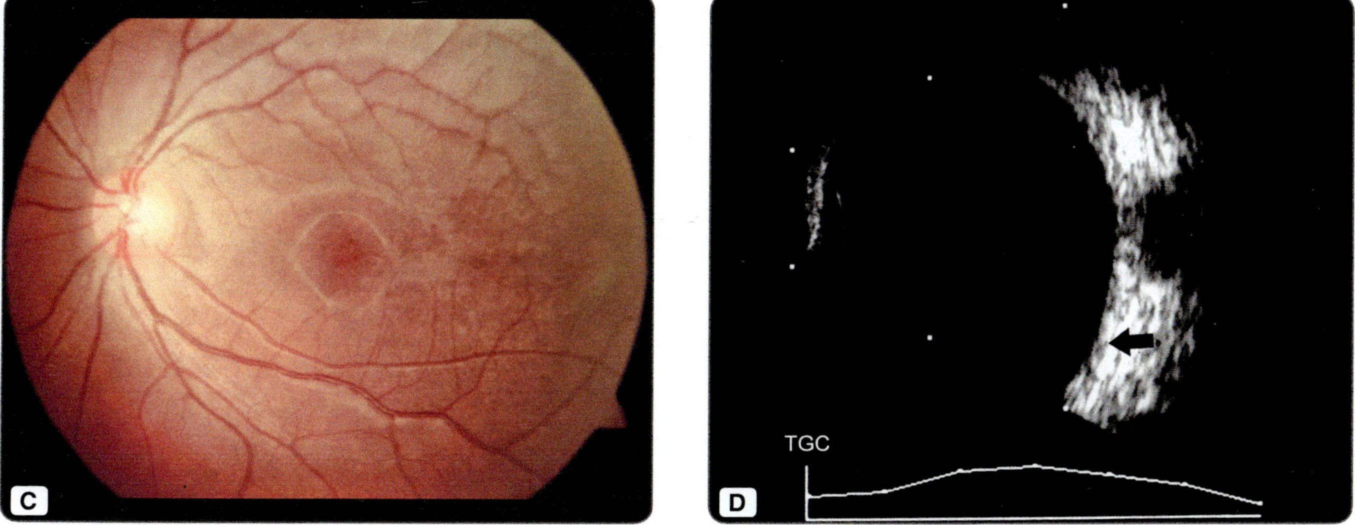

Figures 13.7C and D: The color photograph and B scan image showing complete resolution 2 months after corticosteroid therapy.

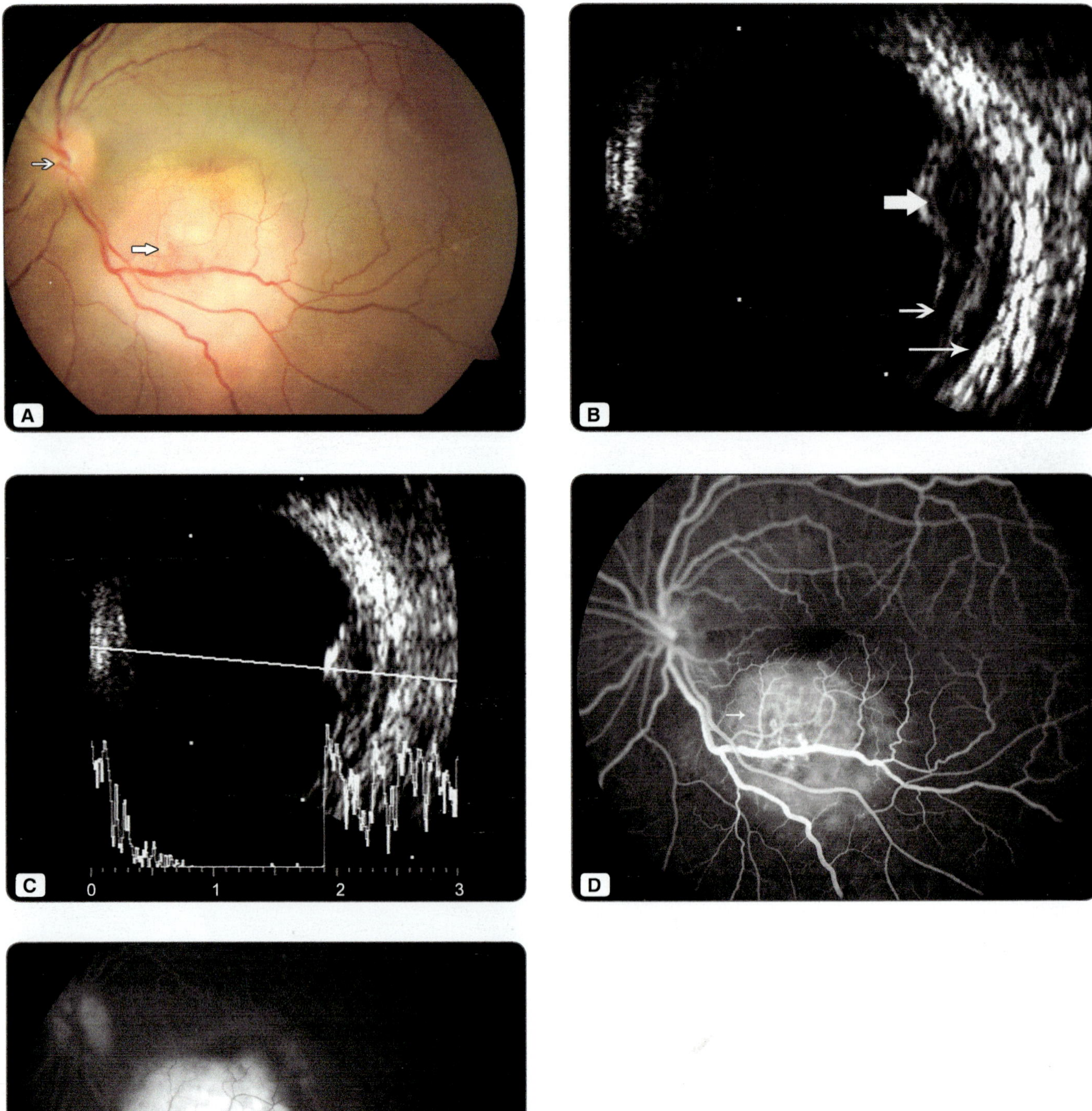

Figures 13.8A to E: A 24-year-old patient with tuberculosis of the hip presented with loss of vision in the left eye. Fundus revealed a subretinal mass with hemorrhages and secondary retinal detachment. USG showed a dome-shaped retinochoroidal elevation (broad arrow) with high surface reflectivity and low reflective internal echoes. Secondary RD (thin arrow) was noted around the mass. Sub-Tenon's thickening (long arrow) was noted which was more in extent than the circumference of the mass itself. Fluorescein angiography showed mottled hyperfluorescence with late pooling in the area of the mass.

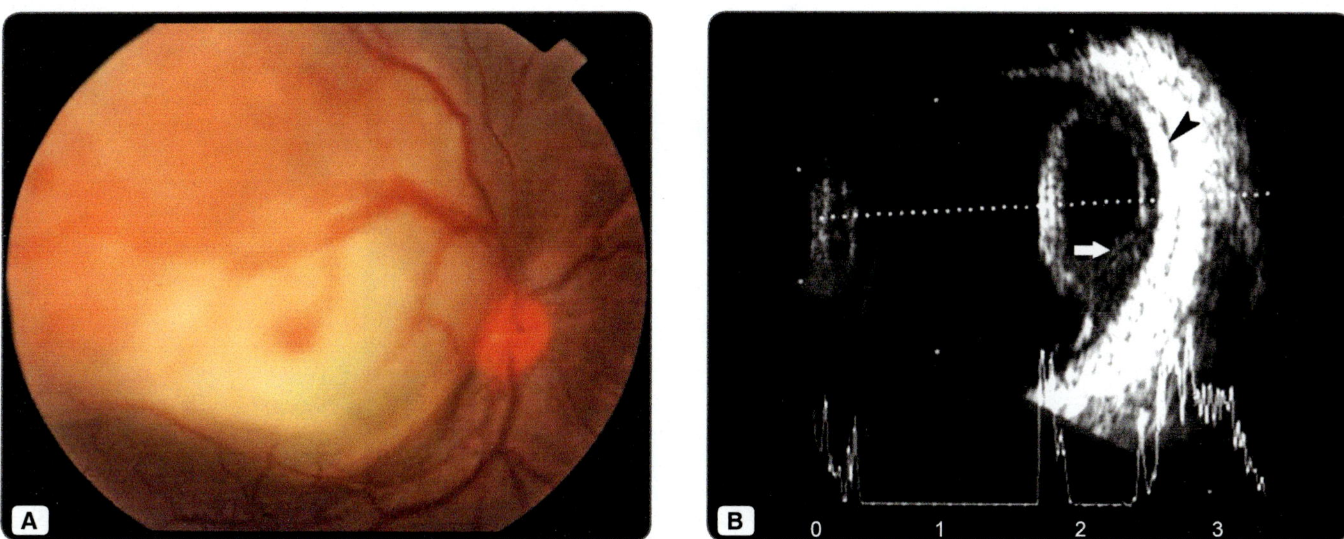

Figures 13.9A and B: Color photograph and B scan images of a patient with a subretinal tubercular abscess. The B scan shows the abscess cavity with a fluid level (arrow). There is Tenon's widening at the base (arrowhead).

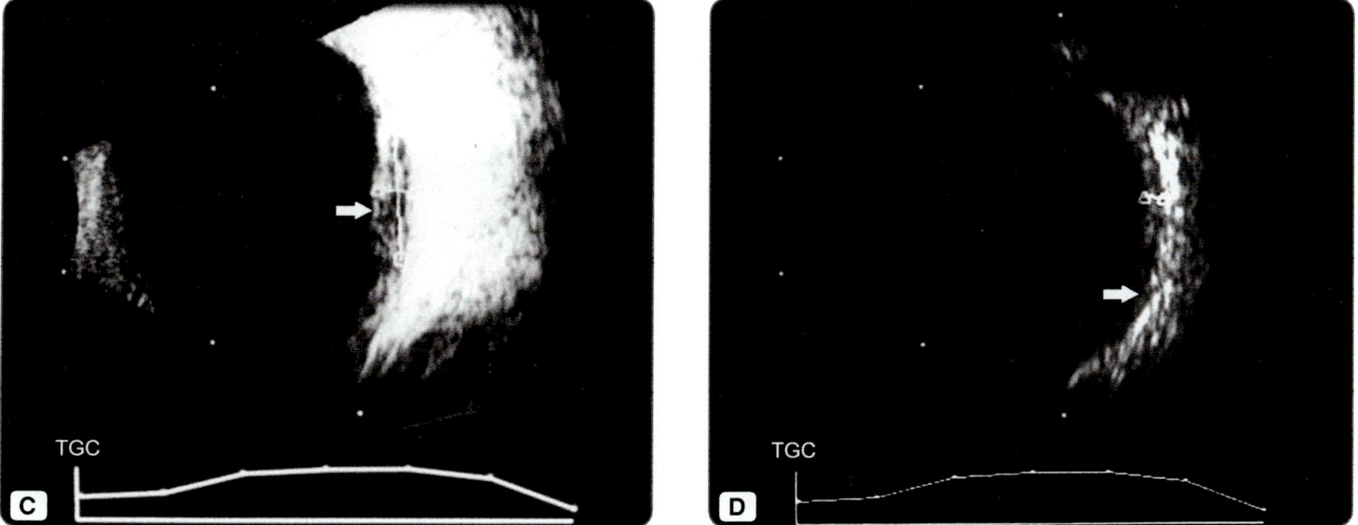

Figures 13.9C and D: The B scan images show progressive resolution of the lesion with antituberculous therapy.

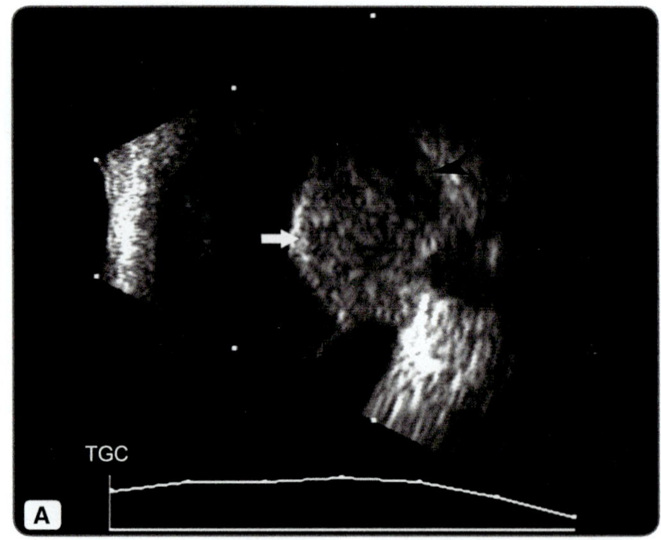

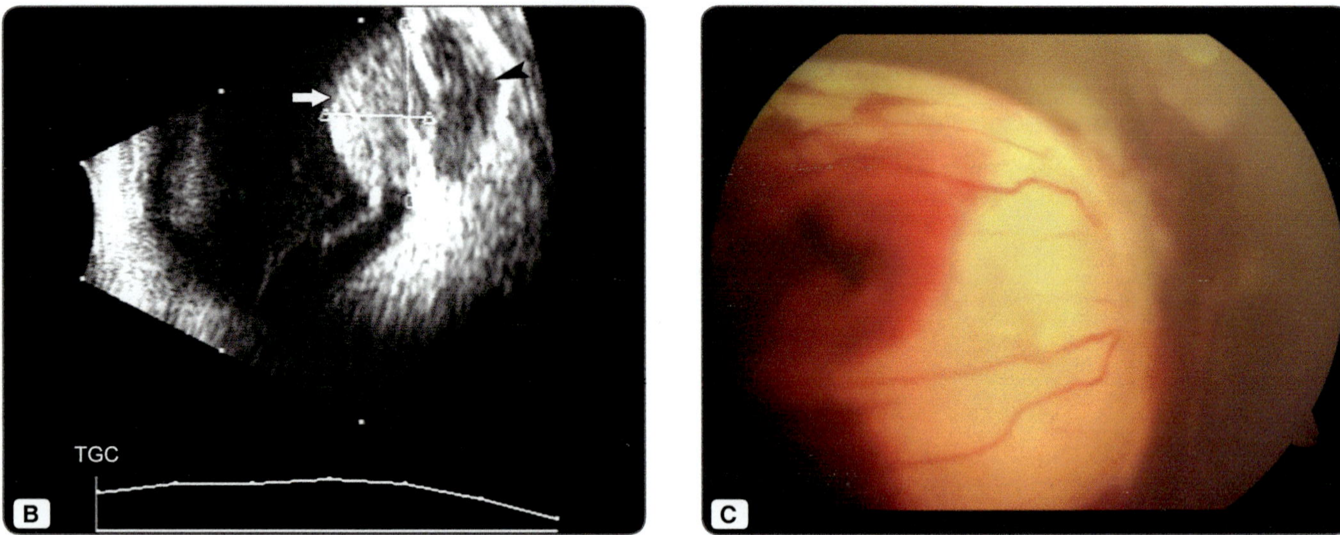

Figures 13.10A to C: B scan images of a young patient presenting with a mass adjacent to and overlying the optic disc. The ultrasound image shows a choroidal mass with secondary retinal detachment (arrow), scleral edema and gross Tenon's widening (arrowhead). The clinical picture is taken after fine needle aspiration biopsy from the mass, showing retinal hemorrhages at the site of biopsy. Biopsy was positive for *M. tuberculosis*.

14 Toxocara Granuloma

CLINICAL FEATURES

- Important in the differential diagnosis of leukokoria.
- Can present as endophthalmitis or a tractional retinal detachment.
- The granuloma is typically peripheral with membranes extending from the mass to the disc, however it can occur at the posterior pole.
- Intraocular calcification can occur.

ULTRASOUND

- The granuloma appears as a mass lesion, commonly peripheral, but can also occur near the disc. This can be high reflective, with a surrounding tractional retinal detachment.
- Traction retinal folds from the mass to the disc.
- Multiple vitreous membranes can be seen, some of which can be high reflective.

NUGGETS

Look carefully for an elevated lesion at the periphery in an eye with multiple vitreous membranes or endogenous endophthalmitis, especially in the younger age group.

A tractional retinal detachment around a mass which looks calcific is suggestive of toxocara.

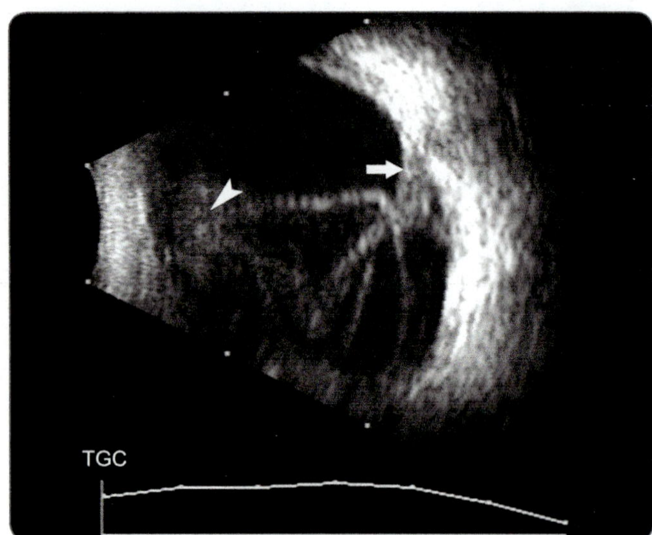

Figure 14.1: B scan image showing multiple vitreous membranes extending from the retrolenticular area toward a peripapillary tractional retinal detachment (arrow). A clump of moderately reflective echoes is seen behind the lens (arrowhead).

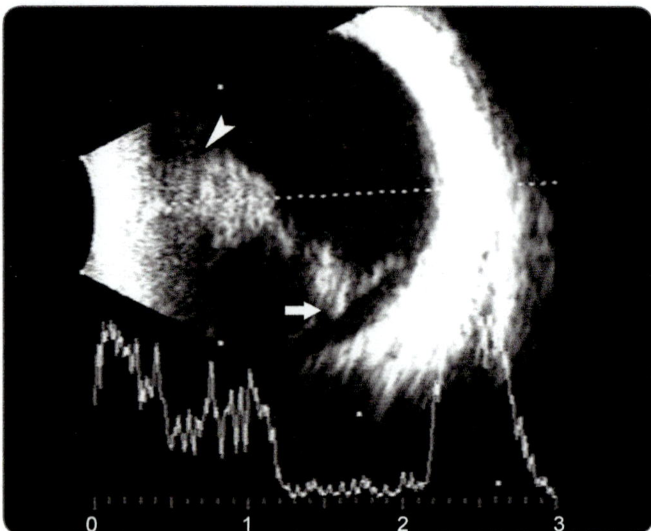

Figure 14.2: B scan with vector A of the peripheral area showing a highly reflective retrolental clump of echoes (arrowhead). These are seen to extend to the peripheral retina causing a tractional retinal detachment (arrow).

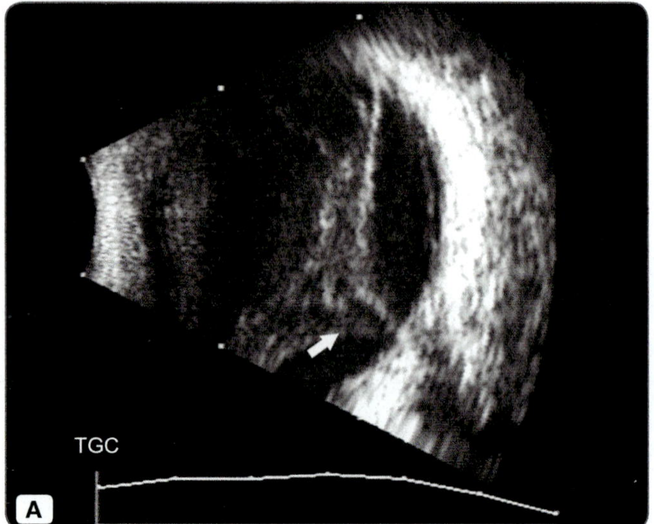

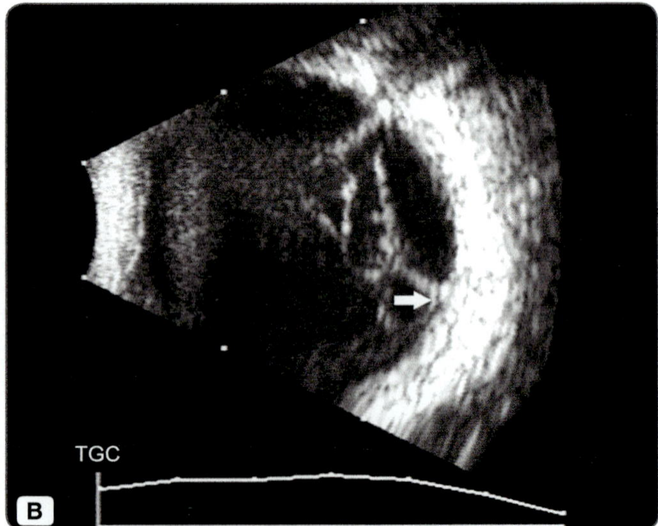

Figures 14.3A and B: B scan images of an eye with multiple vitreous membranes attached to the optic disc (arrow). In the second image, the membranes are seen to attach to an area of low to moderate reflectivity in the mid periphery (arrow) suggestive of a granuloma.

15 Ocular Cysticercosis

CLINICAL FEATURES

- Cysticercosis is caused by *Cysticercus cellulosae*, the larval form of pork tapeworm, *Taenia solium*
- Although posterior segment involvement is the most common, cysticercosis may affect any part of the visual system from orbit to visual cortex. The common route of entry into the eye is through the short posterior ciliary arteries
- The live cyst does not cause inflammatory signs; these are seen after the cyst is dead
- The patient may initially complain of a floater in case of intravitreal cysticercosis. The presenting complaint may be decreased vision in case of a subretinal cyst causing either a retinal detachment or a submacular cyst.

ULTRASONOGRAPHY

- Well outlined round to oval echolucent cyst with an echo dense nodule adjacent to inner wall of cyst representing the scolex
- The cyst wall in case of a live cyst is seen to undulate on exposure to light. The scolex also exhibits spontaneous movements, well seen on kinetic echography
- Extensive vitreous echoes, membranes and retinal detachment can develop in response to inflammation caused by the dead cyst.

NUGGETS

It is important to rule out neurocysticercosis if ocular or orbital cysticercosis has been diagnosed.

Spontaneous movements of the scolex and cyst wall are diagnostic.

Mimicking conditions include dislocated crystalline lens, retinal cysts in long standing detachments and congenital vitreous cysts.

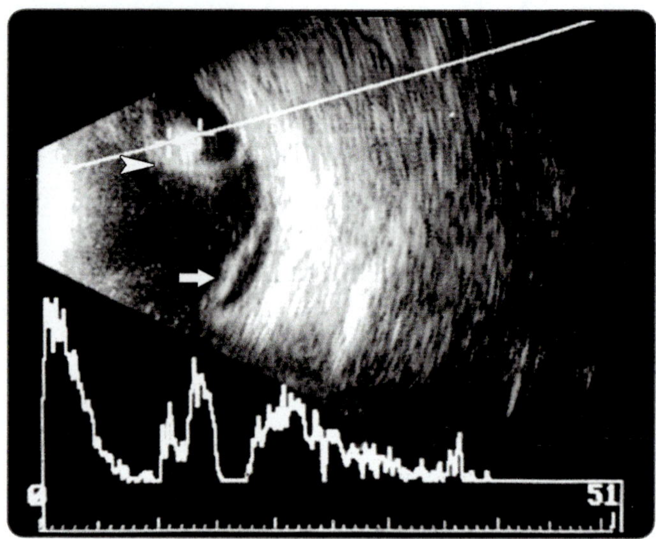

Figure 15.1: B scan with vector A scan showing a cystic lesion (arrowhead) in the upper half of the image and a high reflective membrane (arrow) in the lower half. Note the high reflective scolex attached to the inner wall of the cyst confirming the diagnosis of cysticercosis. The membrane represents a retinal detachment. The vitreous cavity is relatively clear and does not show presence of inflammatory membranes suggesting that this is likely to be a live cyst.

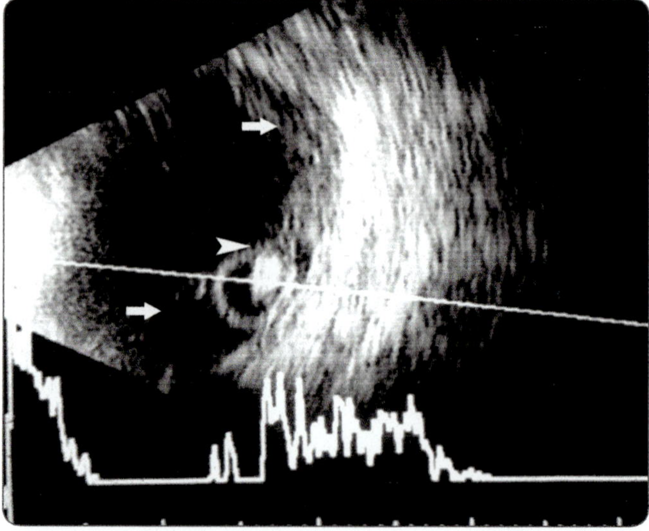

Figure 15.2: B scan with vector A showing a cyst with scolex in the vitreous cavity (arrowhead). Note the presence of vitreous echoes and membrane formation (arrowhead) indicative of an inflammatory response.

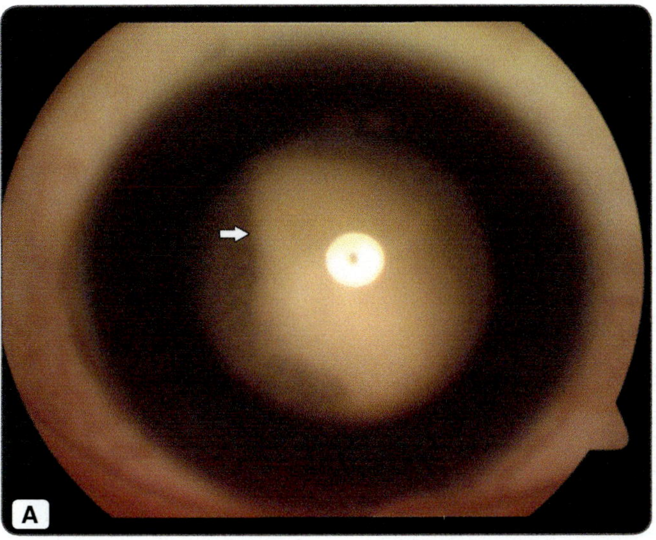

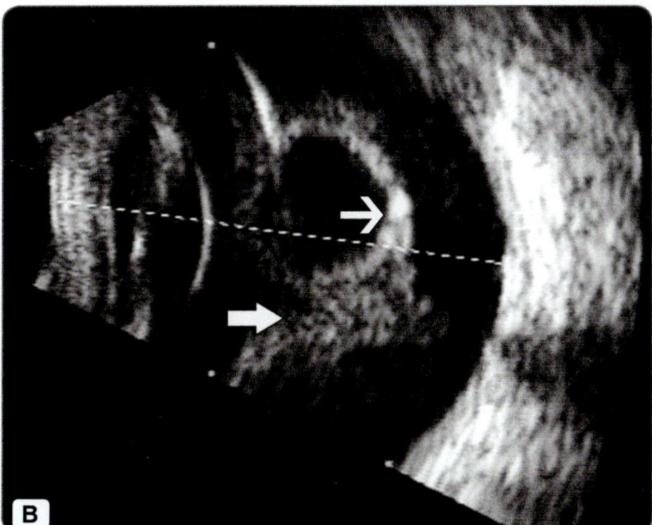

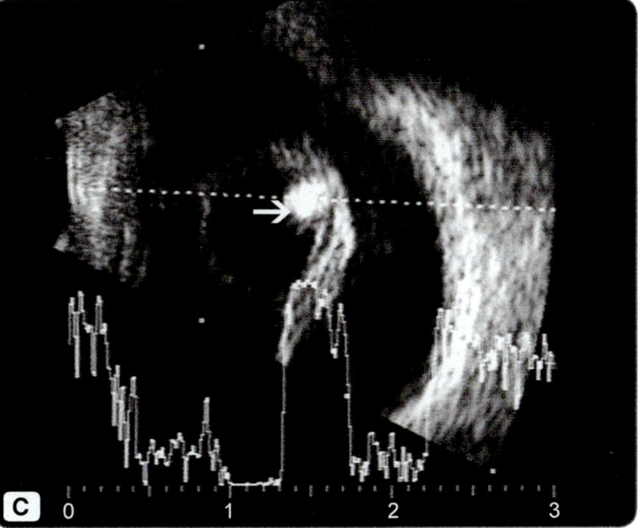

Figures 15.3A to C: Anterior segment photograph and B scan images of the right eye of a 12-year-old boy who presented with a painful decrease in vision for 3 months. Total retinal detachment with retrolental proliferation was seen clinically (Fig. A). B scan ultrasound showed the highly reflective membrane (broad arrow) with cyst formation (thin arrow) attached to the optic nerve (Fig. B). The cyst is seen to have a localized clump of high reflective echoes suggestive of a scolex arrow in Figure C. The cyst was removed surgically and confirmed to be cysticercus.

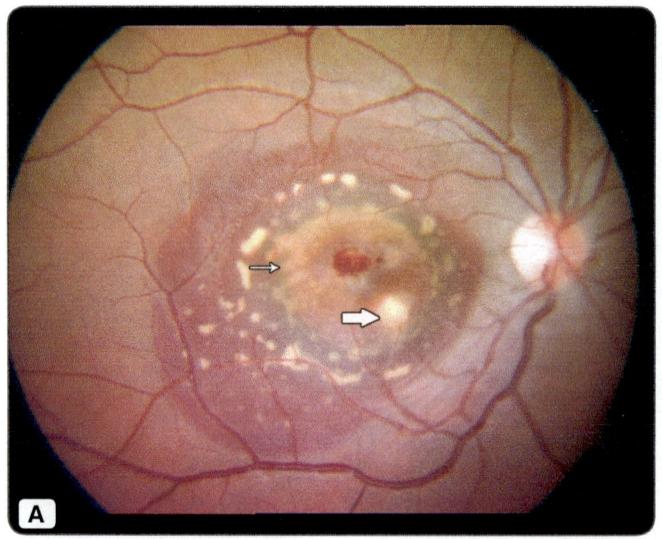

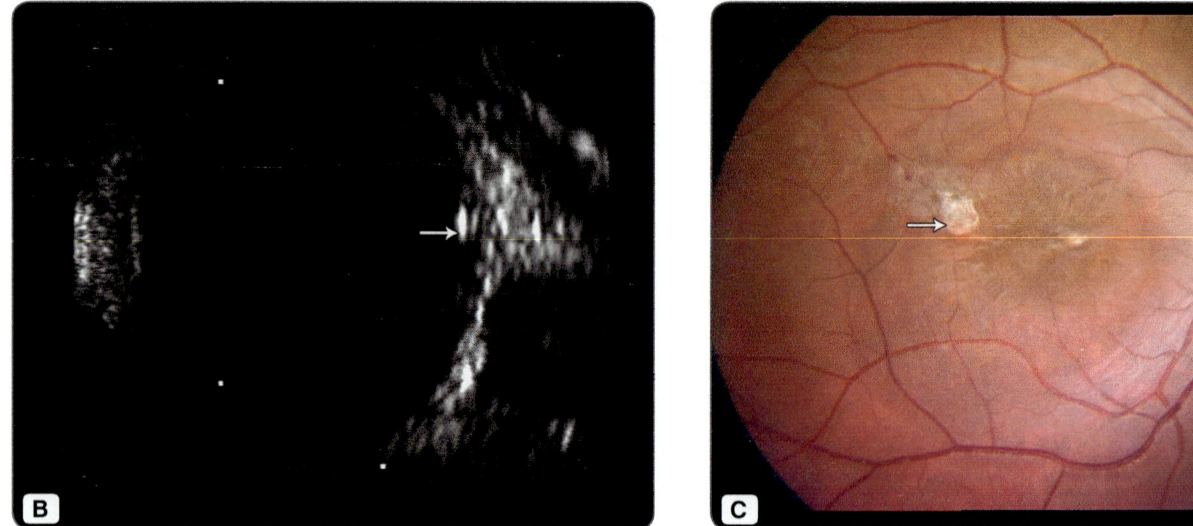

Figures 15.4A to C: A 14-year-old male presented with decreased vision in OD for the past 1 month (BCVA 3/60). Fundus examination (Fig. A) showed a subfoveal cyst (thin arrow) with scolex (thick arrow) moving in response to light and multiple subretinal exudates. Ultrasound B scan (Fig. B) showed a localized elevation in the macula (arrow) with a clump of high reflectivity suggestive of a scolex. CT brain showed oval calcification in the left temporal lobe. The patient underwent successful cyst removal after pars plana vitrectomy. Postoperative fundus shows clearing of the macular lesion with a small scar at the site of retinotomy.

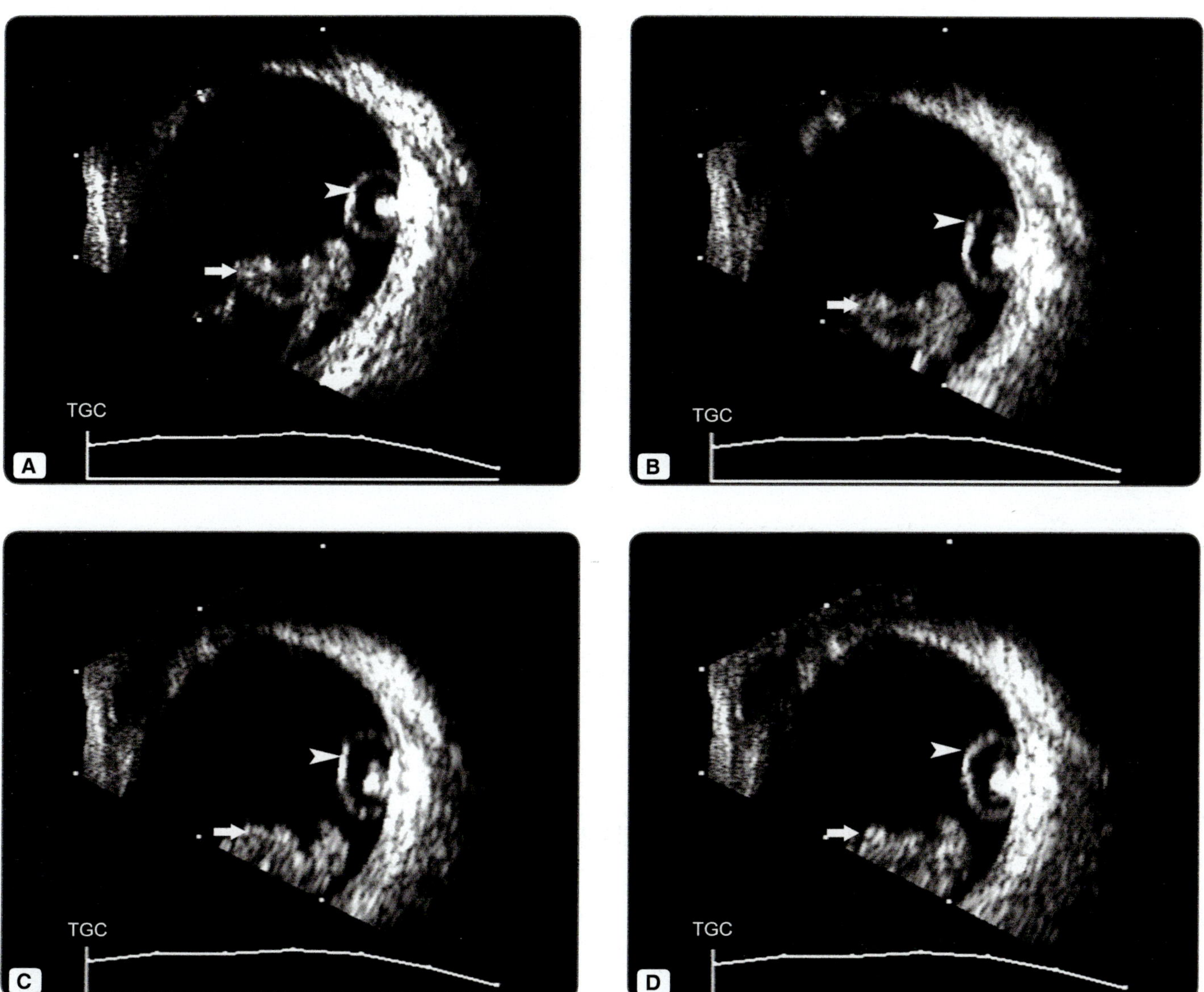

Figures 15.5A to D: Serial B scan images of an eye with a live cysticercus cyst (arrowhead) and a giant retinal tear (arrow) that occurred during attempted removal. Note the timer at the lower right corner of the image. The cyst wall changes contour and the scolex is seen to change its position with the passage of time. The movement of the cyst wall and the absence of vitreous echoes are indicative of the presence of a live cyst.

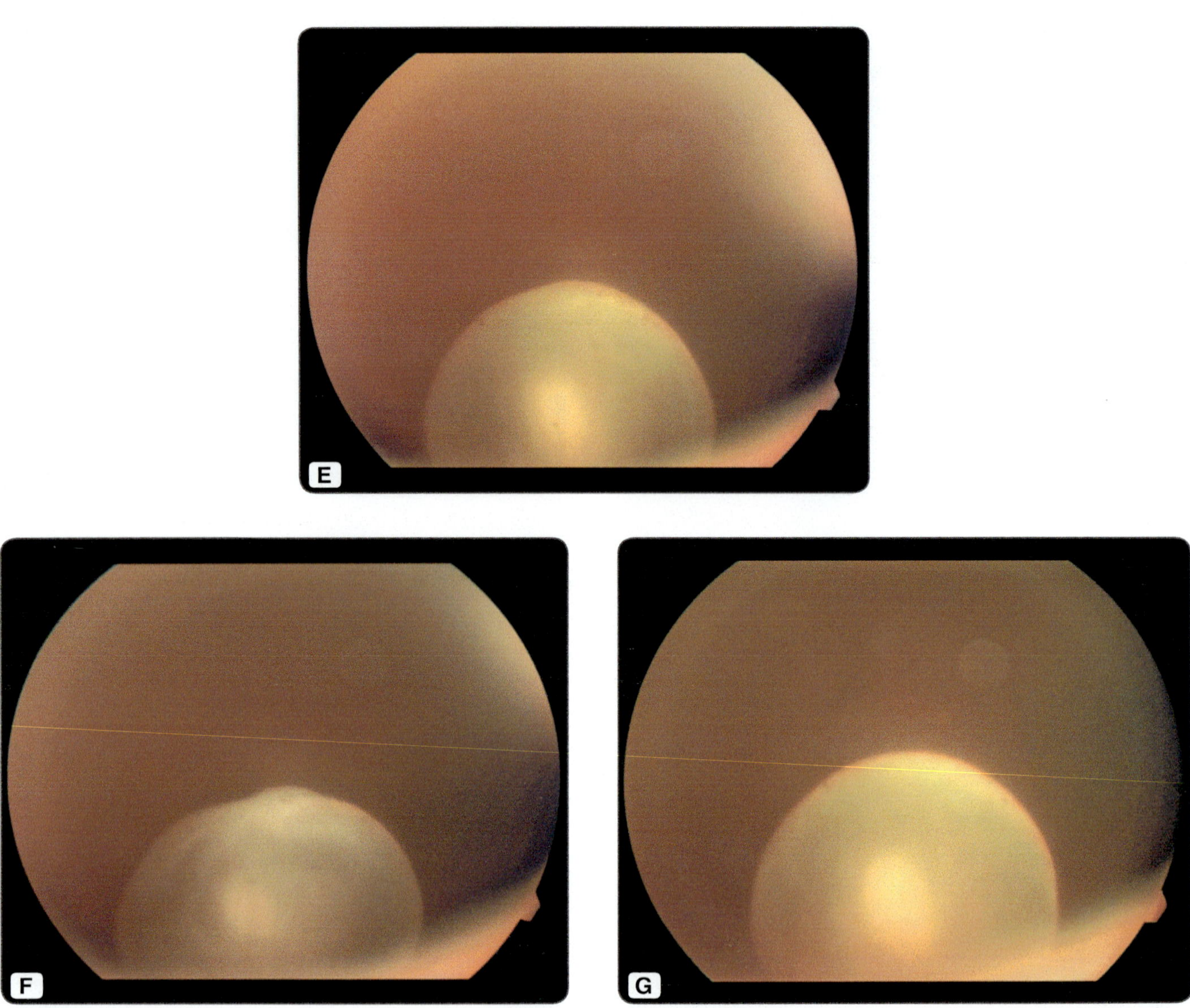

Figures 15.5E to G: Clinical photographs of the same case showing the change in contour of the cyst wall.

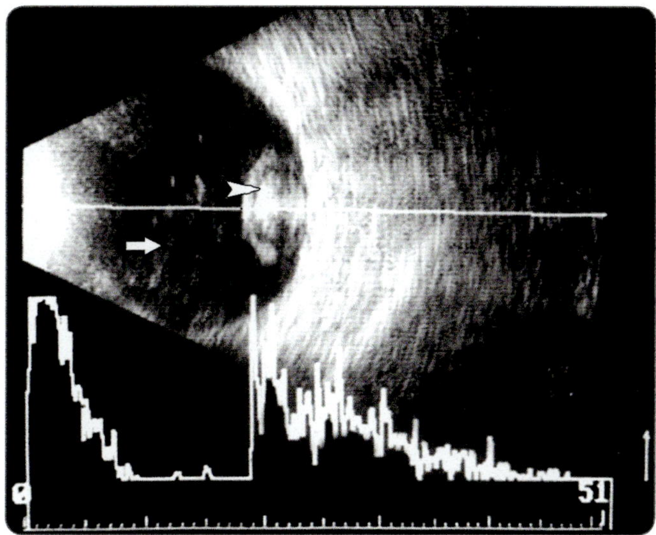

Figure 15.6: B scan with vector A showing a globular lesion at the posterior pole. The intralesional echoes are very high reflective, but are seen to fill the entire lesion (arrowhead), which differentiates it from a scolex. The vitreous shows low reflective dot echoes (arrow). This is a case of dislocated cataractous lens with vitreous inflammation.

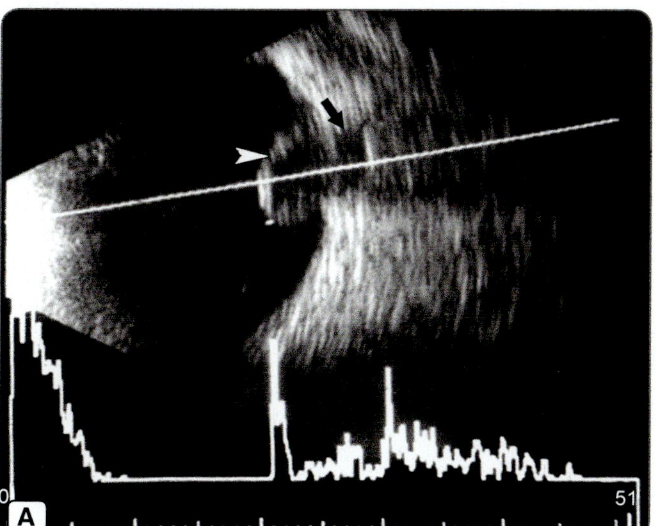

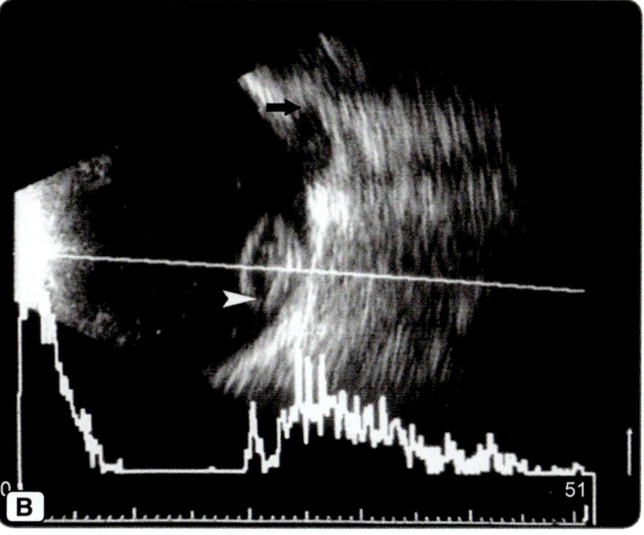

Figures 15.7A and B: B scan with vector A of an eye with occlusio pupillae and chronic uveitis. The B scan shows a globular lesion (arrowhead) over the optic disc with an area of high reflectivity in the center. In Figure B, taken in an erect posture, the globular lesion moves inferiorly. This is a case of dislocated crystalline lens with optic disc coloboma (black arrow).

Section 5

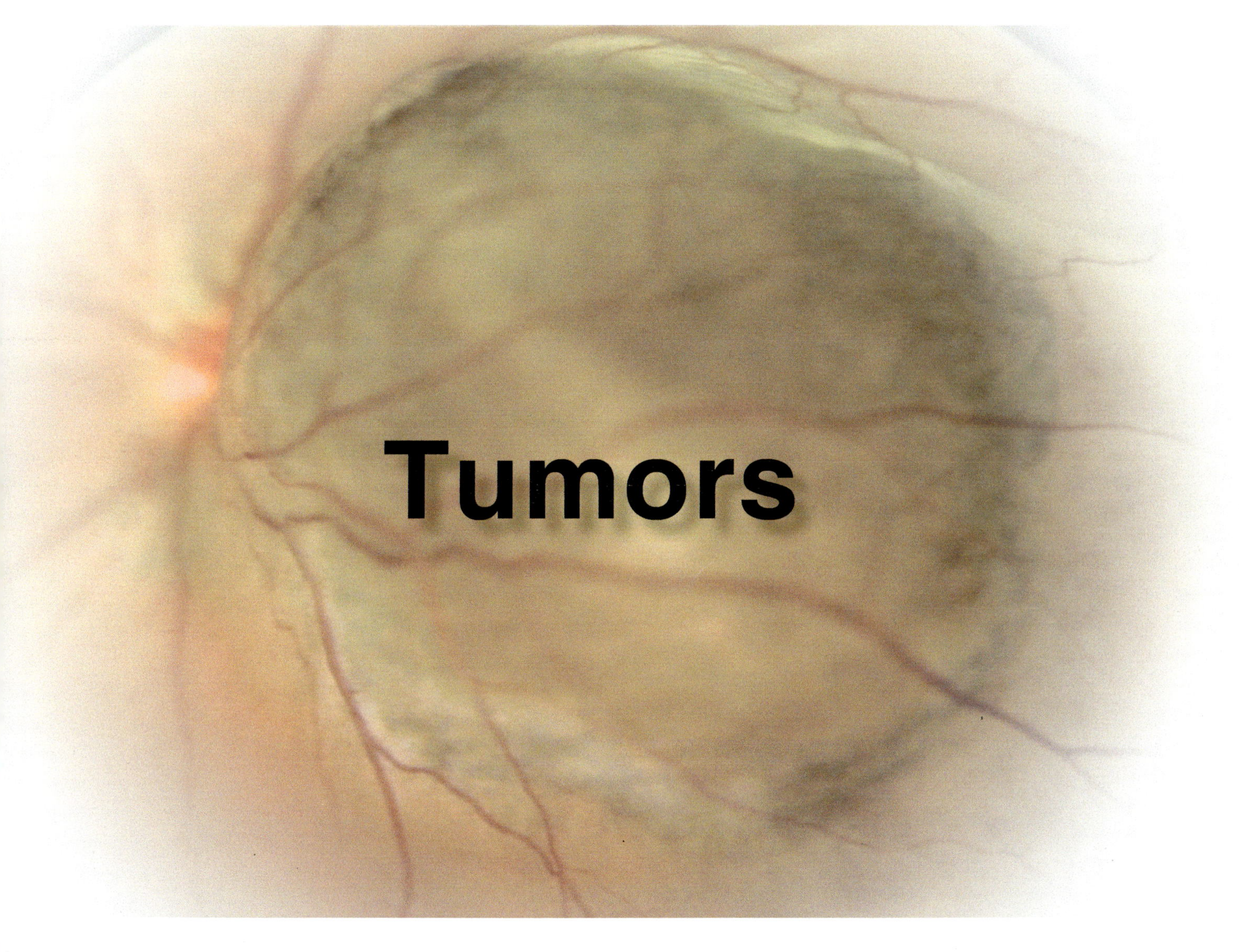

Tumors

16 Ultrasound in Tumors

- Noninvasive imaging tool
- Detection of tumors in opaque media
- Characterization of the lesion in clear media
- Differentiation from mimicking conditions
- Three-dimensional measurements
- Assessment after treatment and at follow-up.

REQUIREMENTS FOR A GOOD ULTRASOUND ASSESSMENT

1. Detailed clinical findings
2. Minimum elevation above the surrounding normal tissues of approximately 1 mm for detection.
3. Minimum tumor height of 2 mm for quantification
4. Modification of technique, such as use of immersion or standoff for demonstration of anterior tumors with the 10 or 12 MHz probe
5. Higher frequency systems are needed for better examination of smaller tumors, especially if they are located anteriorly
6. An ultrasonologist familiar with the clinical and ultrasound features of tumors.

FEATURES TO BE NOTED IN ALL TUMORS

1. Number (of tumors)
2. Shape
3. Surface
4. Location, and layer involved
5. Presence, extent and location of RD
6. Reflectivity of lesion compared to sclera
7. Measurements—base-vertical and horizontal, height
8. Presence of extrascleral extension, optic nerve extension, orbital soft tissue involvement, orbital bone destruction, remodeling
9. Presence of tumor vascularity
10. Associated inflammatory signs.

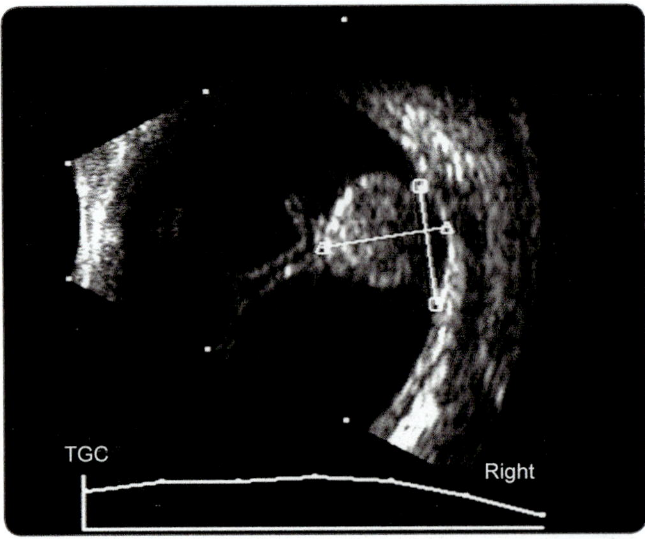

Figure 16.1A: B scan image of a mushroom shaped choroidal melanoma. Note the points used for measuring the tumor dimensions. The maximum tumor height is measured from the apex of the mass to a point perpendicular to it on the inner scleral surface. The maximum lateral dimensions are measured at the base of the tumor.

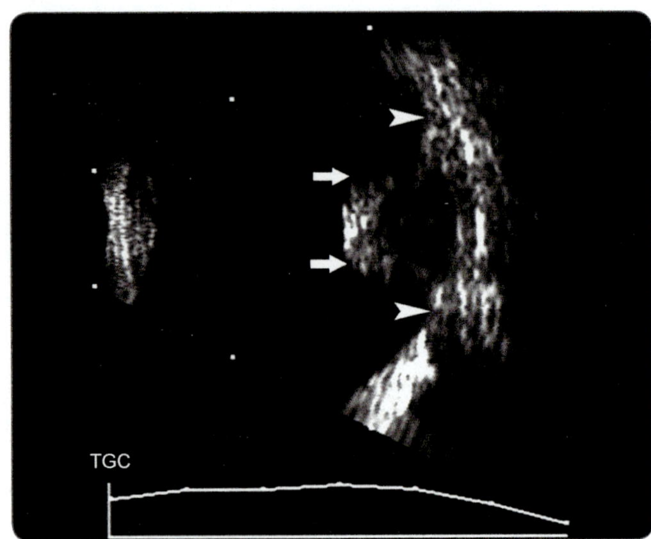

Figure 16.1B: B scan image of a mushroom-shaped melanoma. The arrows mark the maximum tumor extent at the surface. However, the true tumor extent is seen to be much greater when measured at the base (arrowheads).

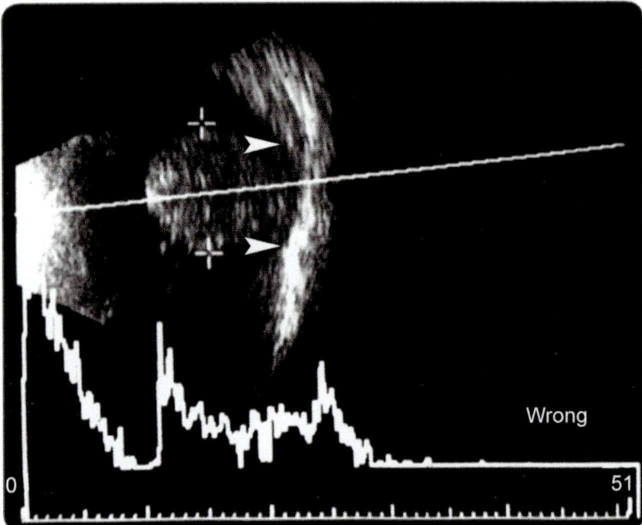

Figure 16.2A: B scan with vector A scan showing the cursors placed at the maximum tumor width which does not correspond to the tumor base. This is an erroneous reading and is not useful to follow the response of the tumor to treatment. The arrowheads mark the actual tumor base.

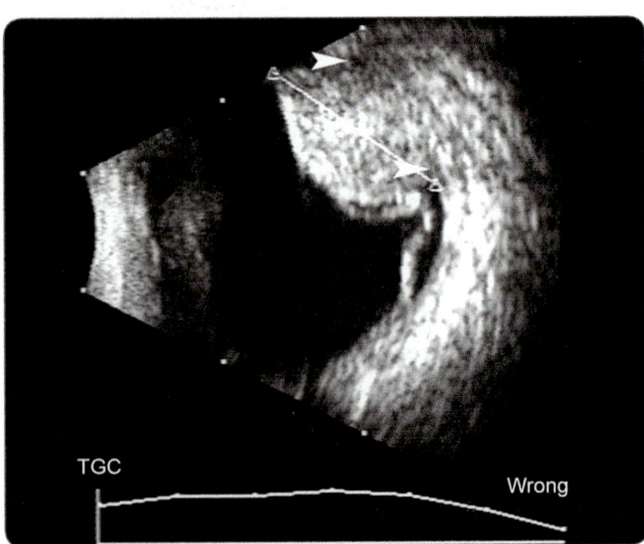

Figure 16.2B: B scan image of a peripherally located tumor. Here, the measurement has been taken obliquely and does not represent the true dimension of the tumor. The arrowheads mark the actual tumor base.

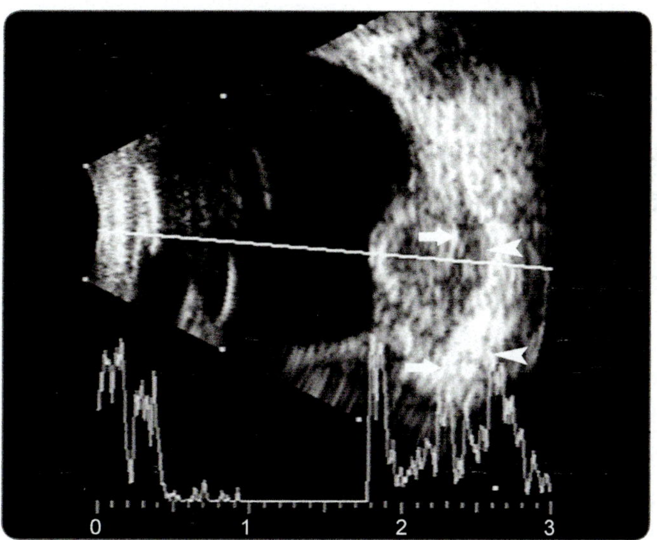

Figure 16.3: B scan image with vector A scan showing a melanoma post plaque therapy. Note the scleral edema caused by the plaque. The tumor height in this situation should be taken till the inner sclera (arrow) and not the outer sclera (arrowhead).

17 Choroidal Melanoma

CLINICAL FEATURES

- Malignant tumor of the melanocytes of the choroid. Most tumors are believed to develop from pre-existing melanocytic nevi.
- The most common primary intraocular tumor in adults.
- Seen typically as a dome-shaped mass which can range from purely amelanotic to darkly pigmented. The overlying RPE changes are seen as drusen or orange pigment.
- As the tumor enlarges it can break through the Bruch's membrane giving rise to a mushroom or collar button shape.
- Secondary retinal detachment may be seen.
- About 30–50% of patients with medium to large choroidal melanoma die within 10 years after diagnosis and treatment; usually secondary to distant metastases.
- Ultrasound is necessary to confirm the diagnosis and also to monitor response to therapy on follow-ups. Diagnostic accuracy with ultrasound is as high as 95%.

ULTRASONOGRAPHY

Classical Features

- Solid mass.
- Dome shaped or mushroom collar button configuration due to tumor growth through a ruptured Bruch's membrane.
- Regular internal structure on B scan .
- Low to medium internal reflectivity on A scan.
- Demonstrable internal blood flow seen as flickering spikes on the A scan.

Additional Features

- Sound attenuation due to the densely homogeneous nature of the tumor. This is seen as acoustic hollowing toward the tumor base on B scan and a rapid decay of spikes on the A scan described as a steep angle kappa. Very dense tumors may also produce orbital shadowing.
- Choroidal excavation. This is an appearance produced by the contrast between the normal high reflective choroid surrounding the tumor and the low reflectivity of the densely homogenous tumor mass.
- Exudative retinal detachment indicates tumor activity, and is classically seen away from the mass rather than over it.
- Increased scleral concavity or posterior scleral bowing at the tumor base has been described in younger patients. The histologic features in most of these cases suggest a more indolent variety.
- Rarely vitreous and/or subretinal hemorrhage can occur secondary to tumor growth.

UNUSUAL OR ASSOCIATED FEATURES

- Irregular structure with high internal reflectivity seen in very large tumors suggesting hemorrhage and necrosis
- Cystic cavities may sometimes be seen within a tumor. These may either represent areas of necrosis or hemorrhage. Differences in tumor pigmentation or a nodule of non-reflective tissue within a solid mass may cause a pseudocystic appearance.
- Calcification may sometimes be seen on the surface.
- Scleritis, inflammatory infiltration or orbital inflammation has also been noted. This along with a transient increase in tumor size may be seen after local treatment such as brachytherapy.
- A diffuse variety of malignant melanoma is seen in about 5% of cases. This may simulate choroidal metastases, and is of lower height (15% of horizontal extent) and considerably larger circumferential extent than is described for a classical choroidal melanoma. The internal reflectivity, however, continues to be low. This usually occurs in the midperipheral or peripheral choroid.

FEATURES INDICATIVE OF LOCAL SPREAD

- Scleral infiltration may be seen near the tumor base as an area of low reflectivity.
- Extrascleral extension is commonly noted as a small nodule or occasionally as a mass larger than the intraocular part itself.
- Tumor spread may be seen along the vortex veins into the orbit without any direct evidence of scleral discontinuity.

MIMICKING CONDITIONS

- Melanocytomas—typically occur on the optic nerve head and are very highly reflective.
- Choroidal nevi. These are relatively flat or minimally elevated and highly reflective. They need to be followed diligently for development of malignancy.
- Collar button or mushroom shape—rarely seen in metastases, has also been described as a rare finding in hemangioma.
- Choroidal excavation is also seen in choroidal hemorrhage.
- Posterior scleral bowing has been described in choroidal schwannoma.
- Posterior pole granulomas (TB, fungal) may present with homogenous low reflectivity. It is important to took for features such as scleral thickening and Tenon's widening which suggest inflammation.

NUGGETS

A choroidal melanoma rarely causes direct scleral invasion, and extrascleral extension along a vessel is usually seen with an intact intervening sclera.

Extrascleral extension may be mimicked by congested blood vessels, inflammation in Tenon's space and extraocular muscle underlying the mass.

Always look carefully for a tumor mass in an eye with unexplained vitreous hemorrhage, especially in a blind eye of an older patient.

The combined use of height to base ratio and reflectivity enables a highly significant discrimination between choroidal melanomas and metastases. The former has an increased height to base ratio and lower internal reflectivity than the latter.

Before diagnosing an extrascleral extension of a posterior pole mass lesion, ensure that the echolucency is not due to the inferior oblique muscle that courses against the globe near the macular region.

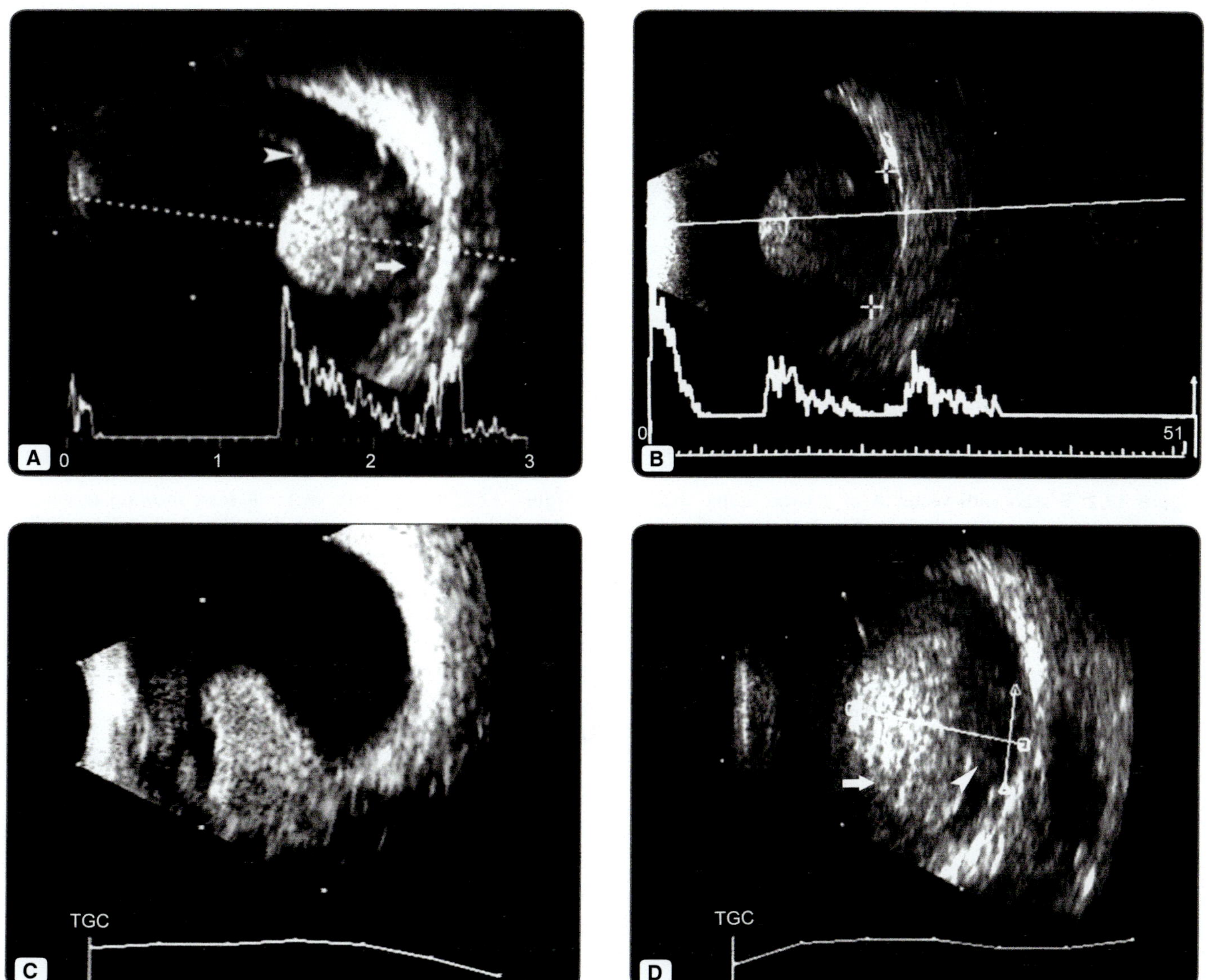

Figures 17.1A to D: Different images of eyes with collar button melanomas. The first image shows a typical mass with high surface reflectivity, acoustic hollowing (white arrow) and choroidal excavation (black arrow). The retinal detachment (arrowhead) is adjacent to, but does not involve the tumor surface. The A scan shows a sharp decay of spikes indicating that the lesion is densely homogenous. Figure B shows a similar lesion without a secondary retinal detachment. Figure C shows a peripheral mass which appears ciliochoroidal and has almost a conical appearance. The height is significantly greater than the base. Figure D is an example of how the lesion (arrowhead) may appear larger than it actually is, because of the wider area anterior to the Bruch's membrane disruption (arrow). Ultrasound is able to give an accurate measurement of the tumor base, which is smaller than the dimensions at the surface.

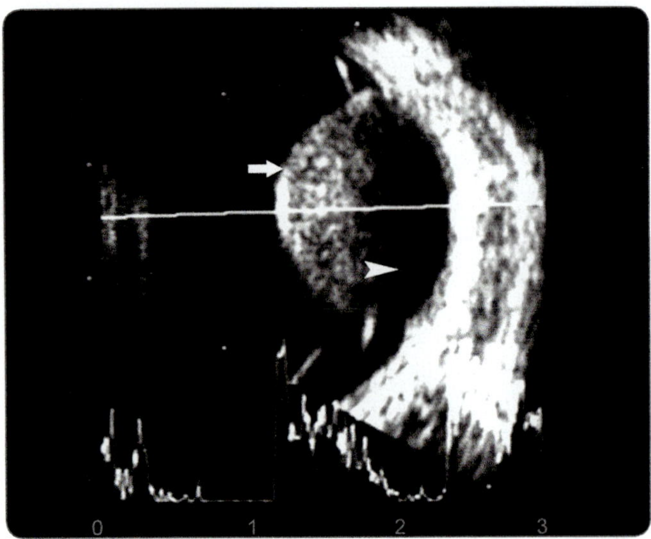

Figure 17.2: B scan with vector A of a large dome shaped melanoma (arrow). Note the significant degree of sound attenuation causing the appearance of acoustic hollowing (arrowhead) at the base with absent spikes on the A scan.

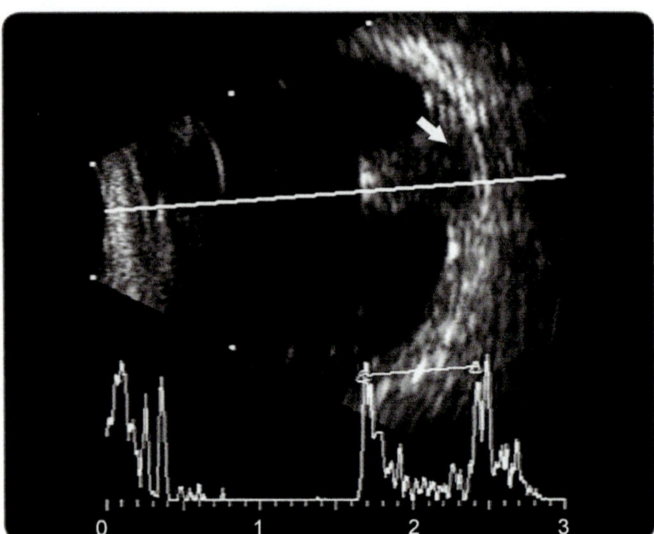

Figure 17.3: B scan with vector A scan showing prominent choroidal excavation (arrow) in this choroidal melanoma. The difference in reflectivity of the choroid at the base of the tumor from the surrounding normal choroid is quite significant.

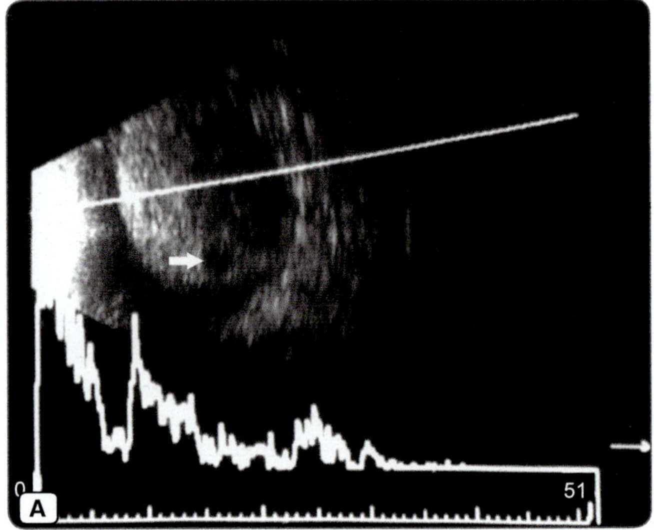

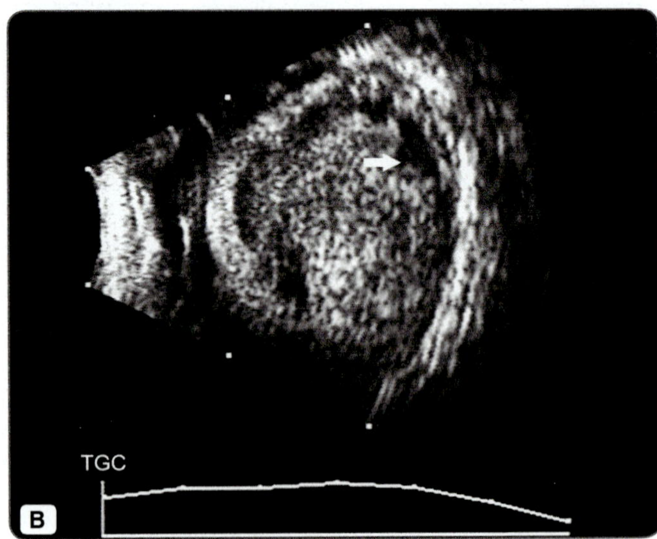

Figures 17.4A and B: B scan images of two large choroidal melanomas. The internal structure shows a small echolucent area (arrow) in Figure A and a large irregular cystic area in Figure B. These changes are believed to represent areas of hemorrhagic necrosis or cavitation and are usually seen in very large tumors.

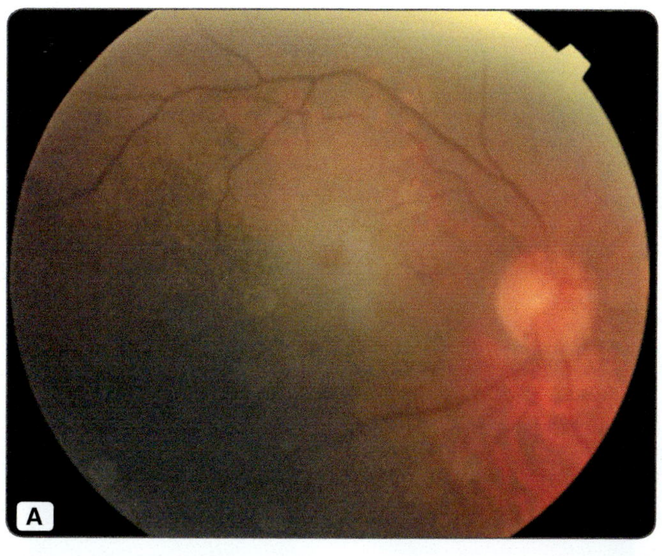

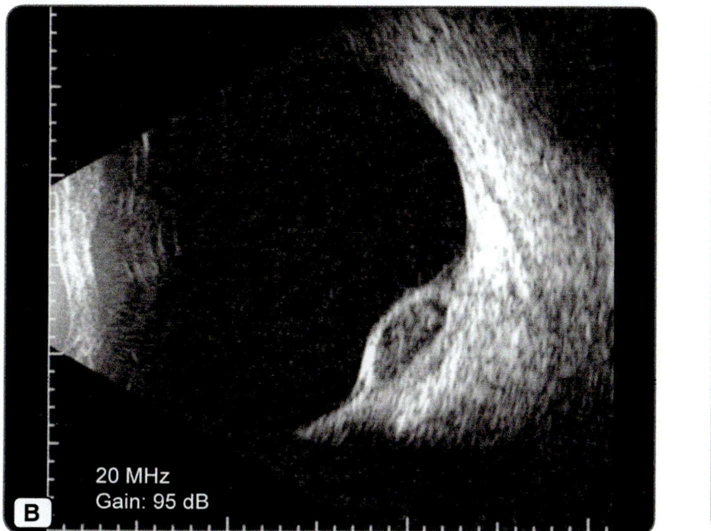

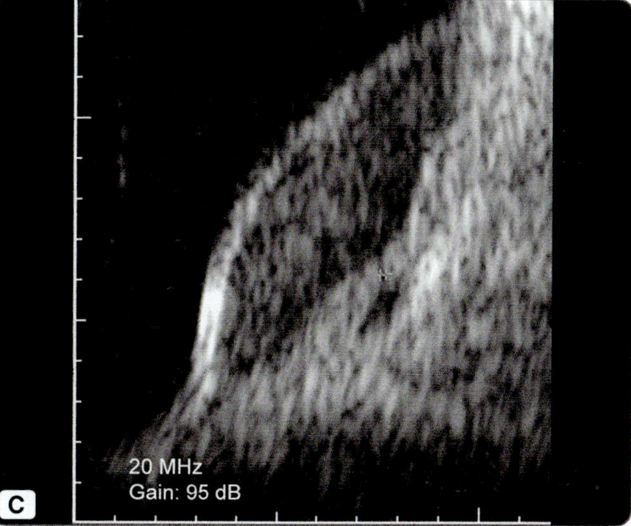

Figures 17.5A to C: Clinical photograph of a patient with a pigmented mass at the posterior pole. The B scan images with 20 MHz probe show a low reflective mass involving the choroid. There is a localized area of echolucency outside the sclera that is suggestive of extrascleral extension. The zoomed up image shows the extrascleral nodule clearly as well as a suspected scleral emissary. *(Images courtesy Dr Vincenzina Mazzeo, Italy)*

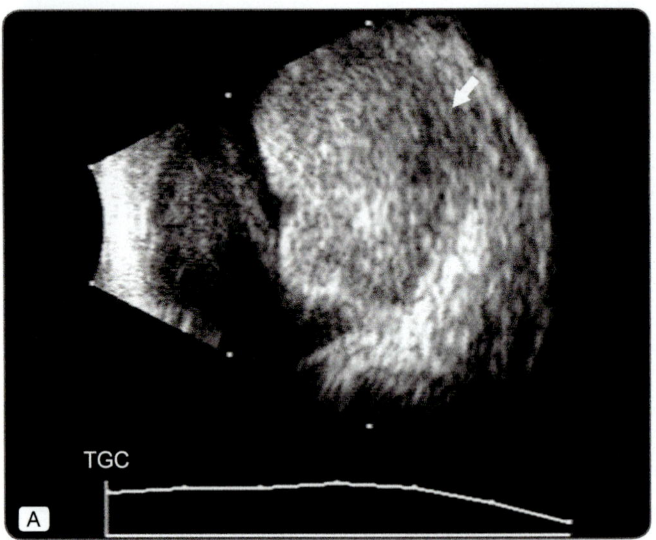

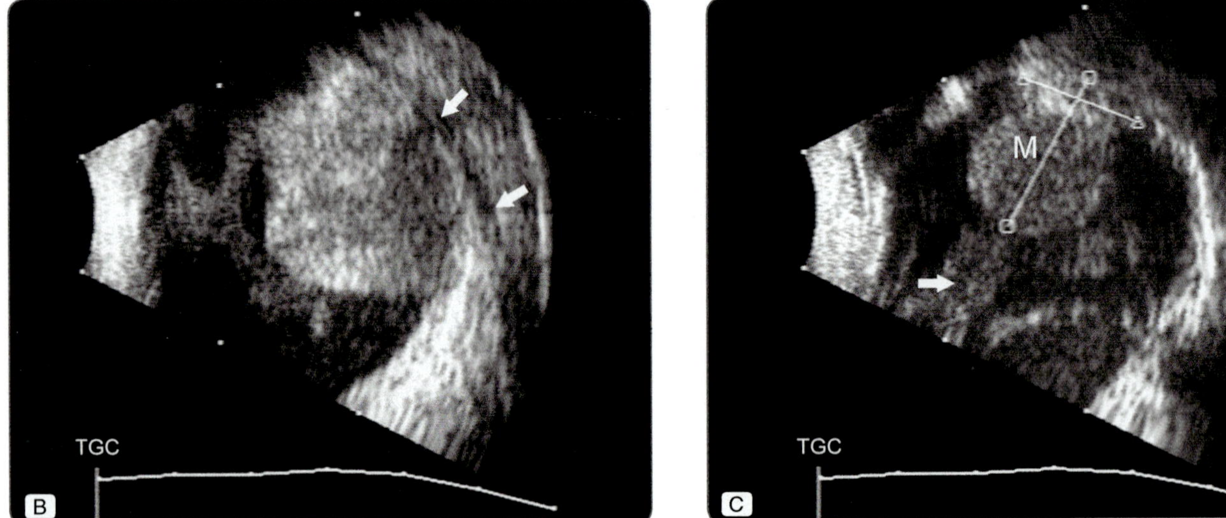

Figures 17.6A to C: These images show some associated features seen in melanomas. Figure A shows a large bilobed melanoma with irregular internal reflectivity and scleral edema (arrow). Figure B shows the tumor overlying a muscle (arrows), which can be mistaken for area of extrascleral extension. Figure C shows a mushroom-shaped mass (M) in an eye with significant vitreous hemorrhage (arrow).

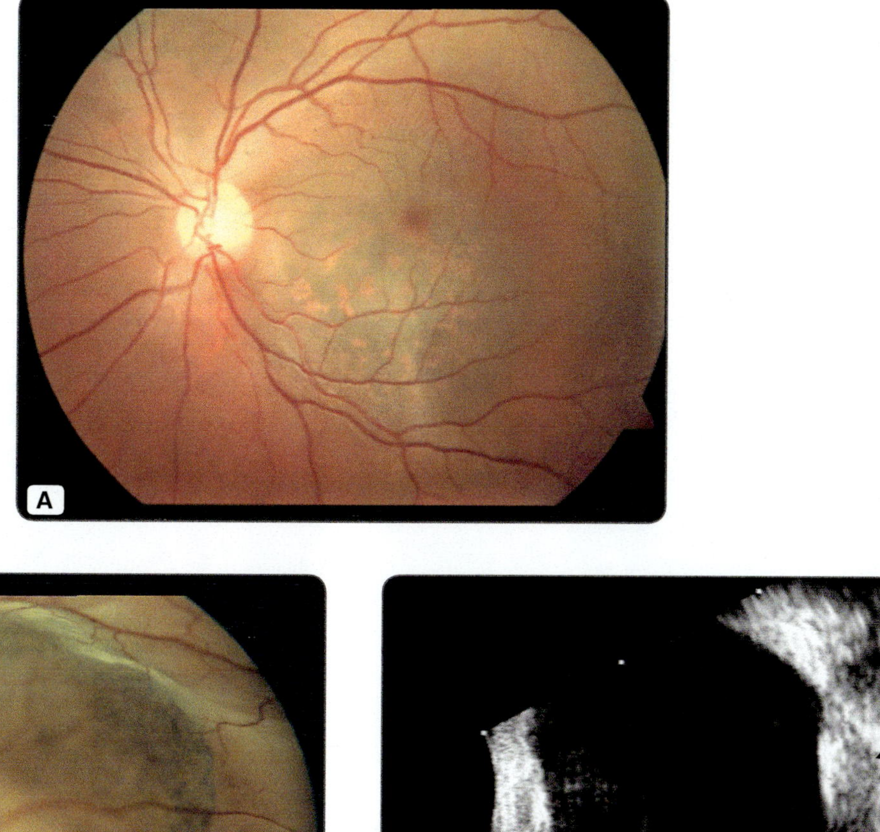

Figures 17.7A to C: The color photographs show the rapid increase in size of a posterior pole tumor over a 4-month period. The elevated mass (black arrow) is adjacent to but not involving the optic nerve. This is better made out on ultrasound than clinically

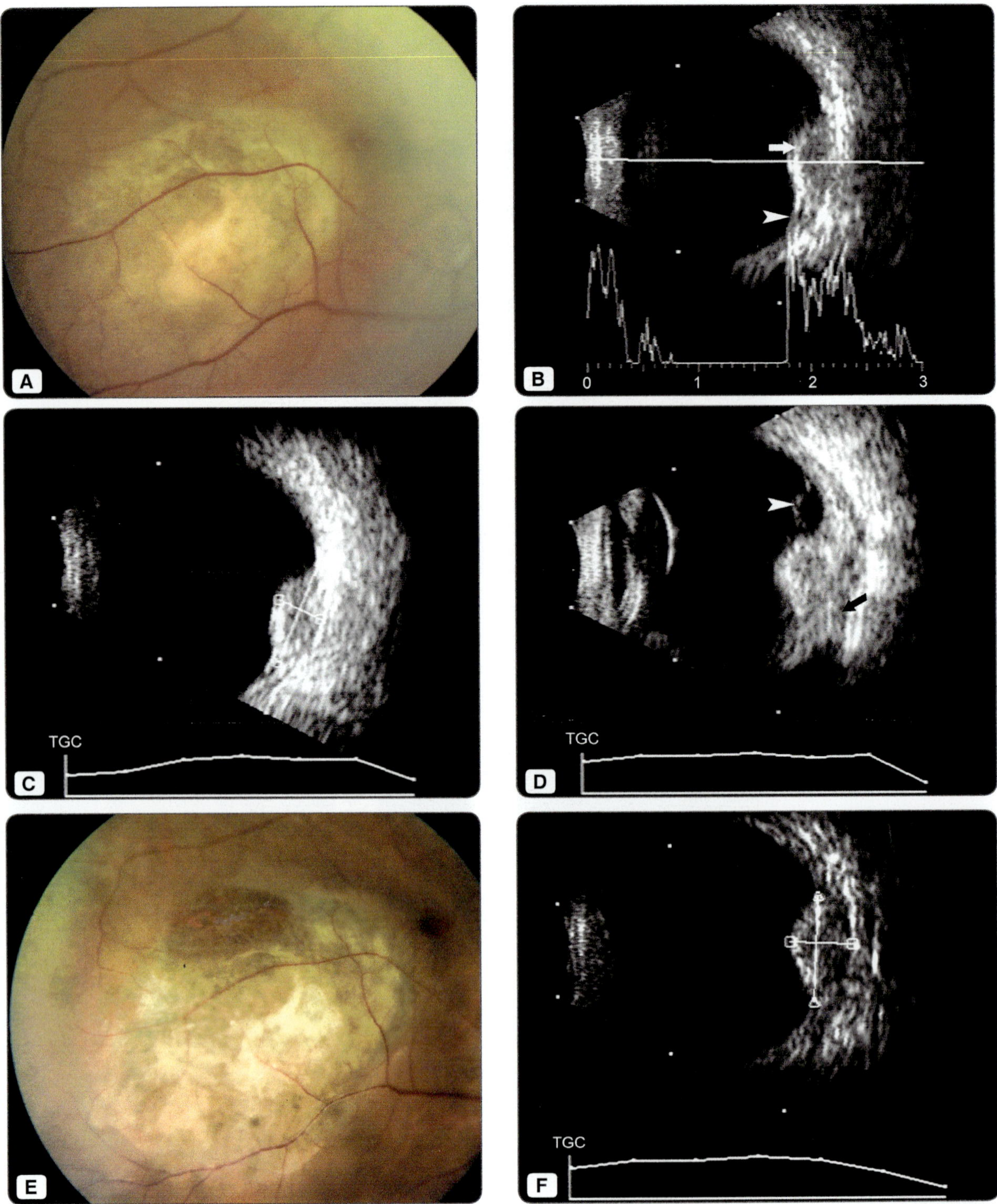

Figures 17.8A to F: This series of images and photographs show a choroidal melanoma before (Figs A to C) and after plaque brachytherapy (Figs D to F). In the pretreatment ultrasound, typical features such as a dome shape (arrow) and low reflectivity are seen. There is a small secondary retinal detachment (arrowhead) adjacent to the mass. The second image shows the tumor dimensions (Fig. C). Figure D shows the mass just after plaque therapy. Note the presence of scleral edema (arrow), an increase in height and increase in retinal detachment (arrowhead). The color photograph three months after treatment shows resolution of the detachment but not much change in size. The ultrasound shows that the scleral edema and retinal detachment have resolved, but there is an increase in the tumor height compared to the pretreatment image.

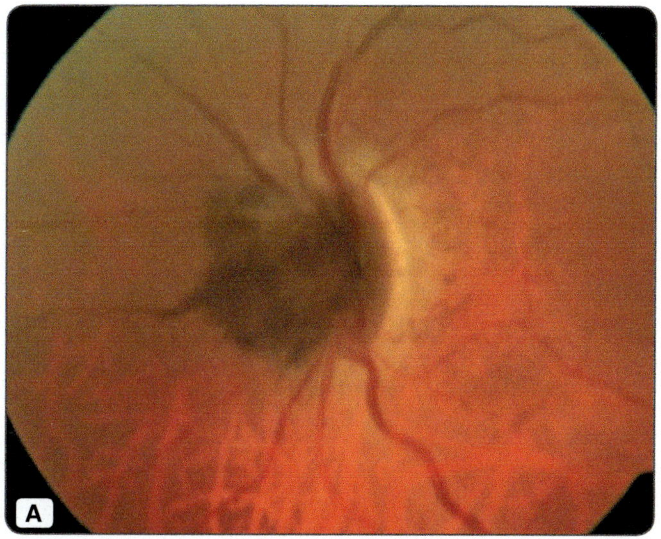

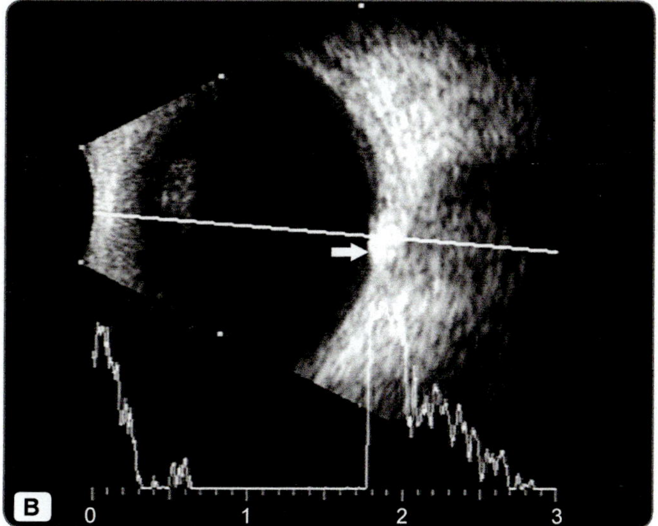

Figures 17.9A and B: Color photographs showing a darkly pigmented mass on the optic disc. The ultrasound B scan with vector A shows a well circumscribed highly reflective mass (arrow) on the disc, typical of a melanocytoma.

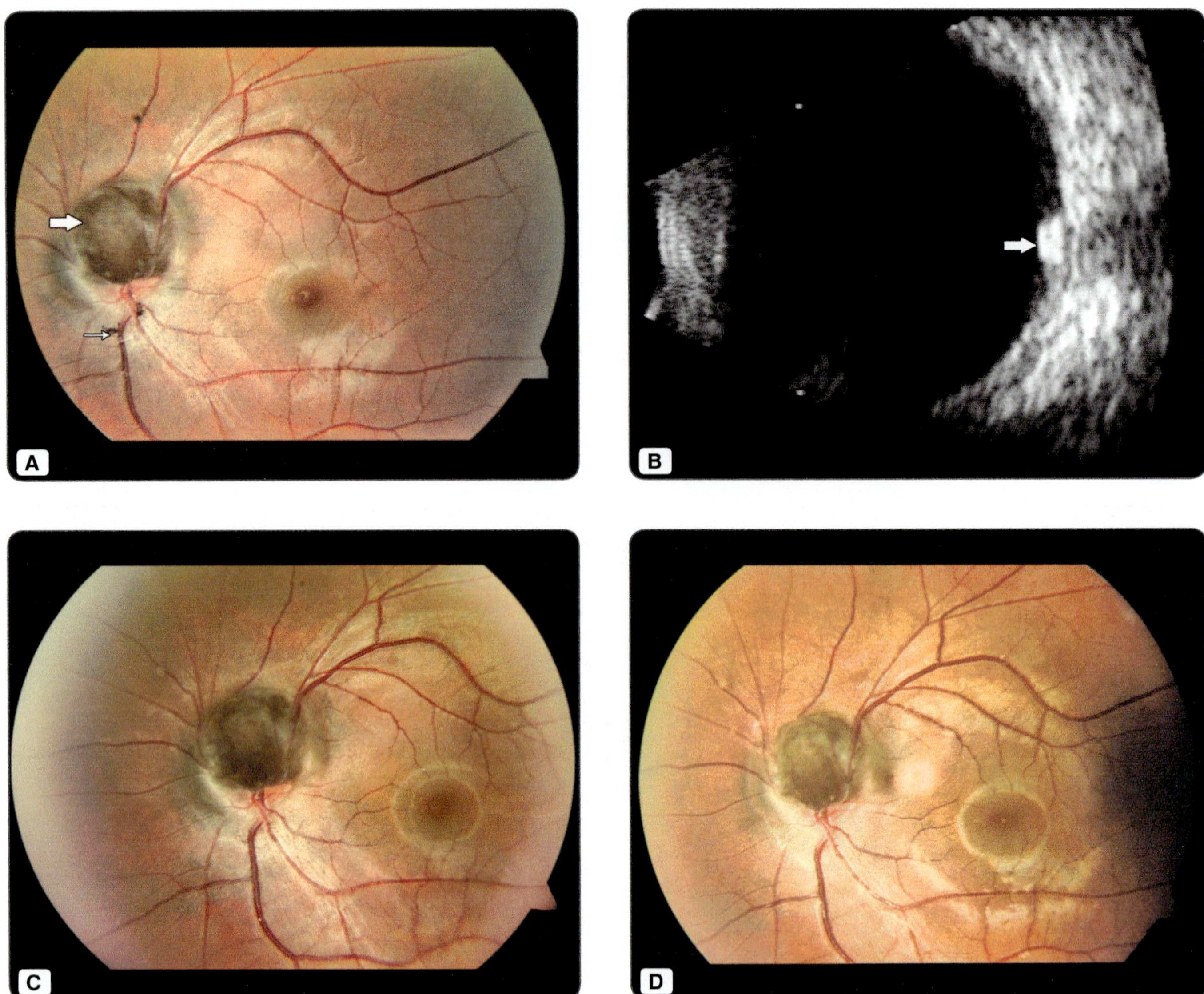

Figures 17.10A to D: Left fundus of a 22-year-old male with accidental discovery of poor vision in the left eye. There is a deeply pigmented globular mass on the optic disc suggestive of ONH melanocytoma (arrow) with pigment dispersion in vitreous cavity (thin arrow). B scan showed a high reflective mass over the optic nerve head (arrow) suggestive of a melanocytoma. Serial fundus examinations showed no change in the lesion at 5 years.

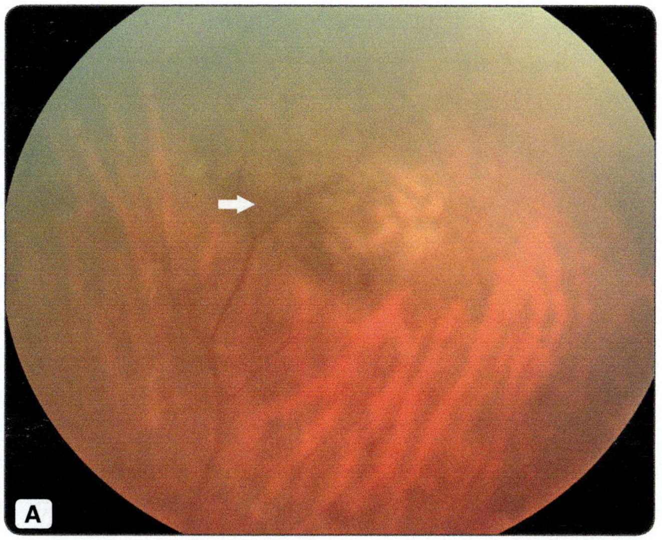

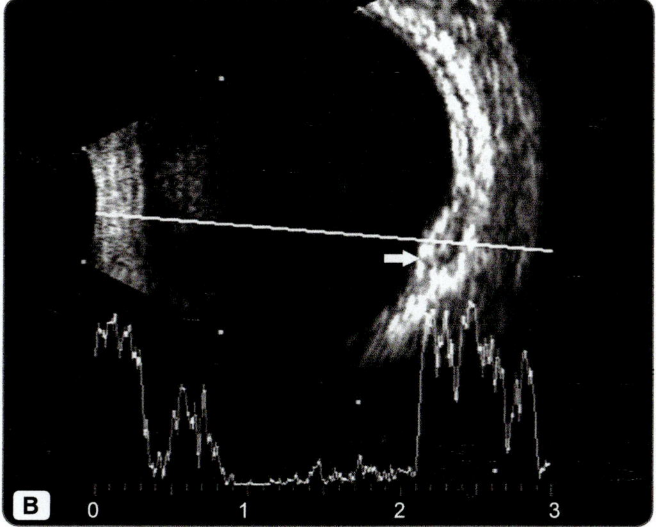

Figures 17.11A and B: Color photographs and ultrasound image of a patient with a minimally elevated lesion (arrow) in the periphery. The lesion shows drusen on the surface and is minimally pigmented. Ultrasound shows that it is arising from the choroid, is minimally elevated and shows high reflectivity (arrow). These features suggest a choroidal nevus.

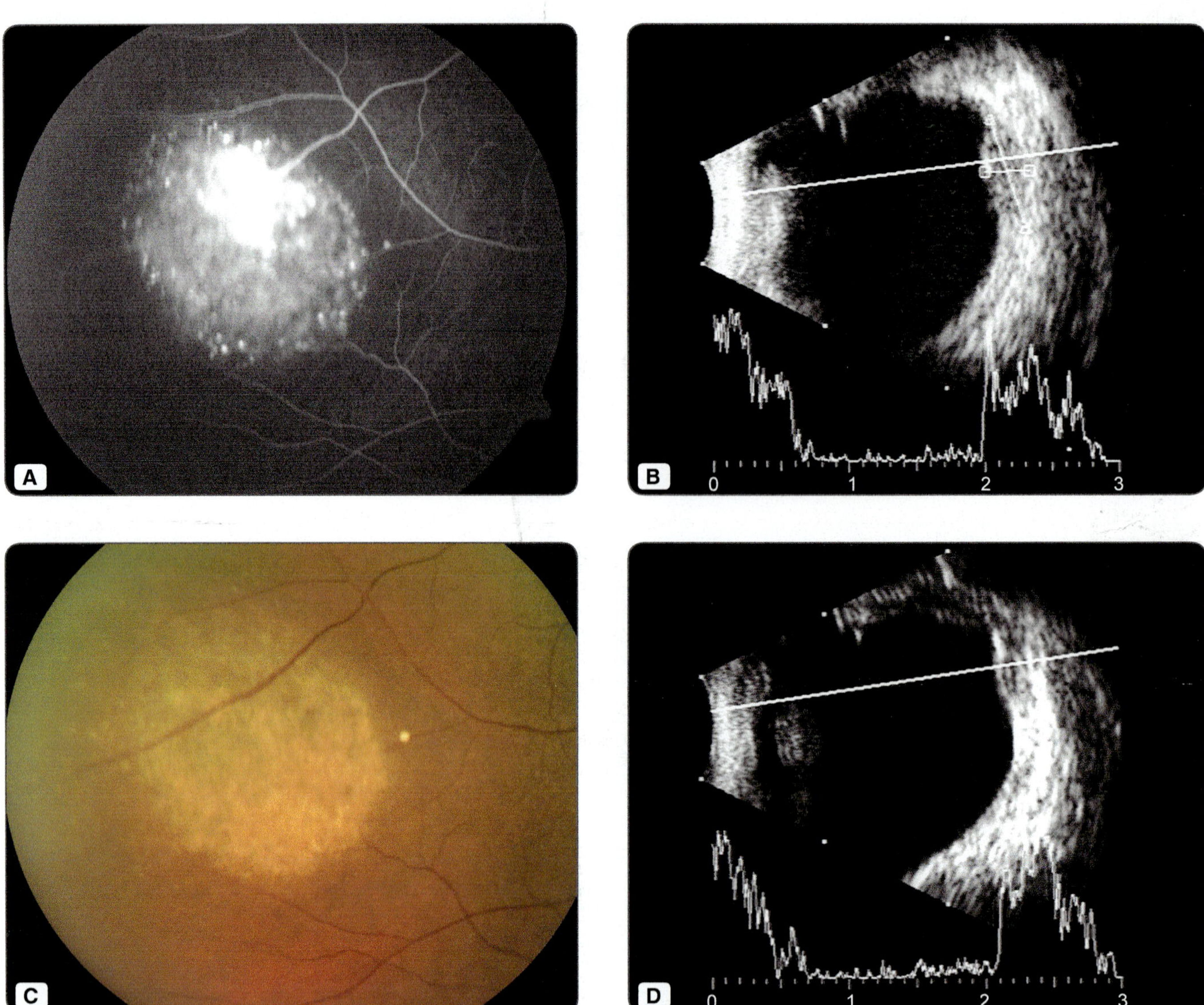

Figures 17.12A to D: Fundus fluorescein angiogram and ultrasound image of a choroidal nevus. Note the lesion size and elevation. Color photograph and ultrasound one year later shows that the dimensions are constant.

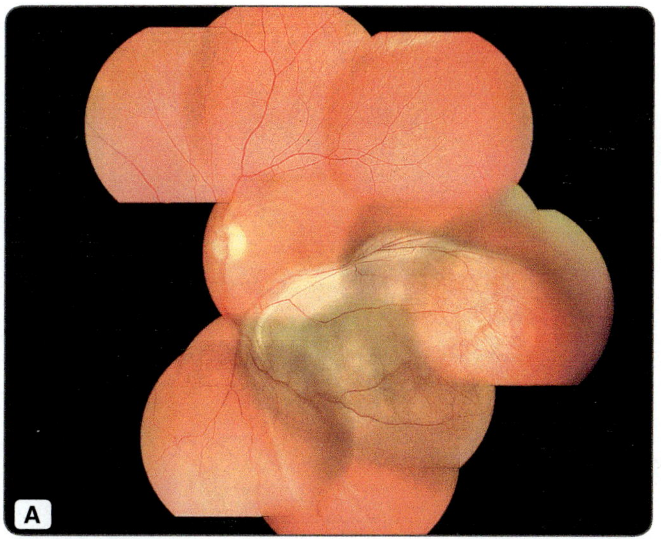

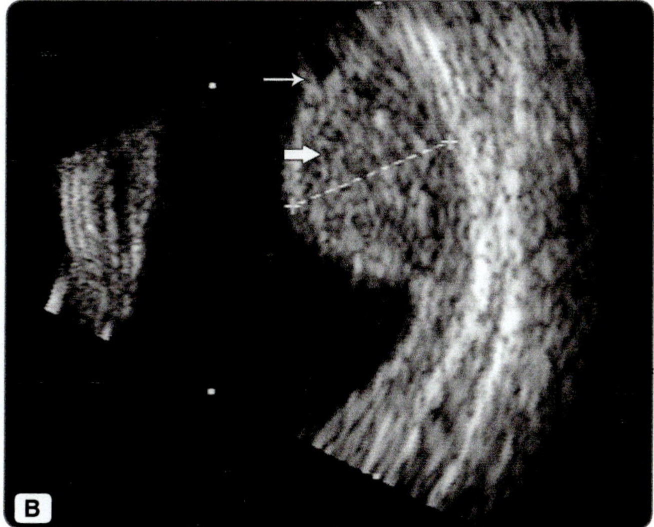

Figures 17.13A and B: A 45 years old female presented with sudden onset drop in vision since a week. Fundus exam revealed choroidal mass lesion inferotemporally with exudative RD. Ultrasound B scan image shows a dome shaped mass lesion (broad arrow) with moderate to high surface reflectivity and uniform moderate internal reflectivity and choroidal excavation. Secondary RD is seen in the upper part of the image (thin arrow). The features suggest a choroidal melanoma.

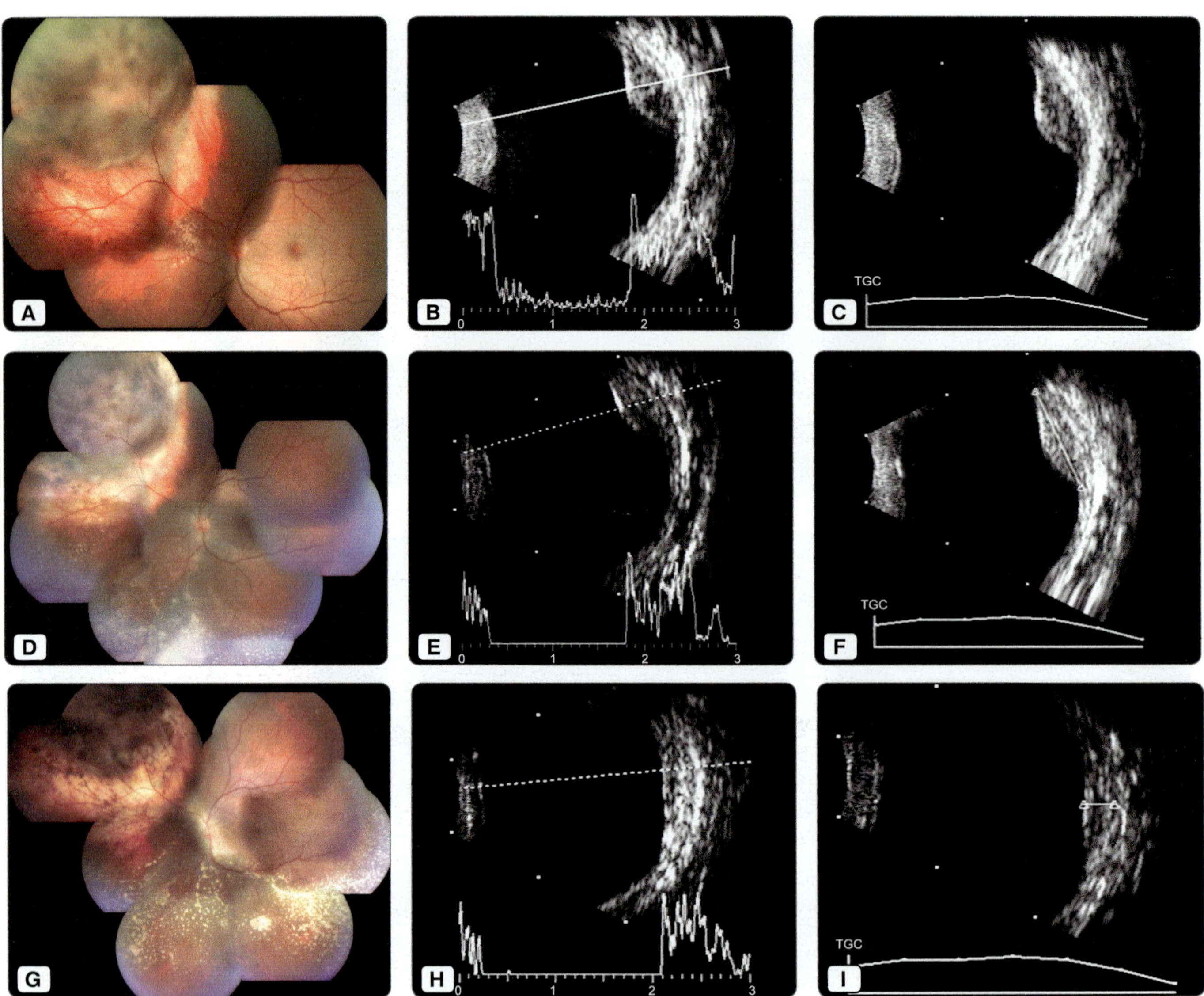

Figures 17.14A to I: Pre- and post-plaque therapy for a malignant melanoma of the choroid (A–C). The tumor is well defined, dome shaped with low internal reflectivity, and with a secondary retinal detachment at the lower border (D–F). Three months after therapy, there is a reduction in size of the mass as well as the secondary retinal detachment (G–I). Repeat ultrasonography 6 months later shows a further reduction in tumor size.

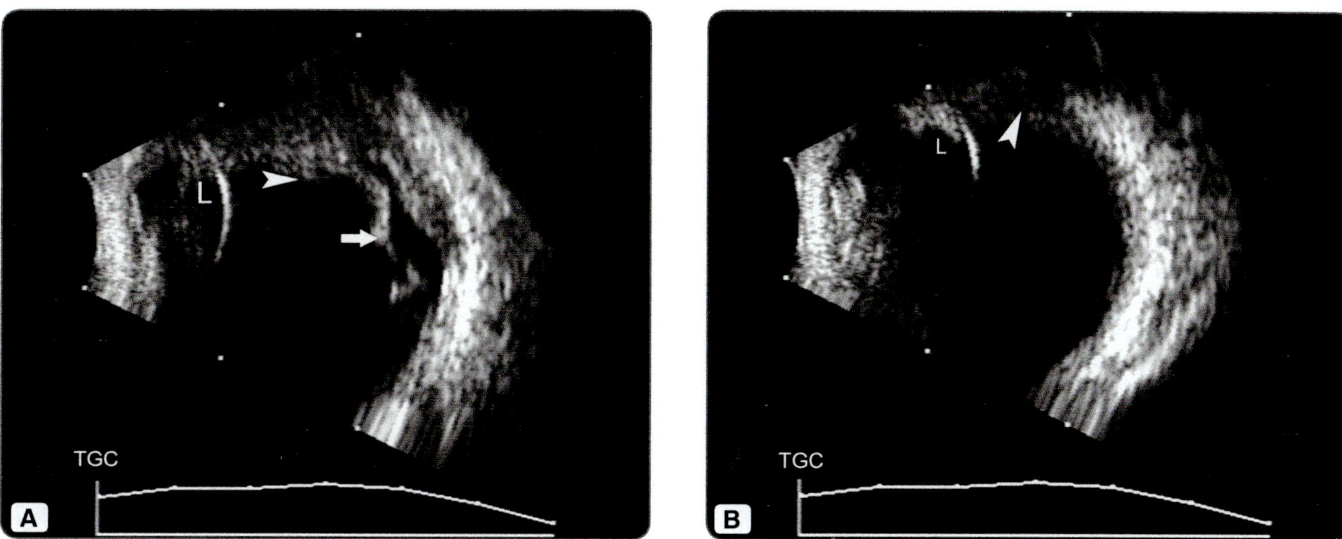

Figures 17.15A and B: B scan images of an eye with suspected ring melanoma of the choroid. There is low reflective choroidal thickening from 4 to 2 o'clock with a prominent mushroom shaped mass (arrowhead) involving the quadrants from 10 to 12 o'clock. In addition there is a secondary retinal detachment (arrow).

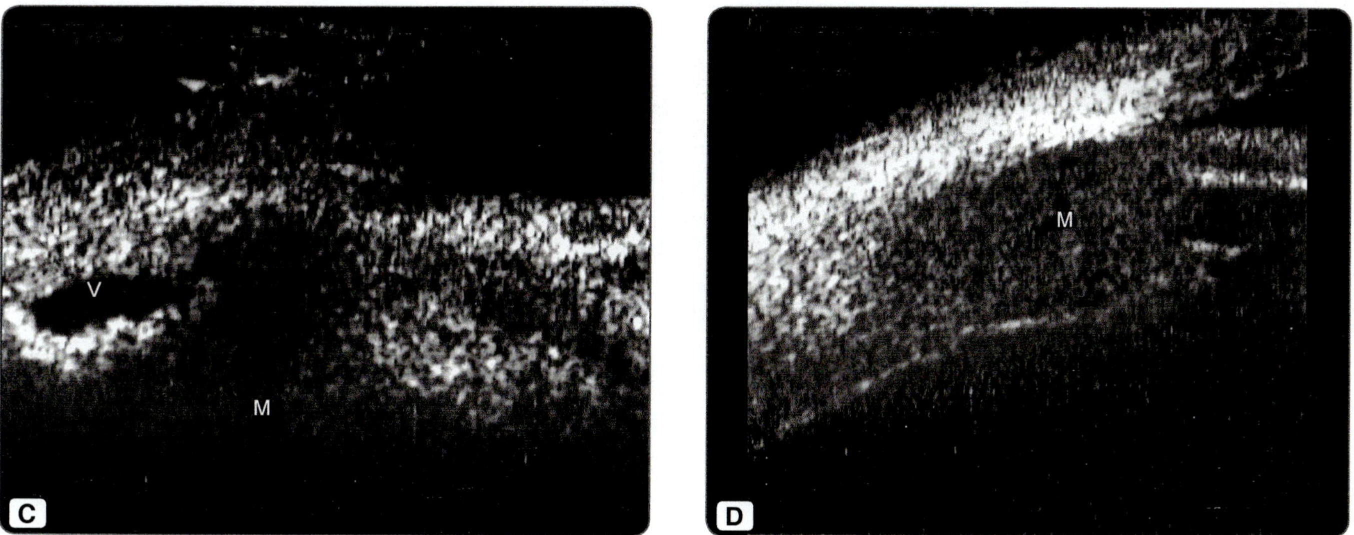

Figures 17.15C and D: UBM images of the same lesion showing a prominent tumor vessel (V) within the lesion (M). There is also involvement of the ciliary body at the 2 o'clock position (M in Figure D).

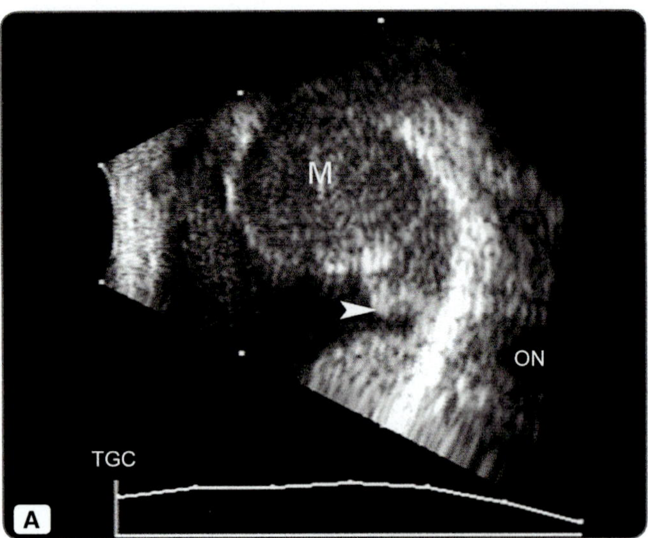

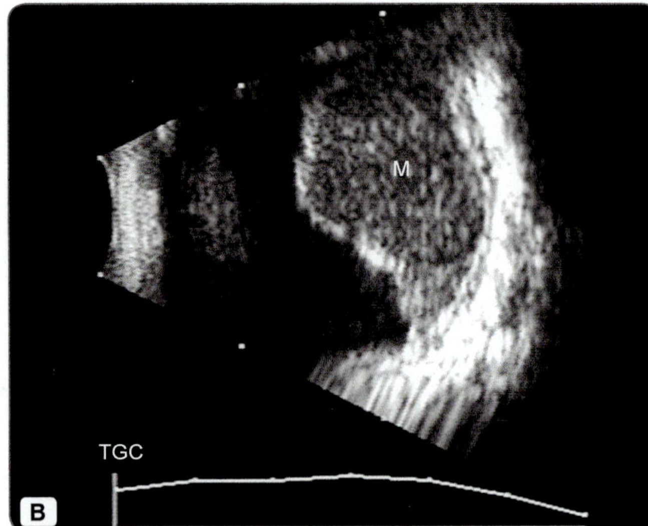

Figures 17.16A and B: Series of images of a 10-year-old boy who reported loss of vision in the right eye after an apparently trivial trauma. The clinical picture showed a solid appearing choroidal detachment. B scan ultrasonography showed a globular mass lesion in the ciliary body region (M) with an associated retinal detachment and subretinal echoes similar to those of the mass (arrowhead).

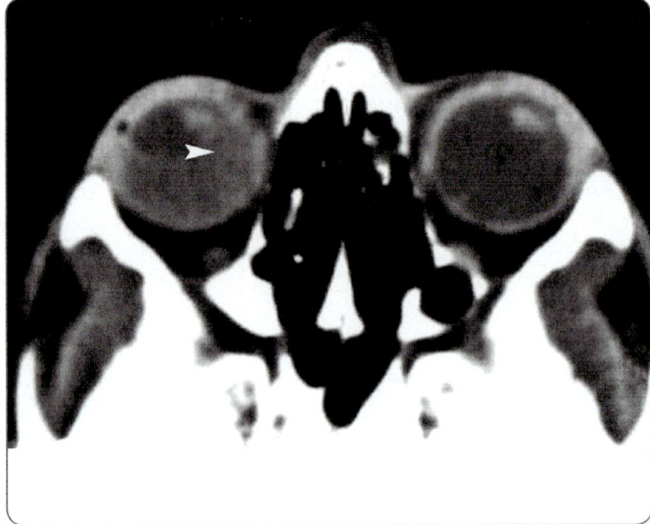

Figure 17.16C: Plain CT scan did not directly delineate the tumor though it showed a membrane with echoes behind it and a suspicious area in the nasal quadrant (arrowhead).

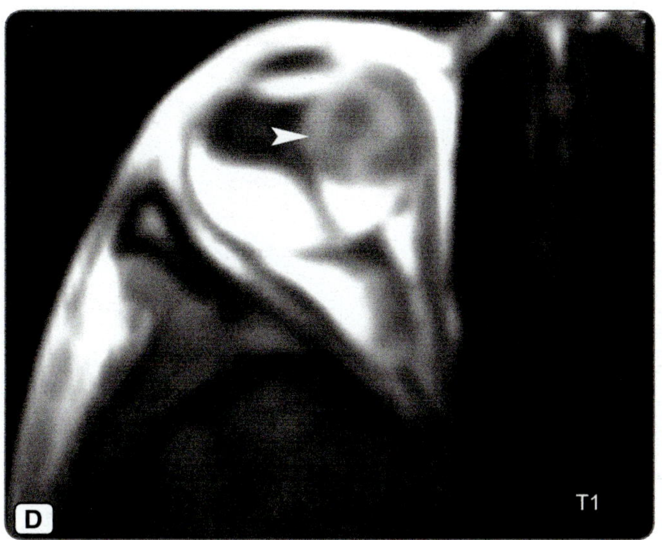

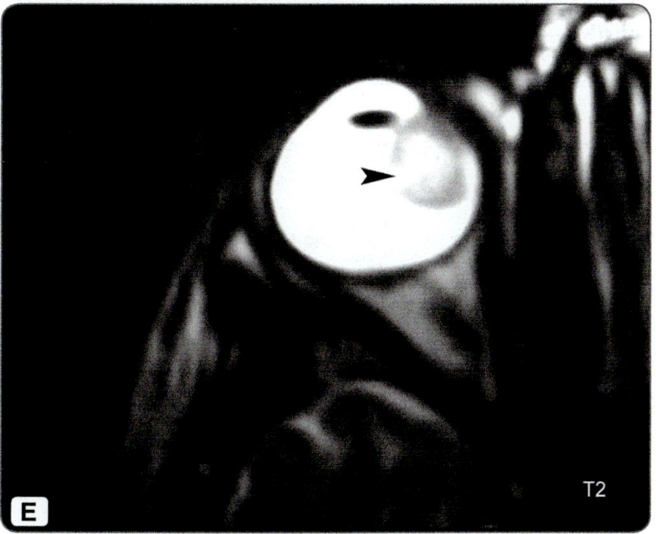

Figures 17.16D and E: MRI images showed a ciliary body tumor (arrowhead), hyperintense on T1 and hypointense on T2 indicating the possibility of a ciliary body melanoma.

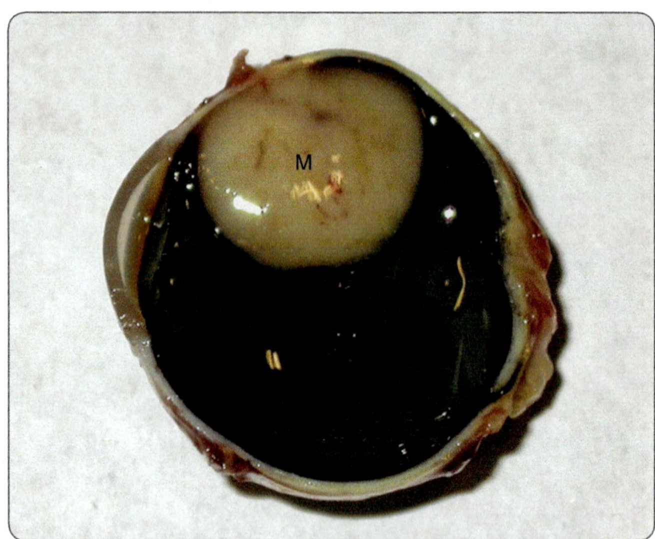

Figure 17.16F: Cut section of the eyeball after enucleation, showing a nonpigmented ciliary body tumor (M). This was shown on histopathology to be an amelanotic melanoma.

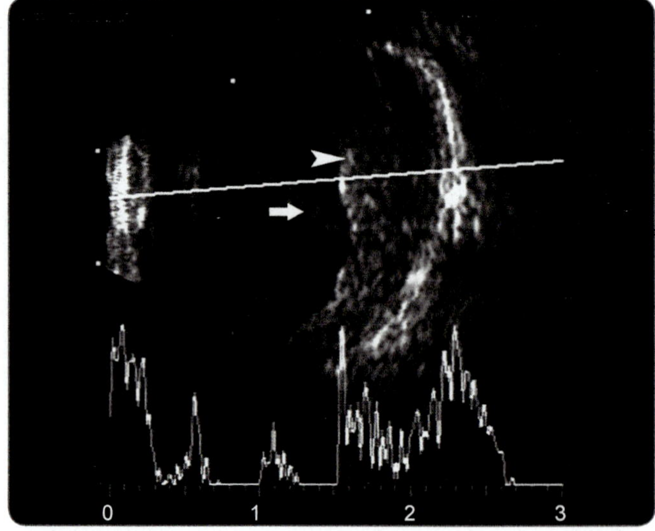

Figure 17.17: B scan with vector A of an eye with a diffuse melanoma (arrowhead) at the posterior pole. Note the lobular appearance and homogenous nature with low reflective internal echoes. A significant additional feature is the bullous retinal detachment (arrow) which is seen only in large or diffuse melanomas.

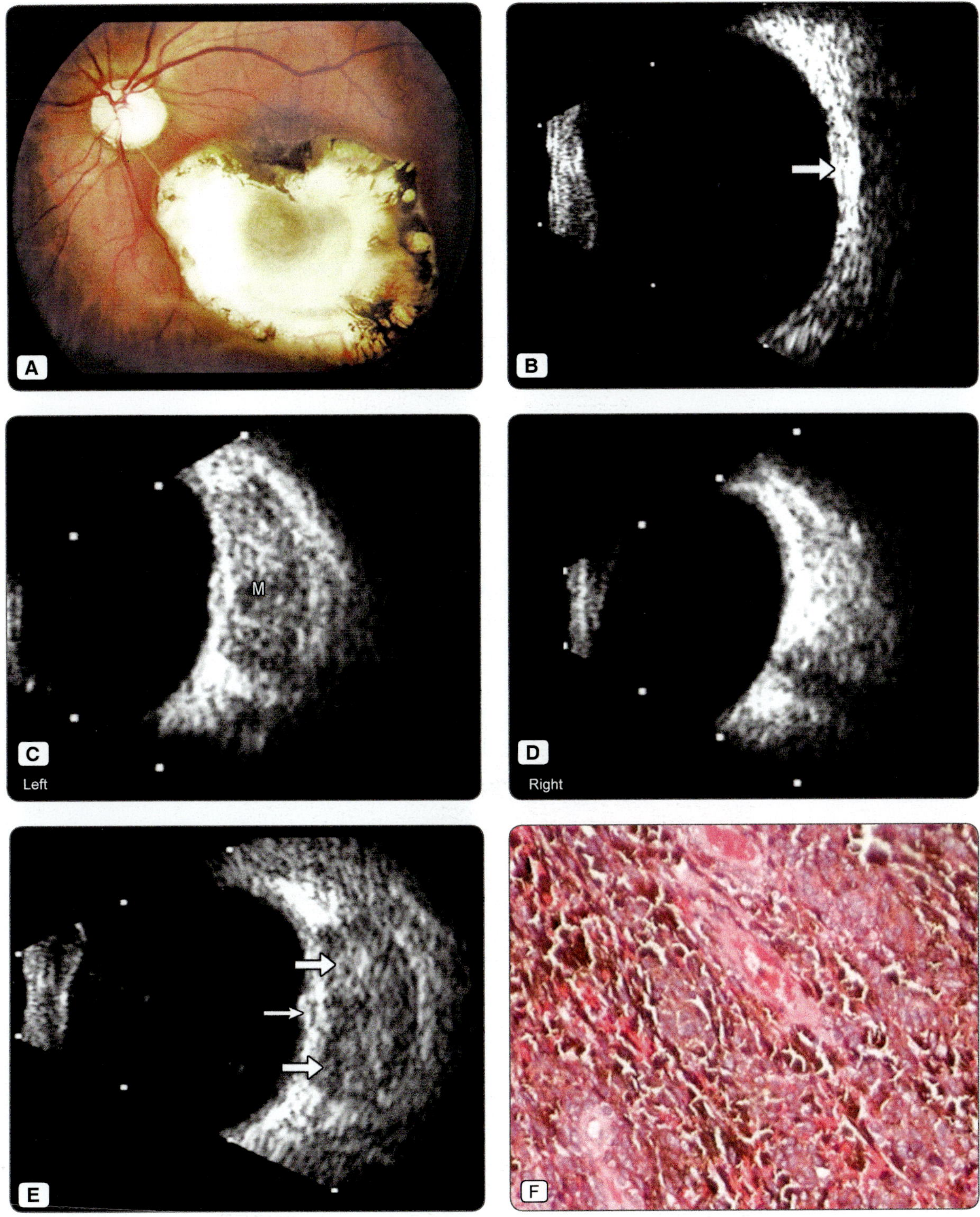

Figures 17.18A to F: Fundus photograph of a patient who had been on regular follow-up after transpupillary thermotherapy for choroidal melanoma. Note the atrophic scar at the site of the tumor previously (A). Ultrasound B scan shows an area of very high reflectivity at the site of the scar (arrow) (B). The dual mode shows the involved left orbit in comparison to the normal right orbit (M = mass). This was diagnosed to be orbital metastasis (C and D). By increasing the depth penetration in Figure (E), what initially appears to be shadowing behind the scar is actually a low reflective, well defined orbital mass molding to the globe wall (arrows). The patient underwent orbital exenteration and a heavily pigmented orbital mass was noted, which on HPE was found to contain melanoma cells (F).

18 Choroidal Hemangioma

CLINICAL FEATURES

- Can occur as a circumscribed tumor or a diffuse lesion. The latter is seen in patients with the Sturge-Weber syndrome
- The circumscribed variety presents as an orange-red subtly elevated lesion at the posterior pole. It can cause loss of vision due to subfoveal location or exudative retinal detachment involving the fovea. Visual loss can also be due to hyperopic amblyopia, or secondary glaucoma.
- Choroidal detachment can occur in the diffuse variety
- Secondary changes of the overlying retinal pigment epithelium (RPE) include fibrous or osseous metaplasia
- The diffuse variety presents as a deep red "tomato catsup" appearance of the posterior fundus. It can be associated with an ipsilateral nevus flammeus in the Sturge-Weber syndrome
- Treatment is indicated when secondary retinal detachment involves the fovea
- Ultrasonography is performed to confirm the diagnosis and monitor treatment response.

ULTRASONOGRAPHY

Circumscribed Hemangioma

- Dome shaped mass at the posterior pole
- Regular internal structure on B scan
- High internal reflectivity on A scan
- No demonstrable internal blood flow
- Secondary retinal detachment can be quite extensive and may even become total
- High reflective plaques on the surface may indicate fibrous or osseous metaplasia.

Diffuse Hemangioma

- Seen as a diffuse high reflective thickening of the posterior choroid that tapers off toward the equator. The elevation is usually less than that seen in a circumscribed lesion
- Occasionally, areas of dome shaped elevation may be seen within this diffuse area
- Secondary retinal detachment can occur
- Thickening of an adjacent extraocular muscle may be seen.

MIMICKING CONDITIONS

Circumscribed Hemangiomas

- High internal reflectivity of the choroid with secondary retinal detachment is seen in metastases, but the choroidal mass is usually lobular in configuration in the latter
- Highly reflective surface plaques are seen in disciform scars, but these usually have an irregular surface and reflectivity. They are also most commonly located at the macula
- Nodular scleritis can present as a dome-shaped high reflective choroidal mass, but it is associated with scleral edema and Tenon's widening.

Diffuse Hemangiomas

- Retinochoroidal thickening in nanophthalmos is more extensive and is associated with other features such as an increased lens-axial length ratio
- Diffuse thickening of the choroid can be present in a variety of other conditions. In inflammations, the reflectivity is usually low.

NUGGETS

It is good to compare with the other eye and look for the ipsilateral port-wine stain in an eye with unexplained unilateral choroidal thickening.

The presence of a dome shaped mass does not rule out a diffuse hemangioma.

Both the diffuse and circumscribed variety of hemangiomas can be bilateral.

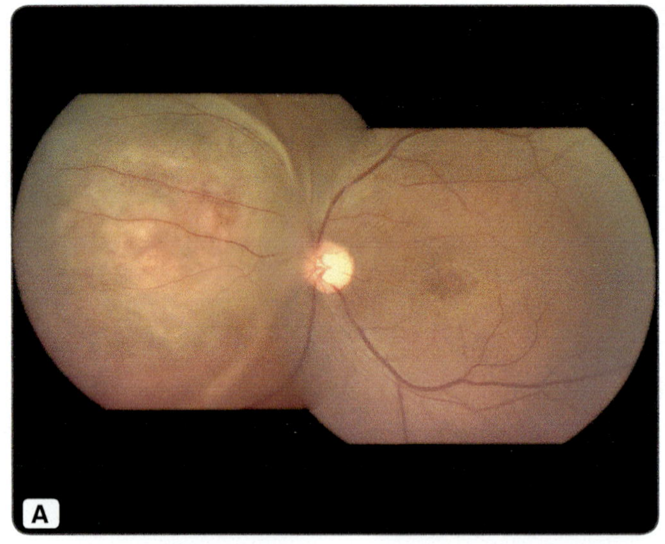

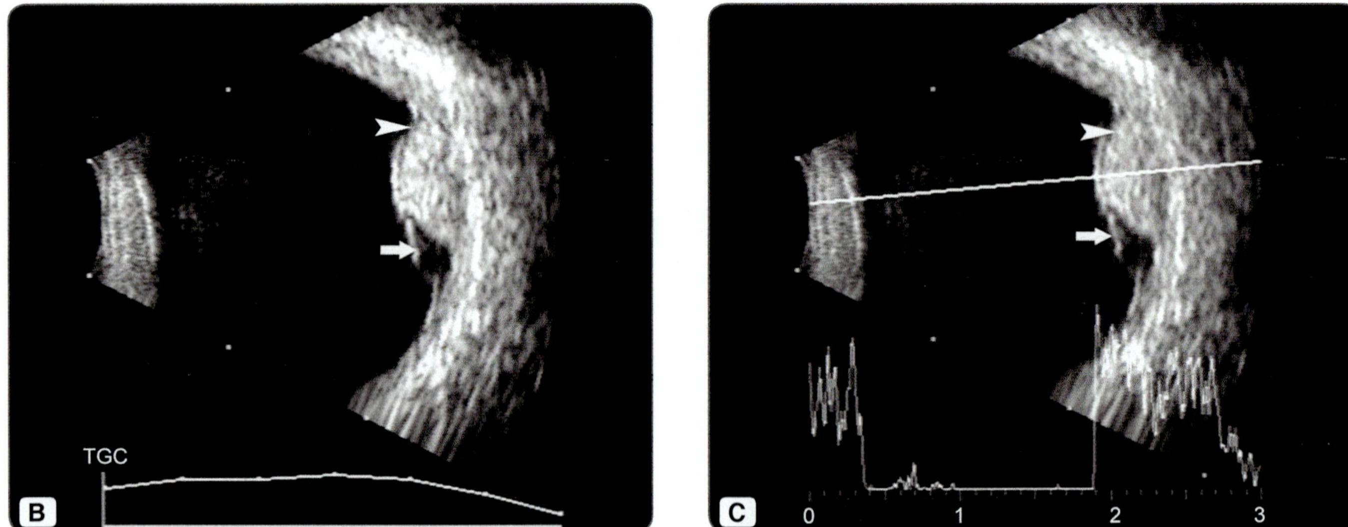

Figures 18.1A to C: Color photograph of a patient with a reddish orange mass nasal to the optic disc with a secondary retinal detachment. Ultrasound B scan with A vector showing a dome-shaped mass (arrowhead). The internal reflectivity is regular as seen on the B scan and of high reflectivity on the A scan. There is a secondary retinal detachment both over and adjacent to the tumor (arrow).

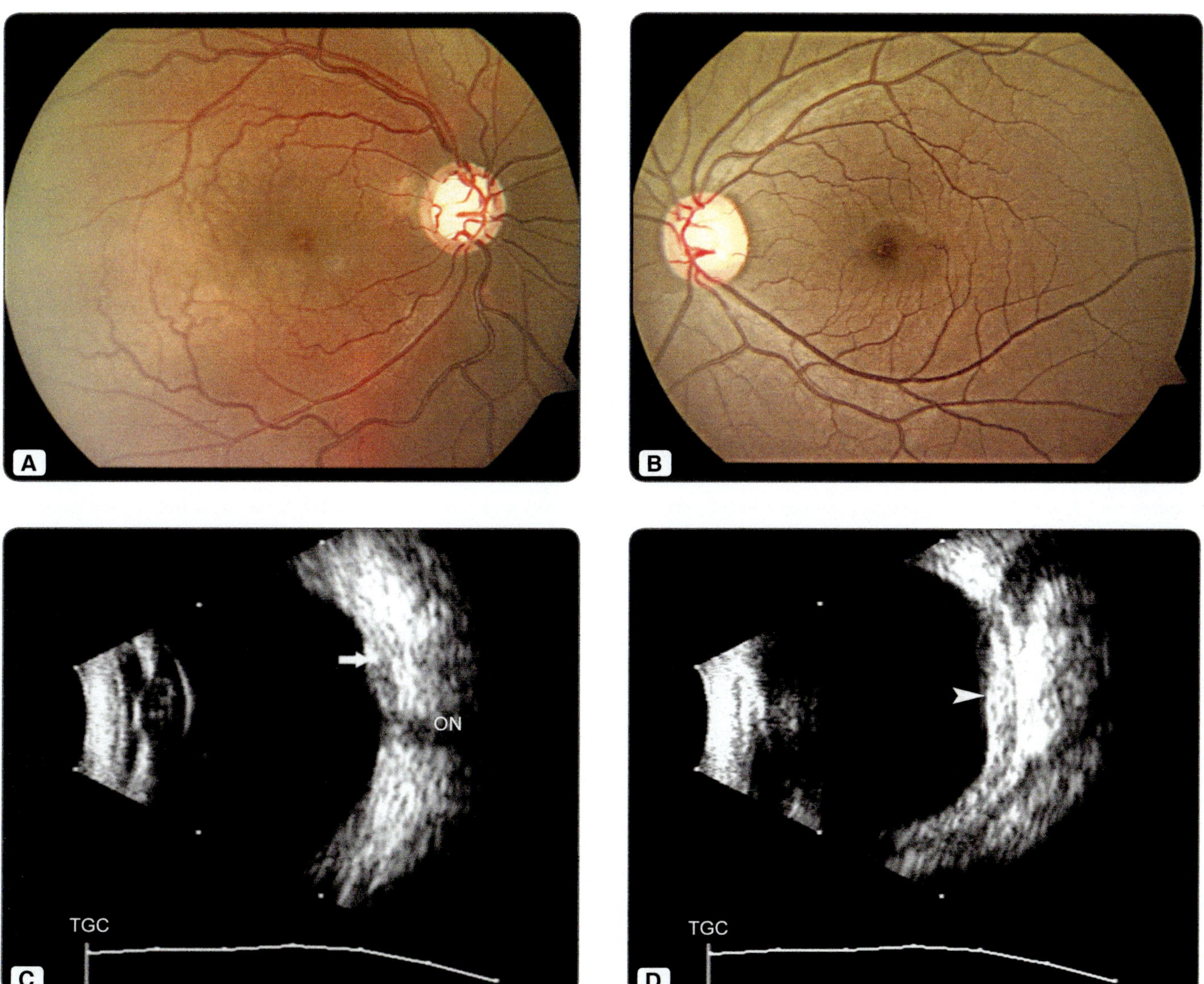

Figures 18.2A to D: Color photographs of a patient with Sturge-Weber syndrome and a diffuse choroidal hemangioma. The right optic disc is cupped and the fundus has a tomato catsup appearance, more evident when compared to the normal left fundus. The B scan shows a very subtle elevated lesion (arrow) just above the optic nerve (ON) in addition to a more uniform thickening of the choroid inferiorly (arrowhead, Fig. B). Such dome shaped elevations can occur within a diffuse hemangioma.

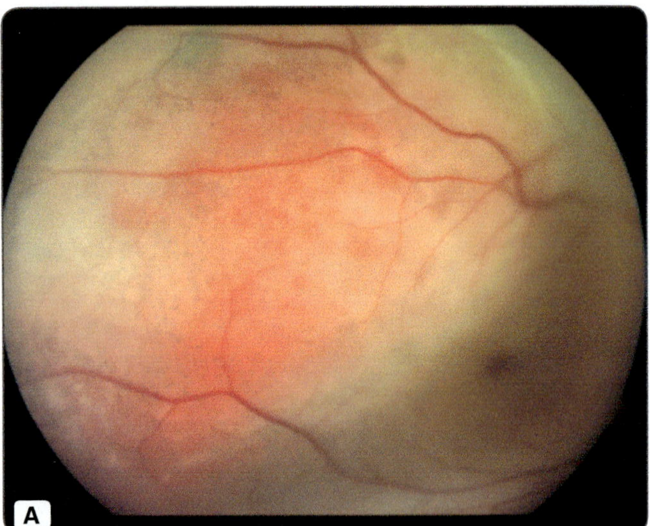

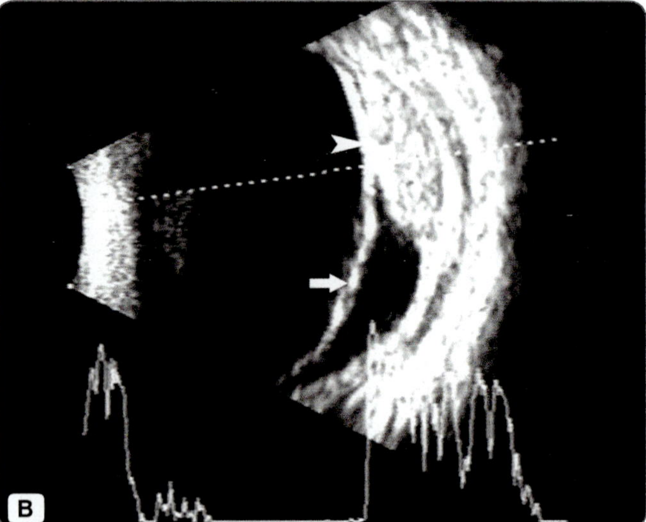

Figures 18.3A and B: Clinical photograph and B scan with vector A shows a circumscribed hemangioma (arrowhead) with extensive secondary retinal detachment (arrow). Note that the retina is detached even on the tumor surface.

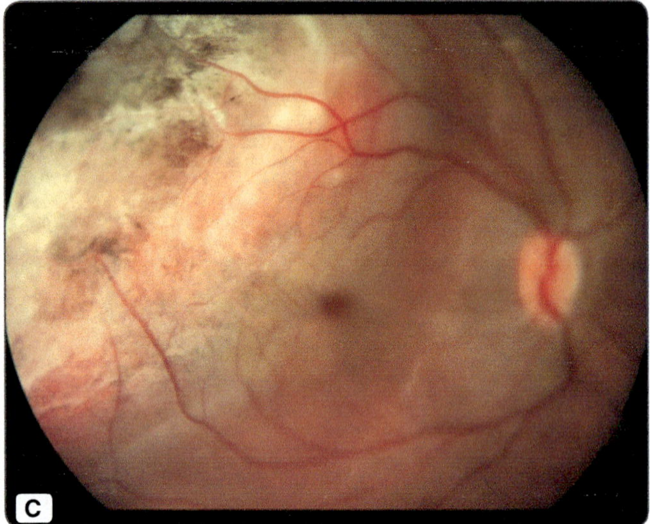

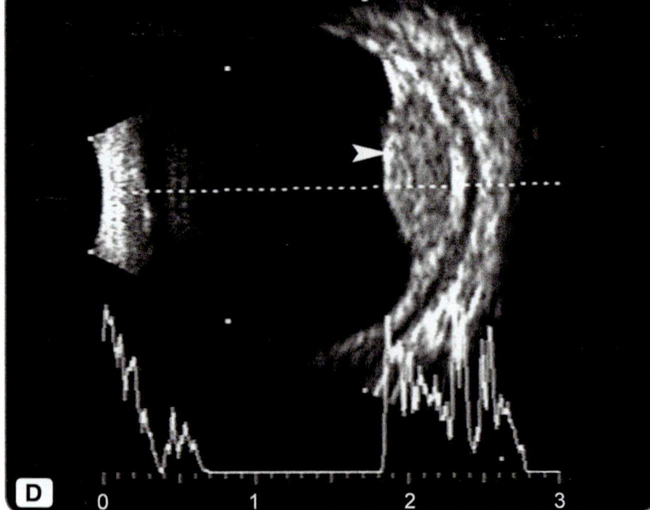

Figures 18.3C and D: The same patient following transpupillary thermotherapy—note the resolution of the retinal detachment. The size of the mass and its characteristics remain unchanged on ultrasound, but the clinical picture shows pigmentary changes as a result of treatment.

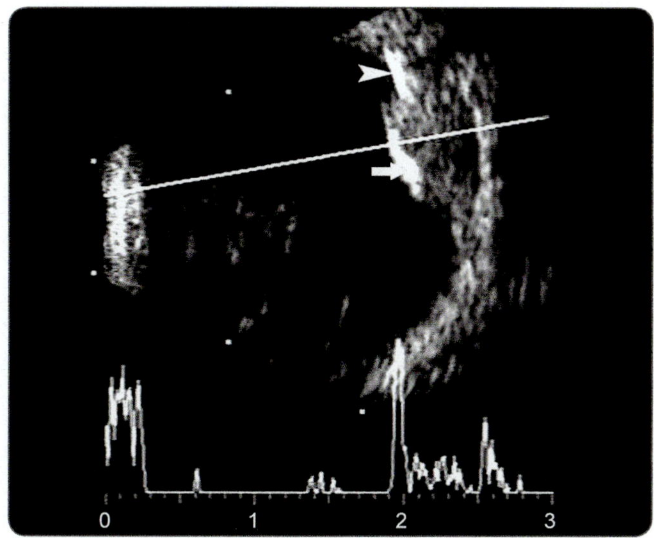

Figure 18.4A: A circumscribed choroidal hemangioma with secondary surface changes. Note the high reflective surface plaque (arrow), causing dampening of the intralesional echoes. A second plaque-like lesion at the upper margin (arrowhead) is seen to cause orbital shadowing behind it, suggesting the presence of calcification.

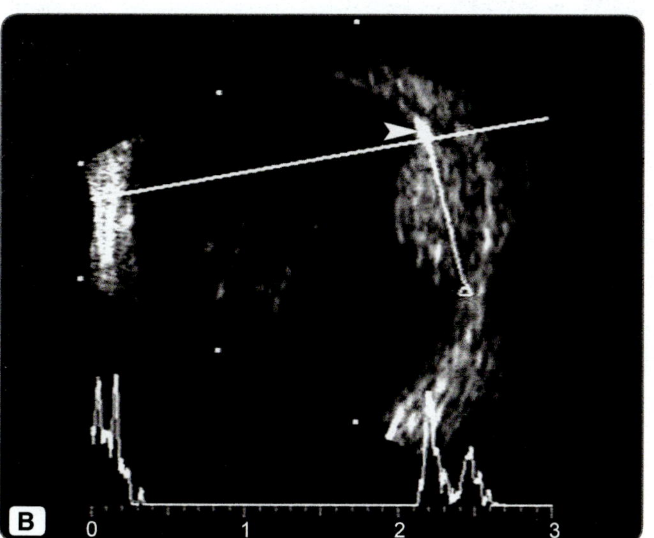

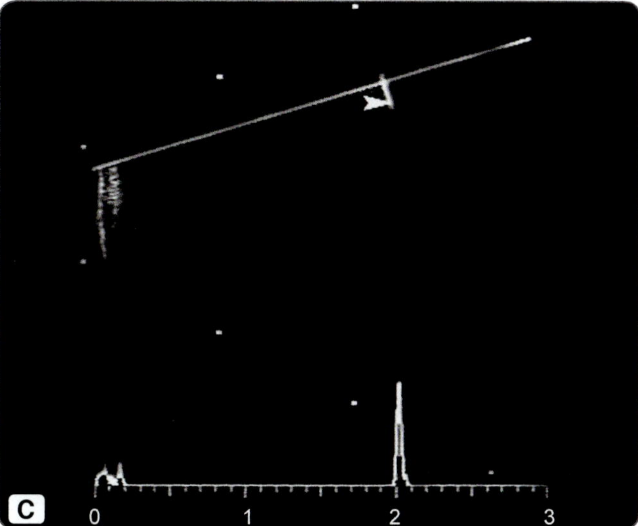

Figures 18.4B and C: The A vector is passed through the high reflective plaque at high and low gain, confirming the presence of calcification.

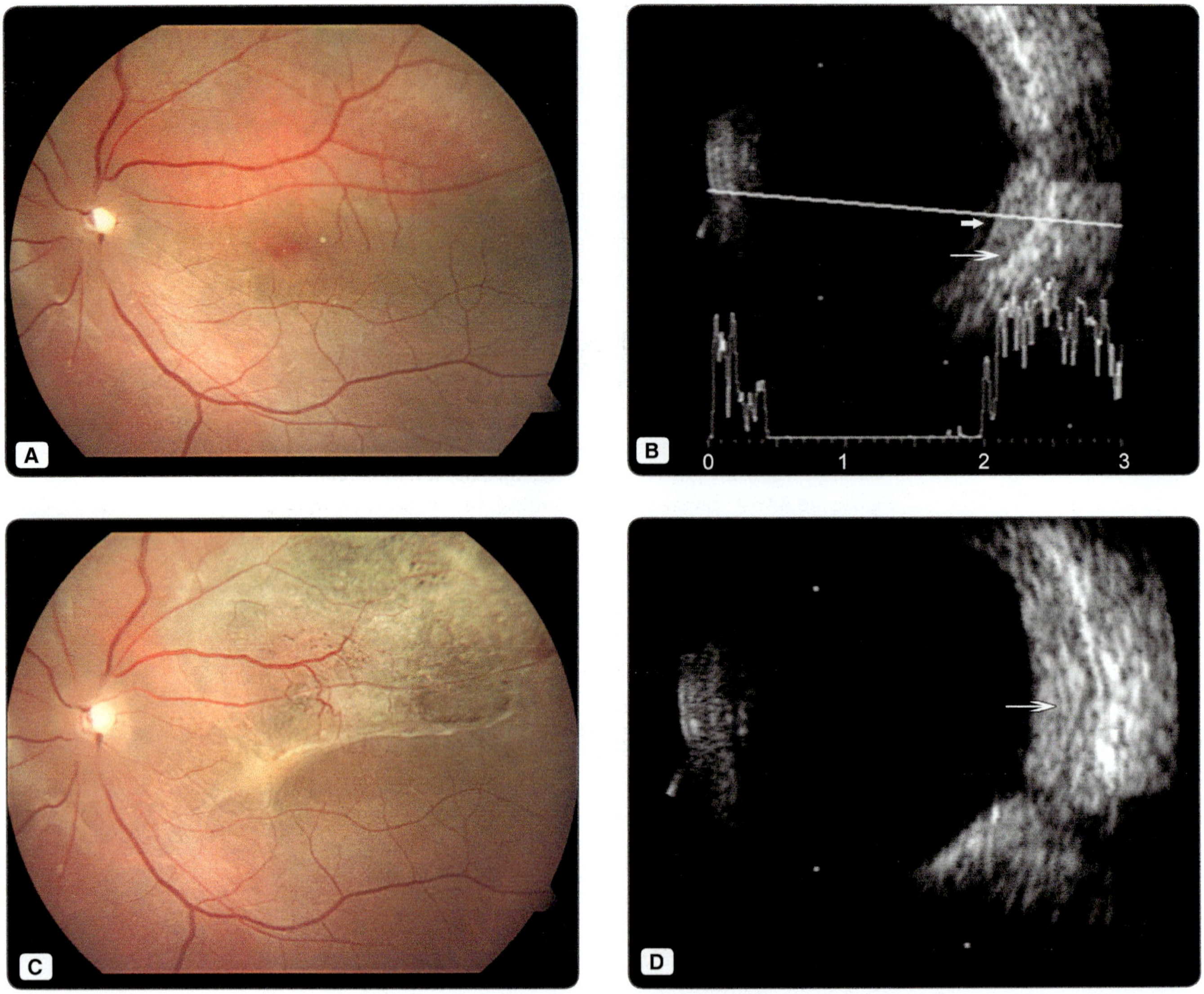

Figures 18.5A to D: An 18-year-old boy presented with decreased vision in left eye. He had a nevus flammeus and unilateral diffuse choroidal hemangioma with secondary RD. Ultrasound revealed a high reflective diffuse choroidal thickening and secondary RD (arrow). The patient underwent transpupillary thermotherapy to the lesion – fundus picture three months later shows the pigmentation that resulted. The ultrasound shows absence of retinal detachment. The choroidal thickening persists.

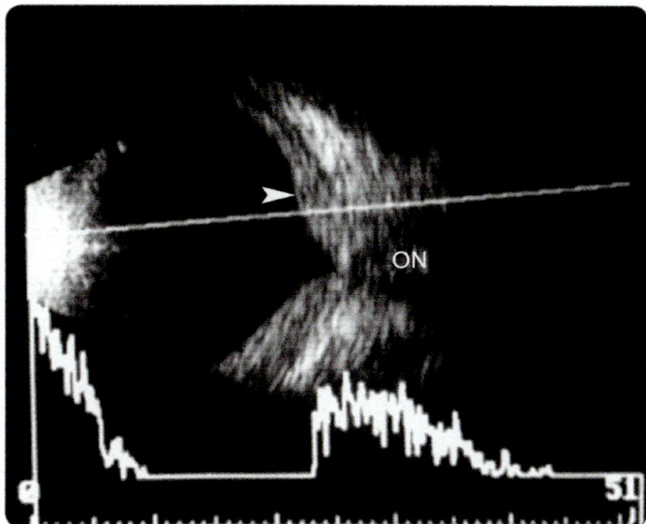

Figure 18.6: An axial B scan with A vector showing diffuse high reflective thickening of the choroid which is most marked posteriorly (arrowhead) and tapers off towards the periphery. This is typical of a diffuse choroidal hemangioma. Note the false appearance of optic disc cupping due to the increased choroidal thickness in the peripapillary region.

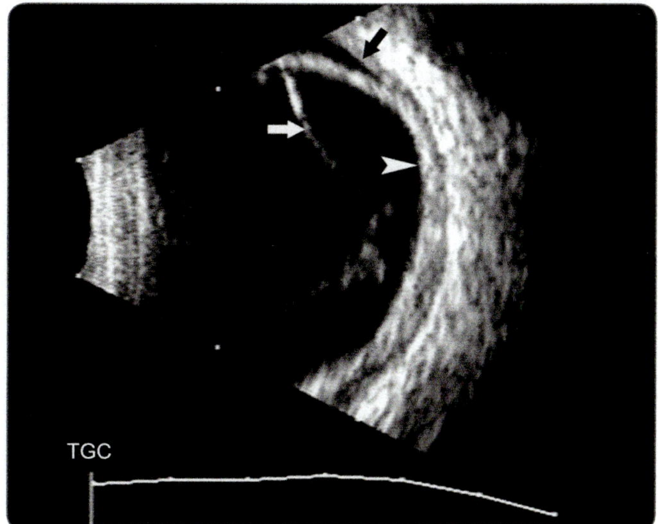

Figure 18.7: B scan image of a young boy with Sturge-Weber syndrome and diffuse hemangioma (arrowhead) who underwent filtering surgery for glaucoma. Postoperatively, the patient developed serous choroidal detachment (black arrow) and secondary retinal detachment due to hypotony. Note the high reflective membrane (arrow) suggestive of a retinal detachment. The serous choroidal detachment is seen in the upper part of the echogram.

19 Choroidal Metastases

CLINICAL FEATURES

- Metastases to the eye are most often due to hematogenous spread from carcinomas
- Commonest site of involvement is the choroid
- Twenty five percent of patients with ocular metastases have no known history of systemic malignancy and 10% eventually have no detectable primary tumor
- Choroidal metastases typically involve the posterior pole and are seen as creamy colored relatively flat lesions
- They may be single or multiple, unilateral or bilateral
- There is typically an associated exudative retinal detachment, which may be quite extensive.

ULTRASONOGRAPHY

Typical Features

- Solid mass at the posterior pole
- Irregular or bumpy contour
- Variable internal structure which can be regular, irregular or have a central excavation
- Moderate to high internal reflectivity on A scan
- No demonstrable internal blood flow
- Extensive exudative retinal detachment usually over the tumor surface as well.

Unusual Features

- Collar button shape has been described in metastatic adenocarcinoma from the lung
- Bullous choroidal detachments
- Low reflective internal echoes and presence of internal vascularity that may mimic a melanoma can be seen in metastatic 'oat cell carcinoma' of the lung

MIMICKING CONDITIONS

- Subretinal hemorrhage in AMD may present with similar features, however, the retinal detachment is usually not so extensive
- Subretinal abscess due to either fungal or tuberculous infection, may present with an irregular mass and extensive retinal detachment. However, these cases also show some degree of scleral edema and Tenon's widening. Occasionally, one may see a fluid level or cystic area in an abscess
- Ocular lymphoma or reticulum cell carcinoma may present as a more diffuse bumpy elevation of the choroid, which has an irregular internal structure. However, these cases may not show extensive retinal detachments. There is also some associated vitreous reaction, which can be seen as low reflective intragel echoes
- A diffuse amelanotic melanoma can present similarly; however, it is usually located more anteriorly and the reflectivity is low.

NUGGETS

A careful ultrasound, sometimes requiring standoff, is necessary in patients with retinal detachments and no visible retinal break. The metastatic lesion may be only minimally elevated and missed on cursory evaluation.

A choroidal metastasis due to a primary melanoma elsewhere can have all the clinical and ultrasound features of a primary choroidal melanoma.

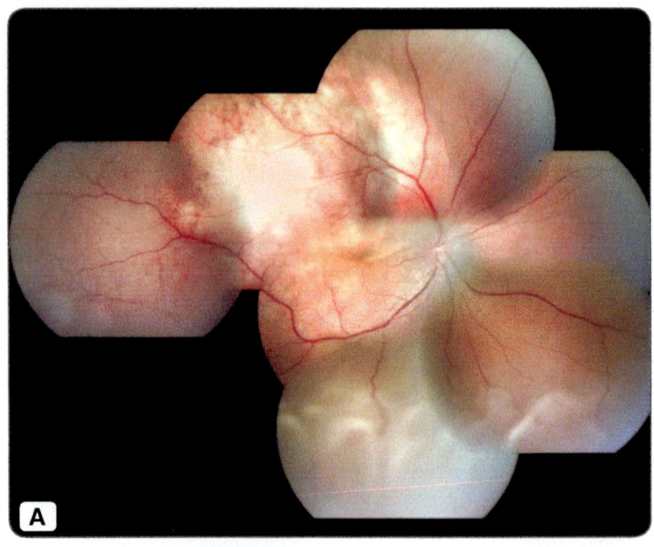

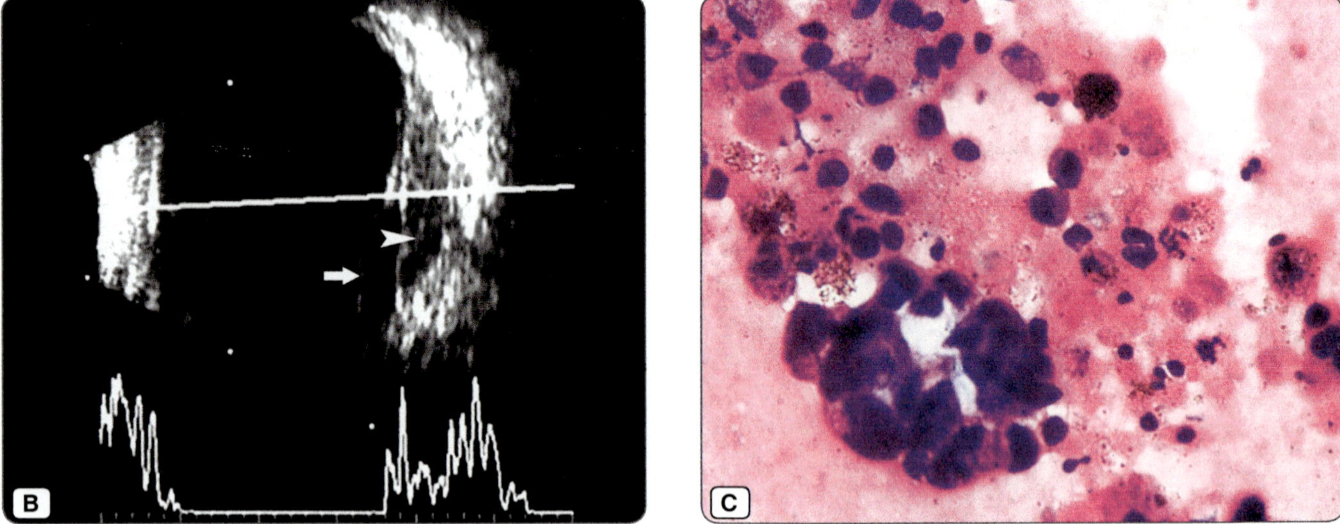

Figures 19.1A to C: Color photograph and ultrasound images of a 30-year-old male with a large choroidal mass and secondary retinal detachment. The B scan with vector A shows a lobulated well-defined mass (arrowhead) with homogenous low to medium internal echoes. There is also a secondary retinal detachment (arrow). Fine needle aspiration cytology showed large cells with hyperchromatic nuclei suggestive of adenocarcinoma. The diagnosis was metastatic adenocarcinoma from an undetected primary tumor.

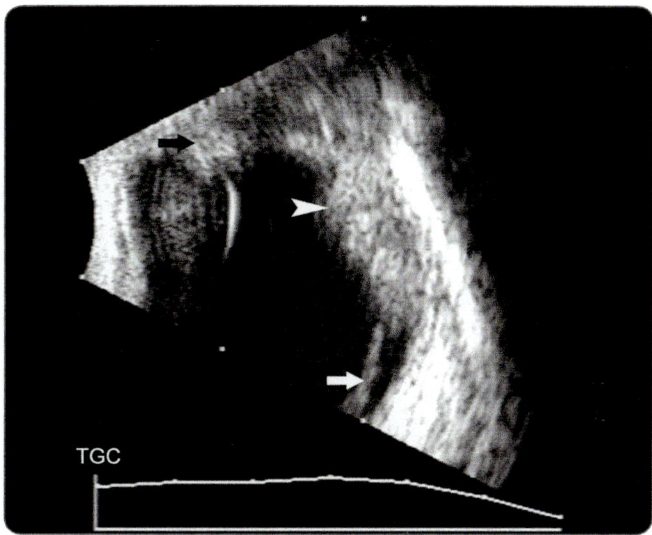

Figure 19.2: B scan image of an anteriorly located choroidal mass (arrowhead). The surface is lobulated and internal echoes are uniform and moderately reflective. There is suspected involvement of the ciliary body as well (black arrow). A secondary retinal detachment (arrow) is seen inferior to the mass.

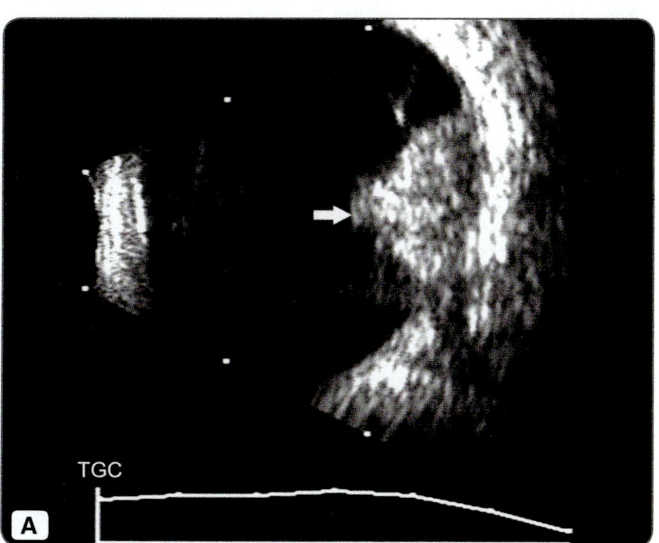

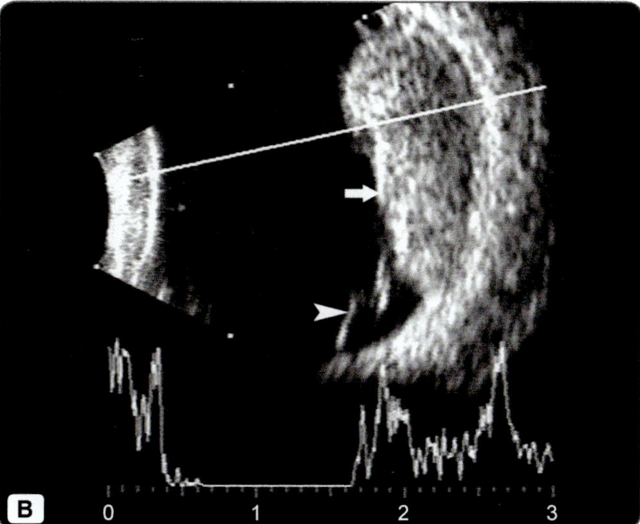

Figures 19.3A and B: Metastatic tumors can sometimes have a collar button appearance (arrow) as seen in this metastatic melanoma. However, the long axis of the mass in Figure B (arrow) shows that the basal diameter is much greater than the height indicating that it is likely to be a metastasis. A secondary retinal detachment is also seen (arrowhead).

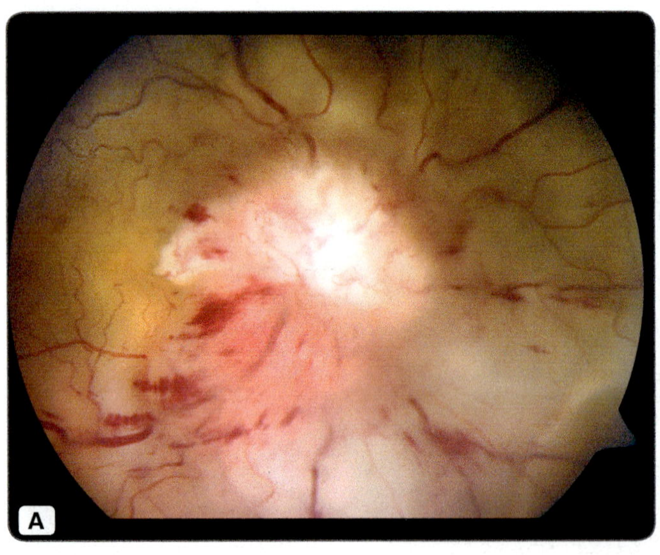

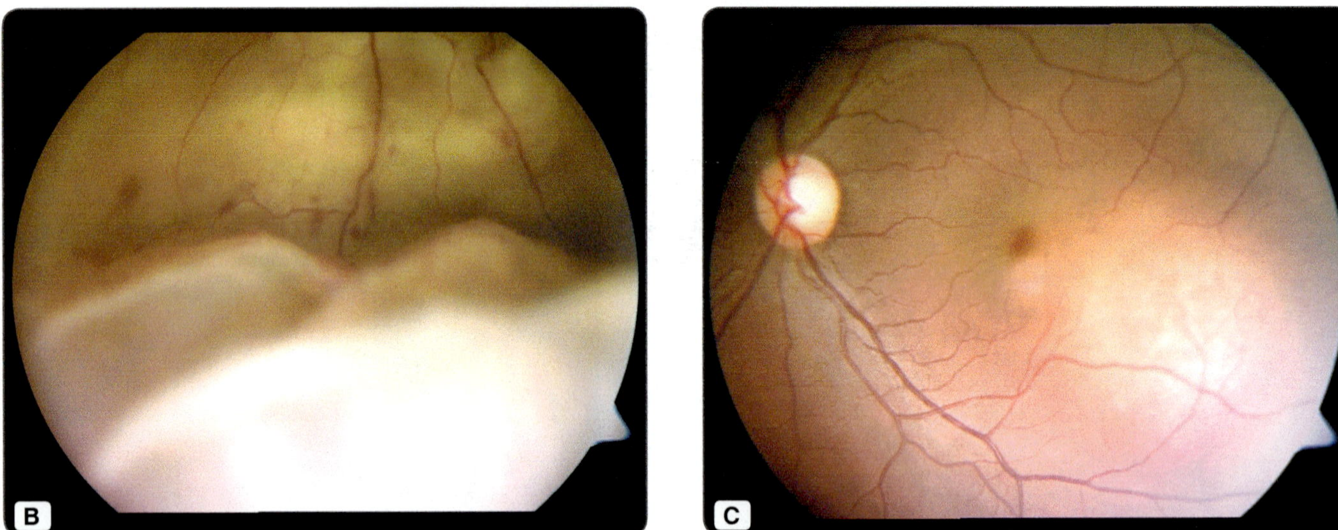

Figures 19.4A to C: Color fundus photographs of the right (Figs A and B) and left (Fig. C) eyes of a patient with multiple systemic metastases from breast carcinoma. The right eye shows a mass infiltrating the optic nerve (Fig. A) and a bullous retinal detachment (Fig. B). The left eye shows a posterior pole choroidal mass (Fig. C) just abutting the fovea.

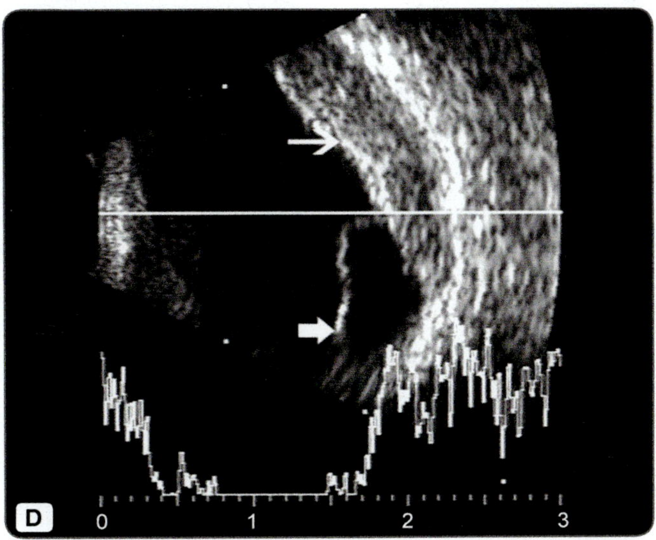

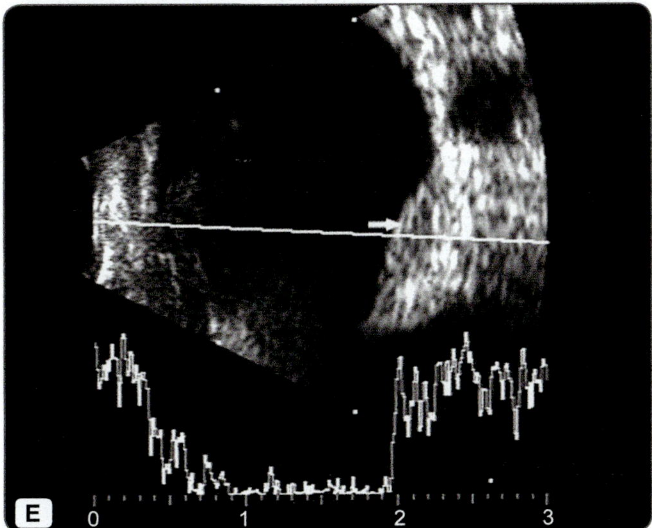

Figures 19.4D and E: Ultrasound B scan with vector A images (Figs D and E) show a choroidal mass with lobulated surface and uniform moderate internal reflectivity. There is a secondary retinal detachment noted in Figure D.

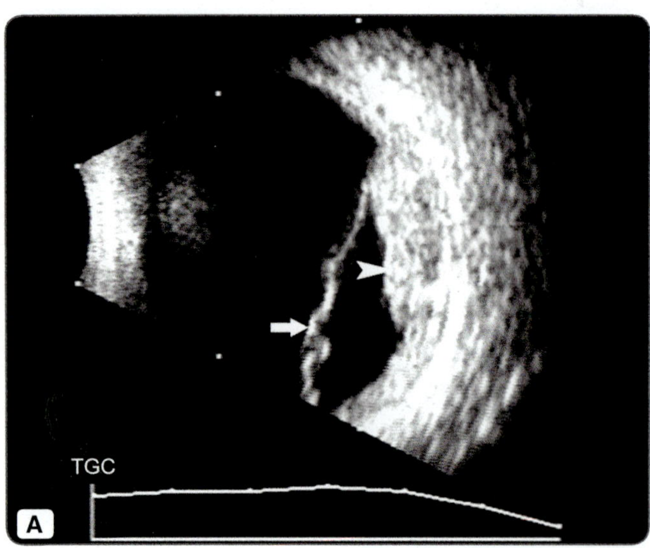

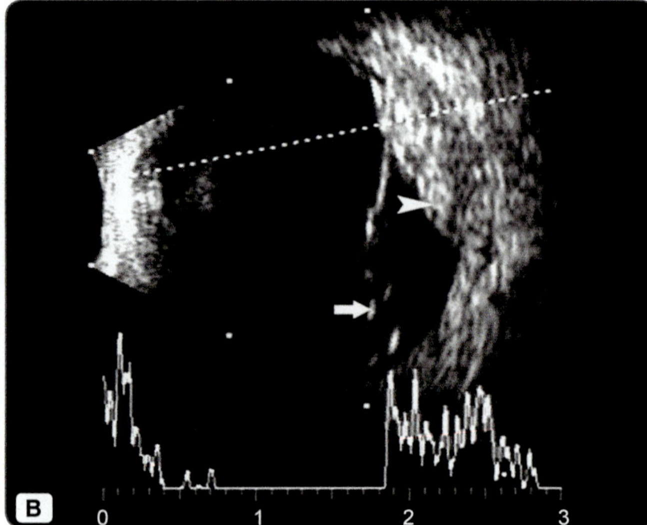

Figures 19.5A and B: B scan images of a patient with choroidal metastases from bronchogenic carcinoma. The mass is lobulated (arrowhead), with moderate internal reflectivity. A secondary retinal detachment (arrow) is seen over the tumor surface.

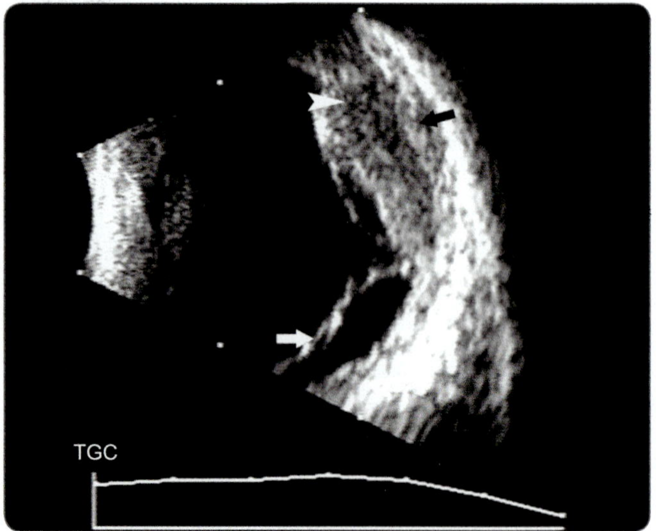

Figures 19.6: Choroidal granuloma. B scan image of a lobulated anterior choroidal mass (arrowhead). The mass has moderate internal reflectivity and a secondary retinal detachment (arrow). What serves to distinguish it from a metastasis is the presence of low reflective scleral edema (black arrow) that confirms the diagnosis of an inflammatory or infective lesion.

20 Retinoblastoma

CLINICAL FEATURES

- Most common malignant childhood tumor occurring 1 in 15–23,000 live births
- Presenting feature is leukocoria in two-thirds of cases
- The tumor could be either endophytic (growing towards the vitreous cavity) or exophytic (growing within the subretinal space). The pattern of tumor growth (endophytic or exophytic) has no significant influence on the prognosis
- The presence of calcium is an important feature, signifying rapid growth
- Extraocular spread of retinoblastoma into the orbit is a poor prognostic factor. Intraocular surgical procedures such as pars plana vitrectomy, inadvertently performed on patients with retinoblastoma, predisposes to orbital extension or metastasis of retinoblastoma. In addition, other factors which indicate a poor prognosis are choroidal invasion, anterior chamber seeding, as well as optic nerve invasion, particularly involvement along the line of optic nerve transection
- Ultrasound is an important diagnostic tool. It also helps to assess treatment response. In addition, one may also need to perform CT and MRI studies to facilitate the diagnosis. UBM helps in evaluation of the anterior extent of the tumor, important in prognosis.

ULTRASONOGRAPHY

- Single or multiple mass lesions in the vitreous cavity arising from the retina
- Irregular high internal reflectivity
- Presence of calcium, seen as high reflective specks or clumps within the lesion, causing orbital shadowing. Ninety percent of retinoblastoma cases show the presence of calcium. The echographic findings depend primarily on the degree of calcification within the tumor and not on any other histological features
- The vitreous cavity can show echoes due to vitreous seeds in an endophytic lesion
- In an exophytic lesion, an exudative retinal detachment may be seen overlying the mass, with subretinal echoes, suggestive of subretinal seeds
- A funnel-shaped total retinal detachment with a thick solid mass with similar shape just behind it may be seen. This can have an irregular internal echo pattern, medium high internal reflectivity, no sign of vascularity and no after-movements. Calcification may be absent. This echographic pattern suggests the diffuse infiltrating variety of retinoblastoma. It is seen in relatively older children and has a poor prognosis

- Very large tumors may show a significant amount of orbital inflammation with all ultrasound features of orbital cellulitis
- The presence of cystic changes in tumors have been described. This can be due to tumor necrosis.

COMMON MIMICKING CONDITIONS

- Coats' disease
- Persistent fetal vasculature
- Toxocara endophthalmitis
- Advanced retinopathy of prematurity (ROP)
- Astrocytoma
- Medulloepithelioma
- Retinal dysplasia.

NUGGETS

The diagnosis of retinoblastoma is highly likely if calcification is seen before the child is 3 years of age. Beyond this, though retinoblastoma would still be the first differential diagnosis, other simulating conditions would need to be considered.

Optic nerve invasion as well as extraocular extension may be missed on ultrasound if there is a large tumor with extensive calcification leading to significant orbital shadowing.

Retinal astrocytoma can show progressive enlargement, retinal detachment, varying degrees of calcification and vitreous seeding, findings that can mislead the clinician toward the diagnosis of retinoblastoma especially in an older patient.

Coats' disease may mimic exophytic retinoblastoma, and here the absence of a mass lesion on ultrasound may help to differentiate between the two. The retina in retinoblastoma appears thicker and is more immobile than in Coats' disease. Calcification though rarely seen in Coats, is a typical feature of retinoblastoma.

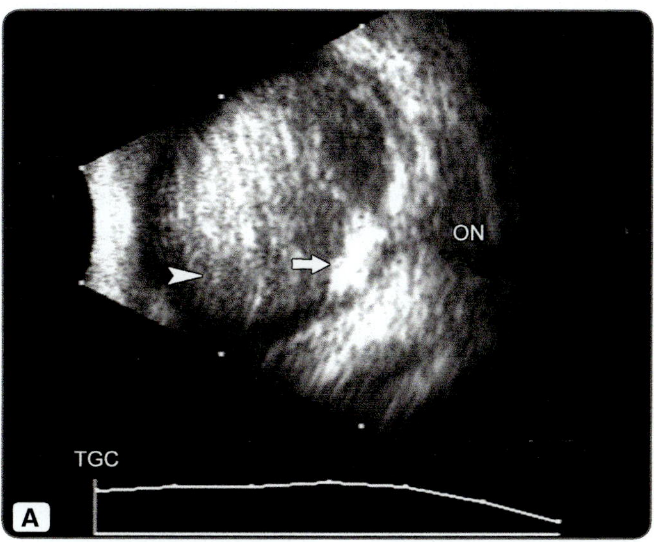

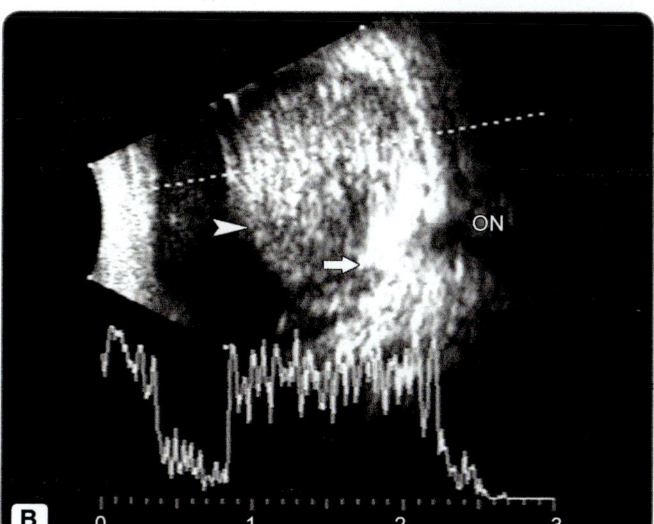

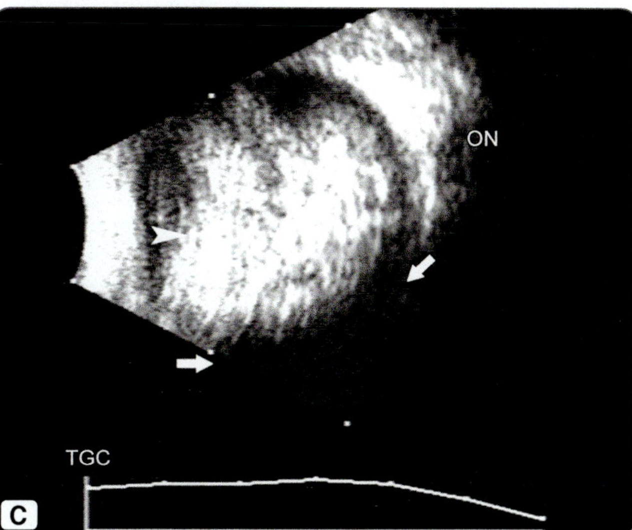

Figures 20.1A to C: B scan with vector A images of a large mass lesion (arrowhead) in the vitreous cavity. This is suggestive of an endophytic mass. The internal reflectivity is irregular and shows areas of calcification (arrow). The calcification exactly overlaps the optic nerve shadow (ON). Figure C shows a mass (arrowhead) with extremely dense calcification with strong orbital shadowing (arrows).

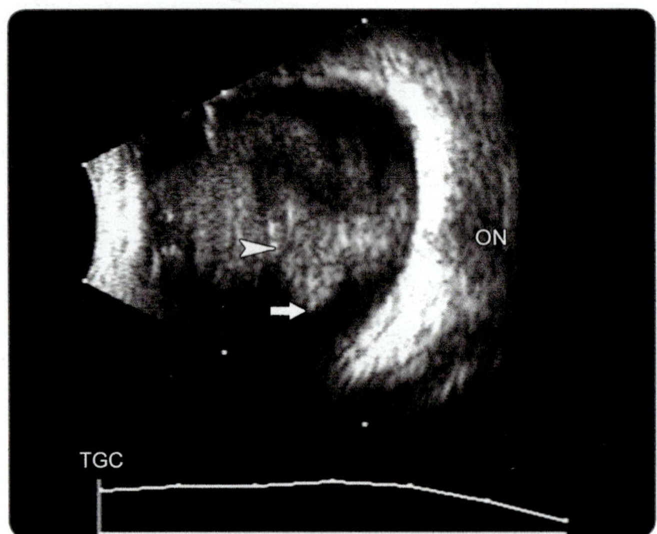

Figure 20.2: B scan of an exophytic retinoblastoma showing a grossly thickened and detached retina (arrow). Few specks of calcification (arrowhead) are seen within this.

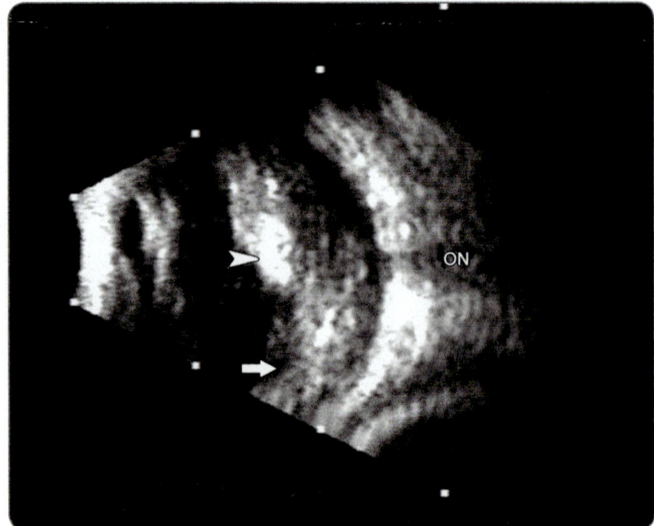

Figure 20.3: B scan image of a diffuse retinoblastoma (arrow) along the posterior globe wall. An area of calcification is seen within the mass (arrow head).

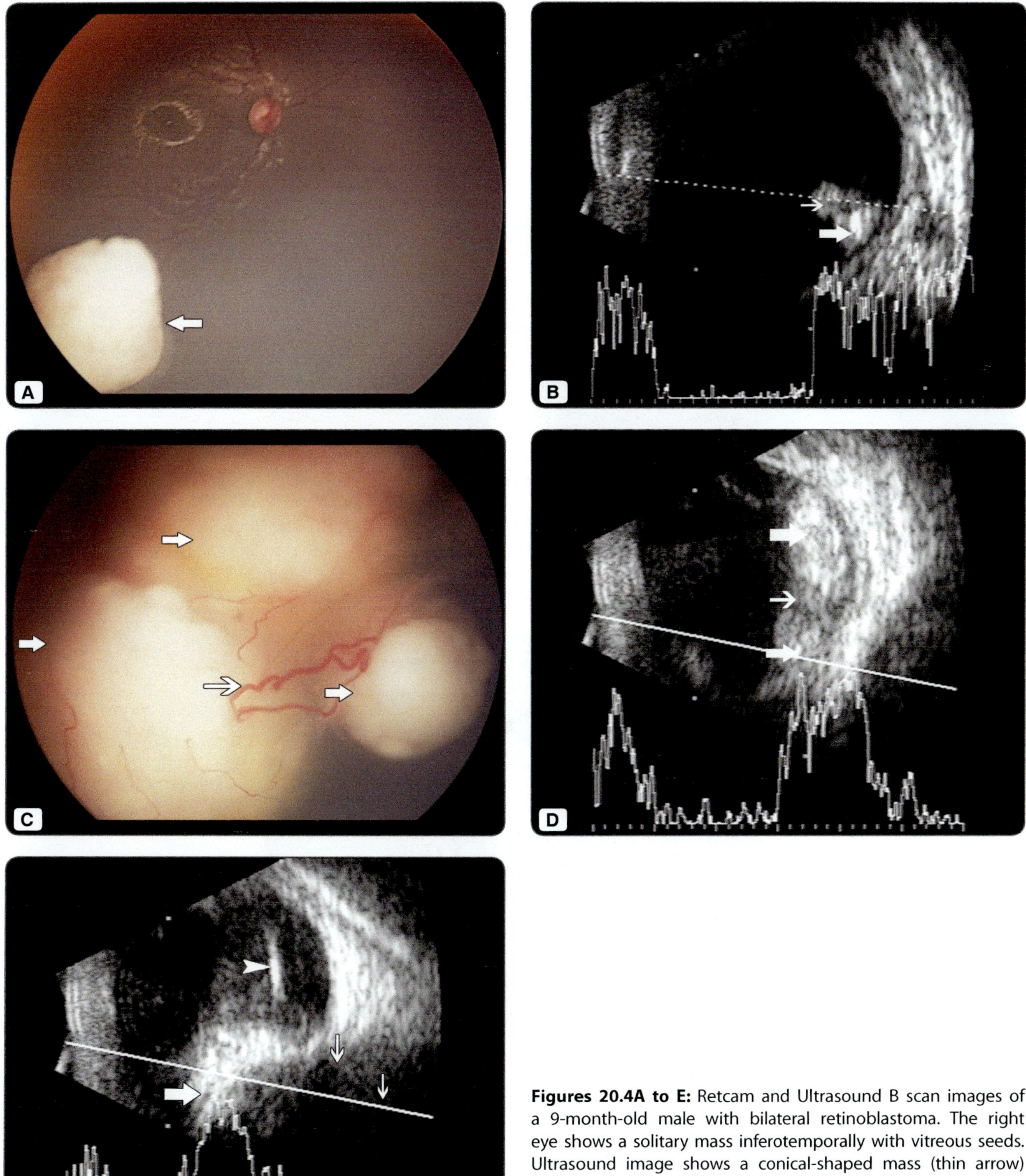

Figures 20.4A to E: Retcam and Ultrasound B scan images of a 9-month-old male with bilateral retinoblastoma. The right eye shows a solitary mass inferotemporally with vitreous seeds. Ultrasound image shows a conical-shaped mass (thin arrow) with a clump of calcification (arrow). The left eye shows a large lobulated tumor (arrows) with a feeder (thin arrow). Ultrasound shows the tumor mass (thin arrow) to be high reflective with areas of calcification (broad arrow). Secondary RD is seen (arrow head).

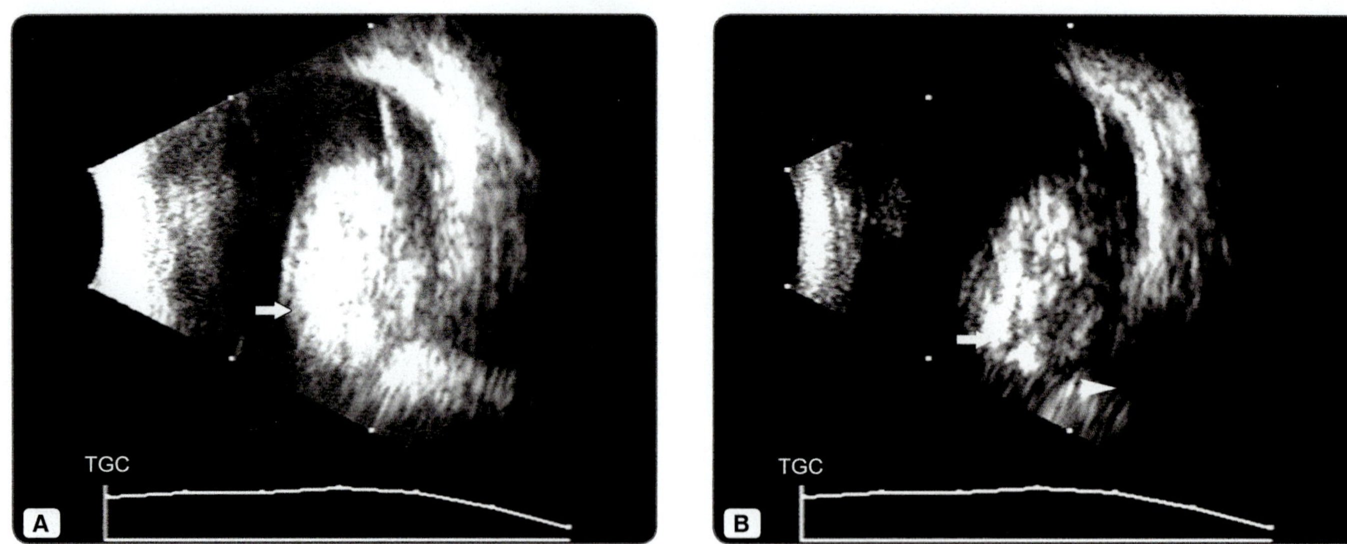

Figures 20.5A and B: B scan images of an endophytic tumor (arrow) with high reflectivity and large amounts of calcification. The calcification and shadowing (arrowhead) are better made out in the second image taken at reduced gain.

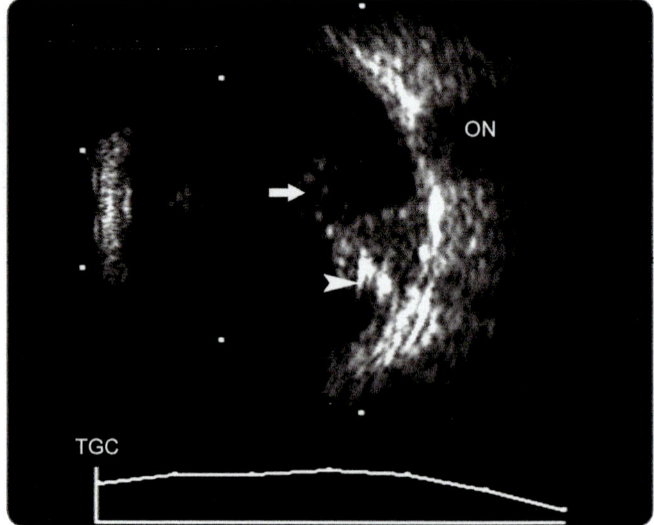

Figure 20.6: B scan image of a small posterior pole retinoblastoma showing tumor calcification (arrowhead). Overlying the mass there are dot-like echoes in the vitreous, which are due to vitreous seeds (arrow).

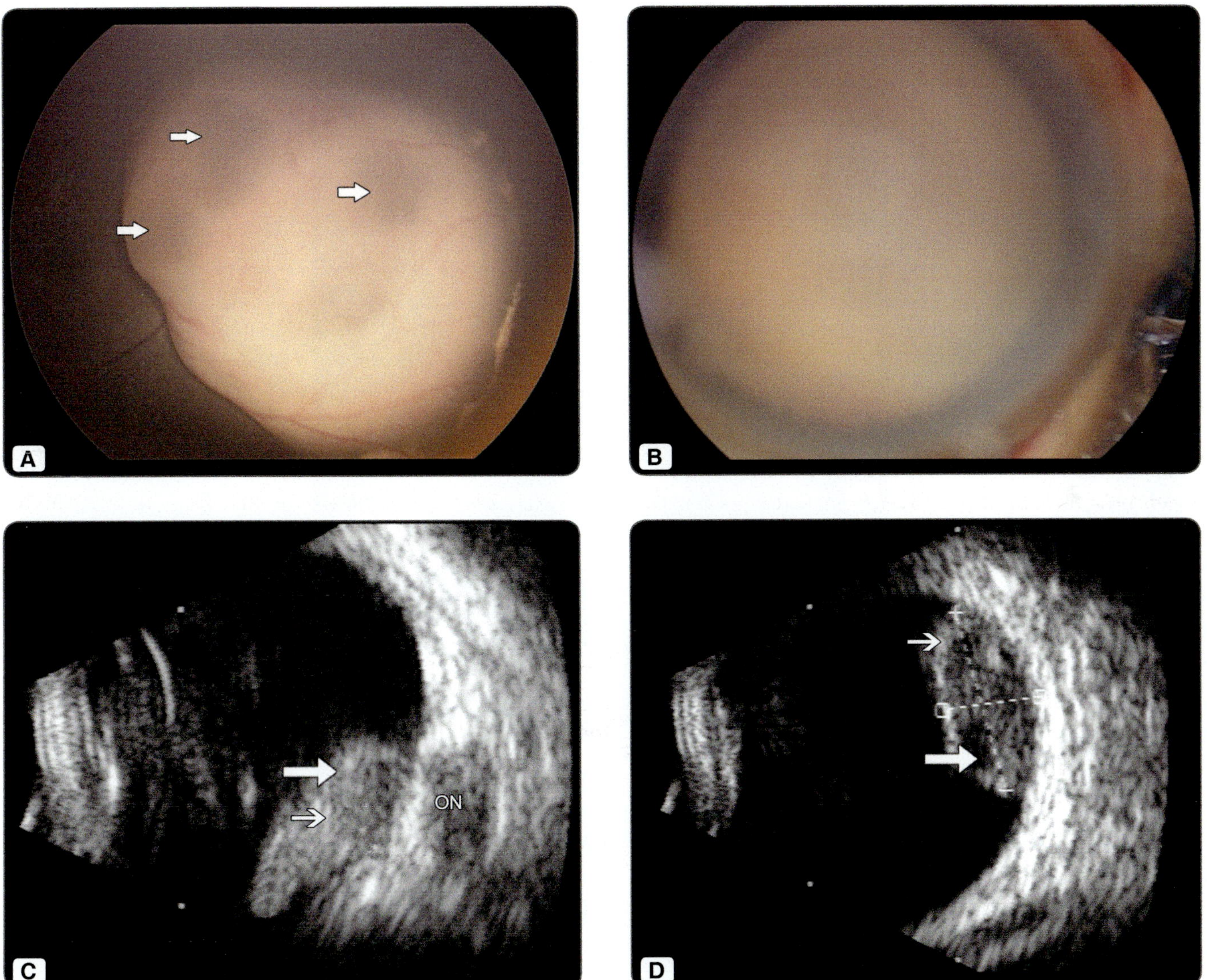

Figures 20.7A to D: Retcam (both eyes) and ultrasound images of the right eye of a 2-year-old child with bilateral retinoblastoma. The left eye shows a large tumor filling the entire vitreous cavity. The right eye shows a large tumor overlying the disc and extending nasally. The dark areas within the mass (arrows) correspond to cysts within the mass. Ultrasound B scan images (Figs C and D) of the right eye shows a well-defined mass lesion with cystic spaces (arrow) as well as specks of calcification (thin arrow). The optic nerve shadow looks enlarged. Cystic changes are known to occur in retinoblastoma.

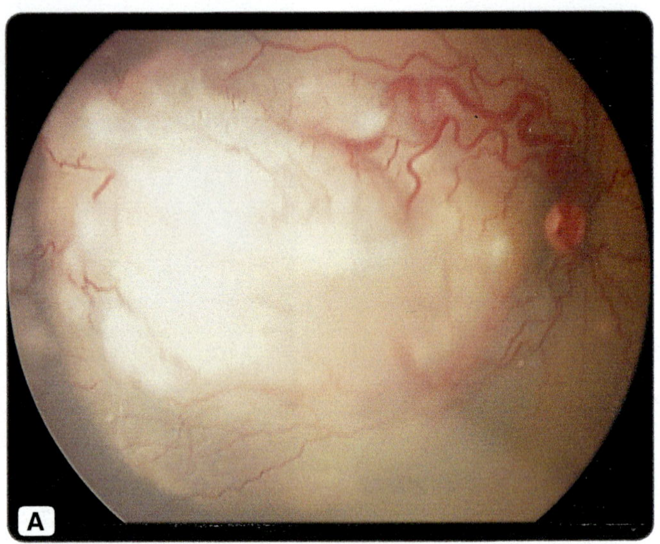

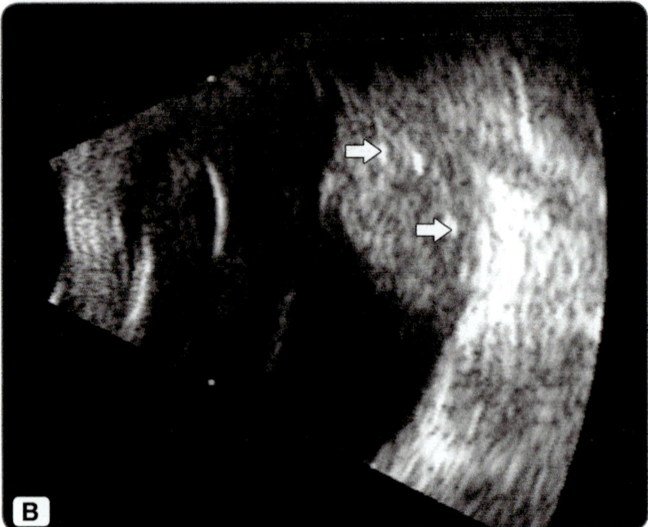

Figures 20.8A and B: Fundus of the right eye of a female child showing exudative RD with a large subretinal tumor and dilated vessels. Ultrasound showed a large mass with specks of calcification (arrows).

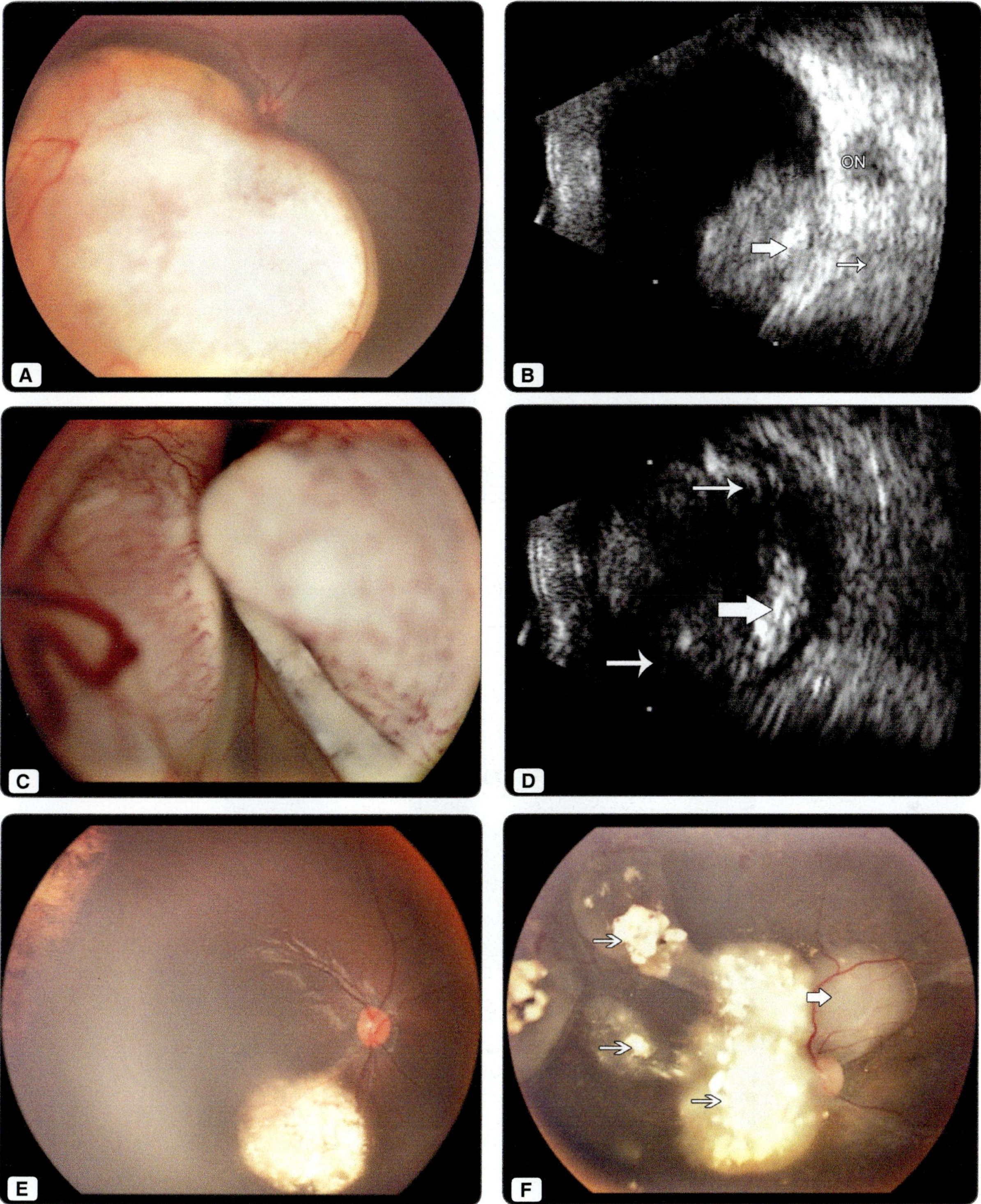

Figures 20.9A to F: Fundus photographs and ultrasound B scan of the right eye of a child with retinoblastoma. Note the large endophytic mass extending below and temporal to the disc. The ultrasound image shows a high reflective mass with calcification (arrow) causing shadowing (thin arrow). Fundus pictures of the left eye of the same patient showing a very extensive subretinal tumor with secondary RD. The ultrasound image shows a thickened detached retina (arrow) with areas of plaque-like calcification (broad arrow). Note that the shadowing obscures the optic nerve view. Figures E and F depict the eye after chemotherapy showing calcific regression with a cottage cheese appearance. The picture of the left eye after chemotherapy showing both cottage cheese (thin arrow) and fish flesh (thick arrow) appearance.

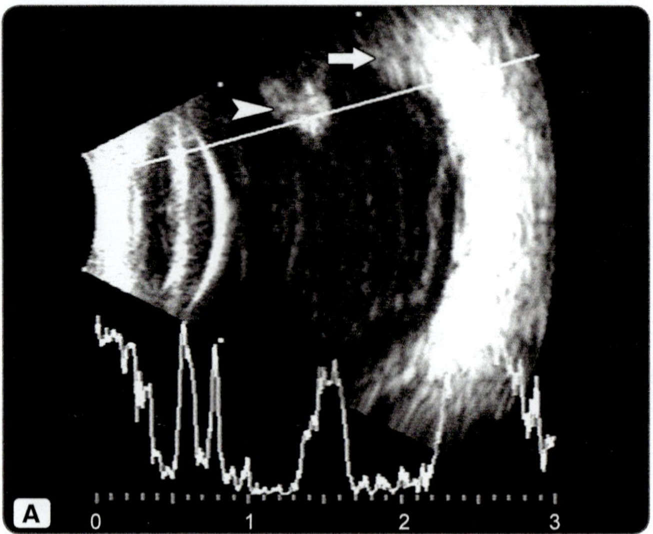

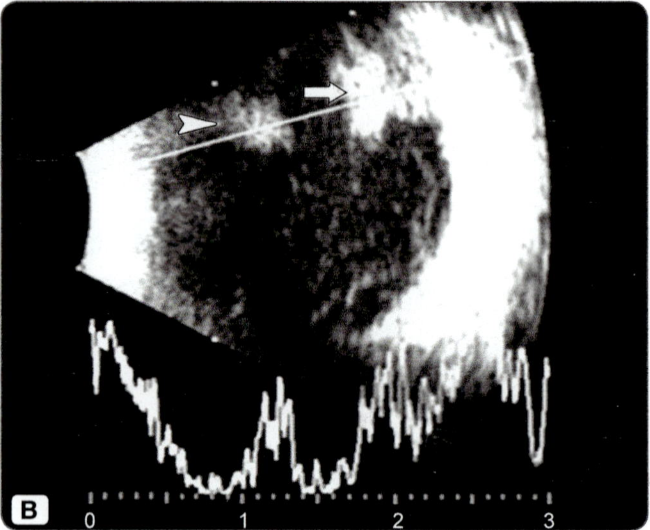

Figures 20.10A and B: B scan with vector A of a patient operated upon for suspected endogenous endophthalmitis. The vitreous shows numerous dot-like low reflective echoes. A prominent rim of uncut gel is seen (arrowhead), behind which is seen a high reflective mass lesion (arrow). A shallow membrane attached to the optic disc is seen, suggestive of a retinal detachment. Figure B shows the mass lesion characteristics better. The dots represented vitreous seeds from a retinoblastoma.

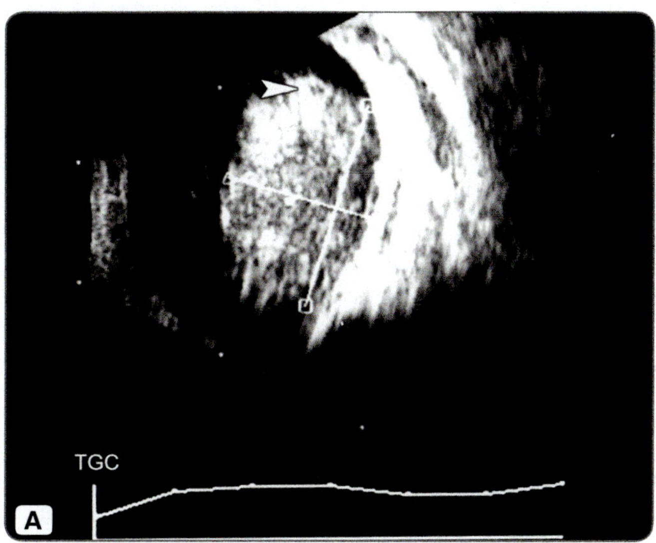

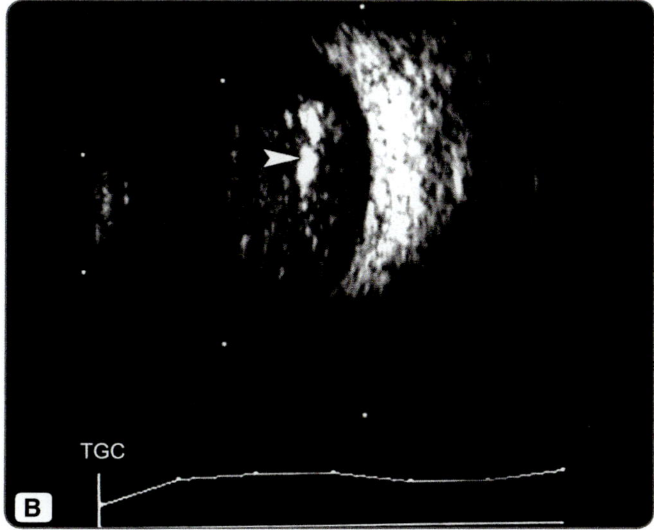

Figures 20.11A and B: B scan images of a 5-month-old child with leukokoria. There is a high reflective mass in the vitreous, which shows clumps of calcium (arrowhead) at reduced gain. The features were suggestive of retinoblastoma, however, the enucleated specimen showed histopathologic features of retinal astrocytoma.

21 Choroidal Osteoma

CLINICAL FEATURES

- Benign tumor of the choroid that is composed of mature bone
- Seen in healthy young females in the second or third decade
- Unilateral in 75–80% of cases
- The patient may be asymptomatic or have varying degrees of visual impairment
- Yellow orange placoid lesion, typically juxtapapillary
- Associated choroidal neovascularization or subretinal fluid may be present.

ULTRASONOGRAPHY

- Useful diagnostic tool
- Very high reflective plaque-like lesion with orbital shadowing.
- "Pseudo-optic nerve" or "double optic nerve" appearance may be seen if the lesion is away from the optic disc.

MIMICKING CONDITIONS

- Ocular coat calcification in phthisical eyes. The eye is usually shrunken and distorted.
- Sclerochoroidal calcification. The high reflective lesions are smaller in size, bilateral and multifocal. Other features of hypercalcemia may be present.
- Calcific changes in a macular scar or secondary calcification in tumors, most commonly retinoblastoma. Here, the lesion may be more elevated and show other features typical of the tumor.

NUGGETS

Look for the linear nevus sebaceous syndrome in a patient with features of a choroidal osteoma.

Calcification occurs on the surface of the tumor in cases of osseous metaplasia in melanomas and hemangiomas. In retinoblastoma, the calcification is seen as specks or clumps within the mass lesion. In osteoma, the entire lesion is calcific and plaque-like.

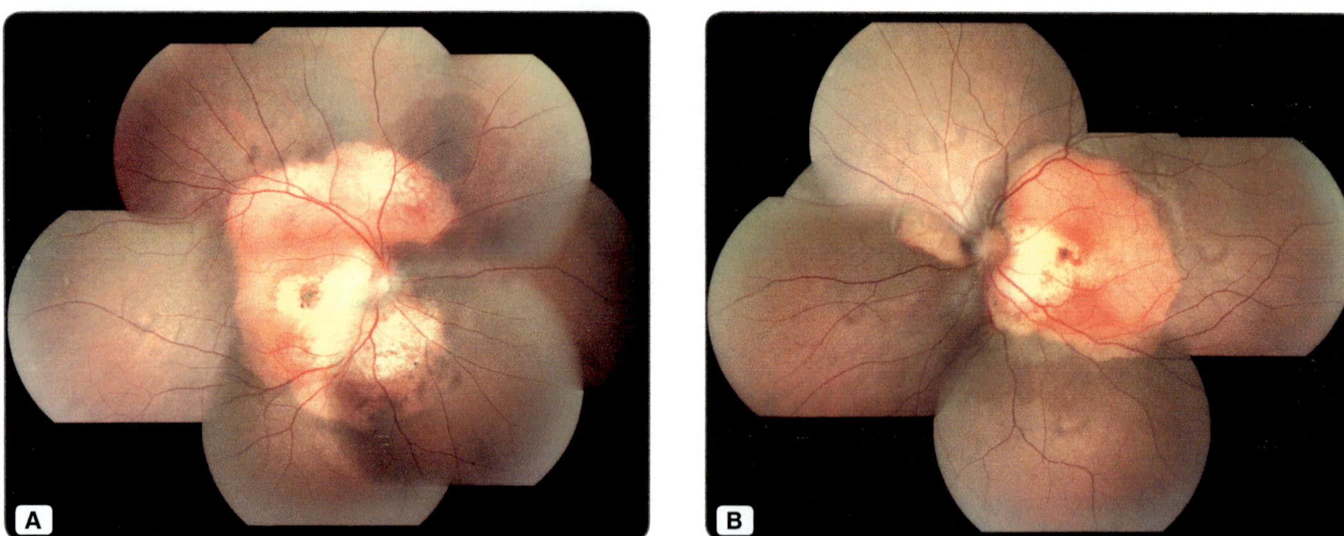

Figures 21.1A and B: Color fundus photographs of a young lady with complaints of decreased vision in both eyes over a couple of months. The posterior pole shows a flat orange-red lesion also involving the peripapillary area. The foveal area shows a subretinal neovascular membrane.

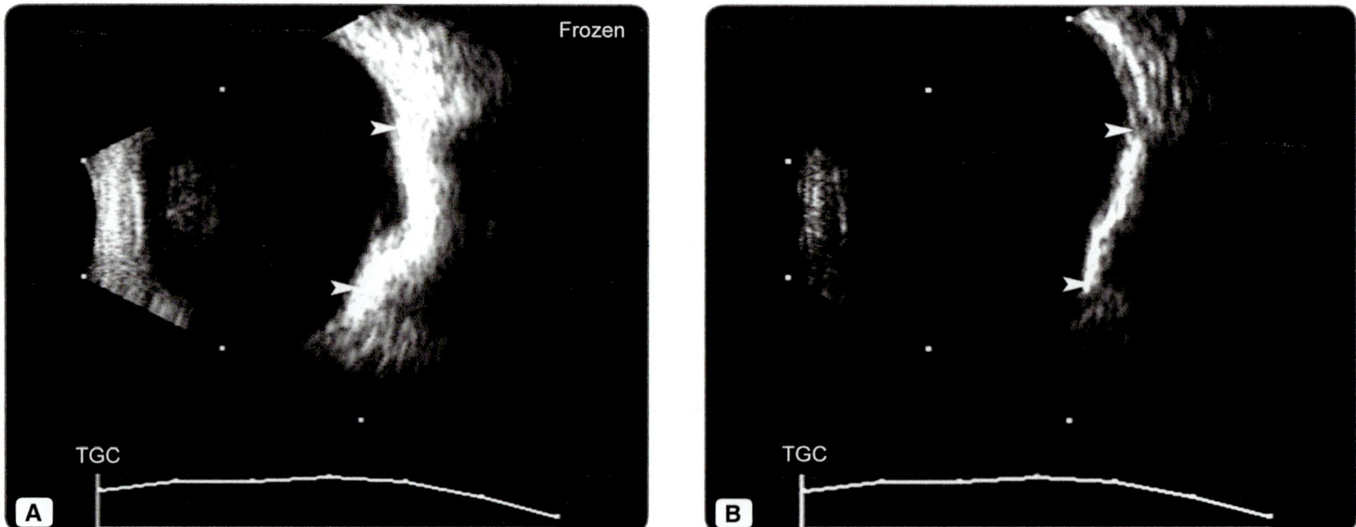

Figures 21.2A and B: B scan ultrasound images of the right eye at high and low gain settings. These show a very high reflective plaque-like lesion (arrowhead) within the ocular coats causing intense shadowing. The optic nerve shadow is not seen separately from the plaque. The feature is typical of a choroidal osteoma.

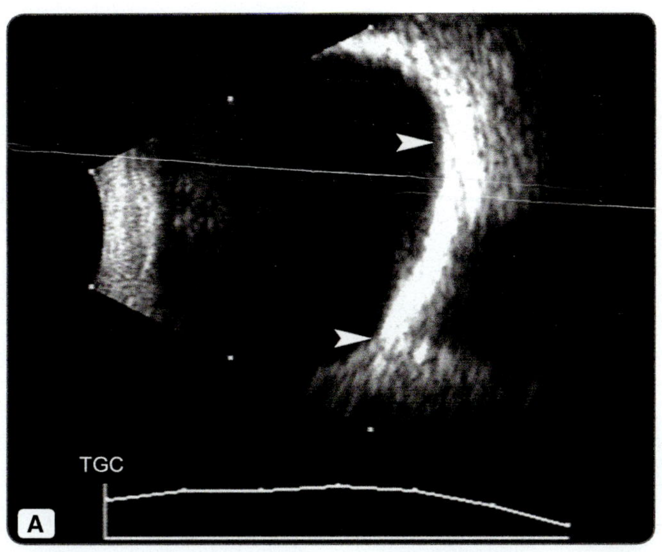

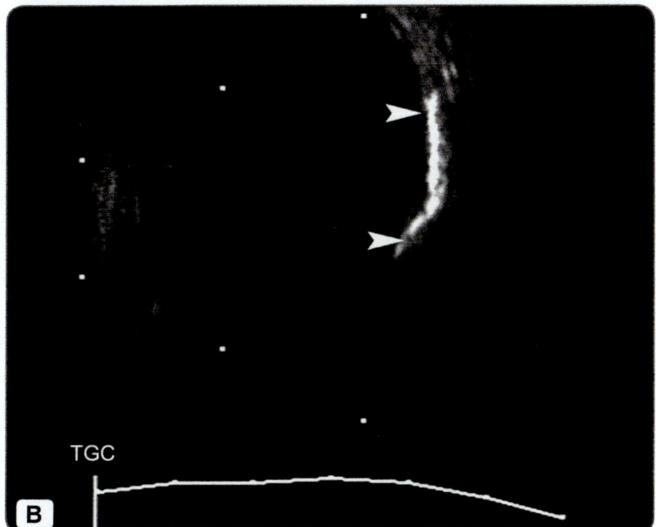

Figures 21.3A and B: B scan images of the left eye showing a plaque lesion with similar features.

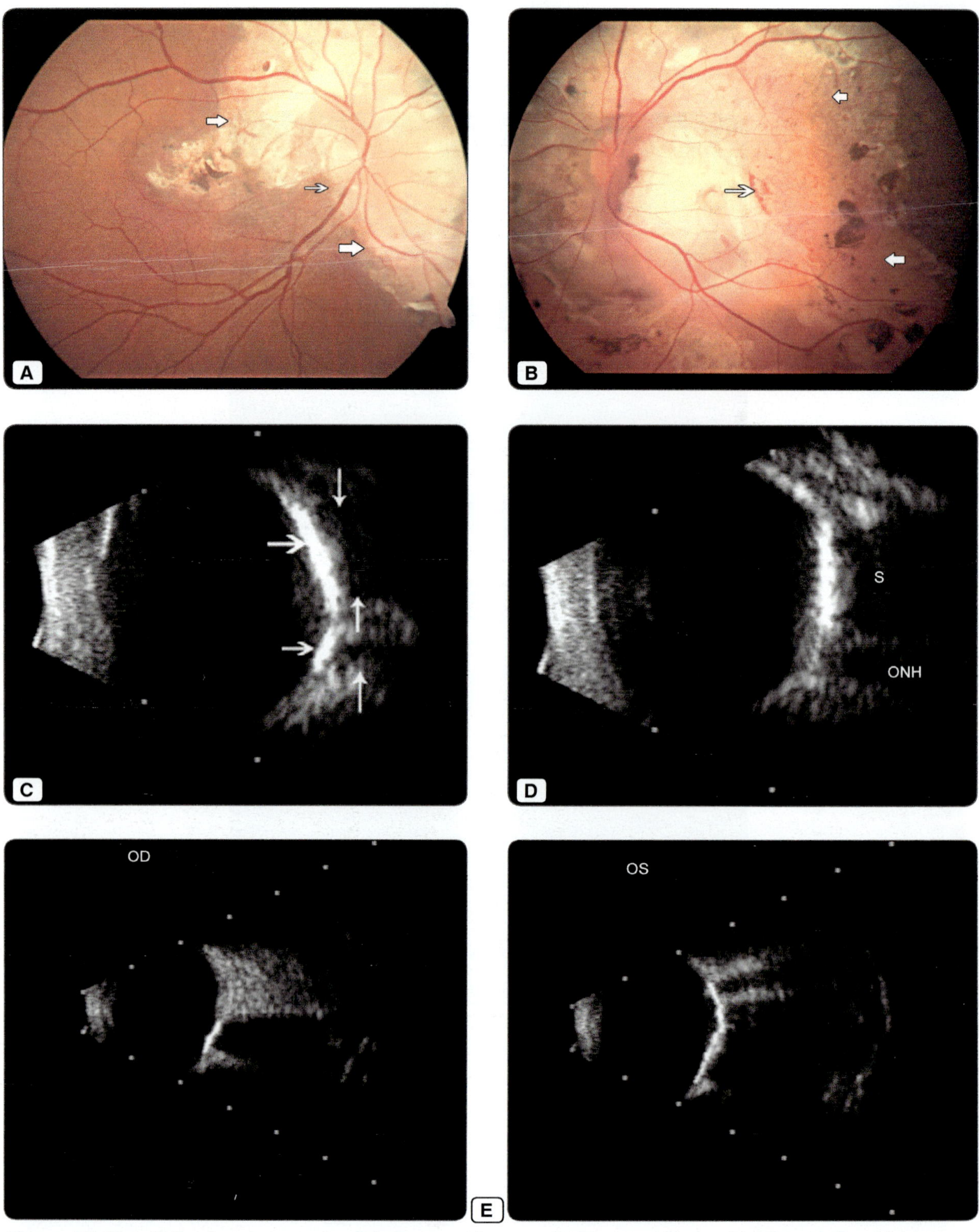

Figures 21.4A to E: Fundus photographs and ultrasound images of a 38-year-old lady with bilateral choroidal osteoma. The right eye shows the lesion to be predominantly nasal to the disc with a small area adjacent to the disc free of the lesion (thin arrow). The left eye shows a more extensive lesion with subretinal hemorrhage indicating CNV formation (thin arrow). Ultrasound shows a plaque like area of calcification in both eyes causing intense orbital shadowing (arrows). Note the double optic nerve–like appearance caused by the shadowing (s = shadow, ON = optic nerve).

Section 6

Congenital Anomalies and Disorders of the Pediatric Age Group

22 Coloboma of the Choroid and Optic Disc

CLINICAL FEATURES

- Colobomas can involve the uveal tract either in part or in entirety.
- The eyes can be microphthalmic and commonly have cataracts and poorly dilating pupils.
- A coloboma of the choroid appears as an excavation of varying depth involving the choroid, optic disc or both
- There may be an associated cystic orbital component as well.
- Breaks in the intercalary membrane stretched across the coloboma are the cause of most retinal detachments associated with choroidal colobomas.
- B scan ultrasonography is commonly indicated to diagnose retinal detachment and also to confirm axial lengths prior to cataract surgery in eyes with coloboma of the choroid.

ULTRASONOGRAPHY

- The coloboma is seen as an excavation of the ocular wall, of varying depth.
- The contour may be smooth or have an outpouching.
- The edge is typically overhanging and sharp or shelved, which helps distinguish it from a posterior staphyloma, which has a smooth edge.
- One may be able to visualize the intercalary membrane stretched across the coloboma, and identify breaks within it, if very large.
- In case of a microphthalmic eye, it is important to look for an orbital cyst, seen as an outpouching from the eye. This may sometimes be larger than the eye itself.
- Scleral fistulas may occur within the coloboma, either spontaneously or after trauma. These can give rise to extreme hypotony. The scleral fistula can be visualised as an echolucent communication between the coloboma and the orbit.

MICROPHTHALMOS/ANOPHTHALMOS WITH CYST

CLINICAL FEATURES

- Refers to a congenital malformation in which the volume of the eye is reduced.
- Microphthalmos may be colobomatous or noncolobomatous. Colobomata are because of failure of closure of embryonic fissure. Congenital cystic microphthalmos and anophthalmos are extreme forms of dysembryogenesis.
- Although microcornea or high hyperopia may be a useful clinical clue, microcornea can occur in the absence of microphthalmos.
- Ultrasonography with precise measurement of anteroposterior axis permits an anatomic diagnosis.

Ultrasonography

- Globe is deformed and microphthalmic.
- The cyst is well outlined and low reflective.
- The cyst may communicate with the globe or may be separated from the globe by a thin membrane.

ANOPHTHALMOS

- Orbital cavity shows an apparently normal soft tissue shadow.
- Globe is not detected.

NUGGETS

Knowing the exact location of the coloboma in relation to the macula is important in taking measurements for axial length.

A posterior staphyloma can sometimes appear as a coloboma. In the latter, there is often an overhanging edge or ridge at the margin. Although colobomata can occur in large myopic eyes, they are more commonly seen in microphthalmic eyes whereas posterior staphylomas invariably occur in high axial myopia.

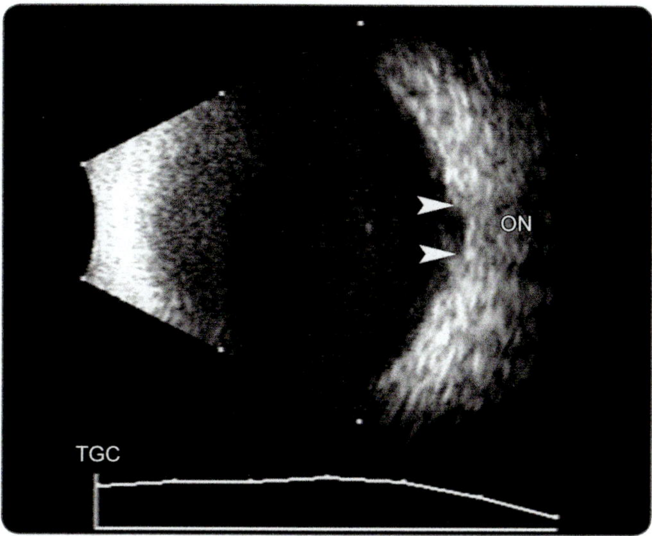

Figure 22.1: B scan image showing a small coloboma of the optic disc. It is seen as a shallow but well demarcated excavation (arrowheads) of the normal optic disc area (ON = optic nerve)

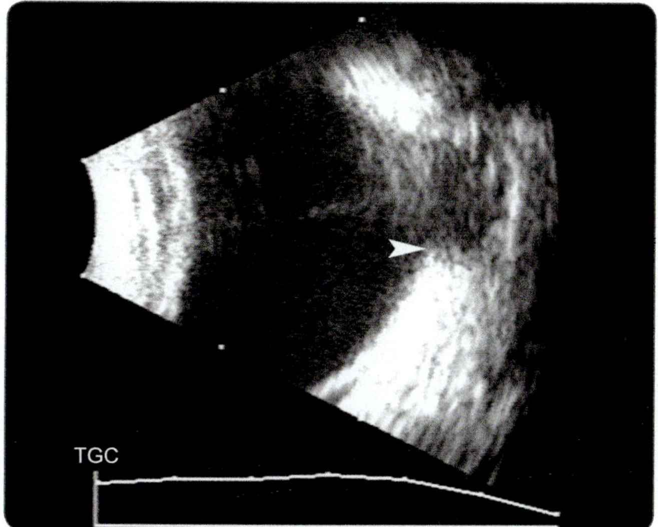

Figure 22.2: B scan image of an eye with a large optic disc coloboma. Note the sharp edge (arrowhead) that separates it from the adjacent choroid.

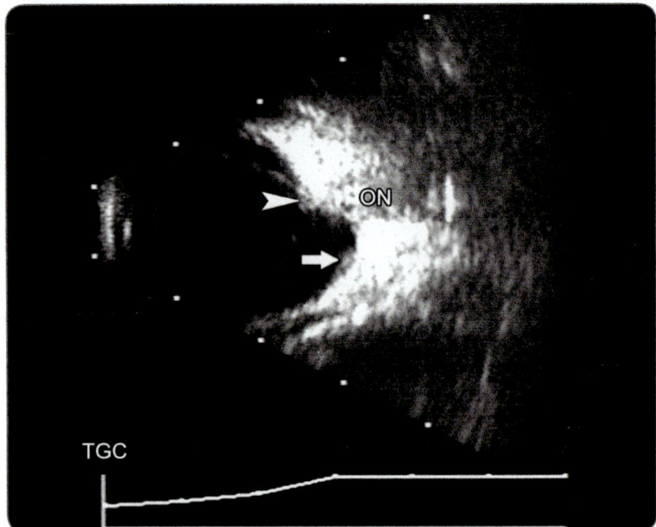

Figure 22.3: B scan image showing a coloboma of the choroid (arrow) involving the lower part of the optic disc (ON). Note the low reflective vitreous membrane attached to the ridge like elevation (arrowhead) at the upper border of the coloboma.

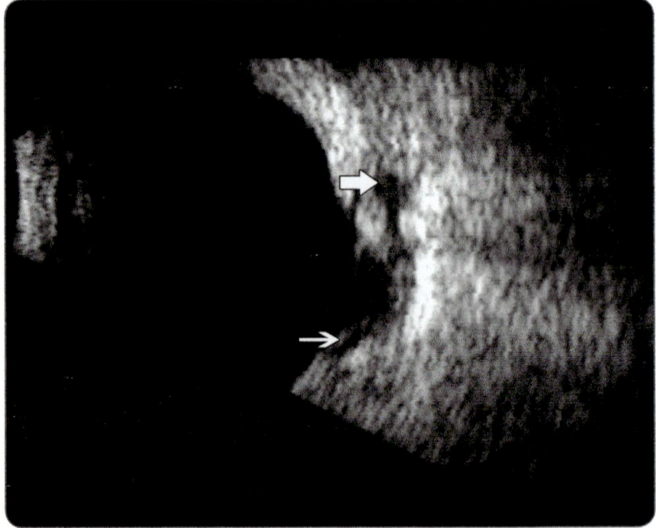

Figure 22.4: Ultrasound B scan of an eye with a choroidal coloboma, detached ICM (thin arrow) and sclera fistula (broad arrow).

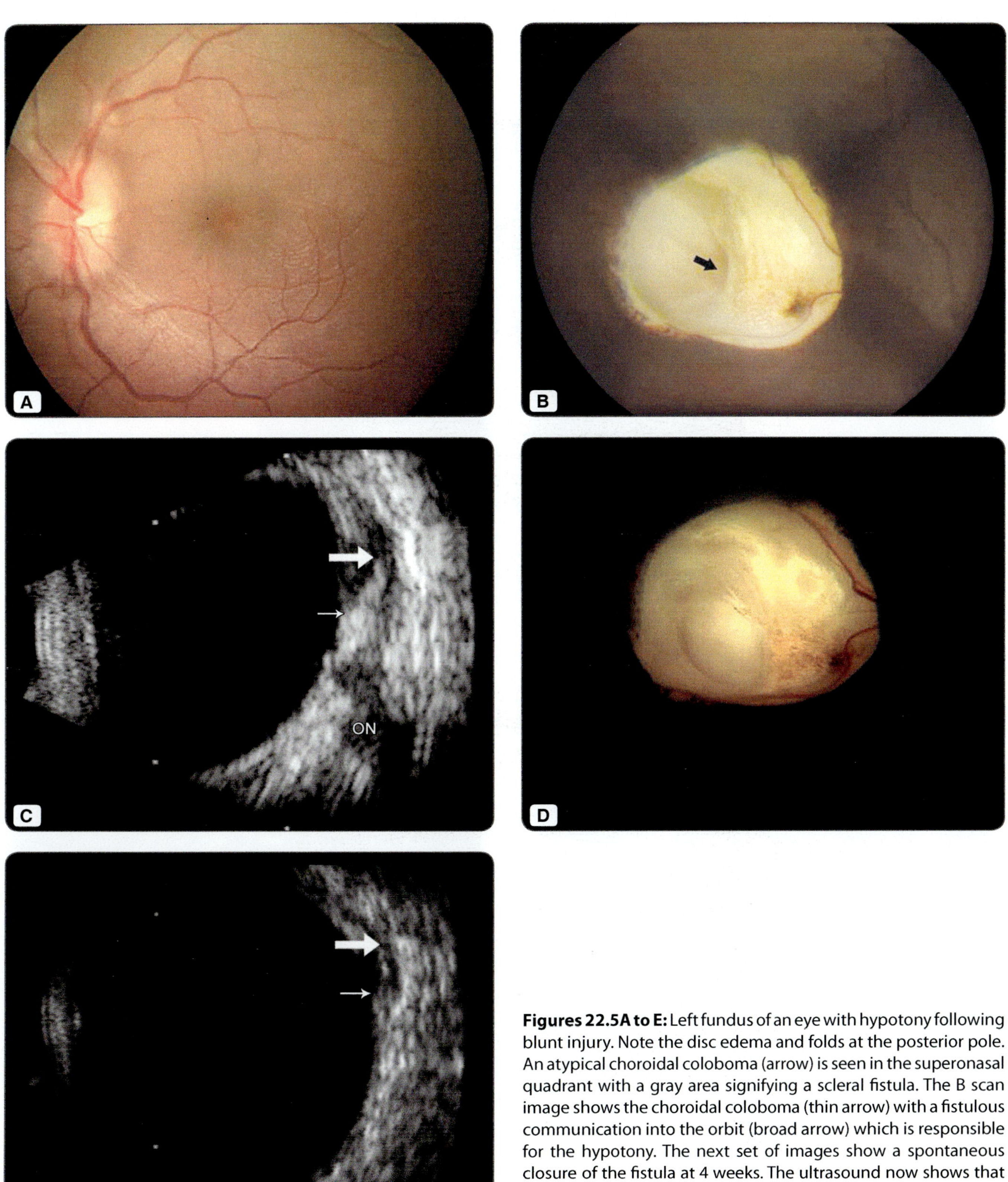

Figures 22.5A to E: Left fundus of an eye with hypotony following blunt injury. Note the disc edema and folds at the posterior pole. An atypical choroidal coloboma (arrow) is seen in the superonasal quadrant with a gray area signifying a scleral fistula. The B scan image shows the choroidal coloboma (thin arrow) with a fistulous communication into the orbit (broad arrow) which is responsible for the hypotony. The next set of images show a spontaneous closure of the fistula at 4 weeks. The ultrasound now shows that the echolucent space in the orbit has disappeared with closure of the fistula (broad arrow). (*Images published by the authors in Retinal Cases and Brief Reports.*)

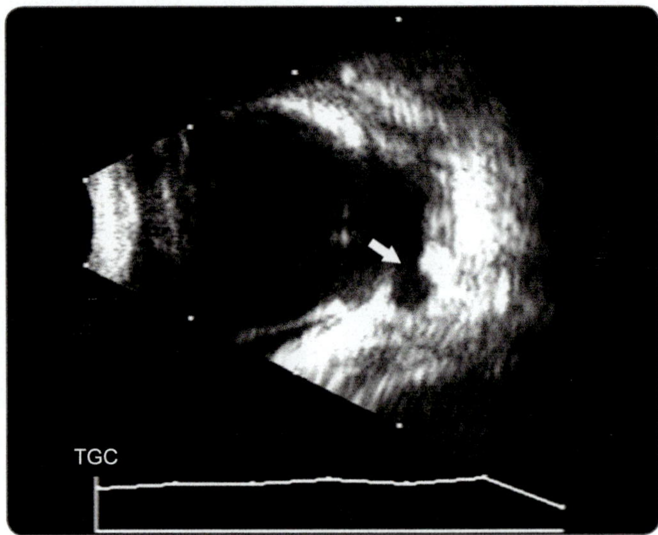

Figure 22.6: B scan image showing an elongated eyeball with a large coloboma of the choroid involving the optic disc area. Note the small cystic outpouching at the lower border of the coloboma. A low reflective vitreous membrane is attached to the edges of the coloboma.

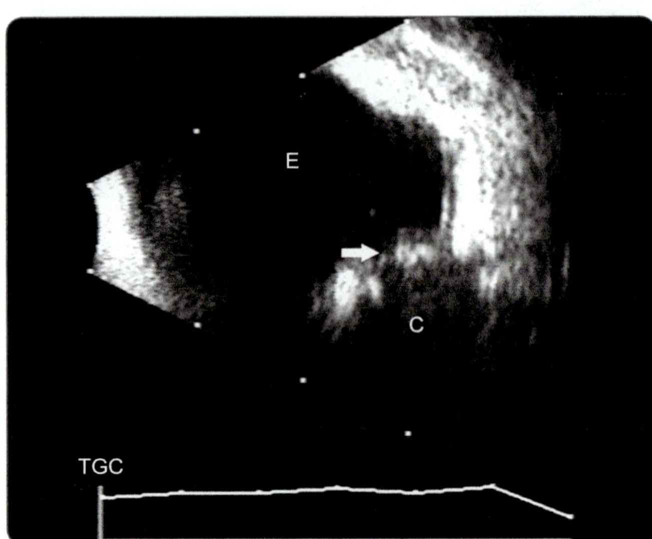

Figure 22.7: A larger cystic outpouching into the orbit (C) from a coloboma of the choroid (Eyeball = E). The communication between the cyst and eyeball is seen (arrow). These cases can present as orbital masses in early childhood.

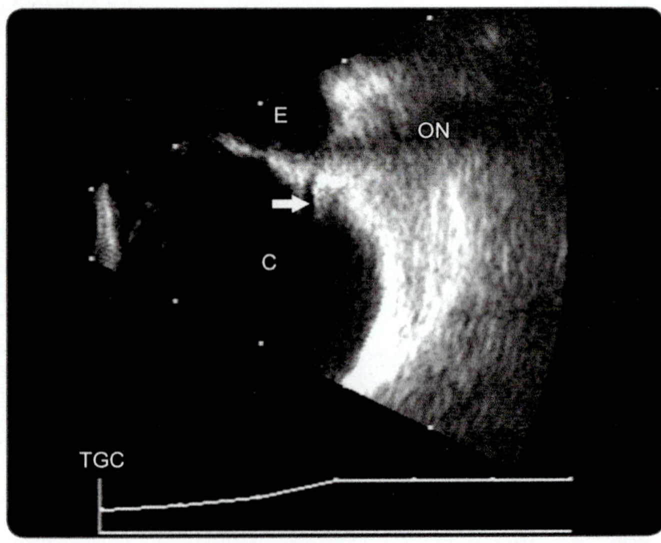

Figure 22.8: The orbital cyst (C) is sometimes larger than the eyeball itself (E) as seen in this B scan image of an eye with microphthalmos and an orbital cyst. The communication between the two is made out (arrow) as well as the optic nerve (ON).

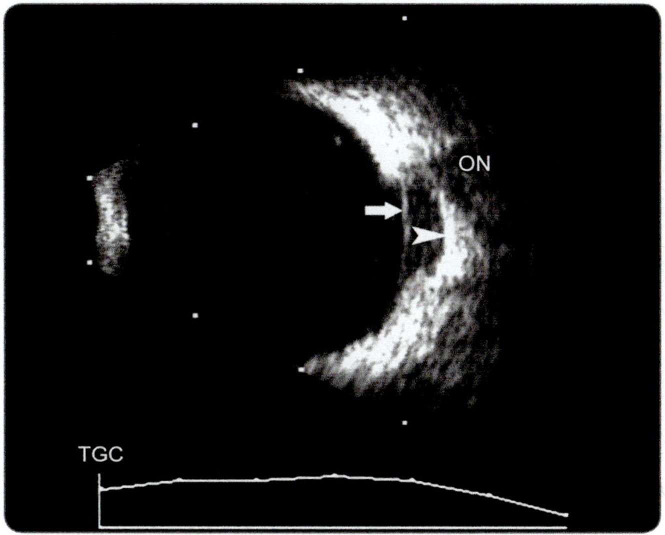

Figure 22.9: B scan image of an eye with a coloboma of the optic disc (ON) and choroid (arrow head). A moderately reflective membrane is seen stretched across the coloboma which represents a detached intercalary membrane (arrow).

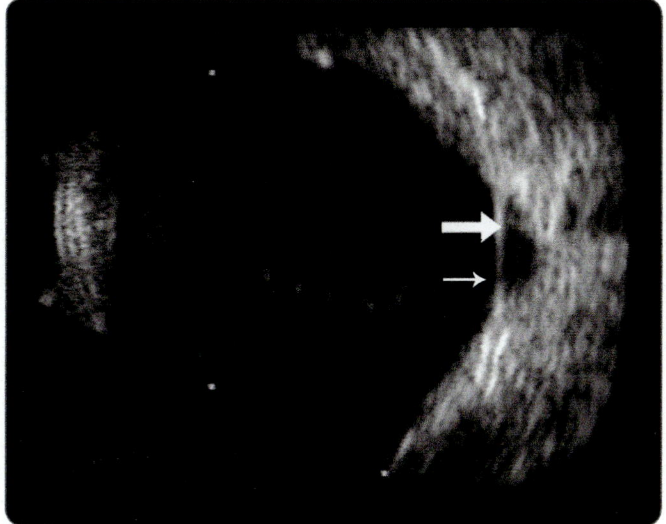

Figure 22.10: Ultrasound B scan of an eye with retinochoroidal coloboma and a detached intercalary membrane (broad arrow). A small break in the membrane is also seen (thin arrow).

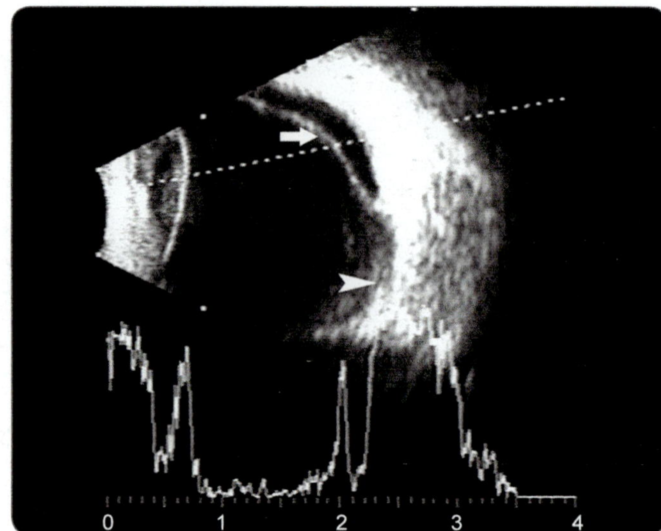

Figure 22.11: B scan with vector A scan of an eye with coloboma choroid (arrowhead) and retinal detachment (arrow). Note that the detachment does not involve the coloboma itself, indicating that the break lies outside the coloboma.

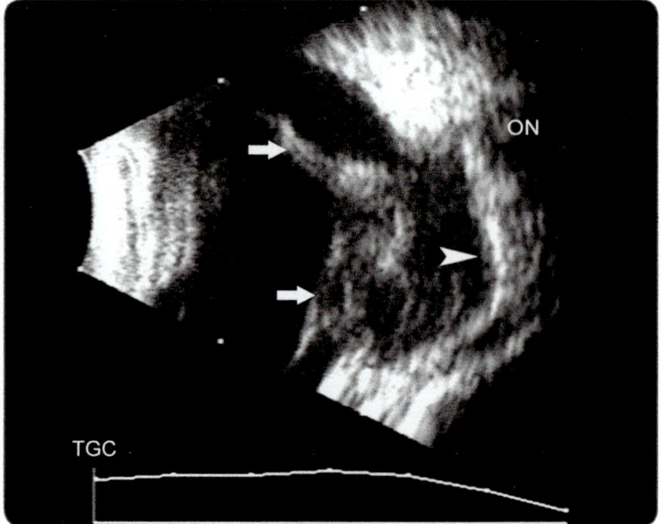

Figure 22.12 : B scan image of an eye with coloboma choroid (arrowhead) and retinal detachment (arrows) involving the coloboma. In such cases, there is likely to be a break within the coloboma itself (ON = optic nerve).

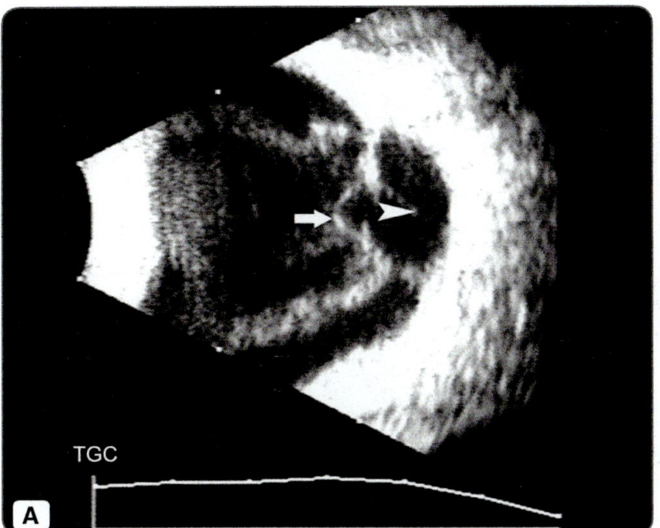

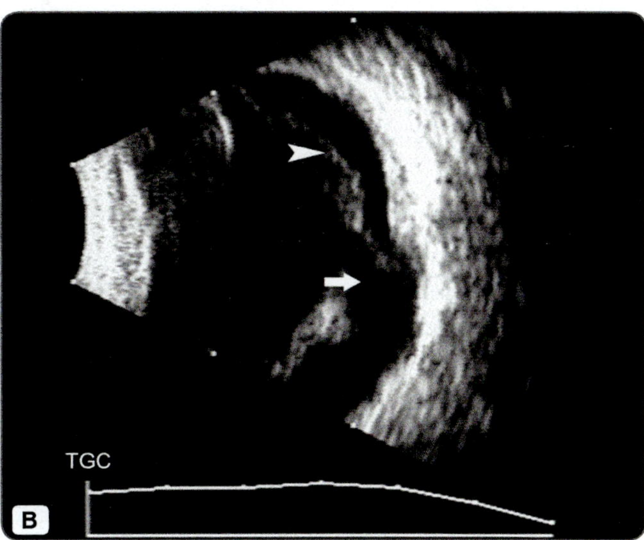

Figures 22.13A and B: B scan image of an eye with coloboma choroid and retinal detachment (arrow) involving the coloboma. Note the taut membranes extending from the base of the coloboma to the detached retina (arrowhead). One often sees these septae within the coloboma. Figure B shows a discontinuity in the retina overlying the coloboma indicating the presence of a break (arrow).

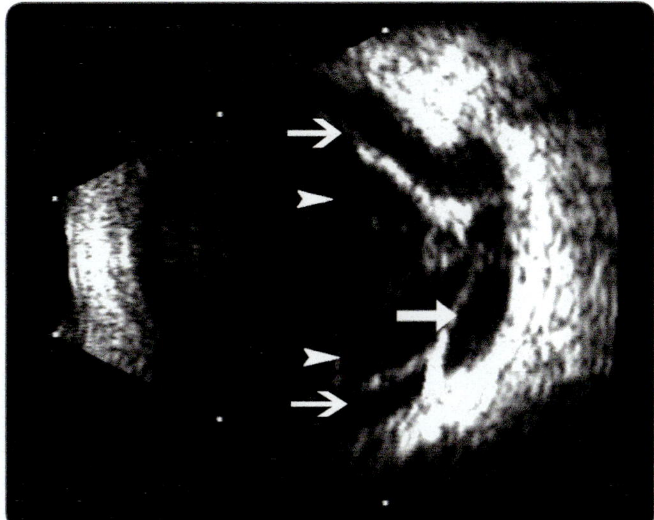

Figure 22.14: Ultrasound B scan of an eye with coloboma choroid and total RD. The vitreous membranes are marked with arrow heads, total RD with thin arrows and the detached membrane with a broad arrow.

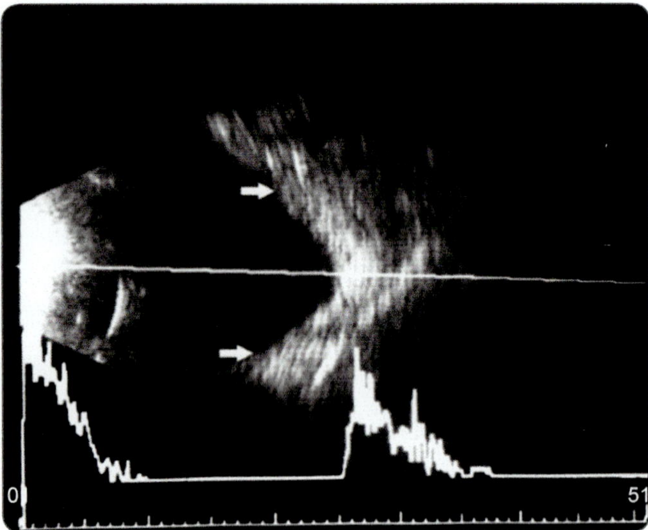

Figure 22.15: An eye with a posterior staphyloma. Note the smooth bowing of the posterior globe wall (arrows) without the sharp overhanging edge seen in a coloboma. Also note the increased axial length.

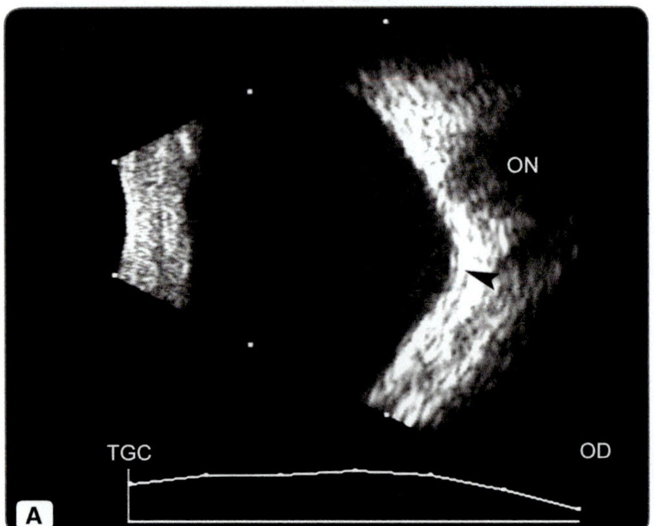

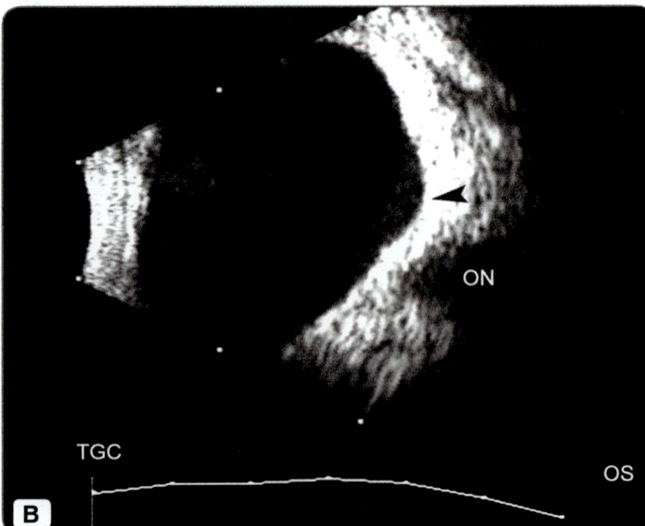

Figures 22.16A and B: B scan images of a young boy with bilateral cataract. He gave history of poor vision and nystagmus since birth. Note the macular colobomas in both eyes (arrowhead). Such colobomas are seen in Leber's congenital amaurosis. The axial lengths were normal.

23 Nanophthalmos

CLINICAL FEATURES

- Occurs due to arrested development of the globe after closure of the embryonic fissure
- Simple, partial, posterior, pure microphthalmos and nanophthalmos are similar clinical entities sharing total axial length and vitreous cavity length reduction
- Essentially a smaller eye (2/3rd of normal volume) with a relatively normal sized lens
- Angle closure glaucoma and exudative retinal detachment due to uveal effusion are known complications.

ULTRASONOGRAPHY

- Reduced axial length in the range of 15.0 to 20.5 mm.
- Relatively normal sized lens. The increased lens-eye volume ratio (16.60 to 37.60%) is classical
- Increased sclerochoroidal thickness (1.37 to 4.00 mm).
- Presence of exudative retinal detachment and choroidal detachment.

NUGGETS

Echography should be used to assess retinal-choroidal-scleral thickness in eyes that are hyperopic and at risk for narrow-angle glaucoma. Thickening may confirm the diagnosis of nanophthalmos and allow careful preoperative assessment and appropriate operative procedures in these high-risk eyes.

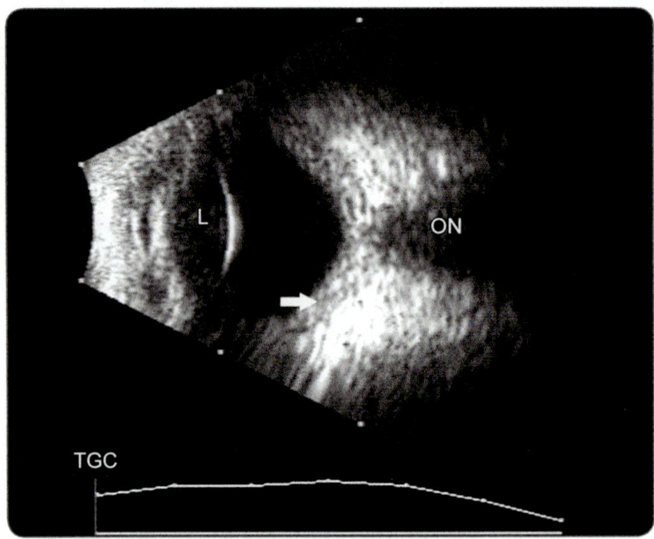

Figure 23.1: Axial B scan image of an eye with reduced axial length showing the relatively high lens-eye volume ratio. The sclerochoroidal thickness (arrow) is also increased (L = Lens, Optic nerve = ON).

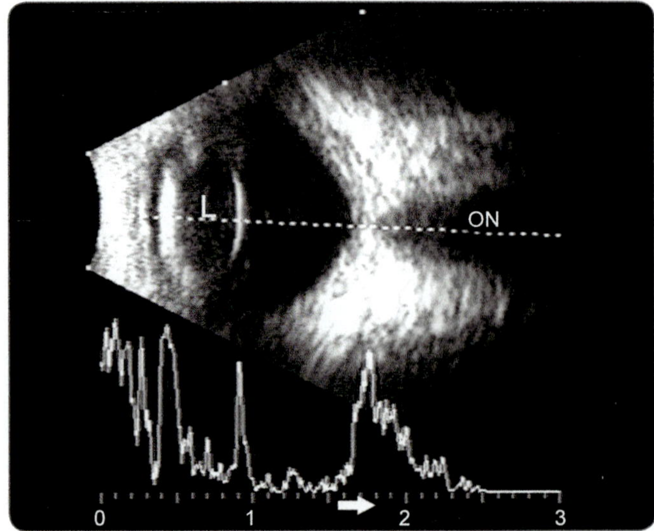

Figure 23.2: B scan with vector A scan showing the reduced axial length (arrow on the caliper).

24 Persistence of Fetal Vasculature (PFV)

CLINICAL FEATURES

- Also known as persistent hyperplastic primary vitreous (PHPV).
- Present at birth, predominantly unilateral (90%).
- Typically a small eye, with localized cataract and prominent ciliary processes.
- Can be purely anterior, posterior or combined.
- Cataract and prominent ciliary processes are features of the anterior form.
- Peripapillary tractional retinal detachments are seen in the posterior form.

ULTRASONOGRAPHY

- Decrease in axial length.
- Thin lens with irregular posterior capsule.
- Retrolental high reflective membrane.
- Vitreous band of variable reflectivity extending from the lens to the optic disc.
- Peripapillary tractional retinal detachment (TRD)

NUGGETS

Always compare axial lengths in an eye with unilateral cataract.

Increase the gain settings to detect a low reflective strand suggestive of PFV, however, the entire extent of the vitreous band may not be visible in all cases.

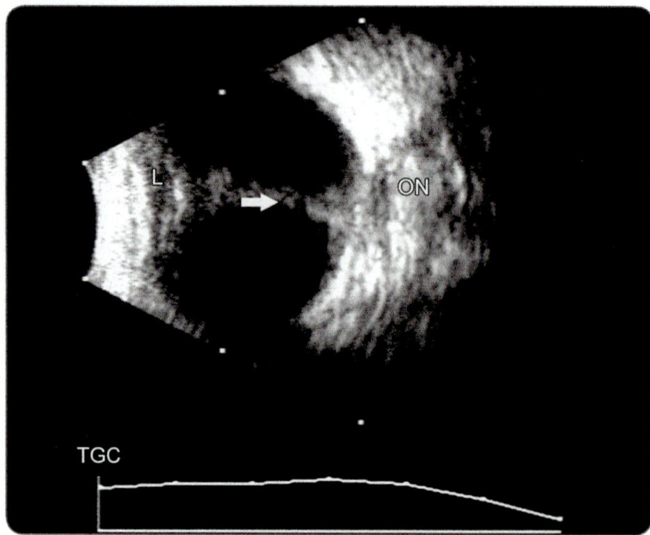

Figure 24.1: Vertical axial B scan image showing a moderately reflective membrane (arrow) stretching from the lens (L) to the optic disc (ON). Irregularity of the posterior capsule is seen as well as a clump of echoes around the optic disc.

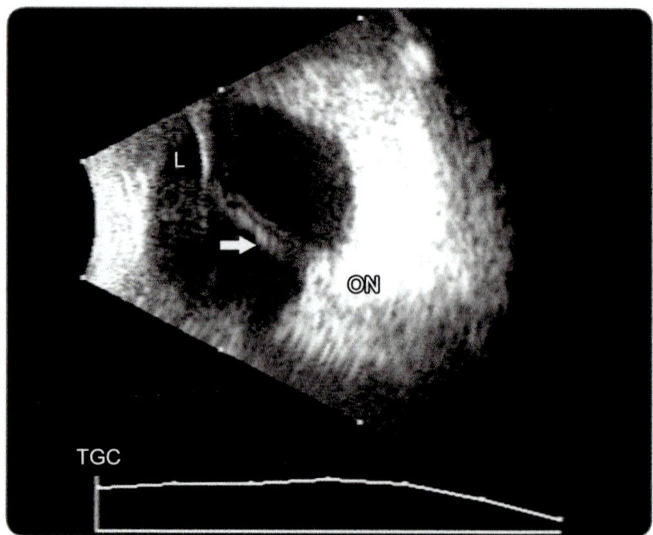

Figure 24.2: Axial B scan image showing a small eyeball and a thick membrane (arrow) extending from the lens (L) to the optic disc (ON).

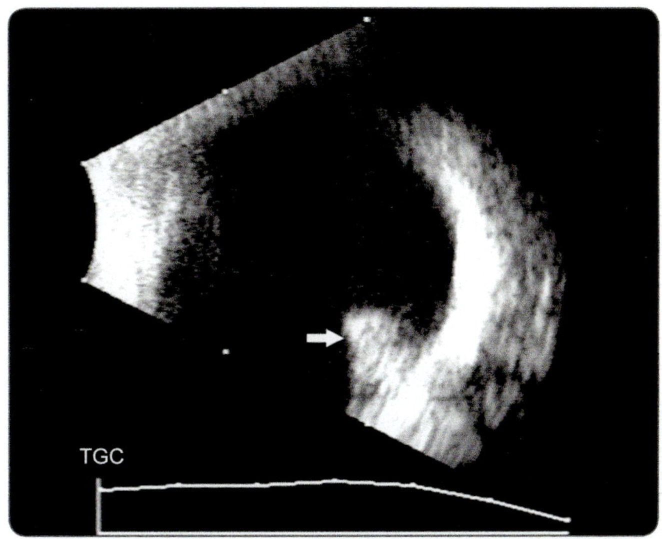

Figure 24.3: Axial B scan image of pure posterior form showing a highly reflective tented membrane in the peripapillary area (arrow).

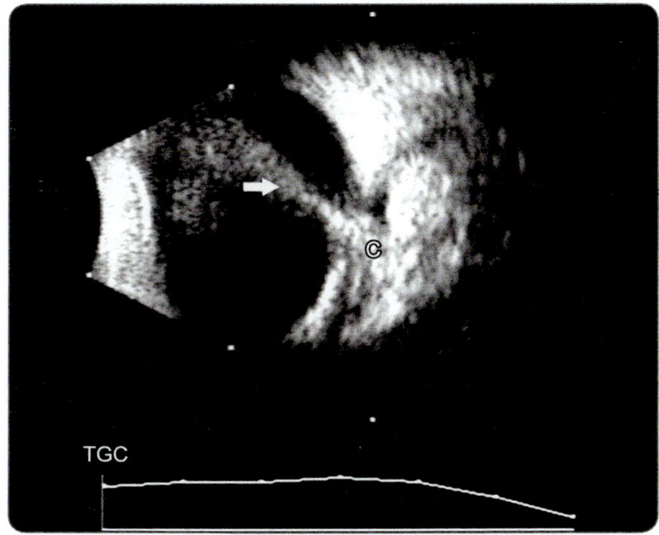

Figure 24.4: Vertical B scan showing a combination of coloboma choroid involving the optic disc (C) along with a high reflective thick membrane suggestive of PFV (arrow).

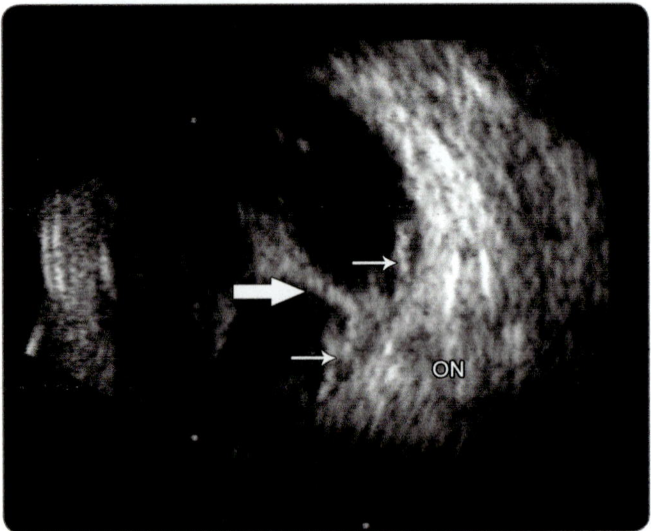

Figure 24.5: Ultrasound B scan shows a thick retinal fold (broad arrow) causing posterior pole traction (thin arrows). The patient was a 6-month-old baby with clinically visible falciform retinal folds.

25 Retinopathy of Prematurity (ROP)

CLINICAL FEATURES

- Bilateral vascular retinopathy
- Seen in low birth weight premature infants with gestational age < 32 weeks and birth weight < 1500 g
- Due to abnormal postnatal growth of retinal vasculature
- Stages 1–5 based on clinical features
- Stage 5 ROP with total retinal detachment presents with leukokoria
- The lens remains clear
- Vitreous surgery is possible but with a very guarded visual prognosis
- Ultrasonography helps to differentiate it from other causes of leukokoria.

ULTRASONOGRAPHY

- Normal or smaller sized eye
- Funnel shaped high reflective membrane attached to the optic disc suggestive of a total retinal detachment
- Shows the exact configuration of the funnel—whether open or closed, either anteriorly, posteriorly or both
- Presence of retinal loops or troughs which should be differentiated from retinal cysts
- Detection of subretinal echoes which could signify blood or cholesterol.

NUGGETS

Presence of subretinal blood or cholesterol signifies a poor prognosis.

Presence and localization of a deep trough would indicate the possible site for starting membrane dissection.

Similar features without the presence of troughs can be seen in retinal dysplasias.

Ultrasound in a small eye can be difficult due to the relatively larger probe dimensions. Significant artifacts can be present sometimes leading to difficulties in imaging the anterior configuration of the retina. Use of larger amounts of gel for a better standoff can overcome this problem.

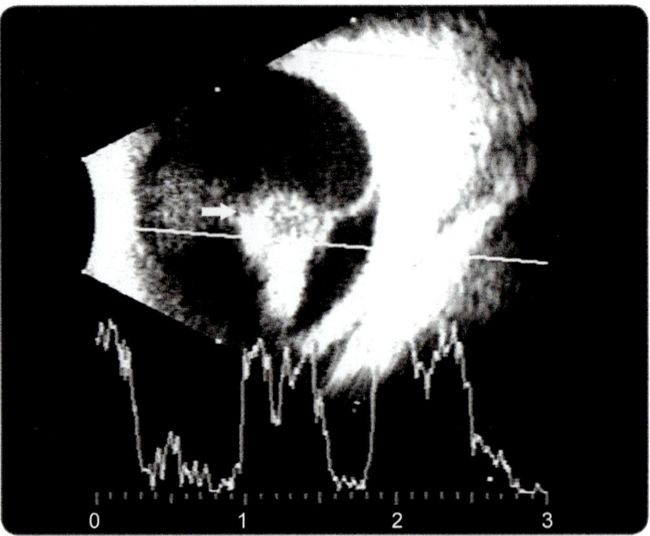

Figure 25.1: Longitudinal B scan with A scan vector showing a clump of high reflective echoes suggestive of fibrovascular tissue (arrow) pulling up the retina in a concave configuration suggestive of stage 4 ROP. Note that the retina in the upper part of the scan is attached.

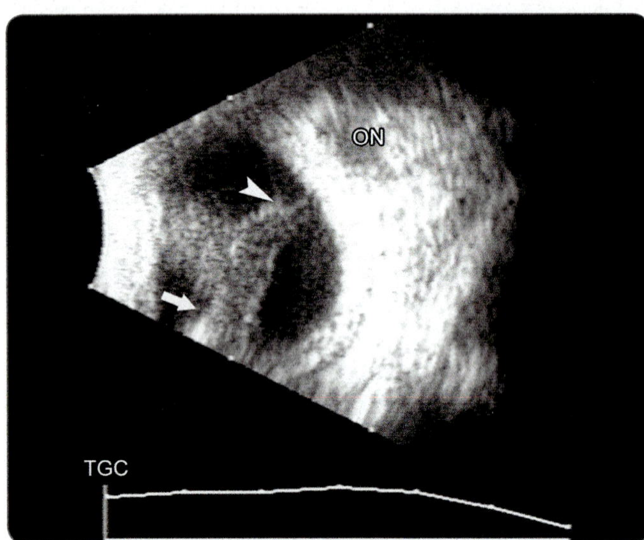

Figure 25.2: Axial B scan image showing a funnel-shaped high reflective membrane inserting into the optic disc. Note the accumulation of echoes in the anterior part suggesting the presence of preretinal fibrous tissue. The membrane is open in the anterior and middle parts (arrow) and narrows (arrowhead) as it approaches the optic disc (ON).

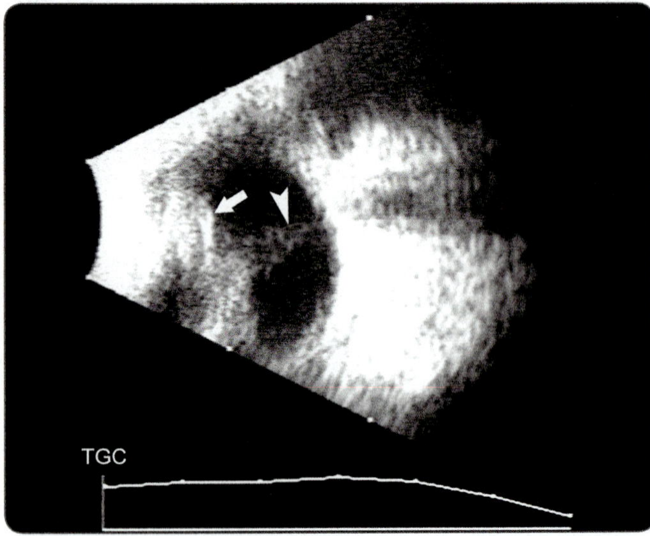

Figure 25.3: Axial B scan image showing a total retinal detachment with open anterior (arrow) and closed posterior funnel (arrowhead). The subretinal space is echolucent.

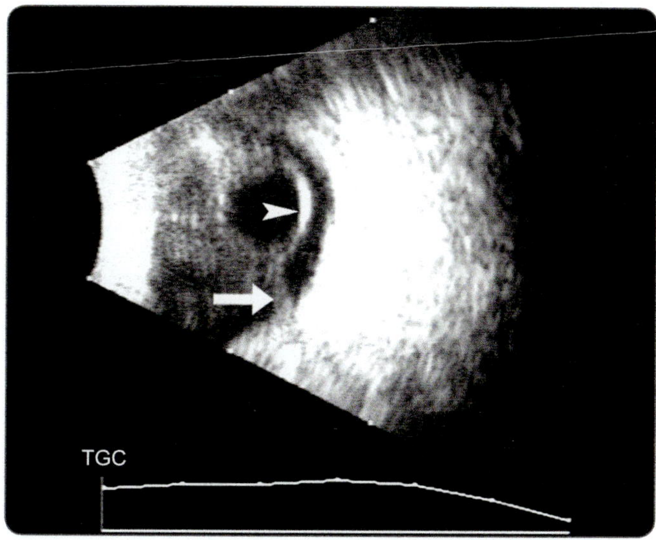

Figure 25.4: Horizontal axial B scan image showing densely packed retrolental echoes. A total retinal detachment with tightly closed posterior funnel is seen (arrow). Note the prominent retinal loop in the superior part of the image (arrowhead).

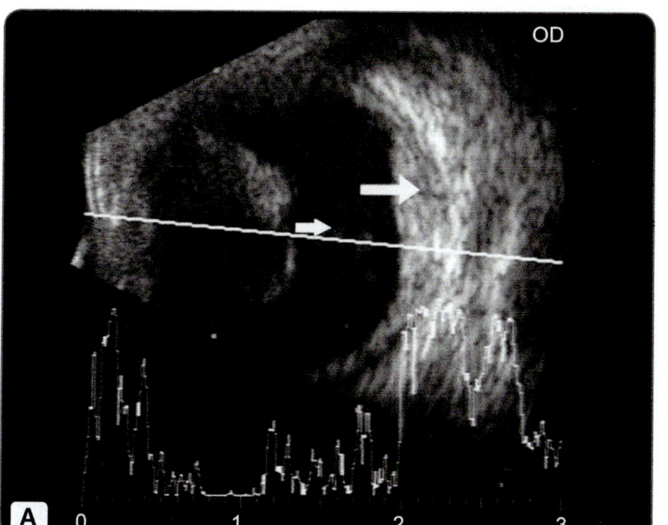

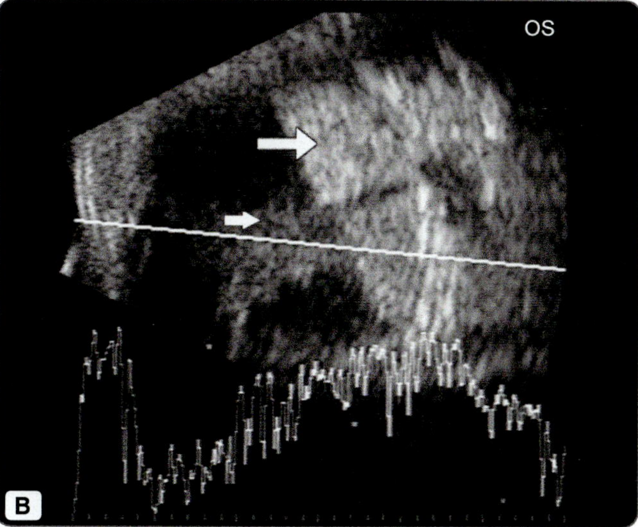

Figures 25.5A and B: Ultrasound images of a 2-month-old premature baby with bilateral retrolental proliferation and total RD. Note the closed funnel RD (arrow) in both eyes and densely layered subretinal echoes (broad arrow) signifying subretinal hemorrhage.

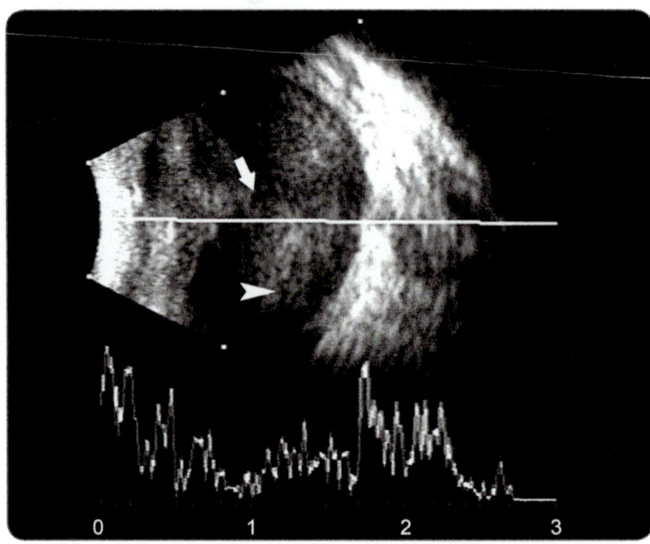

Figure 25.6: Vertical axial B scan image with A scan vector showing a moderately reflective funnel-shaped membrane indicative of a total retinal detachment with tightly closed funnel (arrow). Note the subretinal layering of echoes with moderate to high reflectivity suggestive of subretinal hemorrhage (arrowhead).

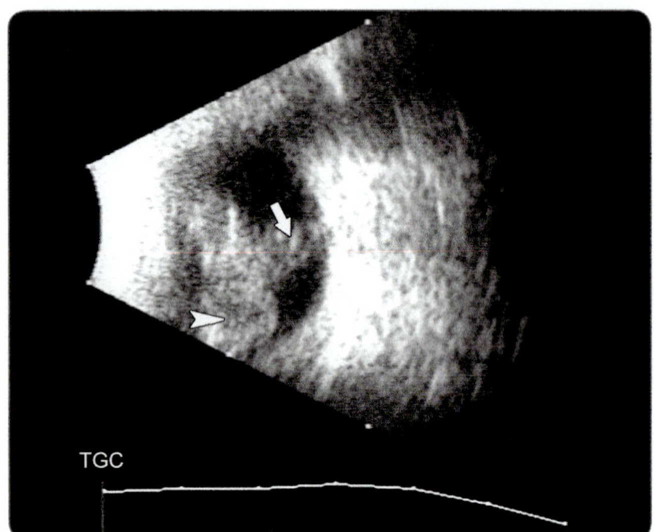

Figure 25.7: Axial B scan image of an eye with stage 5 ROP showing retrolental echoes and a closed posterior funnel (arrow). Shallow retinal loop formation is seen (arrowhead).

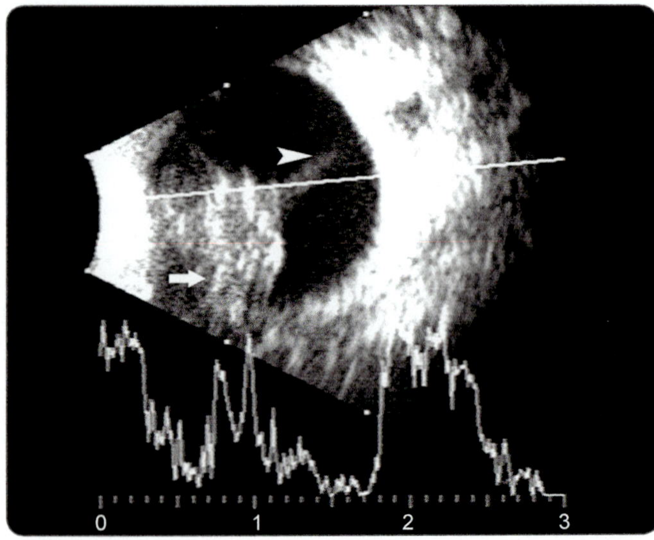

Figure 25.8: Axial B scan with A vector showing advanced stage 5 ROP. The retrolental space shows densely packed echoes suggestive of fibrous tissue (arrow). The retinal detachment assumes a cord-like appearance posteriorly (arrowhead).

26 Coats' Disease

CLINICAL FEATURES

- Common cause of exudative retinal detachment in childhood
- Unilateral in the majority of cases
- Important cause of leukokoria and hence is a differential diagnosis for retinoblastoma
- Ultrasound is indicated to confirm the diagnosis and rule out retinoblastoma.

ULTRASONOGRAPHY

- Localized (in early stages) or total retinal detachment which can touch the lens.
- Occasionally, a plaque of high reflective echoes at the macula may be the only finding, this represents a hard exudate plaque that can be seen in these patients.
- Shifting fluid may not be demonstrable in massive detachments.
- Presence of subretinal echoes signify cholesterol.
- Occasional presence of calcium may cause a diagnostic dilemma.

NUGGETS

Points to differentiate from retinoblastoma are relatively older age group, unilaterality, male predominance, invariable absence of calcification, subretinal cholesterol along with ophthalmoscopic evidence of vascular telangiectasia.

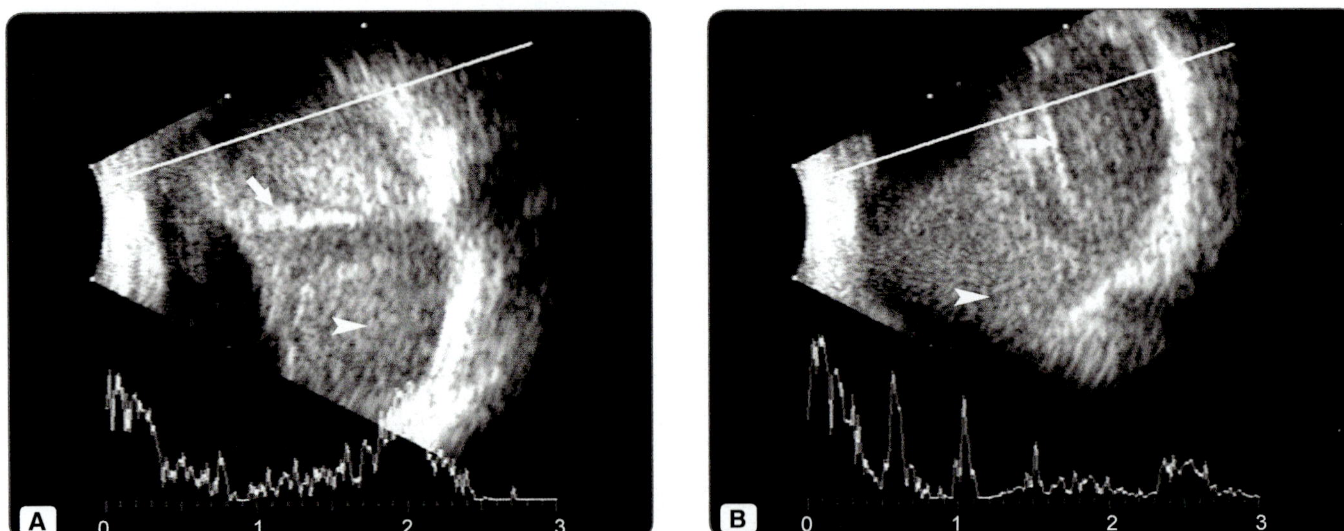

Figures 26.1A and B: B scan with vector A scan showing massive retinal detachment (arrow) with plenty of low reflective subretinal echoes (arrowhead). No mass lesion is seen. The configuration of the detachment does not change with change in head posture.

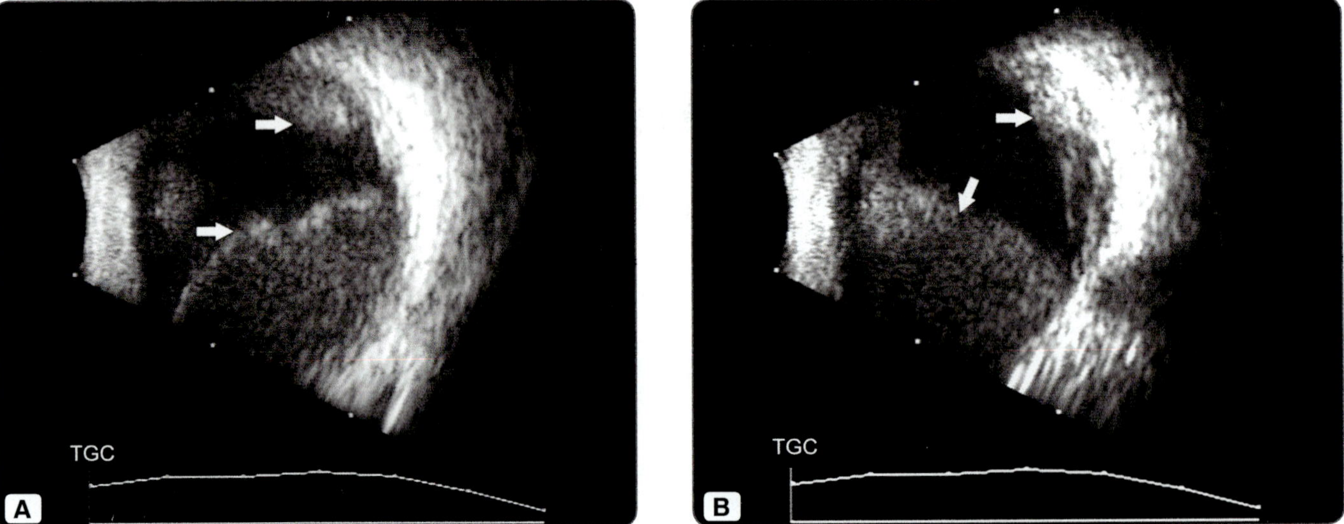

Figures 26.2A and B: B scan images of an eye with exudative retinal detachment due to Coats' disease (arrows). Note the change in configuration of the detachment with change in head position. No mass lesion or choroidal thickening is noted.

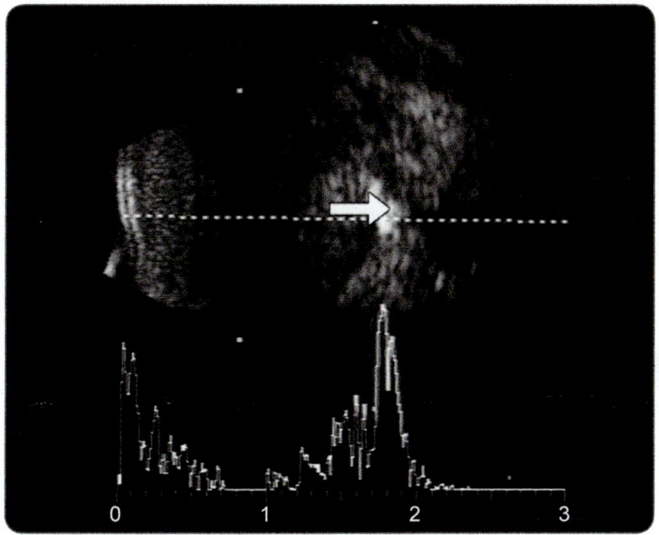

Figure 26.3: Ultrasound image of a 2-year-old male child with neovascular glaucoma and total RD. The posterior pole shows a clump of calcification (broad arrow). The enucleated specimen showed features of Coats' disease.

Section 7

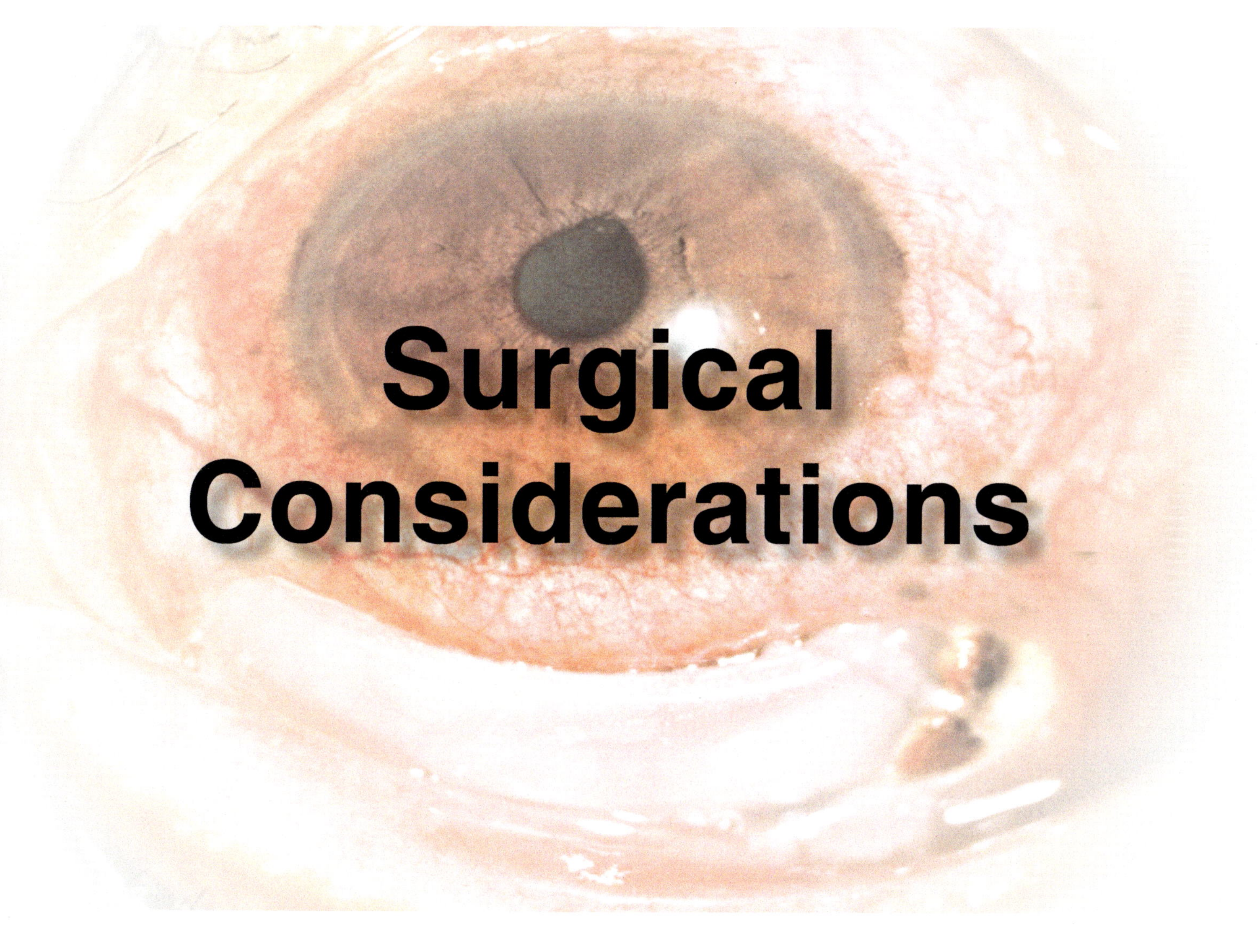

Surgical Considerations

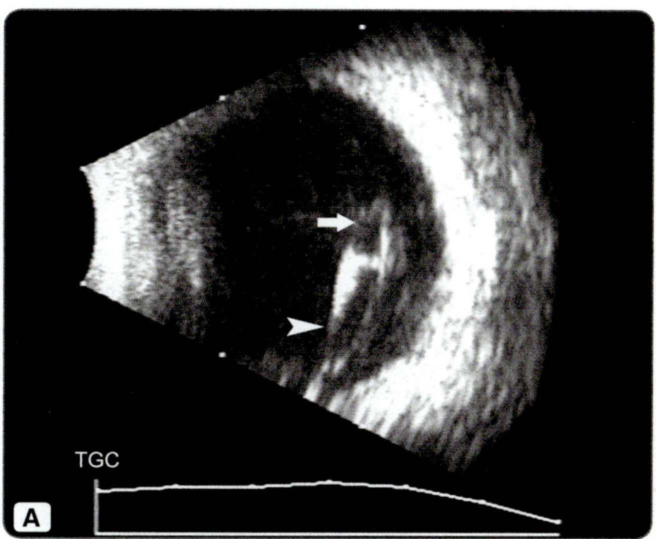

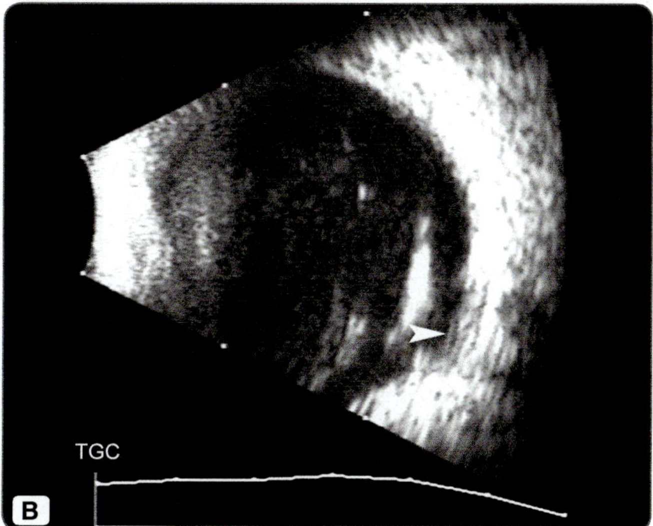

Figures 27.3A and B: B scan image of an eye with a posteriorly dislocated IOL. The image shows the biconvex shape of the IOL (arrowhead) with one haptic touching the inferior retinal surface. Note the low reflective membrane-like echoes around the superior edge (arrow), suggestive of vitreous membranes entangled around the haptic. Figure B shows the shadowing caused by the IOL (arrowhead) when the probe is perpendicular to its long axis.

28 Dislocated Lens Matter

CLINICAL FEATURES

- Usually occurs during cataract surgery.
- Can be a spontaneous occurrence due to pre-existing zonular dehiscence or following trauma.
- Either the entire lens, nucleus, or parts of it can be dislocated into the vitreous.
- Presence of retained lens fragments can cause severe postoperative inflammation.
- Ultrasonography is indicated in cases of significant media opacity.

ULTRASONOGRAPHY

- The features depend on the clarity of the lens.
- The clear lens appears as a globular structure, which is echolucent.
- The cataractous lens appears highly reflective, and the internal echoes vary depending on the amount of cortical hydration.
- A brunescent nucleus causes very high reflectivity with shadowing.
- In cases with a long-standing dislocated lens, it may become calcified and cause dense shadowing.
- Lens fragments appear as high reflective clumps of echoes of varying size.

NUGGETS

If not fixed, a change in head posture results in shifting of the posteriorly dislocated lens and its resulting echoes.

Intralesional echoes vary with the amount of cataract.

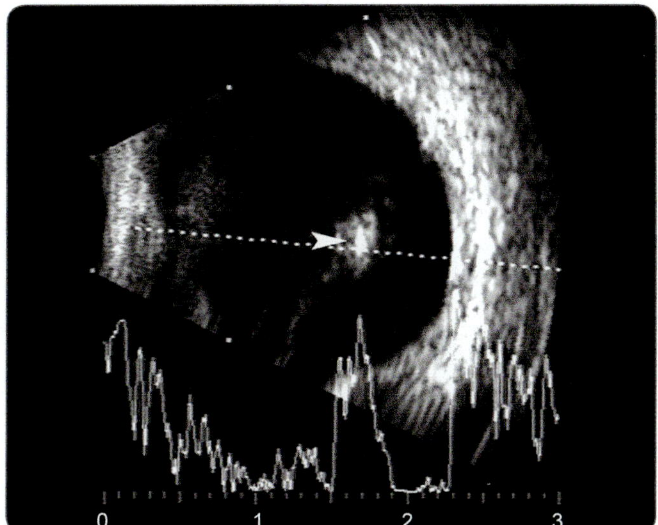

Figure 28.1: B scan with vector A of a patient with severe postoperative inflammation following cataract surgery. The vitreous cavity shows low reflective dot-like echoes. In addition, there is a clump of very high reflective echoes (arrowhead) in the mid-vitreous cavity showing 100% spikes on the A scan. This is suggestive of a nuclear fragment in the vitreous.

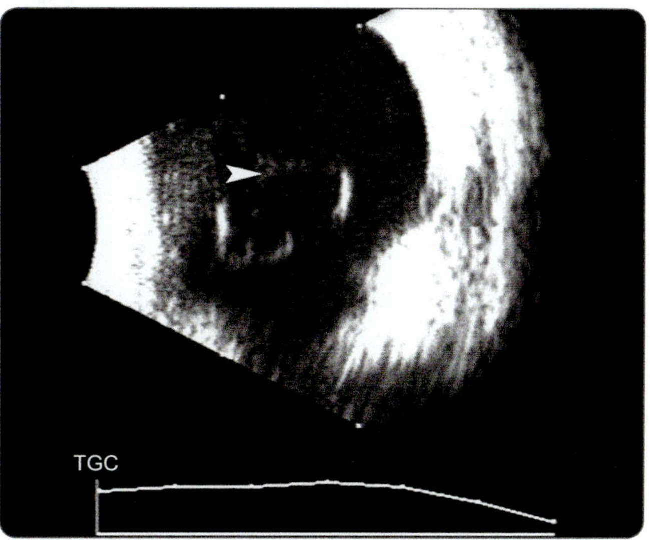

Figure 28.2: B scan image of a dislocated clear lens following blunt trauma. Note the biconvex structure in the mid-vitreous with clear-cut margins and no internal echoes.

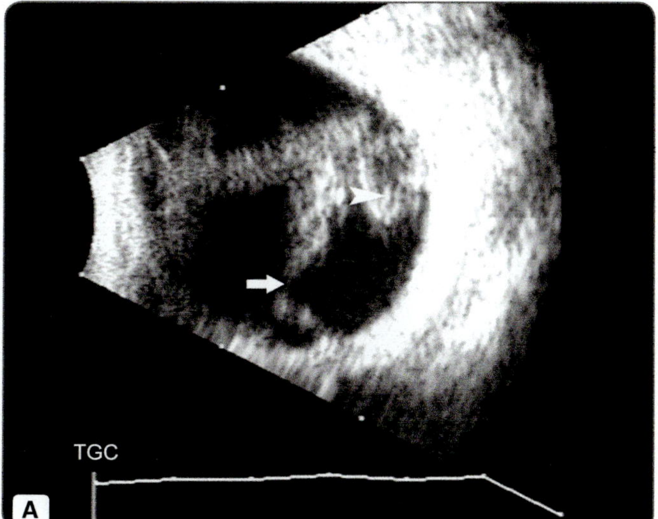

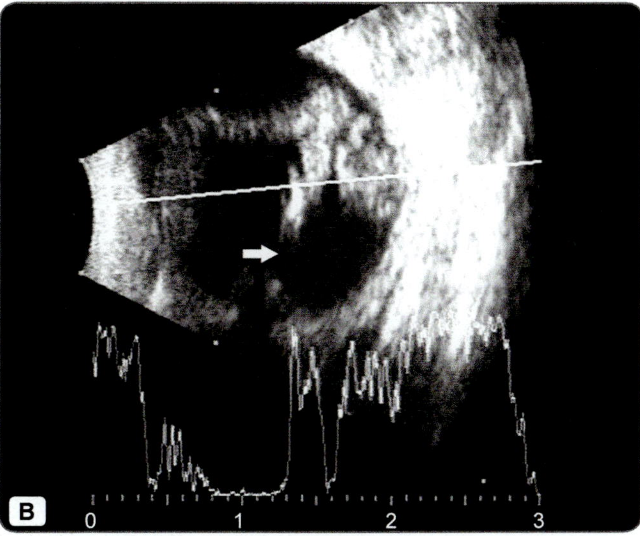

Figures 28.3A and B: B scan image of a case of total retinal detachment following attempted removal of a dislocated nucleus. Note the high reflective membrane attached to the disc suggestive of a retinal detachment (arrow). There is a high reflective biconvex structure behind the membrane, which represents the nucleus (arrowhead). Figure B shows the defect in the lower part of the retinal detachment (arrow) through which the nucleus has gained access to the subretinal space.

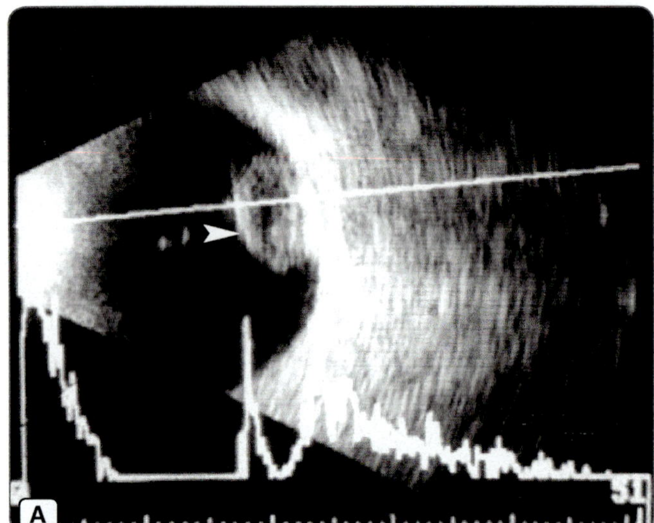
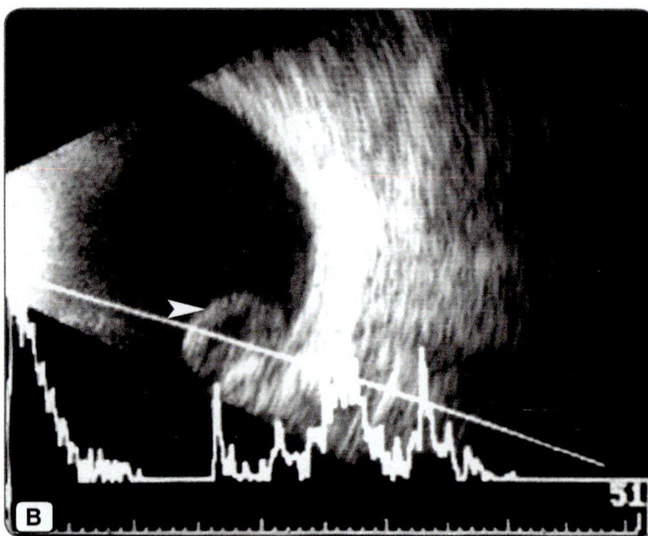

Figures 28.4A and B: B scan with vector of a patient with occlusio pupillae due to chronic uveitis. There is a globular lesion on the optic disc (arrowhead) in Figure A which is seen to move inferiorly with change in head posture, indicating that it is a mobile crystalline lens. There are low reflective echoes within the lens indicative of cataractous changes.

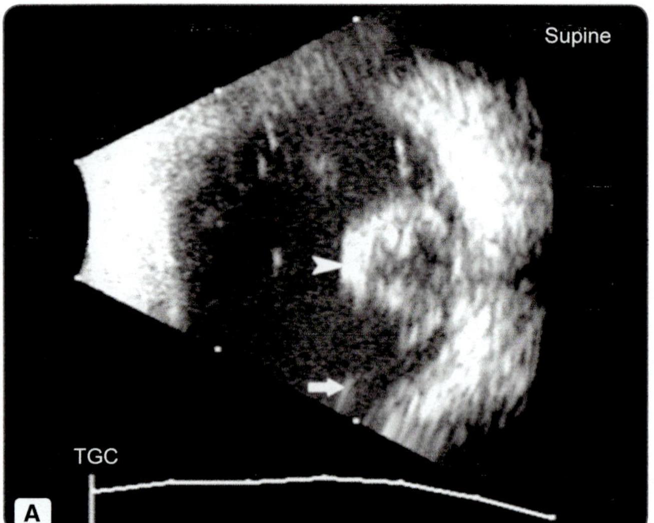

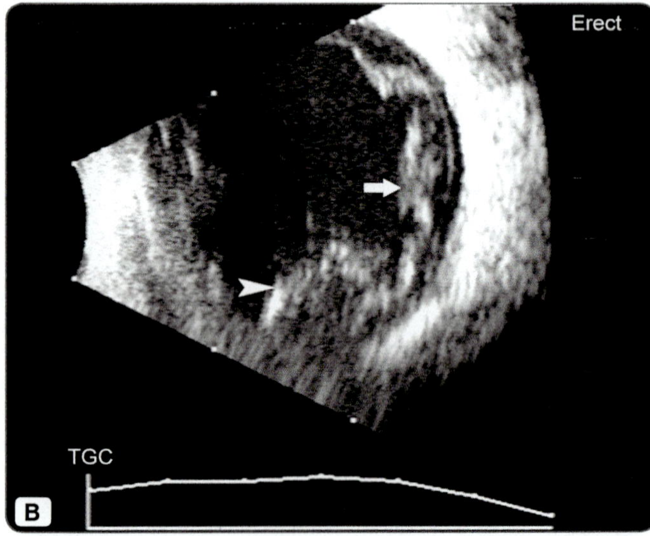

Figures 28.5A and B: B scan images of an eye with a posteriorly dislocated lens (arrowhead) and retinal detachment (arrow). Note the shift in position to the inferior vitreous cavity with change to erect posture. The intralesional echoes within the lens indicate that it is cataractous.

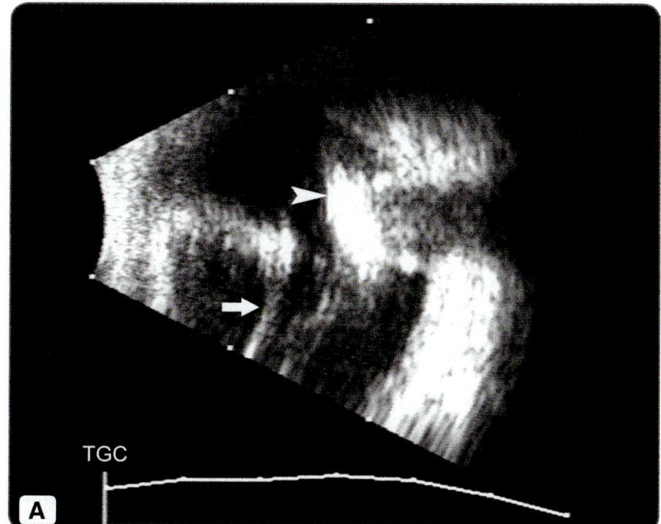

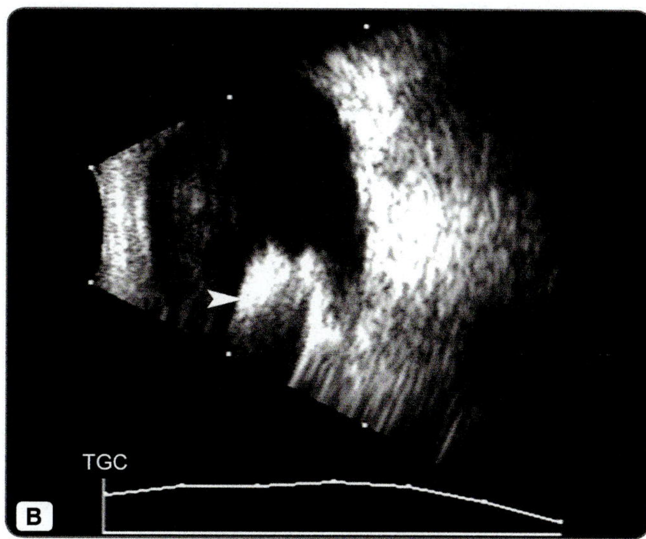

Figures 28.6A and B: B scan images of a patient with clinically diagnosed postoperative endophthalmitis. The vitreous shows significant echoes along with a complete PVD (arrow). There is a very high reflective structure on the posterior globe wall causing dense shadowing (arrowhead). It is seen to move downwards with erect posture. This represents a dislocated hard nucleus.

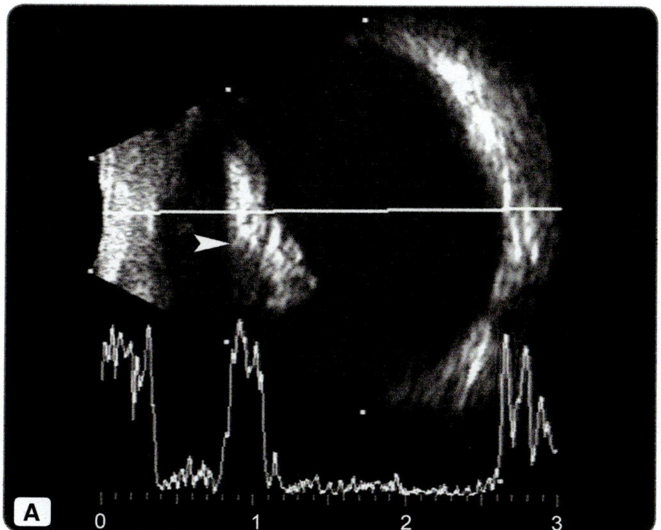

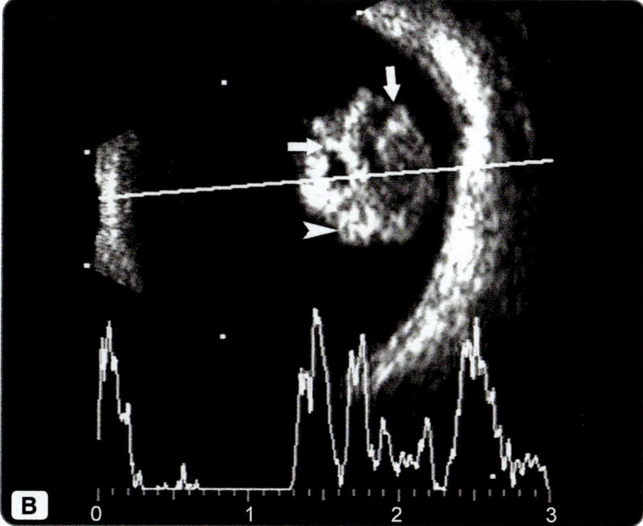

Figures 28.7A and B: B scan with vector A of an eye with dropped nucleus during phacoemulsification. The axial scan shows an irregular high reflective clump of echoes (arrowhead) which appear concave. The transverse scan shows the nuclear fragment (arrowhead) with echolucent areas within it (arrows) indicating the possible sites of trenching during phacofragmentation before the drop occurred.

29 Intraocular Air and Gas

CLINICAL SITUATIONS

Air or gas may be seen in the anterior chamber following trauma, cataract surgery and primary wound repair or in the vitreous cavity following vitreous surgery.

ULTRASONOGRAPHY

- A large air bubble may totally preclude any echographic examination of the posterior segment due to total internal reflection and intense shadowing
- Posterior segment evaluation may also be difficult because of multiple signals or reverberations
- Small air bubbles present as smooth and spherical structures with high surface reflectivity. These spherical shadows are commonly seen to float opposite to the direction of eye movement
- The erect posture may aid in providing some immediate information about the status of the posterior segment in the presence of a large gas bubble.

NUGGETS

Multiple air bubbles may be present and may mimic multiple spherical IOFBs such as air gun pellets.

Repeat ultrasonography 2-3 days later will show a reduction in size of large and possible disappearance of small air bubbles.

In contrast to freely mobile spherical air bubbles, those trapped in the Berger's space may be irregular shaped and relatively immobile.

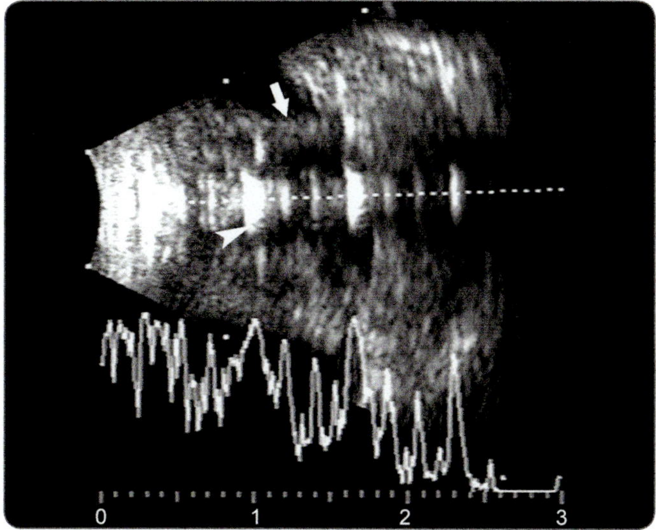

Figure 29.1: B scan image showing multiple echoes of varying reflectivity in the vitreous cavity in an eye with history of penetrating injury and wound repair. The A scan vector is passed through a chain of reverberations (arrowhead). These echoes are of relatively higher reflectivity than the rest of the intragel echoes. Also note the orbital shadowing caused in the path of the echoes. A membrane with echoes suggestive of a choroidal detachment (arrow) is seen superiorly.

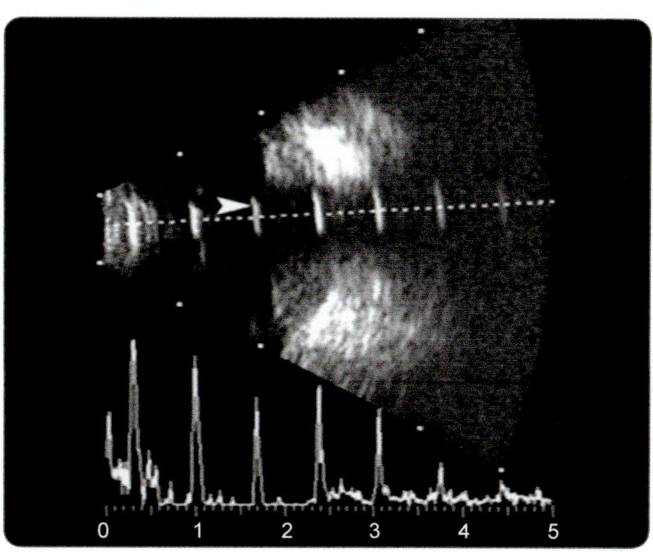

Figure 29.2: B scan image with vector A scan of the same patient after increasing the depth penetration of the probe. The reverberation echoes (arrowhead) are enhanced and are seen to extend into the orbit. The smooth shape of the reverberations, equidistant from each other and the uniform steady decay of the A spike amplitude of each succeeding echo suggest a spherical object such as air.

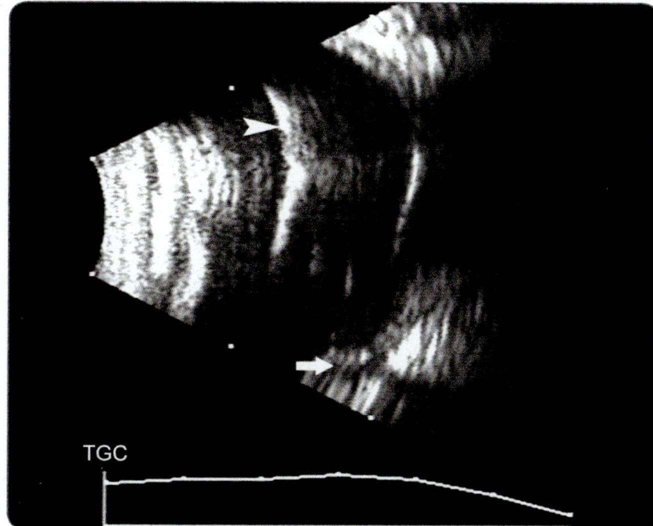

Figure 29.3: B scan image of a patient in the early postoperative period following scleral buckle and gas tamponade. The vitreous cavity shows a high reflective curvilinear echo, which shows reduplication (arrowhead). The echo is seen in the upper part of the echogram with the patient in the erect posture, which suggests that it is a gas bubble that floats up. Note the globe wall indentation inferiorly that is caused by a scleral buckle (arrow).

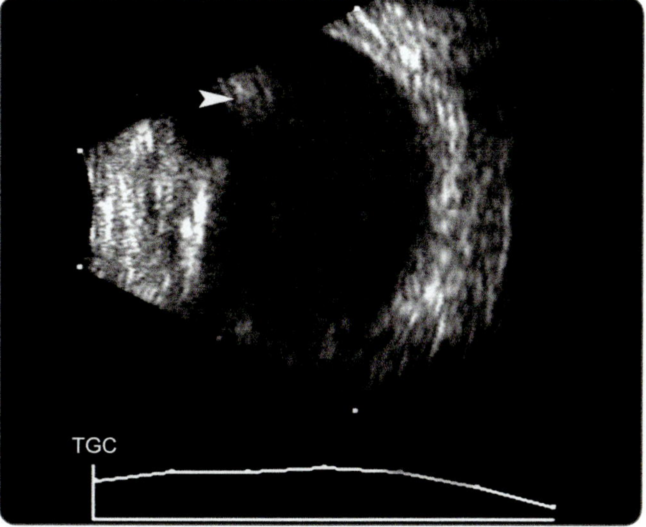

Figure 29.4: B scan image of the same eye 2 days later showing a very small set of echoes on the extreme upper part of the image (arrowhead). The rest of the vitreous cavity is clear. The rapid decrease in the size of the echoes within 2 days is indicative that it is an air bubble.

30 Silicone Oil

CLINICAL FEATURES

- Long-term tamponade used in vitreoretinal surgery for complex retinal detachments.
- Velocity of sound is lower in silicone oil than vitreous.
- Ultrasound may be required to assess the retinal status in silicone oil filled eyes with significant media opacity.

ULTRASONOGRAPHY

- Apparent lengthening of the globe.
- Silicone oil which is not emulsified produces pronounced sound attenuation and difficulty in imaging the retina.
- Emulsified oil presents as high reflective dot-like echoes similar to asteroid hyalosis.
- In the presence of an incomplete fill, the posterior surface of the oil bubble may be mistaken for the retinal surface.

NUGGETS

It is essential to make adjustments for the altered sound velocity of silicone oil (980 m/sec) compared to a normal eye (1,139—1052 m/sec) when calculating the IOL power in a silicone oil filled eye. The adjustments would be different based on the viscosity of the oil.

The depth penetration of the probe should be increased or the orbital settings used to get a better image of the posterior segment of a silicone oil filled eye.

An irregular posterior meniscus could indicate the presence of an underlying retinal detachment.

Performing the examination in an erect posture may give some information about the inferior retinal status as the silicone oil bubble floats up.

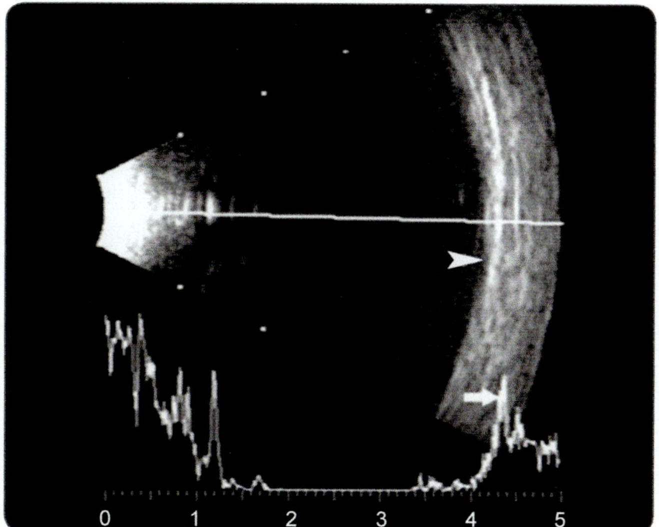

Figure 30.1: B scan image of an aphakic eye with a complete fill of silicone oil. Note the clear vitreous cavity indicating a single bubble. There is apparent lengthening of the eyeball as seen on the scale below (arrow). Also note that the depth has been increased to facilitate visualization of the posterior surface of the bubble (arrowhead) and the eyewall. Due to reverberation artifacts behind the bubble, which is in close contact with the globe wall, it is not possible to adequately assess the retinal status.

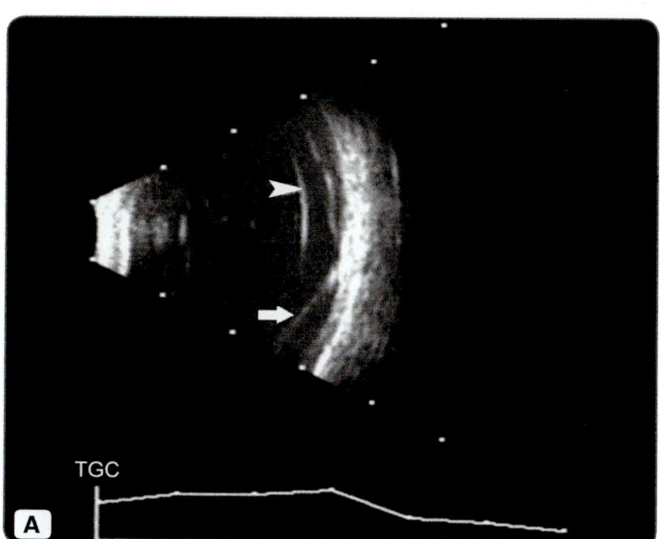

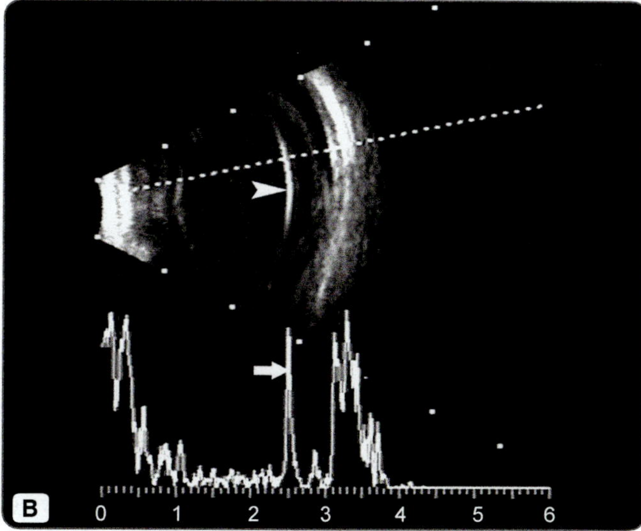

Figures 30.2A and B: B scan image of an eye with incomplete fill of silicone oil. In supine position the oil moves up toward the anterior part of the eye, and behind the meniscus (arrowhead) one is able to see the membrane echoes of a retinal detachment (arrow). In this case as well, it has been necessary to increase the depth penetration to visualize the posterior segment more accurately. In the second image, the 100% spike from the posterior surface of the oil bubble is seen, showing how this could be easily mistaken for the retinal spike if biometry is performed.

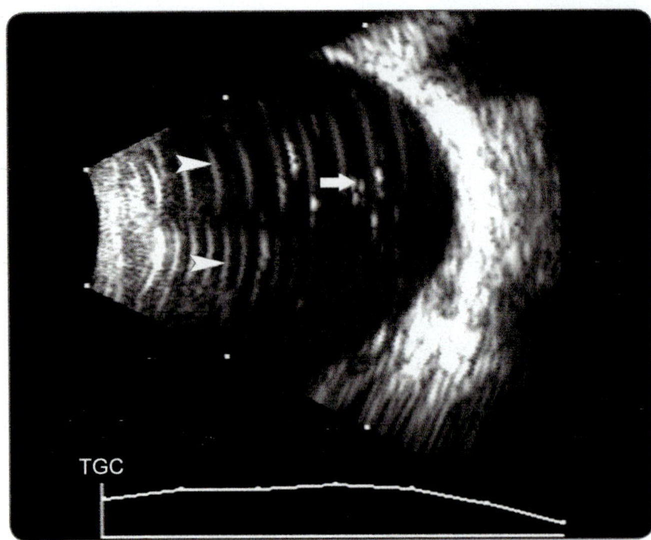

Figure 30.3: B scan image of an eye with residual silicone oil after its removal. Note the two sets of reverberation echoes from the anterior segment (arrowheads). These represent echoes from two bubbles of oil. In addition, there are a few high reflective dot-like echoes corresponding to tiny emulsified droplets (arrow). The shadow of an encircling band is seen inferiorly.

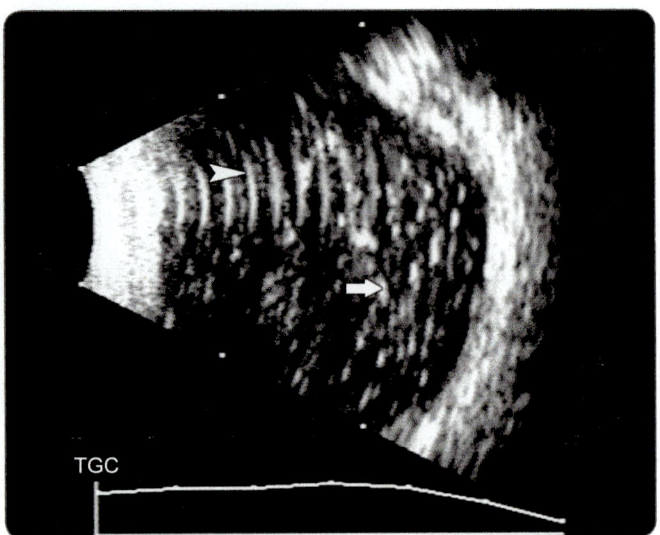

Figure 30.4: Significant residual emulsified droplets (arrow) in an eye following silicone oil removal. In addition, there is a single larger bubble present anteriorly causing strong reverberation echoes (arrowhead). The buckle effect with indentation is seen superiorly.

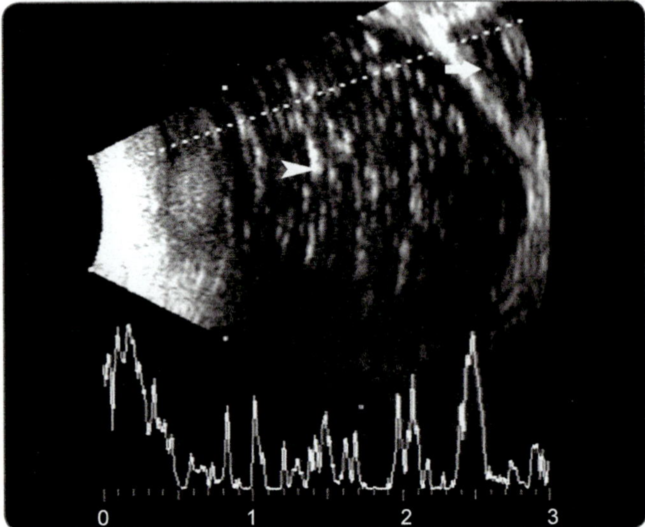

Figure 30.5: B scan with vector A showing the vitreous cavity filled with high reflective echoes (arrowhead) signifying emulsified droplets in an eye following oil removal. The solid silicone buckle effect (arrow) is seen superiorly.

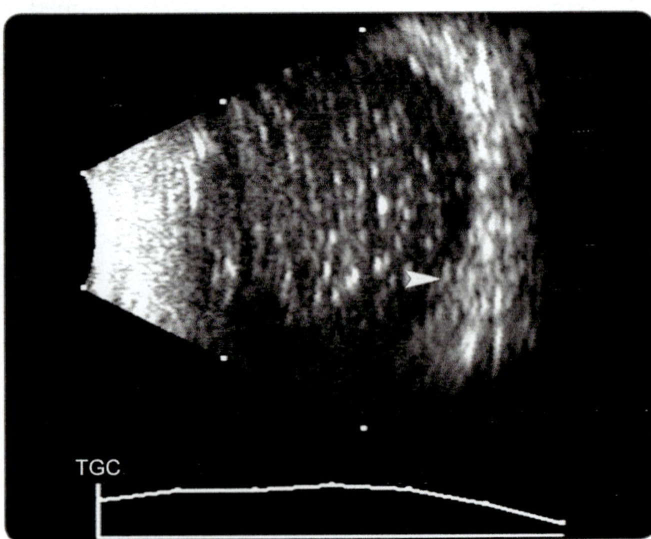

Figure 30.6: B scan showing the vitreous cavity filled with emulsified oil. It is easy to mistake this for asteroid hyalosis; however in this case, there is no echolucent space between the echoes (arrowhead) and the posterior globe wall.

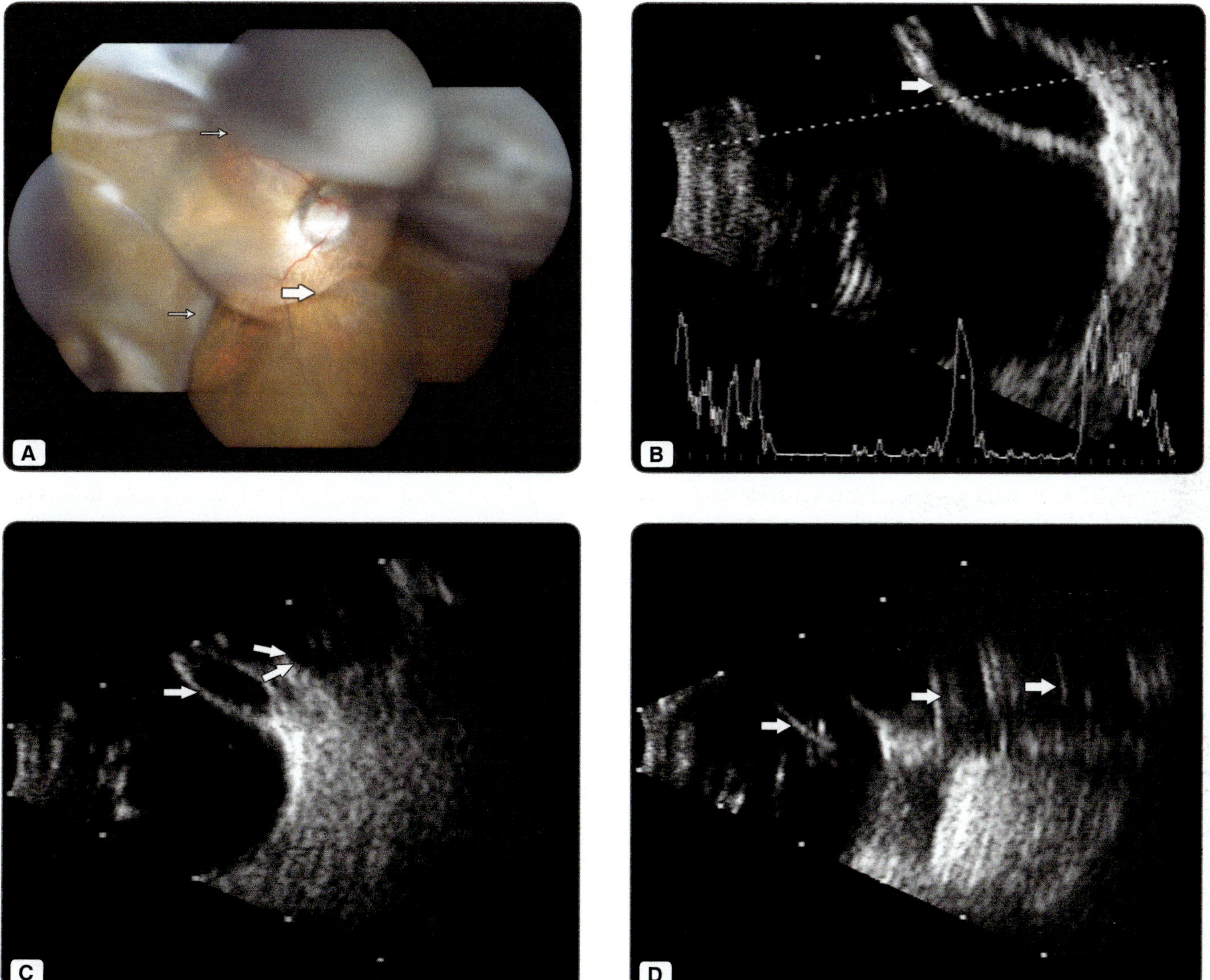

Figures 30.7A to D: Fundus montage of a patient with persistent choroidal detachment 6 months after apparently uneventful vitreous surgery with silicone oil. Note the underfill of oil (arrow) and large choroidal mounds (thin arrows). The B scan ultrasound image shows an echolucent mound corresponding to the choroidal detachment (arrow in Figure B). Figures C and D demonstrate the presence of echolucency in the orbit with reverberations and shadowing (Fig. C and D arrows) caused by the suprachoroidal oil.

31 Scleral Buckle

CLINICAL FEATURES

- A buckle element is often used in retinal reattachment surgery with or without vitrectomy.
- The complications associated with this are mainly exposure, intrusion or infection.
- Ultrasonography may be required to detect the presence of a buckle and note its extent, if surgery details are not available.

ULTRASONOGRAPHY

- Scleral buckles produce a characteristic sonographic picture.
- Indentation is seen all around the globe anteriorly in cases of 360 degree encirclage.
- Local area of indentation is obvious in cases of segmental circumferential buckles.
- These silicone elements show high surface reflectivity with orbital shadowing behind, thus appearing as an echolucent space.
- Silicone sponge has different echographic features. The air filled cavities in these buckling materials give a characteristic hyperechoic shadow.
- It may be possible to distinguish an area of echolucency around the buckle if there is associated scleritis and buckle infection.
- The extent of a buckle can be made out if removal is planned, especially if the primary surgery has been done elsewhere or partial removal has been done and no details are available. This is important as the buckle effect seen internally persists for months to years after removal.

NUGGETS

An encircling band may mimic senile scleral calcific plaques on ultrasound; however, these are usually seen only at the horizontal meridian unlike the band which can be seen all around.

Scleral folds and scleral buckles, especially scleral sponges have similar appearances on ultrasound—in case of scleral folds, other features of severe hypotony will also be present.

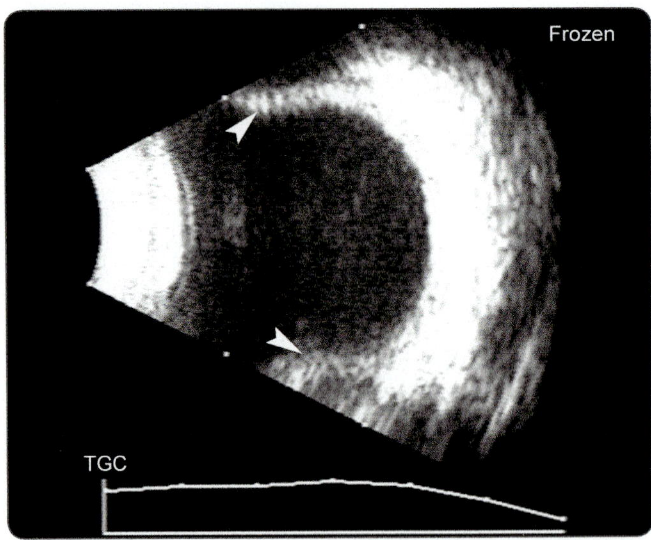

Figure 31.1: B scan image of a patient with a 360 degree encircling band. Note the uniform indentation of the globe caused by the encircling element (arrowheads).

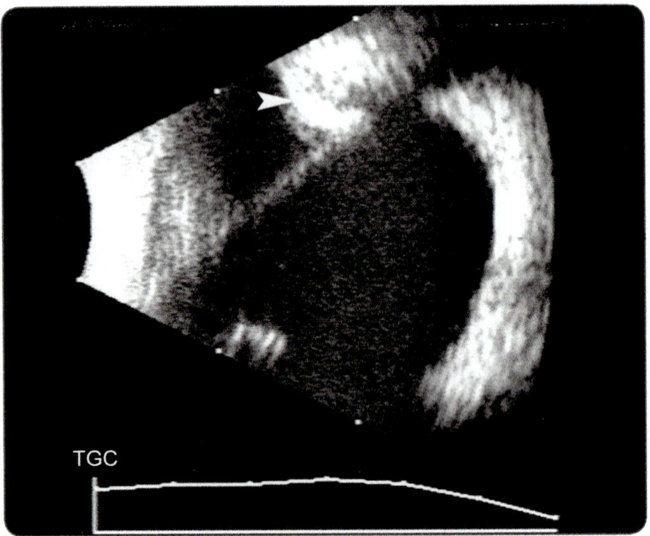

Figure 31.2: B scan image showing globe indentation caused by a silicone sponge. Note the very high reflectivity (arrowhead) due to the presence of air spaces within the sponge. An edge artifact is seen from the lens to the edge of the sponge.

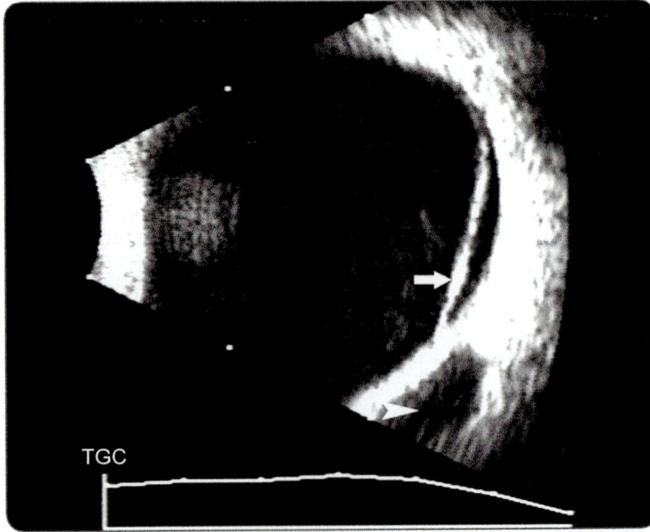

Figure 31.3: B scan image showing a partial retinal detachment (arrow) posterior to a solid silicone buckle. The solid silicone has a high surface reflectivity and very low to absent internal reflectivity (arrowhead) due to the absence of interfaces within it.

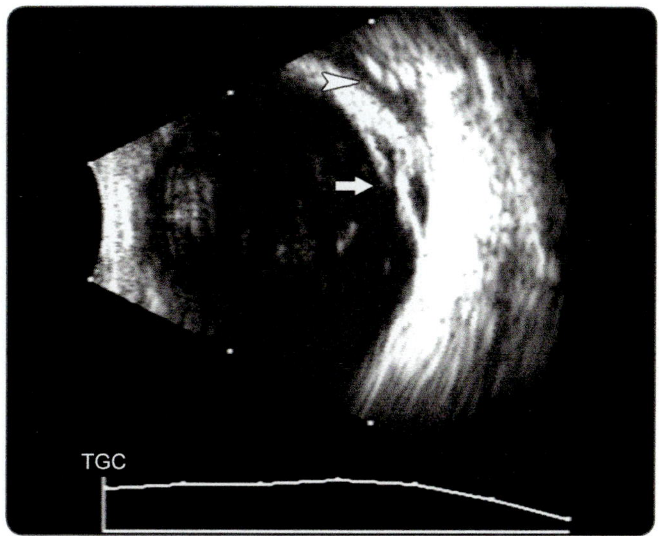

Figure 31.4: B scan image of an eye with a retinal detachment and open break on the surface of a solid silicone buckle (arrowhead). Note the high reflective membrane posterior to the buckle. The break is seen as a discontinuity in the membrane (arrow), which is lifted away from the surface.

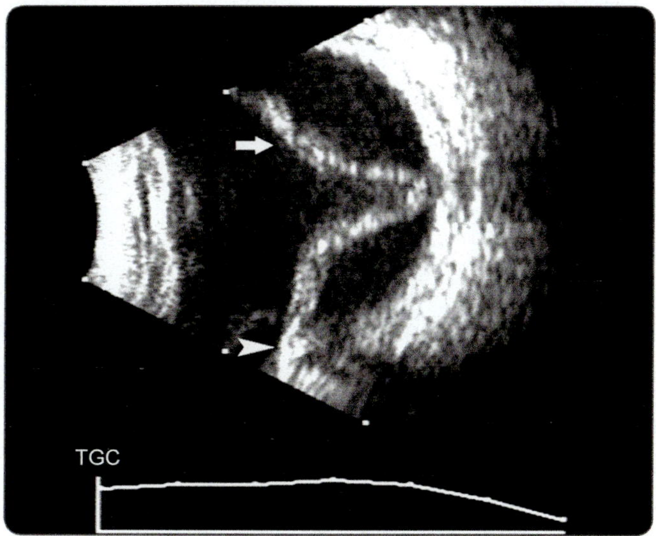

Figure 31.5: B scan image showing a total retinal detachment (arrow) in an eye with an encircling element. Note that the detachment extends anterior to the buckle (arrowhead).

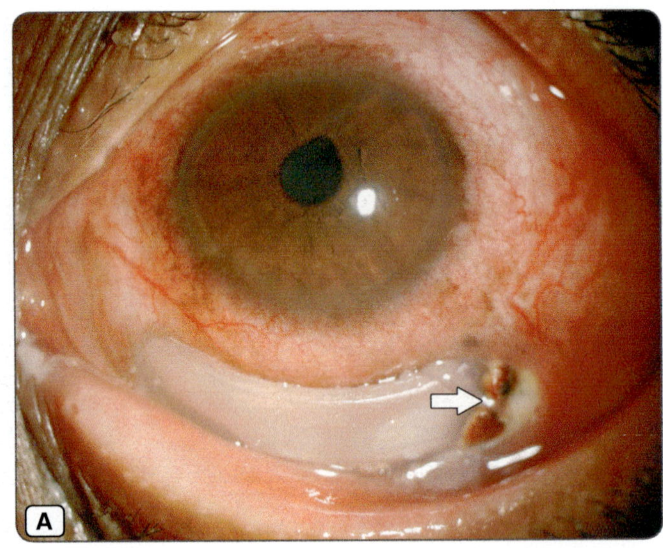

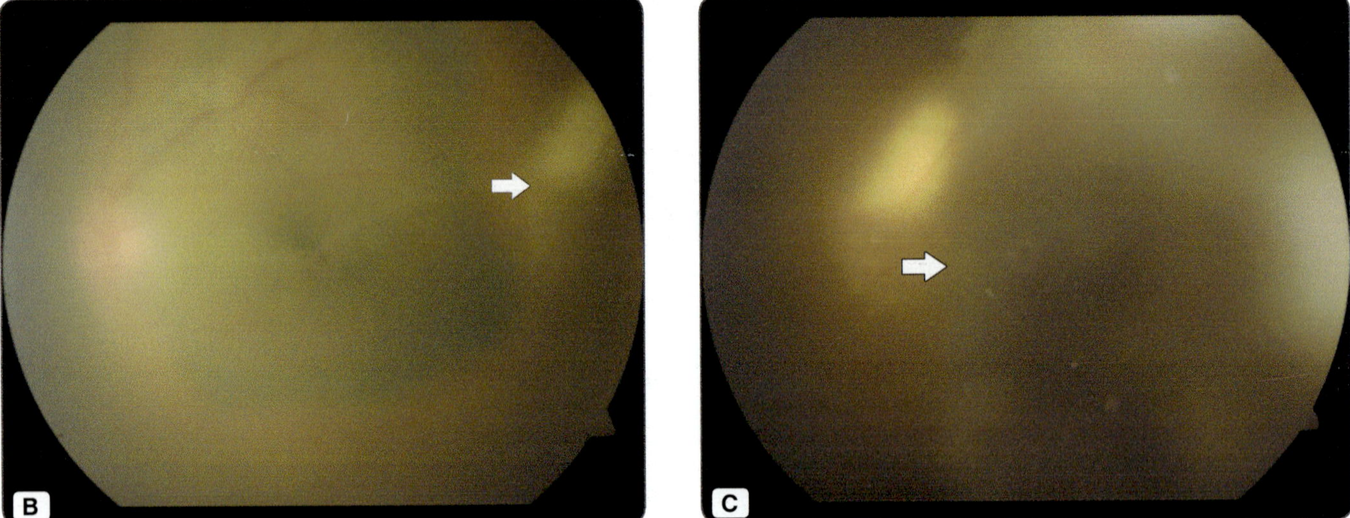

Figures 31.6A to C: External photograph and fundus pictures of a patient with exposed scleral buckle and painful drop in vision seven years after surgery. Note the blackish material at the junction of the exposed and unexposed buckle (arrow). Figures B and C show the vitreous haze with exudation temporally (arrow) and a mass like lesion anterior to it (arrow in Figure C)

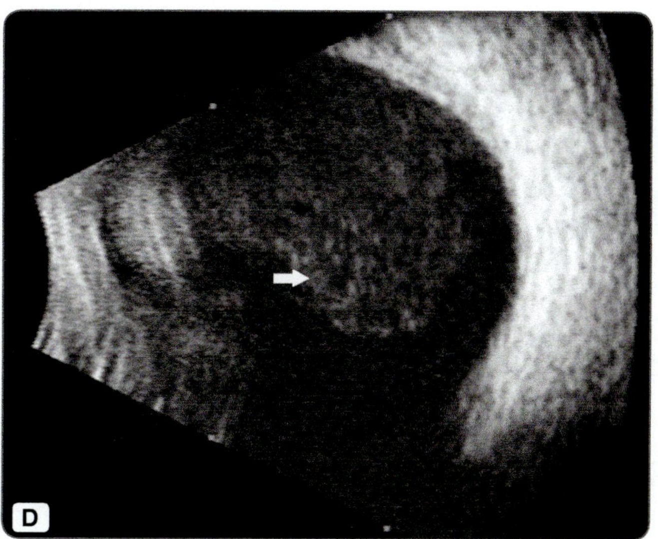

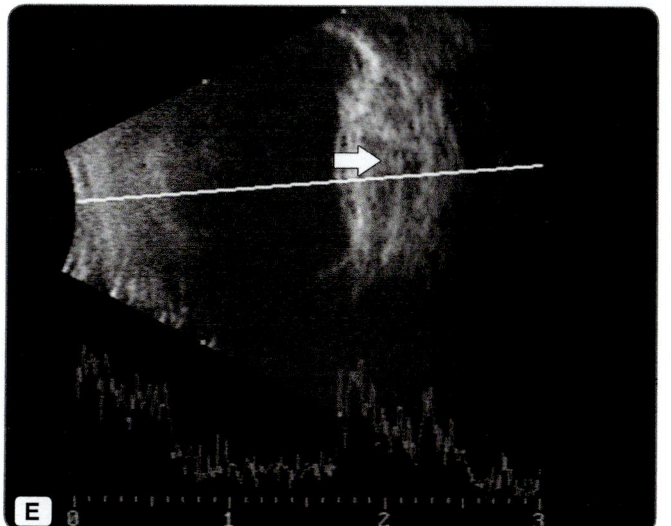

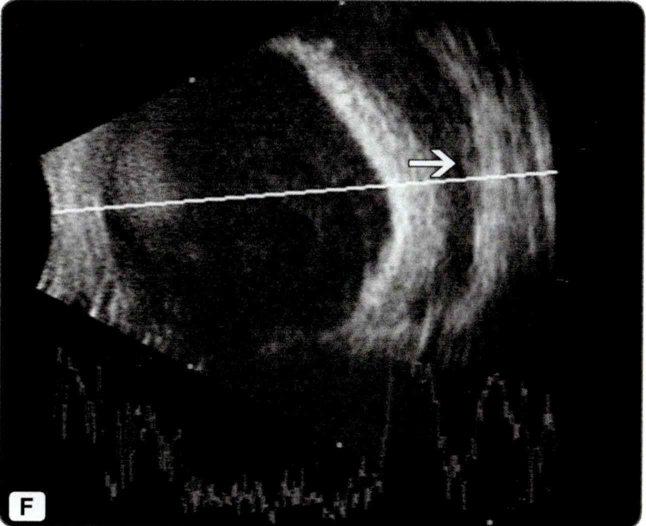

Figures 31.6D to F: B scan images of the same eye showing vitreous echoes suggestive of inflammation (arrow in Figure D). Figure E shows a temporal mass-like lesion of variable reflectivity and an area of echolucency suggestive of the solid silicone buckle element (arrow). Figrue F shows the appearance of the expose segment of buckle – seen as an echolucent structure with no evidence of inflammation or damage to the surrounding areas.

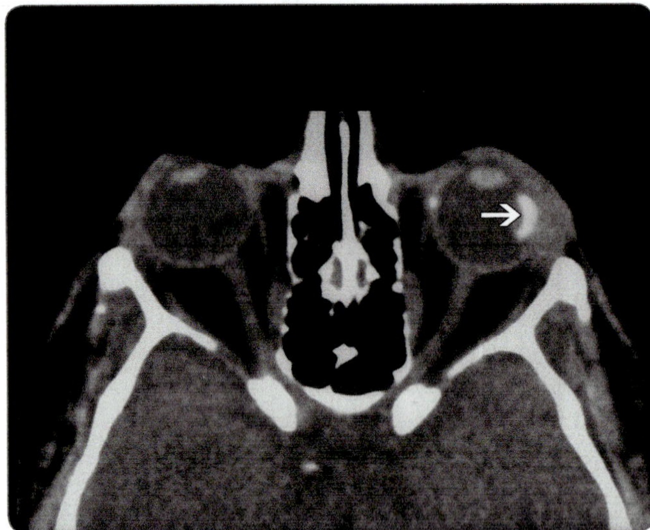

Figure 31.6G: CT scan shows a soft tissue mass around the scleral buckle continuous with the lateral rectus insertion

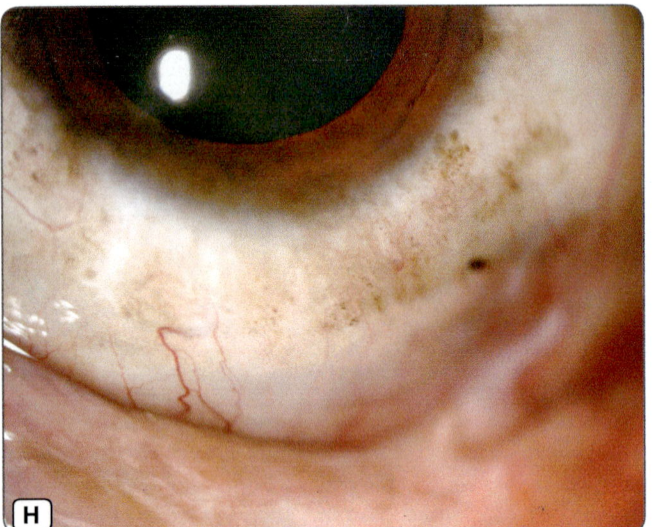

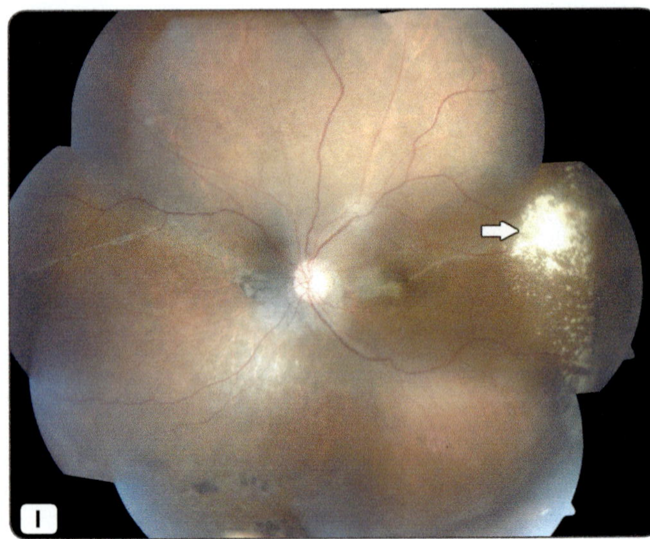

Figures 31.6H and I: The same patient after removal of the buckle and treatment with topical and systemic antifungals (the culture of the buckle element and discharge showed Aspergillus species). The eye is quiet. The fundus montage shows that the media is clear, retina attached with few residual hard exudates (arrow) . The persistence of buckle effect is seen anterior to the exudates (thin arrow)

32 B Scan and Axial Biometry

There are certain situations when axial biometry may result in erroneous or bizarre readings. Here, it may be necessary to perform a B scan evaluation to aid in accurate axial length calculations.

- **Asteroid hyalosis**. The presence of dense asteroids can cause high reflective spikes on the A scan causing an erroneous decreased axial length with the automatic method of biometry. A B scan in the presence of a total cataract or clinical information regarding the presence of asteroids can help in avoiding this problem. Use of the manual method of biometry can also avoid this error.
- **Retinal detachment**. This can be suspected if the retinal spike is weak or there is a significantly shorter axial length compared to the fellow eye in the absence of anisometropia. Here a B scan would confirm the diagnosis.
- **Coloboma choroid and posterior staphyloma**. A B scan would be helpful in localizing the coloboma or staphyloma in relation to the macula thereby confirming the correct axial length. This would also explain a poor retinal spike if the macula lies on the slope of the staphyloma or the edge of the coloboma.
- **Macular lesions** which are elevated may cause a decrease in axial length compared to the fellow eye. In such cases a B scan confirmation is useful, especially if the fellow eye has macular edema or macular degeneration.
- **Silicone oil filled eyes**. In the absence of a positive history and a total cataract, it may be difficult to calculate the axial length. Here a B scan evaluation could provide some information regarding the presence of intraocular silicone oil and enable the appropriate velocity adjustments for biometry.
- **Intraocular air.** This is particularly important if cataract surgery is planned in an eye with traumatic cataract that has recently undergone a wound repair with injection of air to make up the volume. A B scan confirmation would help in assessing the retinal spike and avoiding an erroneous decrease in the axial length.
- Serial axial length measurements are performed in eyes with **congenital glaucoma** - this also serves to differentiate between progressive myopia and glaucoma. B scan can be done without anesthesia; it can rule out a posterior staphyloma which can be the cause of the increased axial length. B scan can also be used to diagnose optic disc cupping in an eye with a hazy cornea or cataract.

NUGGETS

Confirm axial lengths with a B scan in an eye with unilateral cataract and decreased axial length on biometry—it may have an underlying retinal detachment.

Take a detailed history regarding anisometropia, injury or previous ocular surgery before performing biometry.

Always compare biometry readings with those of the fellow eye.

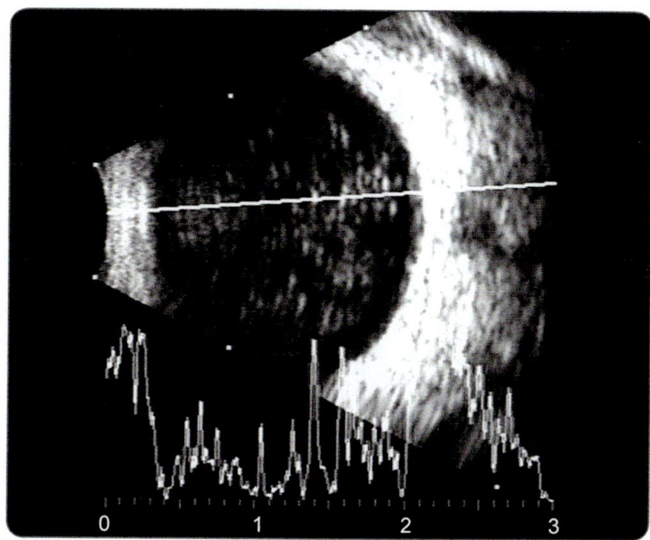

Figure 32.1: Axial B scan with vector A of an eye with asteroid hyalosis. Note the high reflective point like echoes in the vitreous cavity with corresponding 100% reflective spikes on the A scan. Any of these high spikes may be mistaken for the scleral spike during A scan biometry, thus giving a falsely reduced axial length.

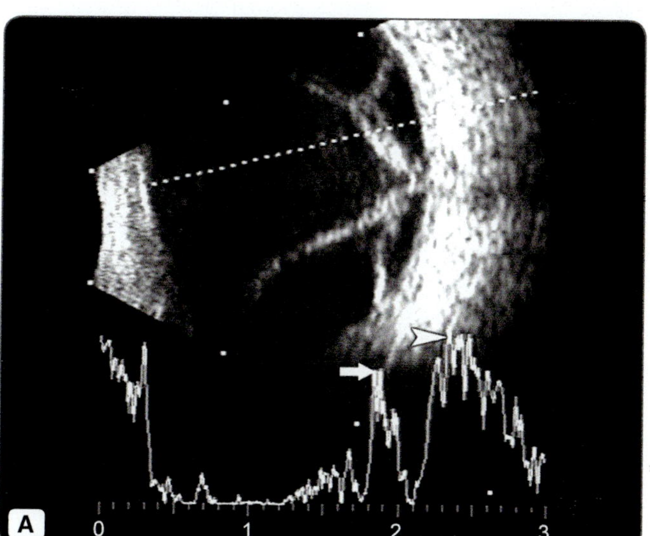

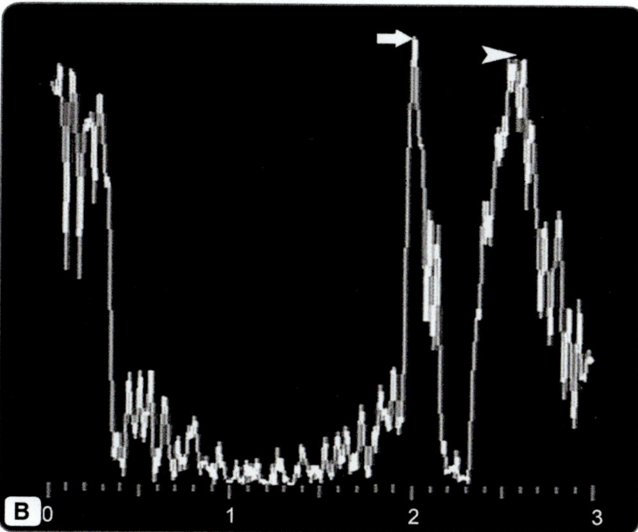

Figures 32.2A and B: Axial B scan with vector A in an eye with a posterior pole tractional retinal detachment. The A scan spike through the detachment is of high reflectivity (arrow). This can be mistaken for a scleral spike when biometry is performed. The correct scleral spike is shown as an arrowhead.

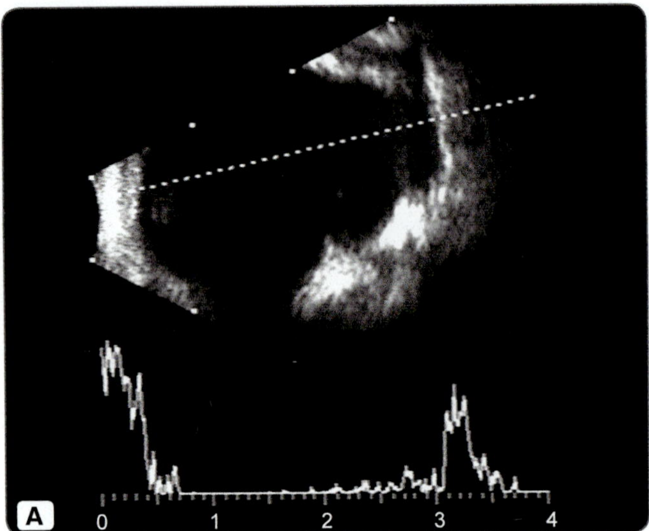

Figure 32.3A: Axial B scan image in an eye with a large choroidal coloboma. Note the irregularly rising poor A scan spike from the scleral surface.

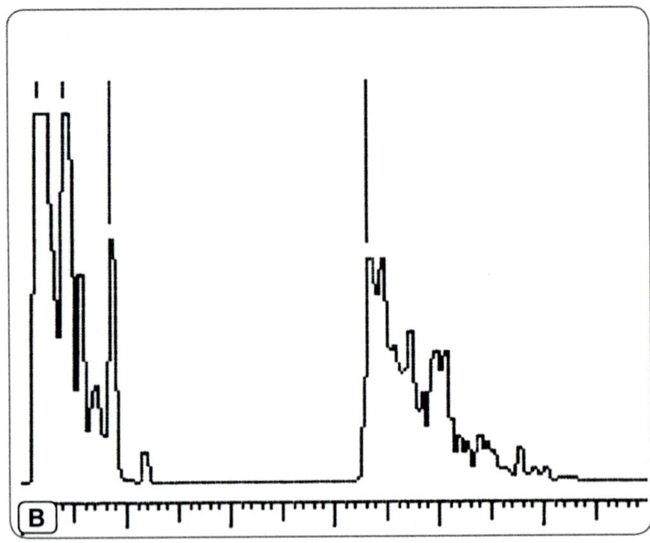

Figure 32.3B: A scan biometry reading from an eye with myopia and a posterior staphyloma. Note that the retinal spike is not as high as expected. Also note the increased axial length.

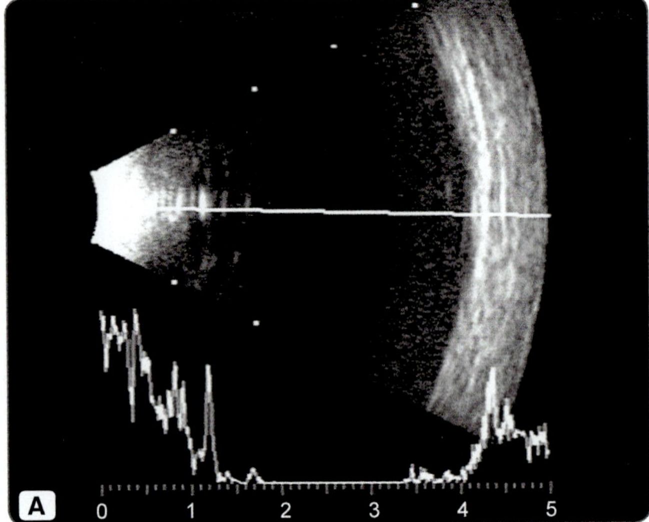

Figure 32.4A: Axial B scan with vector A of an aphakic eye with complete silicone oil fill. Note the apparent increase in axial length and an absence of clear echoes from the globe wall.

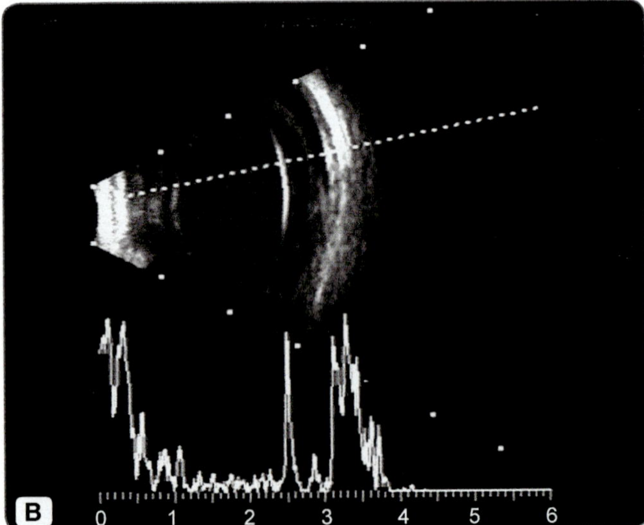

Figure 32.4B: Axial B scan with vector A in an eye with an incomplete fill of silicone oil. The A vector shows a high spike corresponding to the posterior surface of the oil bubble with the patient in supine position. There is a second high reflective spike from the globe wall seen beyond this. This can give a false value if picked up on biometry.

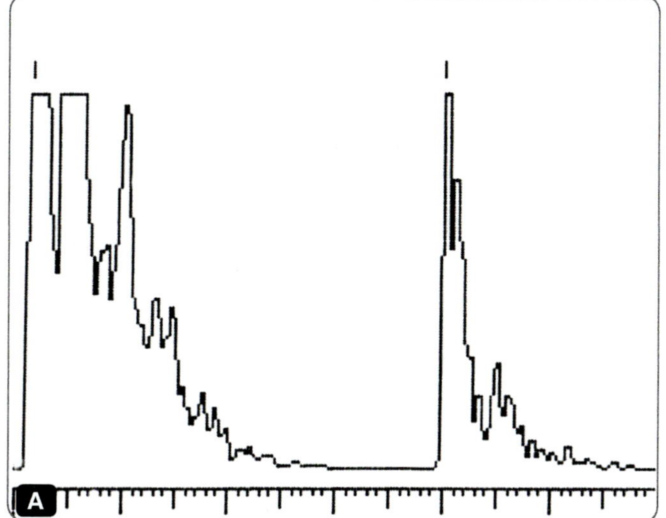

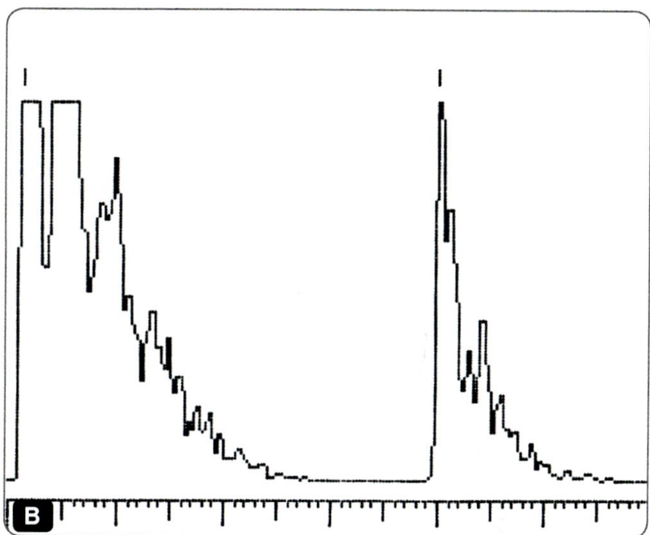

Figures 32.5A and B: Biometry readings of an aphakic silicone oil filled eye. Note the grossly increased axial length if the standard sound velocity is used. Figure 32.5B shows the corrected value when the velocity reading is changed to 980 m/sec for silicone oil.

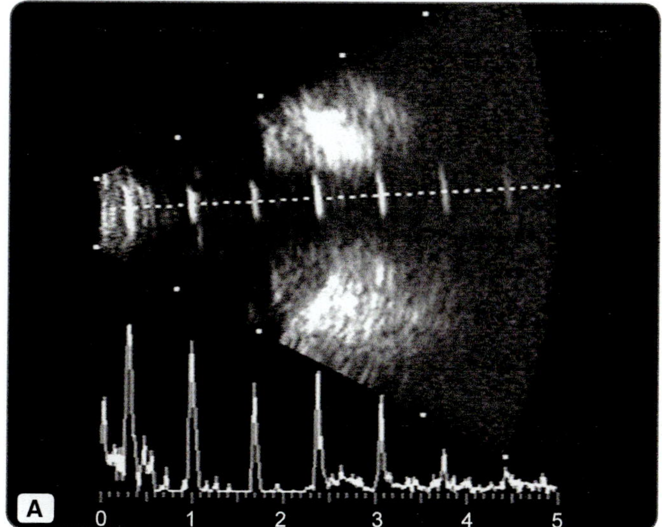

Figure 32.6A: B scan with vector A of an eye with intraocular gas. Note the high spikes in the vitreous cavity caused by the reverberations from the gas bubble.

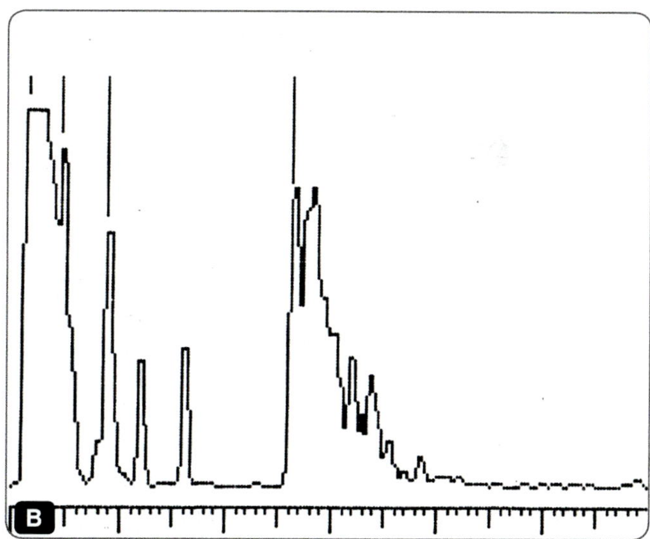

Figure 32.6B: Biometry tracing of an eye with intraocular gas. There are moderate reflective spikes in the vitreous from the gas bubble.

Section 8

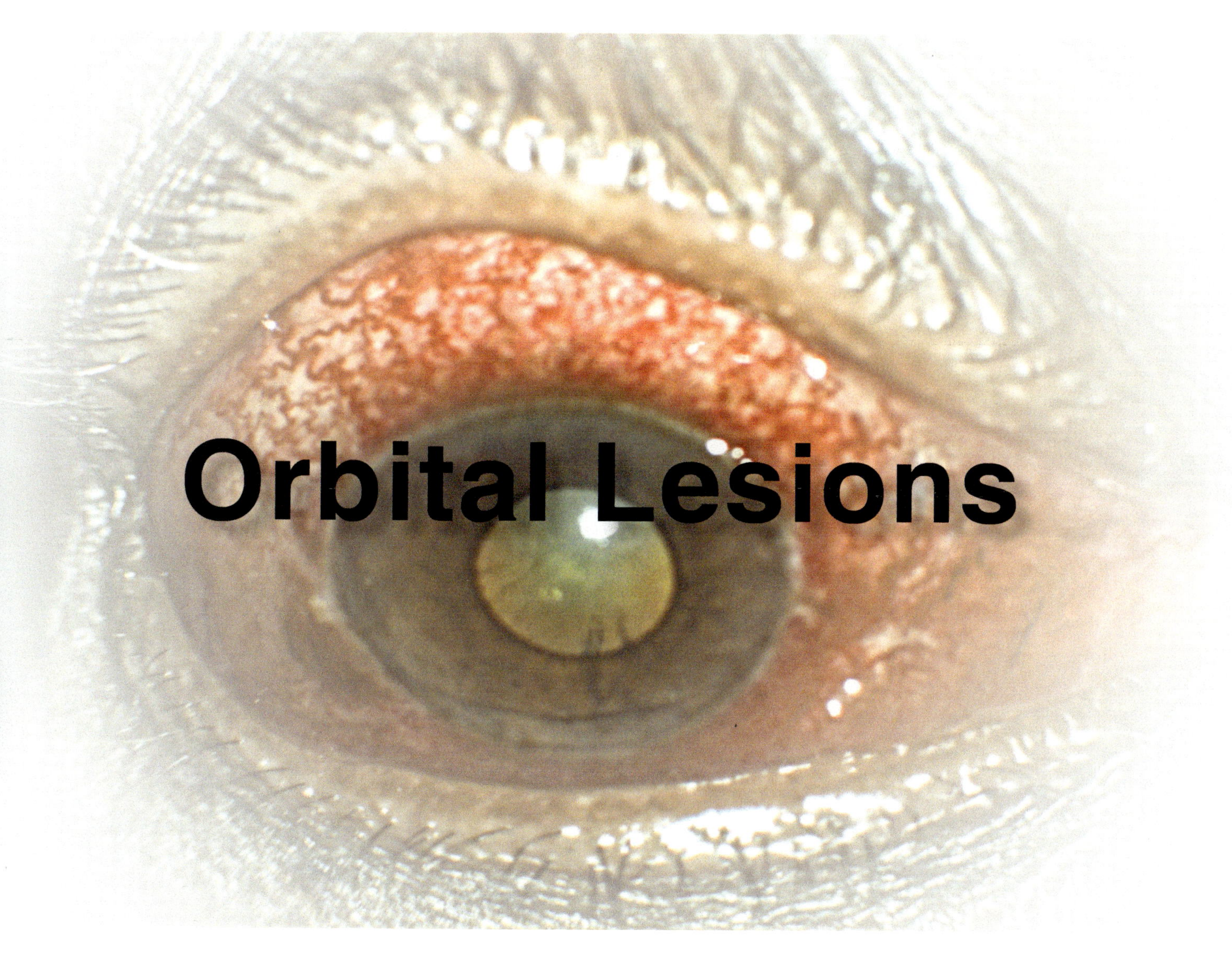

Orbital Lesions

33 Disorders of Extraocular Muscles

INDICATIONS

- Detection of extraocular muscle thickening is probably the most common indication for orbital echography.
- Echography is a useful tool for differentiating causes of muscle enlargement.
- Helps follow-up of even subtle changes in muscle thickness, and identifies a localised pathology if present.

COMMON CAUSES OF EOM ENLARGEMENT

- Grave's orbitopathy
- Idiopathic orbital myositis
- Congestion
- Tumors (e.g. metastatic carcinoma)
- Hematoma.

THYROID RELATED ORBITOPATHY (TRO)

Clinical Features

- The most common cause of unilateral or bilateral proptosis.
- Can occur either in the presence (90%) or absence (6%) of detectable thyroid dysfunction.
- Bilateral but asymmetrical in most cases.
- Females are 6 times more affected than males.
- Clinical features are due to soft tissue swelling and infiltration, myopathy, apical compression, abnormalities of lid position and corneal changes.
- Lid retraction is the most frequent clinical sign.
- Myopathy typically affects the muscle belly thus involving the middle and posterior orbit.
- Apical compression leading to optic nerve dysfunction and severe proptosis leading to exposure keratopathy are ophthalmic emergencies.

Ultrasonography

- Helps confirm the diagnosis and is useful in following the response to therapy.
- Characteristic fusiform thickening of the muscle belly is seen which typically spares the tendon.
- The earliest muscle involved echographically is the superior rectus–LPS complex.
- The thickened muscle is highly reflective due to deposition of hydrophilic mucopolysaccharides. This, along with inflammatory edema creates interfaces within the bundles of muscle fibers which themselves are infiltrated by inflammatory cells.
- Increase in the amount of orbital fat, enlargement of the lacrimal gland and dilatation of the superior ophthalmic vein due to apical crowding are other features.

NUGGETS

Look carefully for enlarged SR-LPS complex in a patient with lid retraction.

Reduce the gain to delineate the high reflective muscle sheath from the high reflective orbital tissue.

Examine and measure all muscles on both sides for comparison as findings are typically asymmetrical.

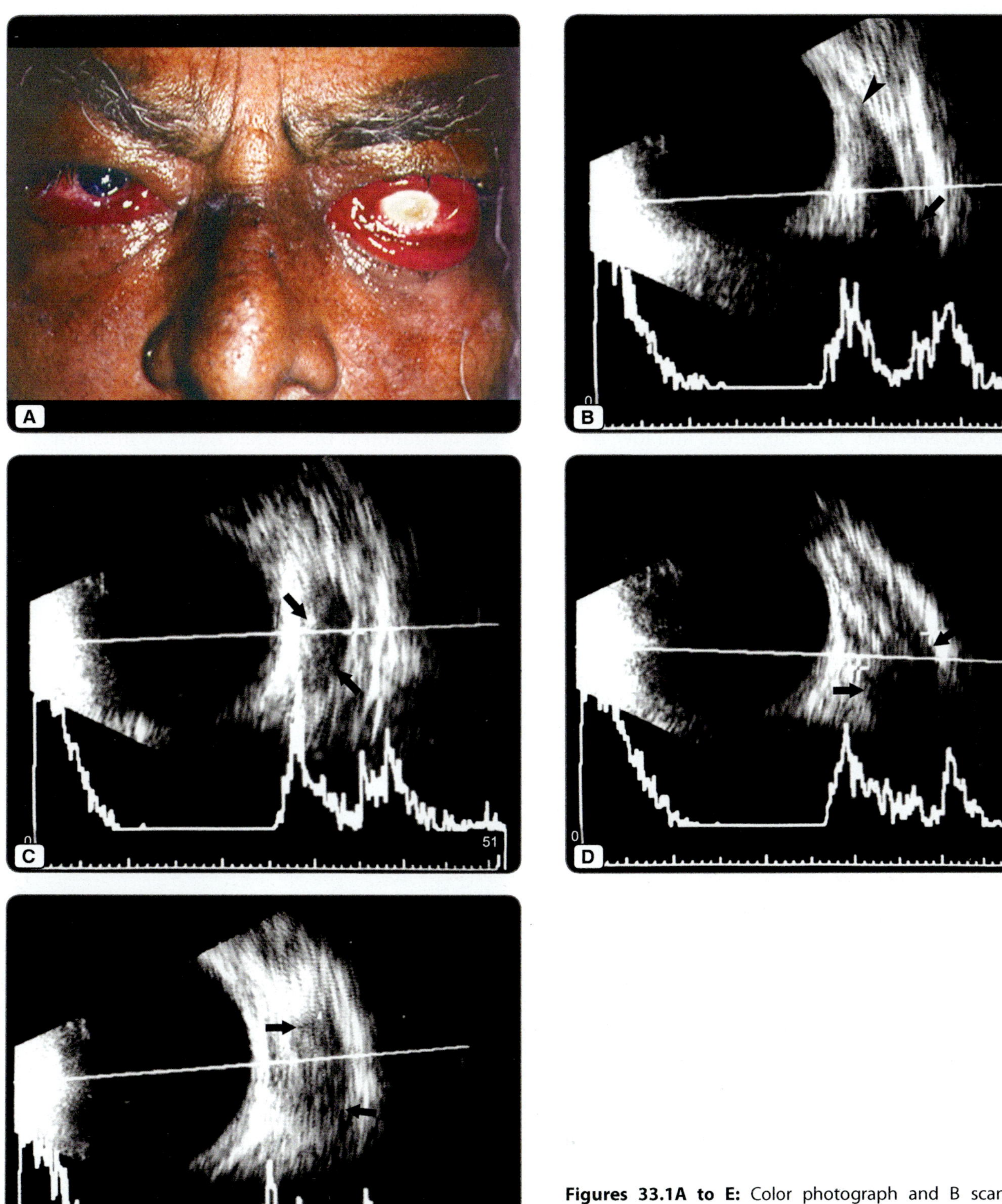

Figures 33.1A to E: Color photograph and B scan images of a patient with severe thyroid orbitopathy and exposure keratopathy in the left eye. Longitudinal and transverse images of the medial rectus muscle (Figs B and C) and superior rectus–LPS complex (Figs D and E) show thickening of the muscle belly (arrow). The tendon appears normal (arrowhead).

IDIOPATHIC ORBITAL MYOSITIS

Clinical Features

- Important cause of painful proptosis
- Unilateral or bilateral, acute or chronic
- Can be isolated, or associated with other features of orbital or ocular inflammation
- Ultrasound is indicated to diagnose the condition and differentiate it from muscle enlargement in thyroid orbitopathy.

Ultrasonography

- Diffuse thickening of one or more extraocular muscles
- Involvement of the tendon and belly is characteristic
- Internal reflectivity is homogenous and low, due to diffuse infiltration of the muscle fibers by inflammatory cells
- Adjacent involvement of the episclera in the form of Tenon's widening may be seen
- In addition, lacrimal gland enlargement and optic nerve thickening may occur.

NUGGETS

Always measure the thickness of the muscle at the site of maximum enlargement.

Ensure that the same location is chosen on subsequent visits.

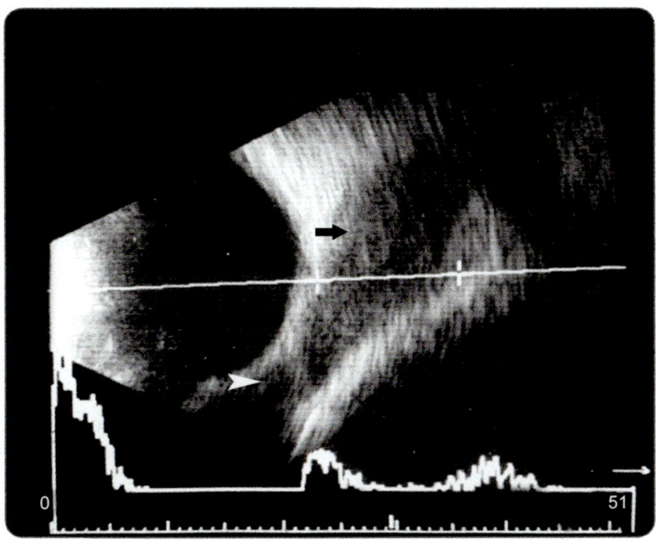

Figure 33.2: B scan with vector A scan showing low reflective muscle thickening in an eye with idiopathic myositis of the medial rectus muscle. Note the involvement of the entire extent of the muscle (arrow = muscle belly, arrowhead = tendon) including tendon.

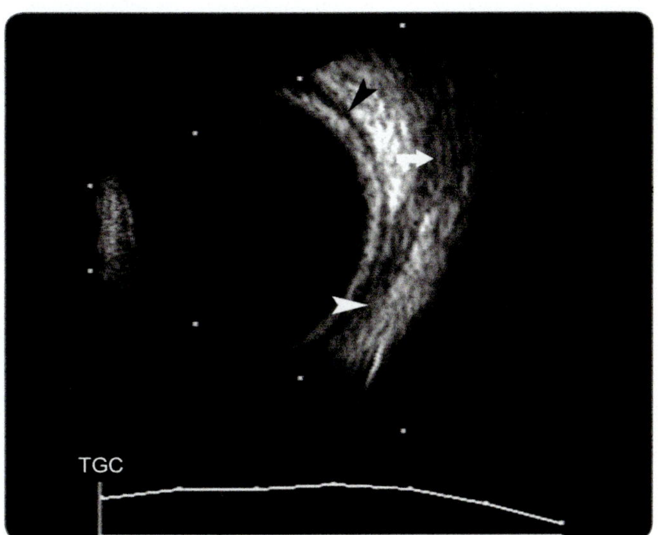

Figure 33.3: B scan image showing thickening of the muscle belly (arrow), tendon (white arrowhead) and episclera (black arrowhead) in an eye with idiopathic orbital inflammation. Note the Tenon's widening along with low reflective thickening of the tendon, in contrast to TRO.

METASTASES TO EXTRAOCULAR MUSCLES

Clinical Features

- Breast and lung cancers account for the majority of orbital metastases
- Present with pain, proptosis, inflammation, bone destruction or ophthalmoplegia
- Twenty five percent are from an undetected primary tumor
- Extraocular muscles are the most commonly involved structures in the orbit
- Fine needle aspiration biopsy (FNAB) can often confirm the diagnosis.

Ultrasonography

- Unilateral or bilateral involvement
- Commonly involves the muscle belly
- Homogenous structure with uniform low to medium reflectivity.

NUGGETS

Metastases may often present with pain, in which case they may be confused with pseudotumor. However, in the latter, other features of inflammation may be present.

Prostate metastases may exactly resemble pseudotumor on ultrasound, so a high index of suspicion is necessary.

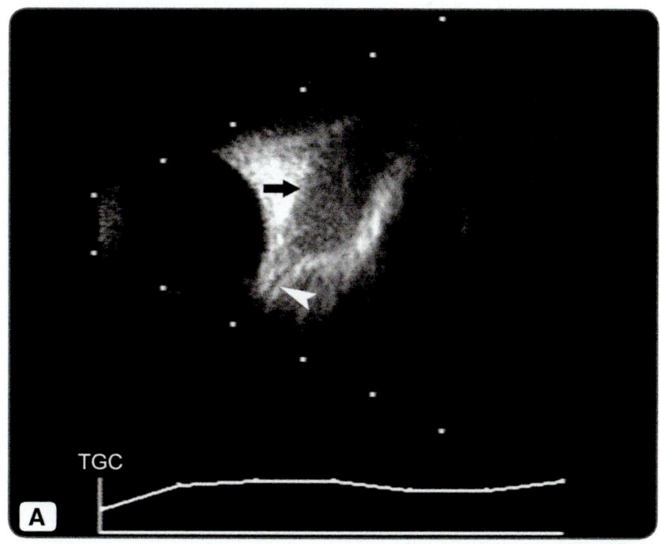

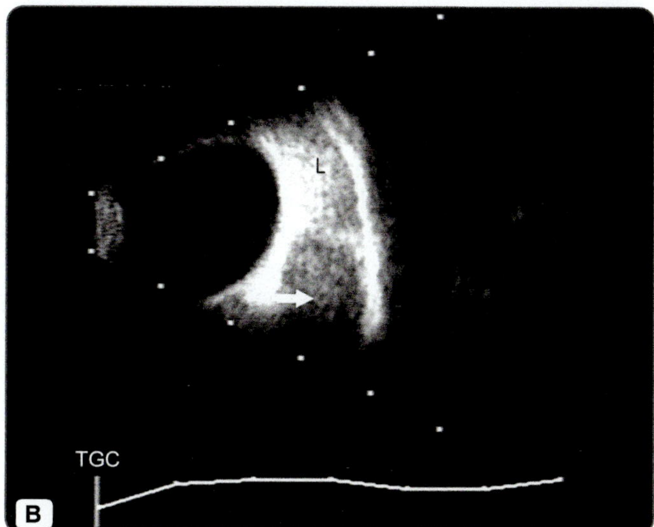

Figures 33.4A and B: B scan images of a patient with orbital metastasis from carcinoma breast. Figure A shows the homogenous thickening of the muscle belly (arrow) of the lateral rectus. The tendon (arrowhead) is uninvolved. In addition, the patient also had enlargement of the lacrimal gland (L). Biopsy specimen confirmed the presence of metastasis.

34 Orbital Cysticercosis

CLINICAL FEATURES

- Cysticercosis is caused by *Cysticercus cellulosae*, the larval form of the pork tapeworm, *Taenia solium.*
- Although posterior segment involvement is the most common, cysticercosis may affect any part of the visual system from orbit to visual cortex.
- Orbital cysticercosis can present with painful restriction of ocular movements or diplopia. It may also be present as a subconjunctival mass.

ULTRASONOGRAPHY

- Well outlined round to oval echolucent cyst.
- Echo dense nodule adjacent to the inner wall of the cyst representing the scolex.
- Preferentially involves the muscle belly, but can involve the orbital soft tissues as well. The shape of the cyst wall is irregular and may mould to the globe contour in case of soft tissue involvement.
- The scolex is the first to disappear with adequate medical therapy with albendazole, followed by the cyst itself.
- Serial ultrasounds can be performed to note the treatment response.

NUGGETS

Cysticercosis of the orbit is almost always unilateral and unifocal, though bilaterality has been described.

It is important to rule out neurocysticercosis if ocular or orbital cysticercosis has been diagnosed.

With response to therapy, the scolex becomes less highly reflective and smaller in size before it disappears.

Cysticercosis of the superior oblique muscle is difficult to diagnose as the trochlea itself may mimic a scolex. This is important if myositis involves the superior oblique.

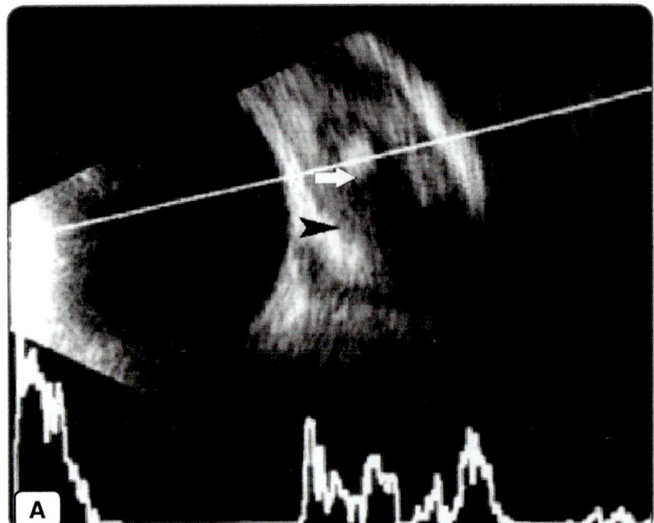

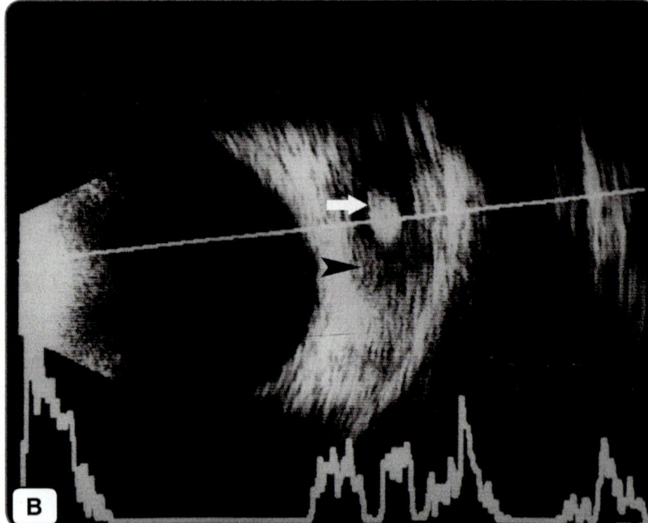

Figures 34.1A and B: B scan with vector A scan images showing a case of extraocular muscle cysticercosis and its resolution with albendazole therapy. Figures A and B are the longitudinal and transverse views before starting therapy. The cyst is seen as an oval echolucent area within the muscle belly (arrowhead). The scolex is seen as a very highly reflective nodule within the cyst (arrow).

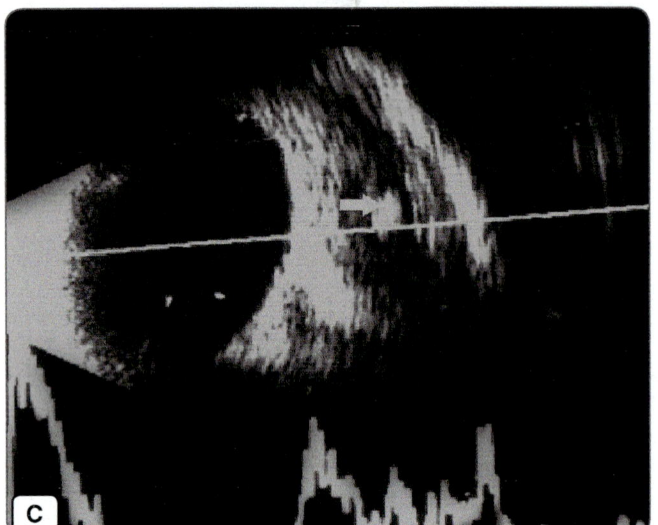

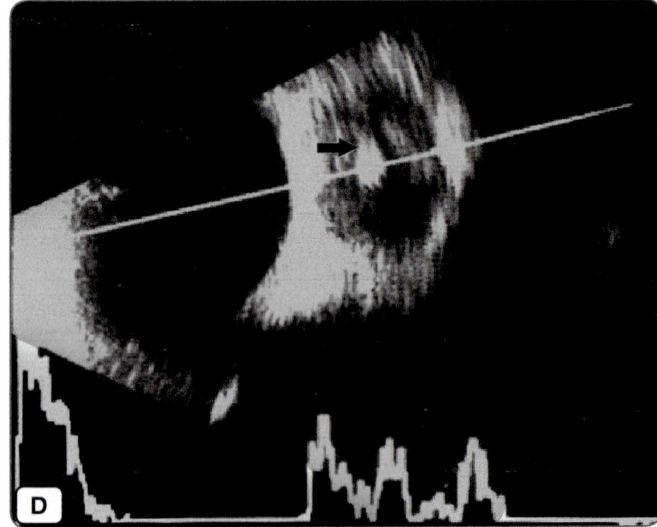

Figures 34.1C and D: There is not much change after two days of therapy.

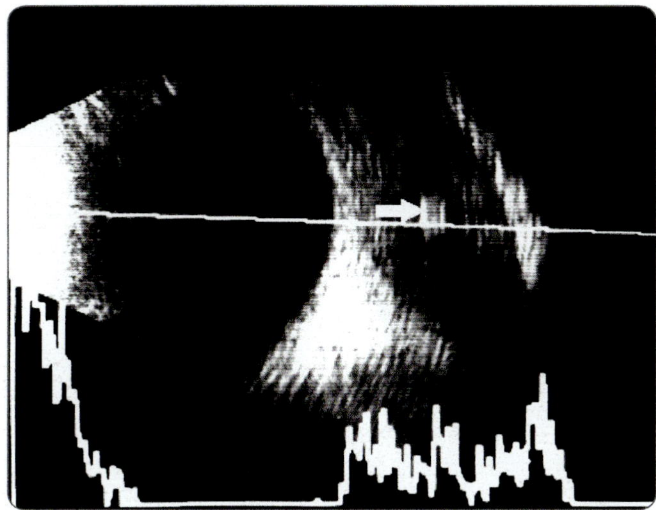

Figure 34.1E: The scan image on the fourth day shows a decrease in size and reflectivity of the scolex. The cyst wall is also not well outlined.

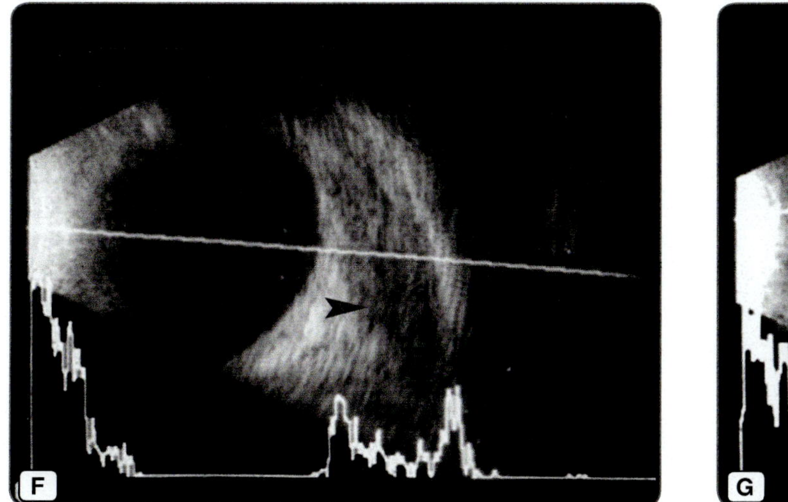

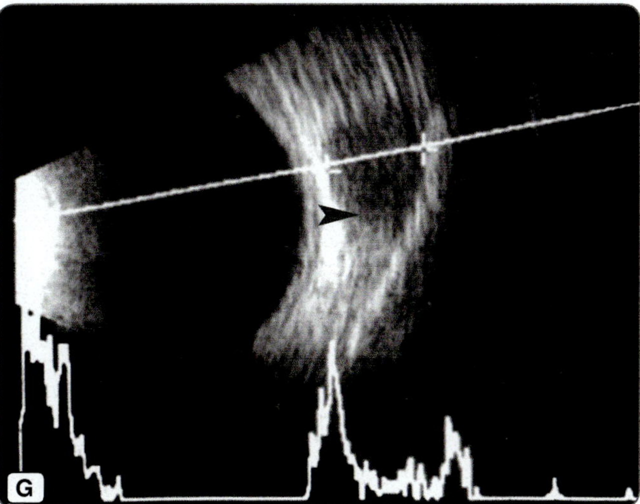

Figures 34.1F and G: At the end of one month, the muscle belly is thickened (arrowhead) with no evidence of cyst or scolex.

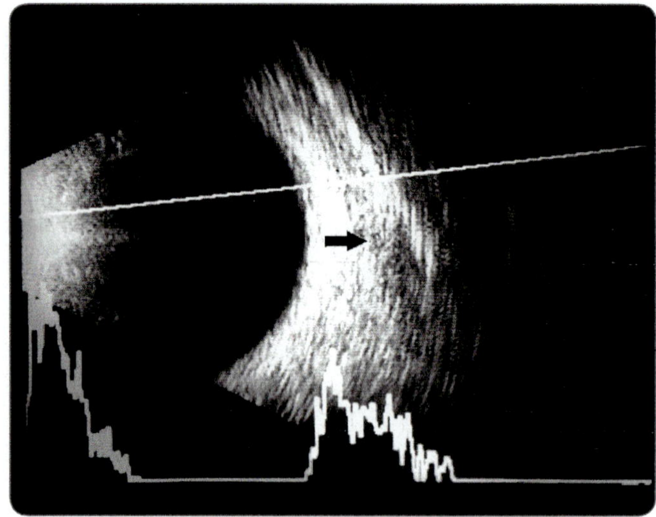

Figure 34.1H: One year later the muscle (arrow) looks normal in all respects.

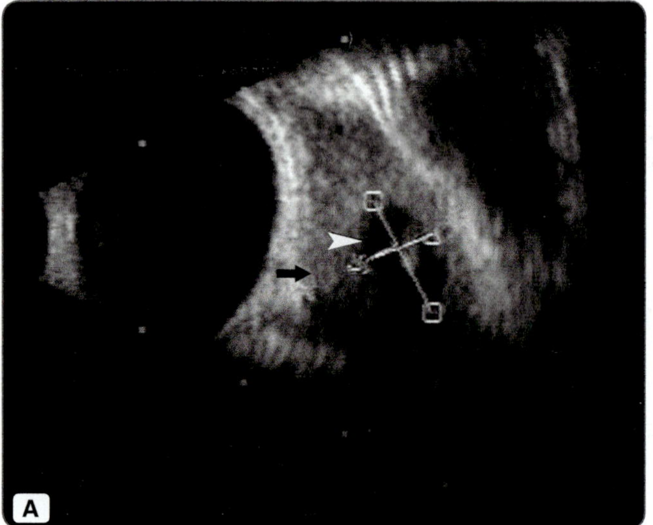

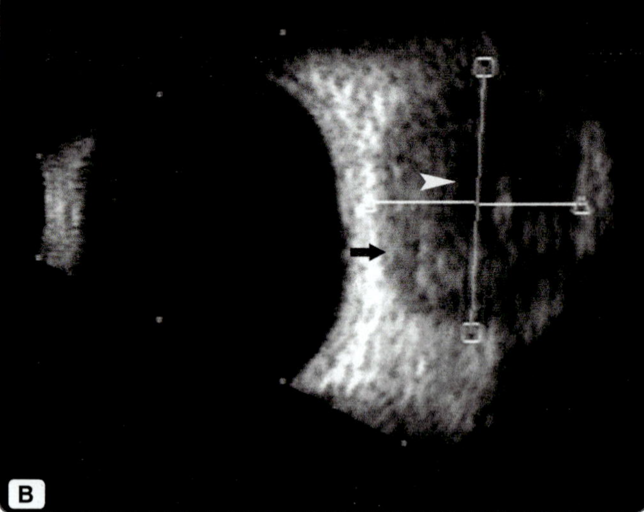

Figures 34.2A and B: B scan images of an eye with cysticercosis of an extraocular muscle. Note the relatively small size of the cyst (arrowhead) when compared to the grossly thickened muscle belly (arrow).

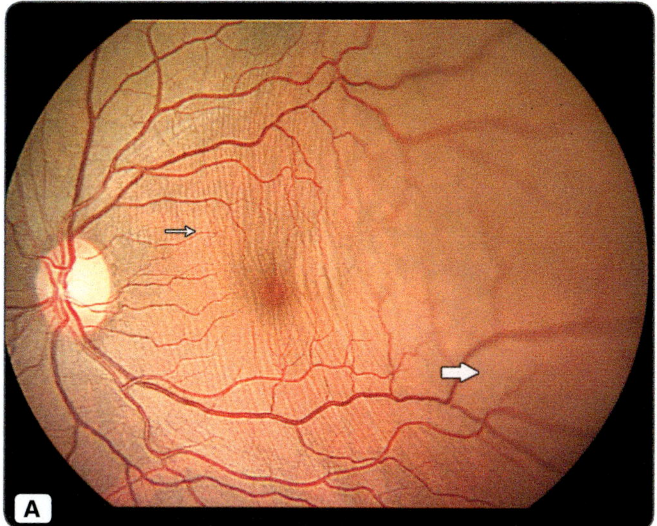

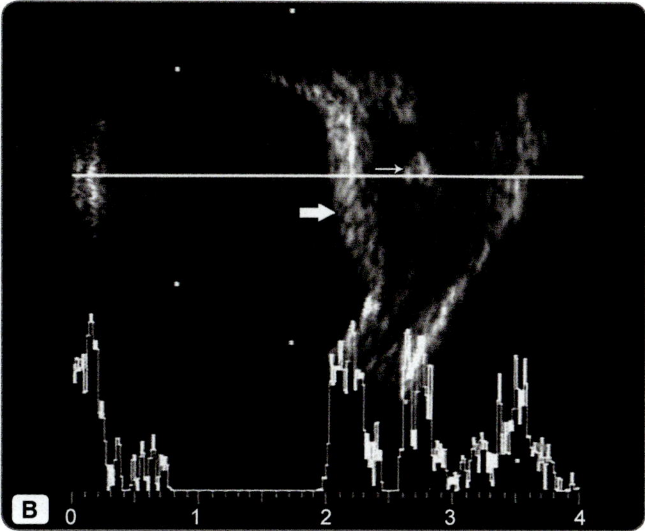

Figures 34.3A and B : Fundus photograph and ultrasound image of a 36-year-old male with blurring of vision, proptosis and restricted movement of the left eye. Fundus showed globe indentation involving the macula and area temporal to it (arrows). Ultrasound B scan with a vector shows the globe wall indentation (arrow). There is an echolucent area with a high reflective clump within the superolateral orbit (thin arrow) suggestive of a cysticercus cyst with scolex.

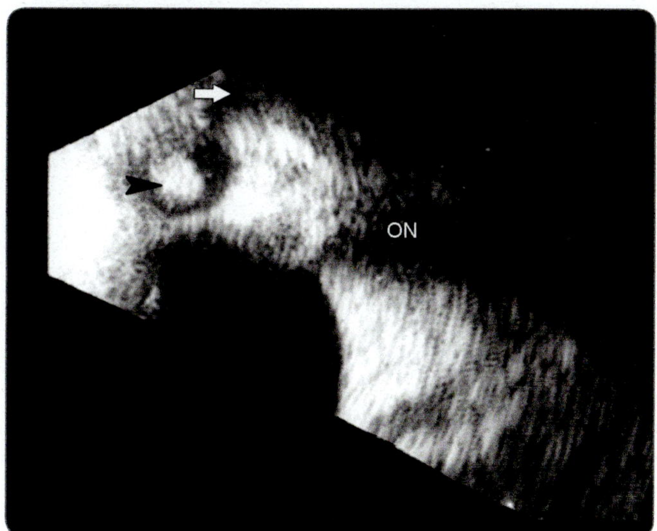

Figure 34.4: Cysticercosis involving the subconjunctival space (arrowhead) anterior to the insertion of the lateral rectus (arrow). ON = Optic nerve

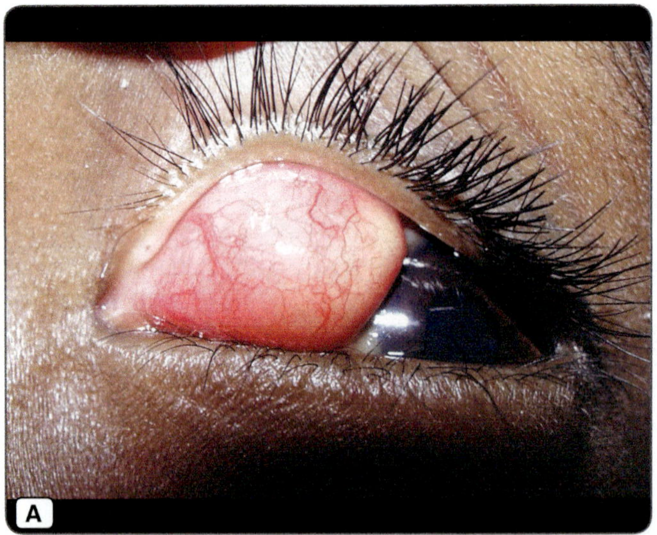

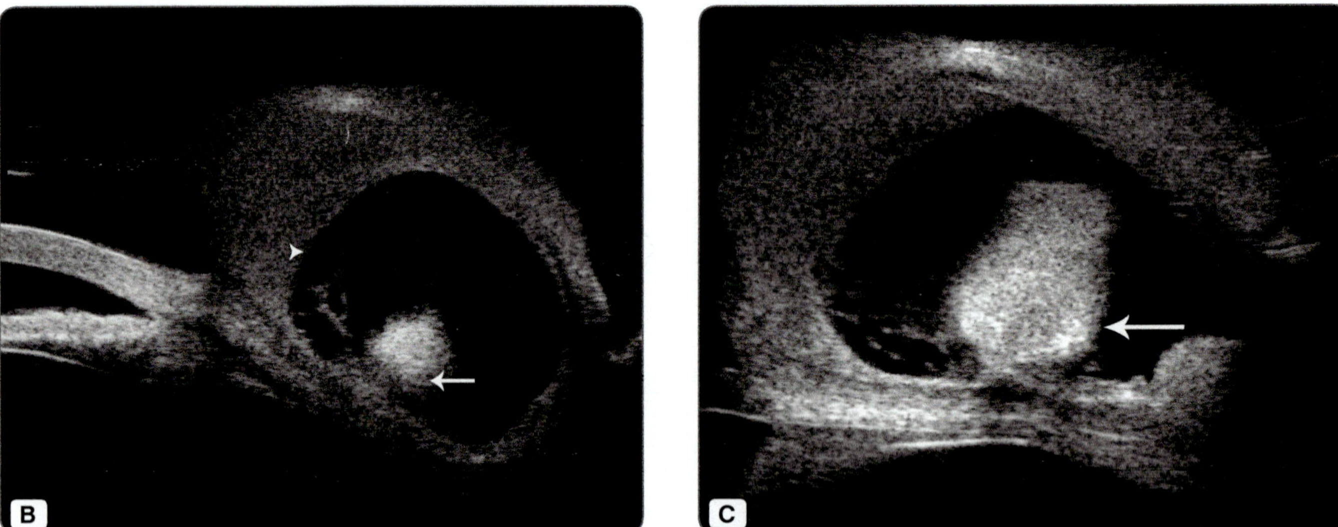

Figures 34.5A to C: Clinical photograph of the left eye of a young male showing a large subconjunctival cyst involving the superonasal quadrant. Figures B and C are UBM images showing a well defined cystic lesion in the subconjunctival space (arrowhead), with a high reflective clump of echoes attached to the inferior cyst wall (thin arrow) suggestive of a cysticercus cyst with scolex. Figure C gives a magnified view of the cyst showing the origin of the scolex from the cyst wall.

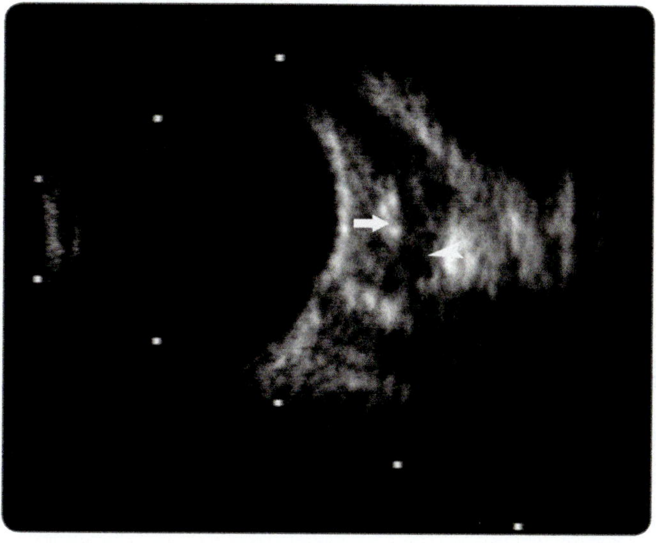

Figure 34.6: Cysticercosis of the orbital soft tissue showing moulding of the cyst wall to the globe. The high reflective scolex (arrow) is seen within the irregular shaped cyst (arrowhead). Note the absence of muscle involvement.

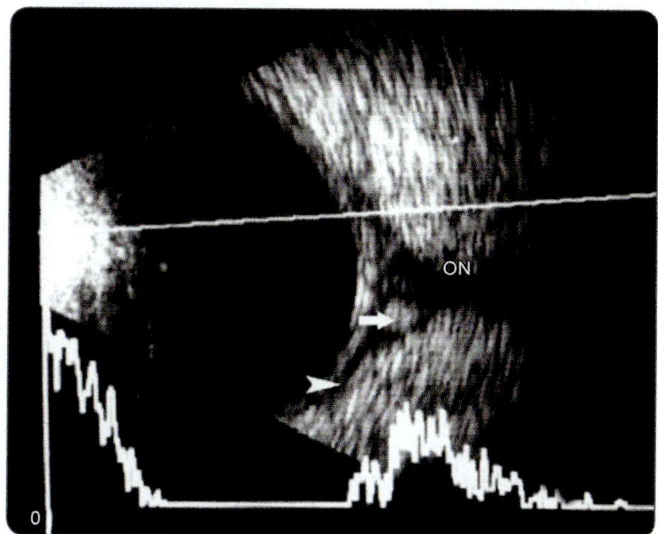

Figure 34.7: B scan image of a case of cysticercosis (arrow) adjacent to the optic nerve head (ONH). Note the adjacent globe wall flattening and Tenon's thickening (arrowhead).

35 Orbital Varix

CLINICAL FEATURES

- Nondistensible venous malformation.
- Slow or no flow in the well defined venous channels.
- Positional proptosis is characteristic with a demonstrable increase in size with Valsalva maneuver.
- Can develop phleboliths due to thrombosis within the venous channels.
- After repeated episodes of thrombosis, the varix may cause enophthalmos rather than proptosis due to adjacent fat atrophy.

ULTRASONOGRAPHY

- To demonstrate the venous channel.
- Echolucent or very low reflective lesion.
- May require Valsalva or prone position for detection.
- In case of a phlebolith, the reflectivity may be irregular with some areas that are high reflective. In such cases the lesion may not change in size with the Valsalva maneuver.
- A thrombosed varix may also appear as a large low reflective mass lesion.
- Other orbital contents like EOMs and optic nerve appear normal.

NUGGETS

Prone position of the patient with the examiner sitting below may demonstrate the varix better.

Always repeat the ultrasonographic evaluation utilizing various maneuvers such as Valsalva and positioning whenever a mass is suspected but not visualized initially.

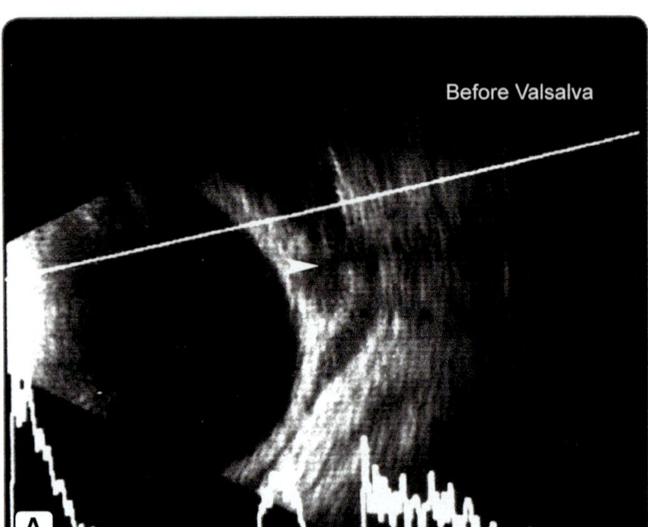

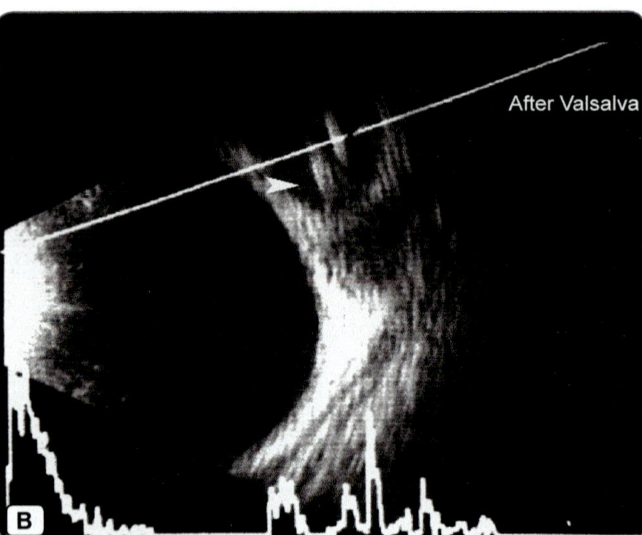

Figures 35.1A and B: B scan images showing an irregular echolucent tubular lesion (arrowhead) in the orbit that has increased in size after Valsalva maneuver.

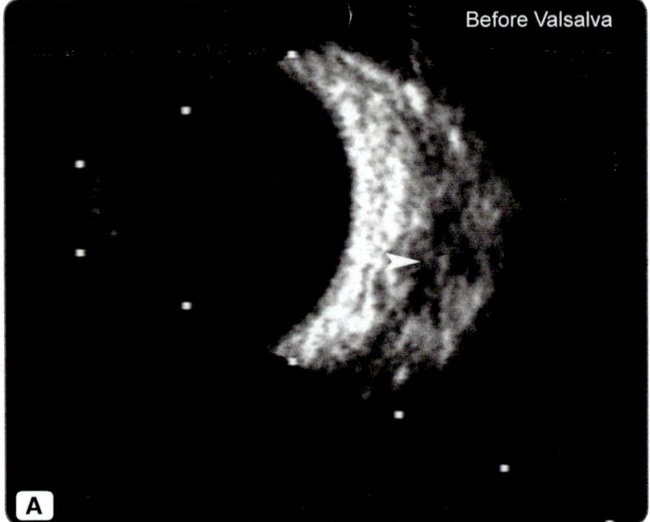

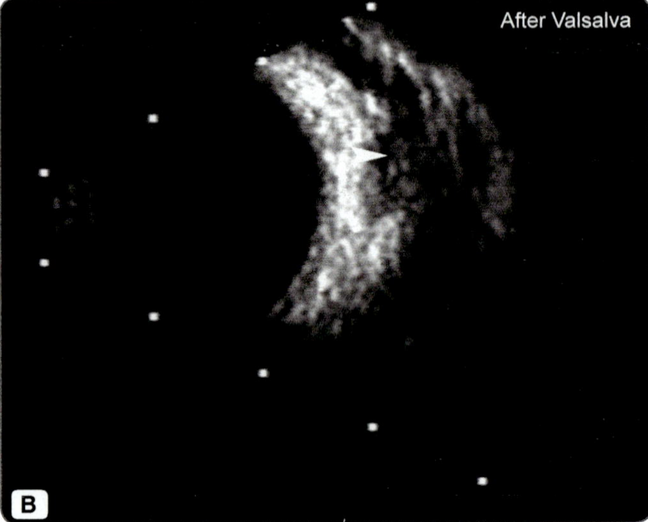

Figures 35.2A and B: B scan images of a coiled echolucent orbital lesion (arrowhead) increasing in diameter with Valsalva maneuver.

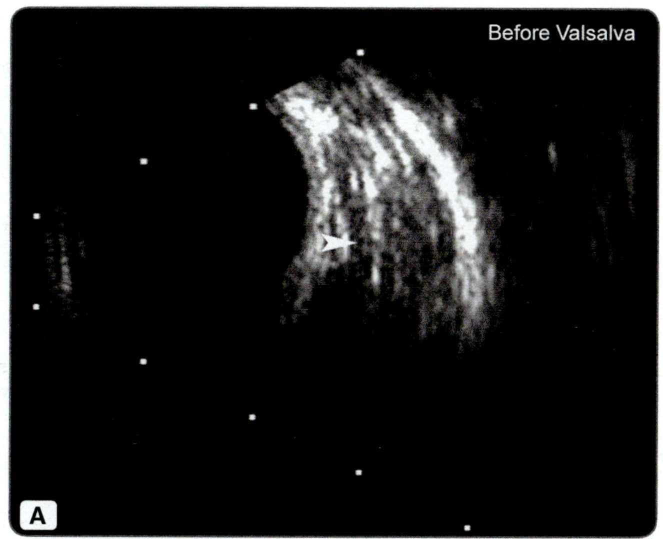

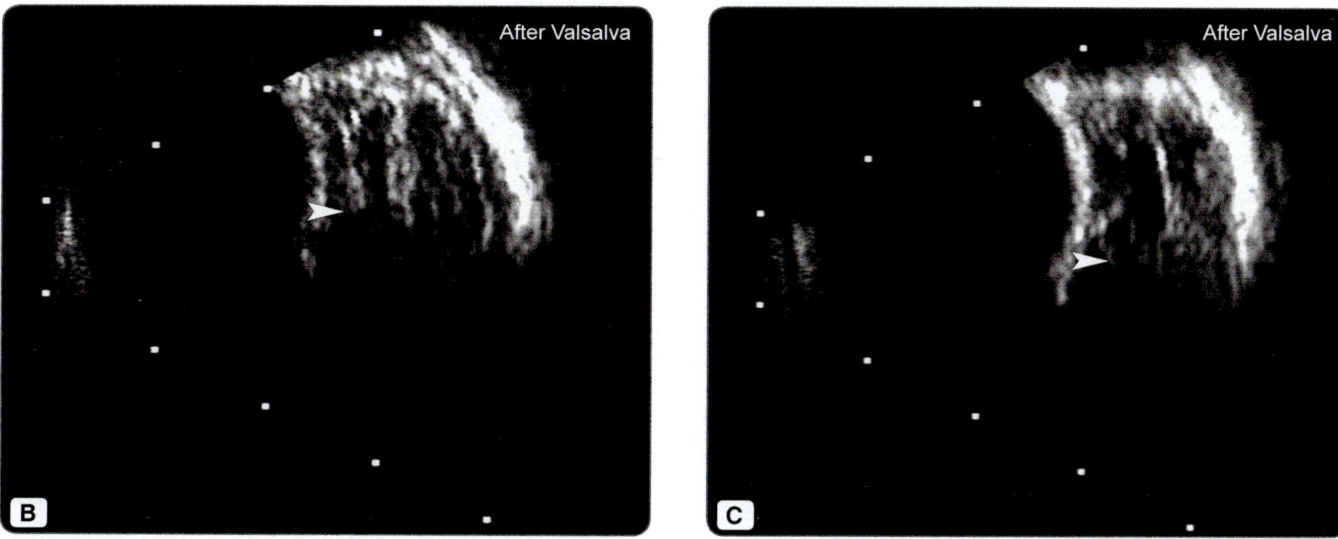

Figures 35.3A to C: The B scan images showing progressive increase in size of an echolucent tubular orbital mass (arrowhead) with continuing Valsalva maneuver.

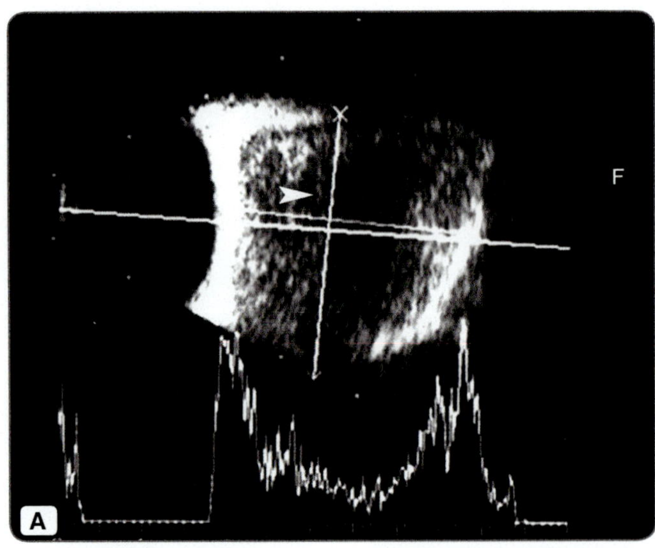

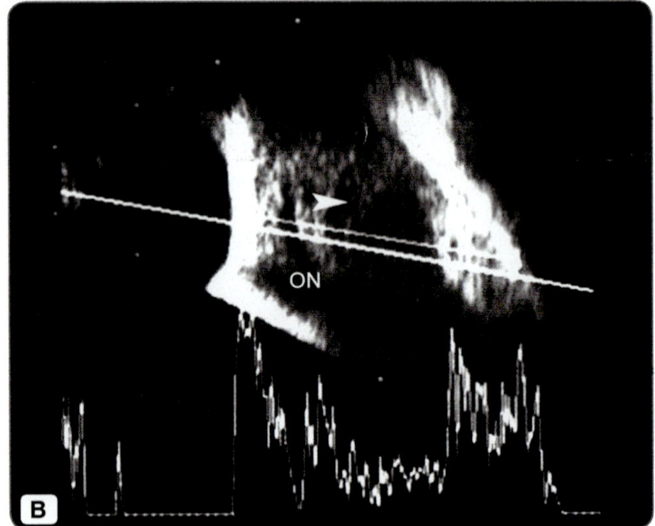

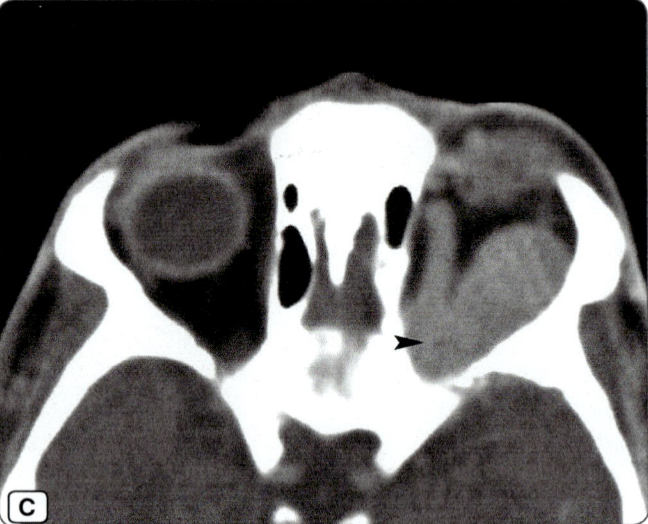

Figures 35.4A to C: Transverse and longitudinal B scans with A vector scan showing a large well defined orbital mass in the lateral orbit with high reflective margins and low to absent internal reflectivity (arrowhead). This suggests a fluid filled lesion that was confirmed to be a thrombosed orbital varix. In this case the Valsalva maneuver is negative. The CT scan shows a mass lesion in the posterior orbit curving from the medial to the lateral aspect.

36 Dilated Superior Ophthalmic Vein

CLINICAL SITUATIONS

- This is a major vein draining from the orbit. It courses obliquely backwards from the superonasal quadrant, crosses over the optic nerve from medial to lateral and reaches the orbital apex.
- It is dilated in cases of arteriovenous malformations involving the orbital and cavernous sinus areas, in inflammations and tumors involving the orbital apex and thrombosis of the cavernous sinus.
- High flow caroticocavernous fistulas are seen most often after severe head trauma. These cause pulsatile proptosis, chemosis, an audible bruit and marked dilatation of the superior ophthalmic vein.
- Slow flow dural cavernous sinus fistulas are typically seen in middle-aged women, and are characterized by a red eye, mild proptosis, raised episcleral venous pressure and features of orbital congestion.
- Cavernous sinus thrombosis is a medical emergency and can present with toxic signs, proptosis which can be unilateral or bilateral, and chemosis.

ULTRASONOGRAPHY

- The superior ophthalmic vein is imaged with horizontal transverse and vertical axial B scan views
- In case of high flow fistulas, there is marked dilatation of the vein which is seen as a tubular structure with absent or very low internal reflectivity. It is seen to course posteriorly as a 'U' shaped structure when viewed on the horizontal transverse scan. Additional findings such as enlarged extraocular muscles, widened optic nerve and ciliochoroidal detachments may be seen. The pulsations of the vein may be felt with the probe and visualized with kinetic echography
- In case of low flow fistulas, there is mild to moderate dilatation of the vein which may show low to moderate reflective echoes within the lumen. The extraocular muscles on the affected side are usually enlarged
- In case of thrombosis of the vein, the enlarged vein shows medium to high internal reflectivity and absence of pulsations. Tenon's space widening may also be seen.

NUGGETS

Pulsatile proptosis can also be seen in case of structural defects involving the orbital wall such as absence of greater wing of sphenoid. Here there is no evidence of superior ophthalmic vein dilatation.

Other orbital veins may also be dilated in case of caroticocavernous fistulas as well as lesions involving the apex.

The superior ophthalmic vein may be seen even in normal individuals if ultrasound is done with the patient prone.

Other tubular echolucent structures that can be seen on orbital ultrasound are orbital varices and aneurysms. These, however, do not always follow the course of the superior ophthalmic vein.

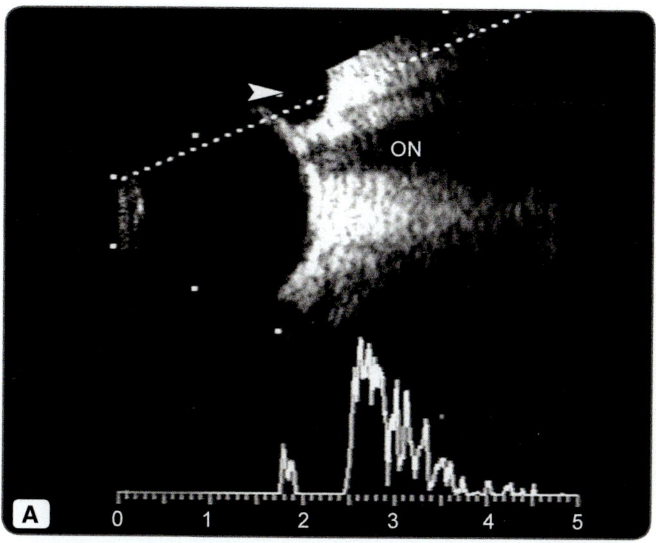

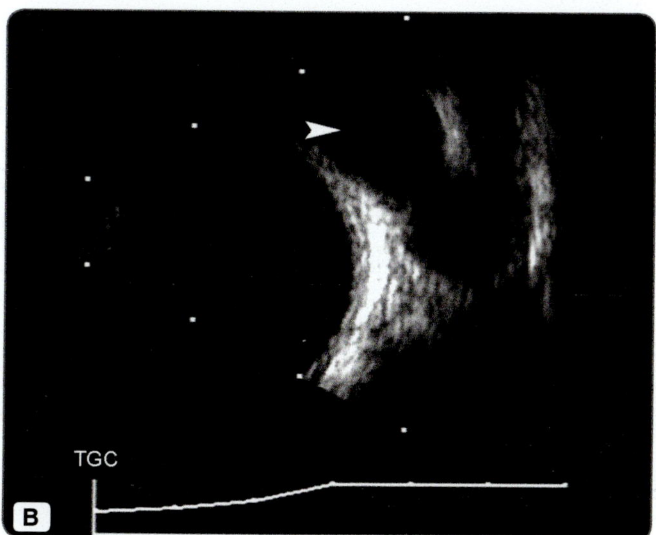

Figures 36.1A and B: Vertical axial (A) and horizontal transverse (B) B scan images of an eye with pulsatile proptosis following head injury. Note the markedly enlarged superior ophthalmic vein in the superior orbit (arrowhead). This, along with echolucency within the lumen is suggestive of a high flow caroticocavernous fistula.

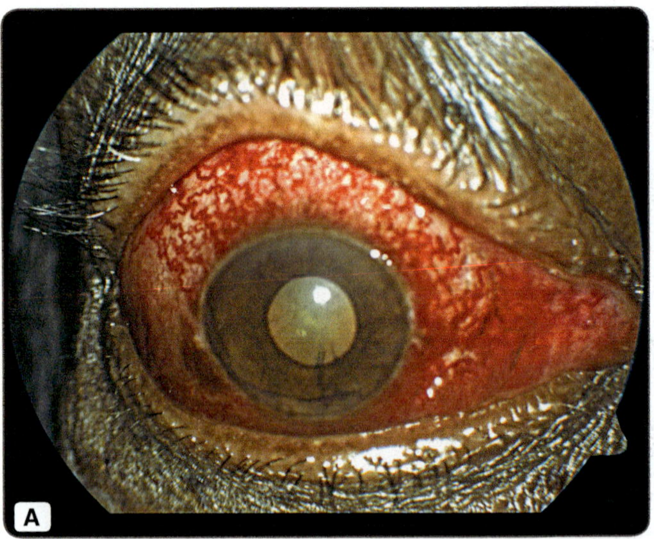

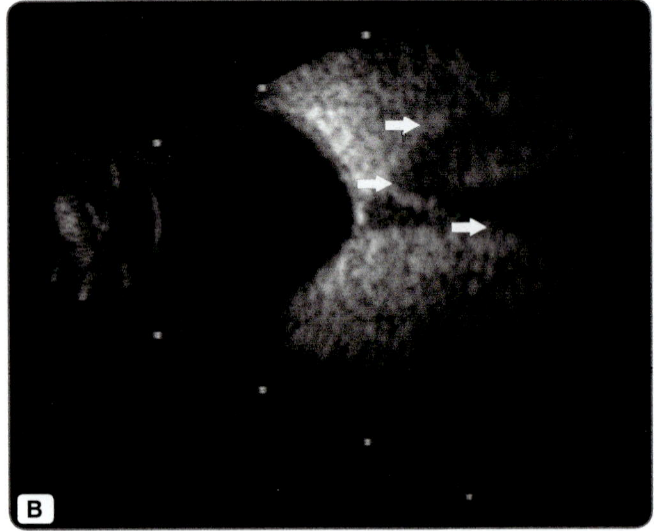

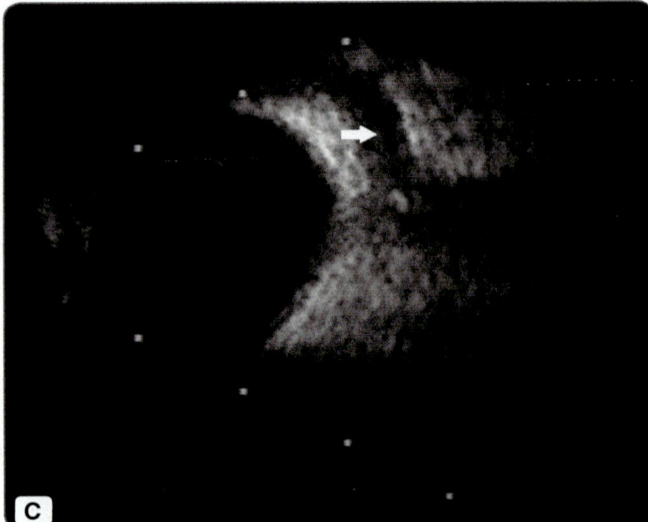

Figures 36.2A to C:

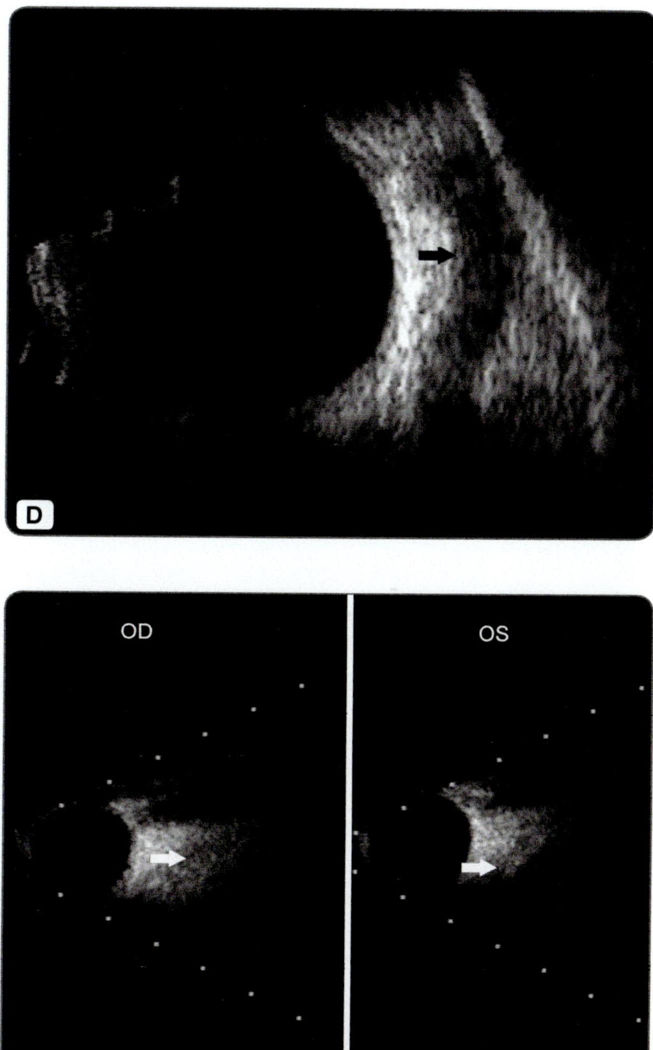

Figures 36.2A to E : Anterior segment photograph of an elderly woman with a traumatic caroticocavernous fistula and right sided proptosis. Note the dilated episcleral vessels. The B scan images show a dilated superior ophthalmic vein seen as a tubular echolucent structure winding along the medial side of the optic nerve (arrows). The dual mode comparing the right and left orbits shows the relative enlargement of extraocular muscles on the affected side, in this case the inferior rectus (arrow).

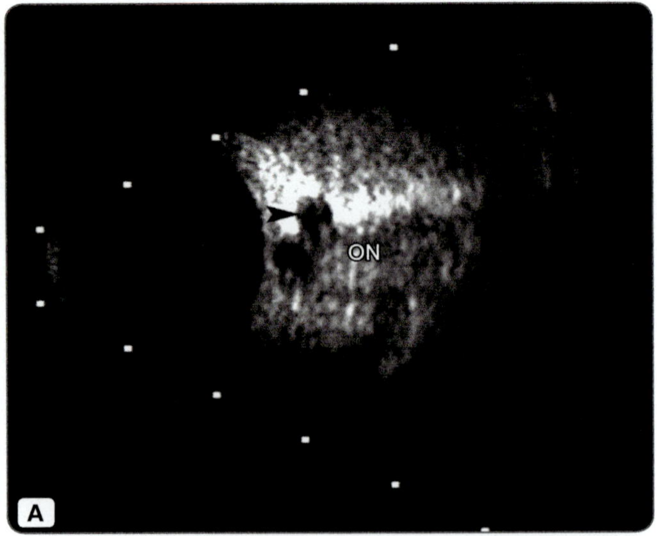

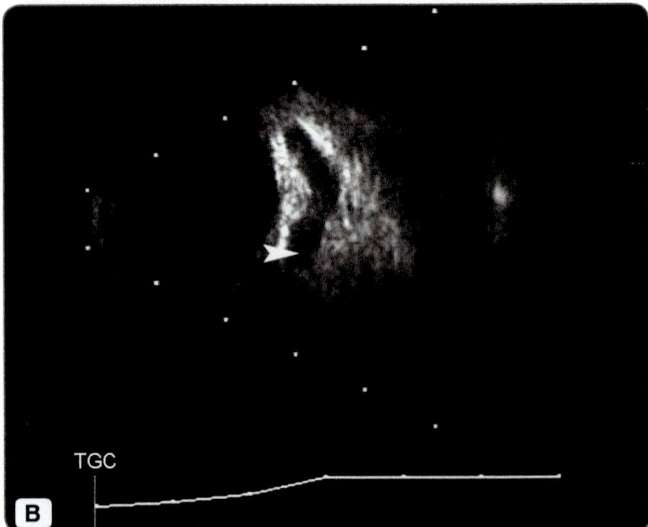

Figures 36.3A and B: Vertical axial and horizontal B scan images of an elderly male treated elsewhere for orbital pseudotumor. The right eye showed mild proptosis and episcleral vein engorgement. Ultrasound showed a dilated superior ophthalmic vein on the right side (arrowhead). MRI scan showed a dilated right superior ophthalmic vein, thrombosed left superior ophthalmic vein with abnormal flow in the left cavernous sinus and intercavernous connecting vessels.

37 Cavernous Hemangioma of the Orbit

CLINICAL FEATURES

- A benign, noninfiltrative slowly progressive tumor.
- Though present at birth, it becomes symptomatic only in adults.
- Usually an intraconal lesion, more commonly in the temporal quadrant.
- Consists of large endothelium lined channels.

ULTRASONOGRAPHY

- Well defined round to oval mass.
- Commonly intraconal, causing globe indentation.
- Moderate to high internal reflectivity with regular acoustic structure.
- Moderate sound attenuation.

NUGGETS

Globe wall indentation and choroidal folds are indicative of a mid or anterior orbital tumor.

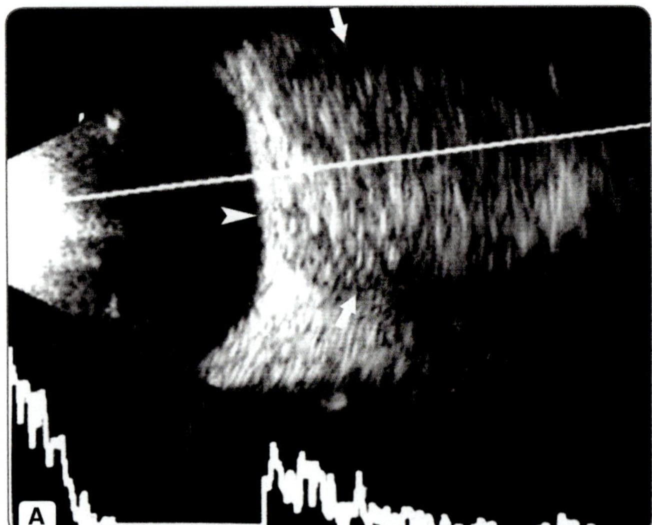

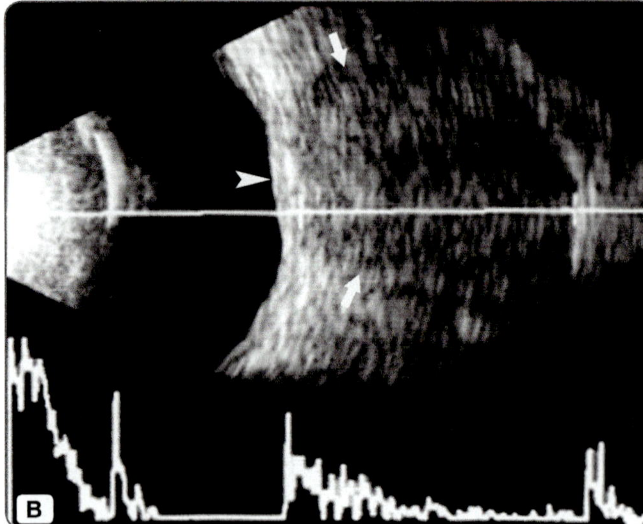

Figures 37.1A and B: B scan echogram in both vertical and horizontal axial views showing a well-circumscribed intraconal mass lesion (arrows) causing globe indentation (arrowhead). The A scan vector shows that the lesion spikes are of high reflectivity, and show moderate sound attenuation. The mass was histologically proven to be a cavernous hemangioma.

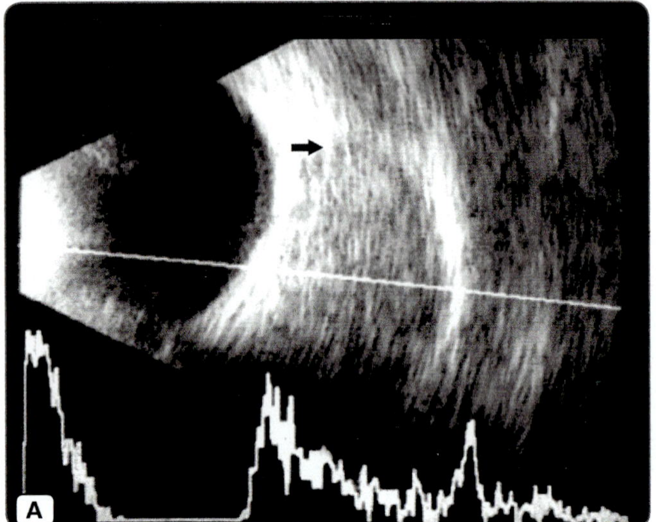

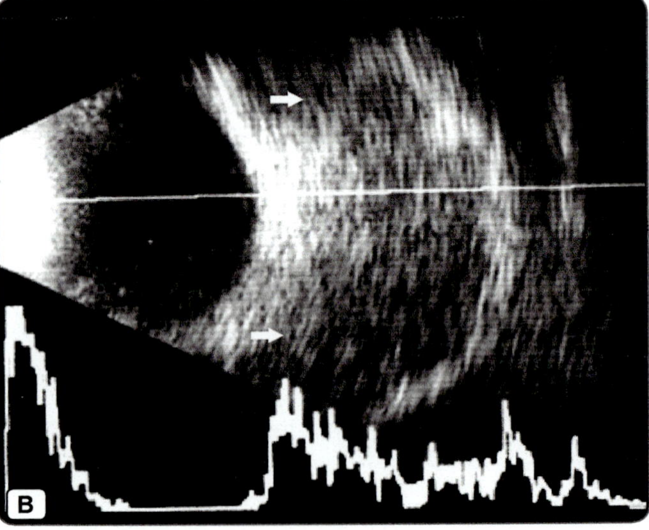

Figures 37.2A and B: B scan with vector A showing longitudinal and transverse views of a large intraconal mass lesion (arrow) with moderate to high reflectivity and moderate sound attenuation. Note the globe wall indentation. The mass was histologically proven to be a cavernous hemangioma with inflammatory changes as well.

38 Orbital Lymphangioma

CLINICAL FEATURES

- Occurs most commonly in the first decade of life.
- Combined veno—lymphatic malformation with relative hemodynamic isolation.
- Consists of serum filled spaces that are lined by flattened endothelial cells.
- Infiltrative, benign, nonencapsulated, compressible.
- Four patterns—superficial, deep, combined and complex.
- Superficial lesions involve the skin and conjunctiva and may present as bluish translucent swellings.
- Deep lesions are characterized by episodes of sudden painful proptosis, due to the occurrence of spontaneous hemorrhage from the interstitial capillaries.
- Increase in lesion size can also occur during episodes of respiratory infection.

ULTRASONOGRAPHY

- Irregular infiltrative mass lesion with evidence of echolucent spaces separated by high reflective septae.
- In case of fresh hemorrhage within the lesion, the spaces may appear dilated and may even show fluid levels.
- The compressible nature of the lesion is lost when hemorrhage occurs and may return at a later date.
- Occasional lesions may show specks of high reflectivity suggestive of calcium and may even show phleboliths.

NUGGETS

Other causes of rapidly developing painful proptosis in a child are:

- Orbital cellulitis
- Metastatic neuroblastoma
- Ruptured dermoid cyst
- Thrombosis within a varix
- Rhabdomyosarcoma
- Chloroma
- Hematic cyst

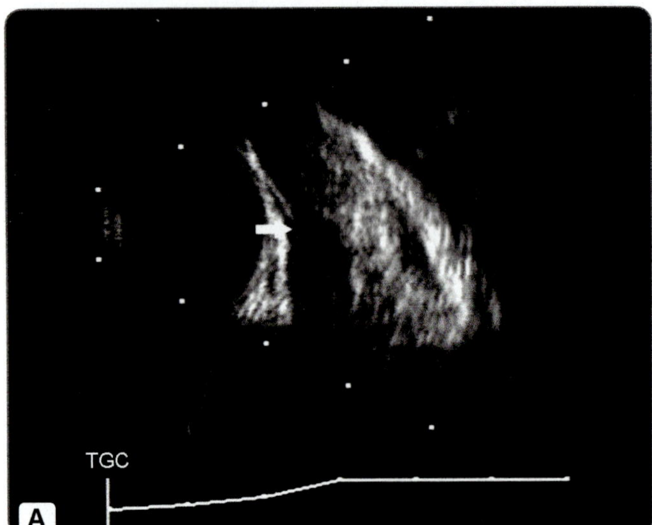

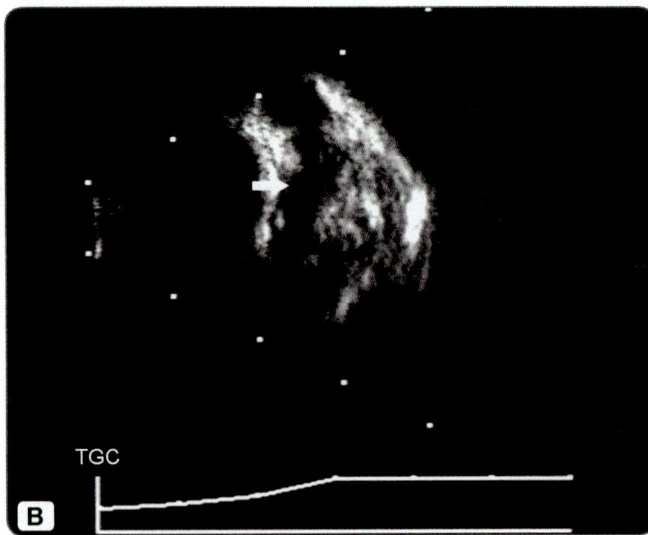

Figures 38.1A and B: Longitudinal and transverse B scan images of the orbit in a 2-month-old baby, showing an ill-defined mass lesion with variable internal echoes. Large tubular echolucent areas (arrows) suggestive of fluid filled spaces are seen. The extraocular muscles are not well seen.

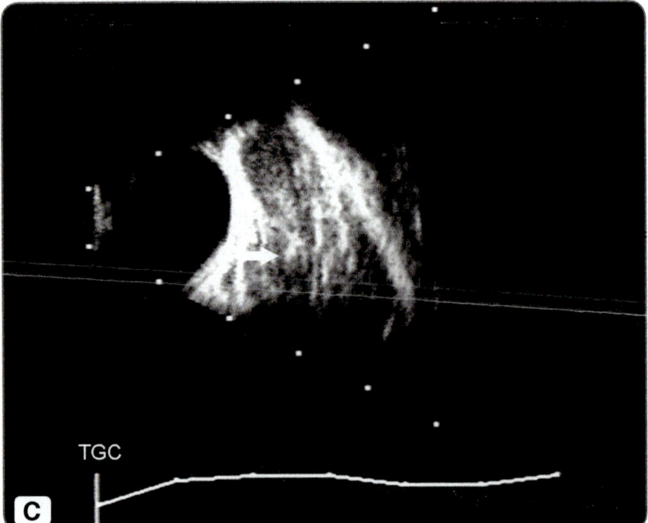

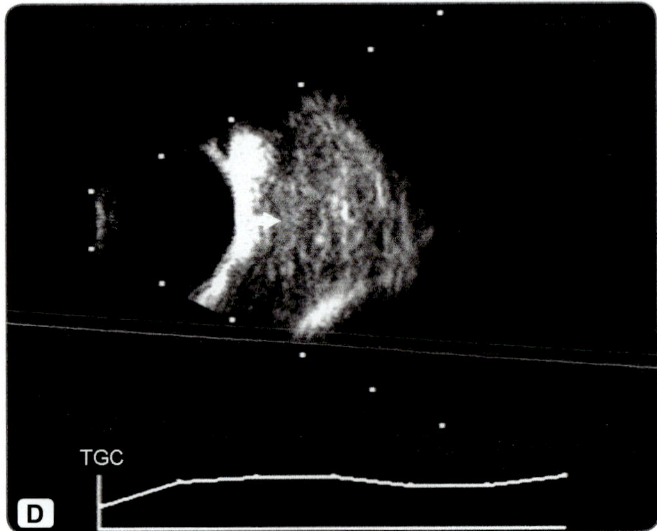

Figures 38.1C and D: Longitudinal and transverse scans in the same patient two weeks later when an increase in the amount of swelling and proptosis was noted. The echolucent spaces are filled with low reflective echoes (arrow) due to hemorrhage within the mass.

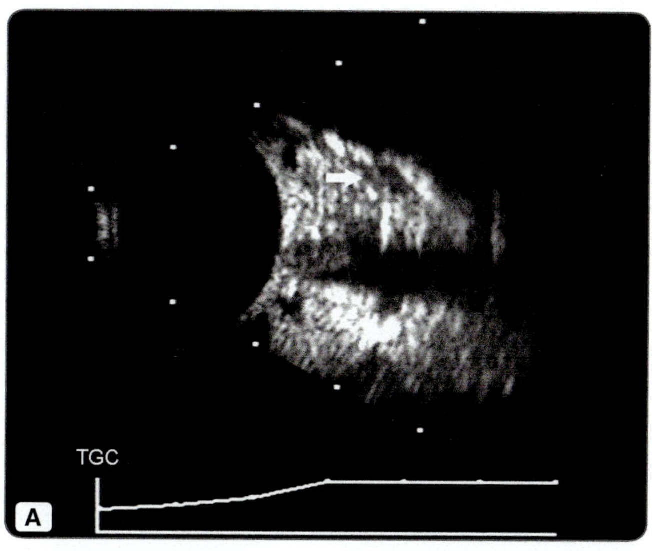

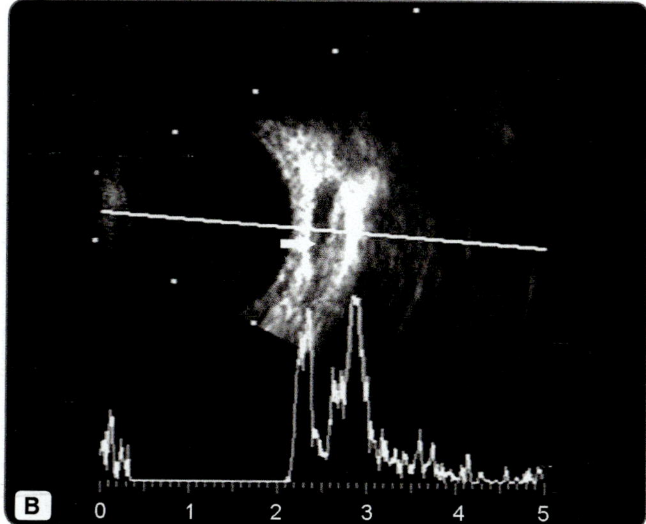

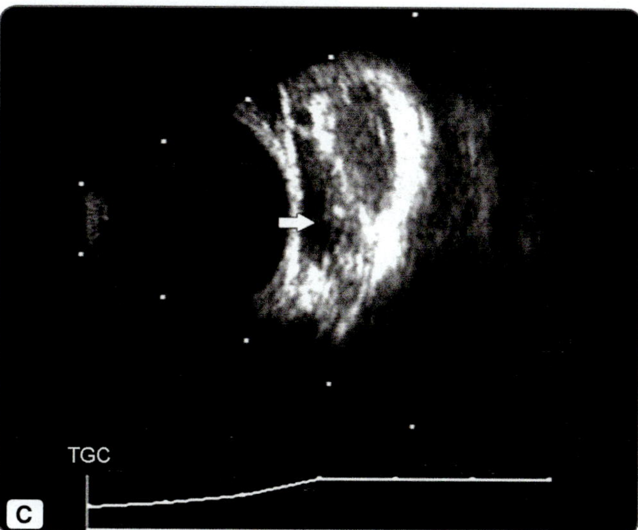

Figures 38.2A to C: Longitudinal axial and transverse B scan images of an eye with lymphangioma. Note the echolucent areas (arrow) within an ill-defined orbital mass lesion. The transverse scans delineate these vascular channels clearly. Layering of hemorrhage is seen as straight levels within these echolucent spaces.

39 Orbital Lymphomas

CLINICAL FEATURES: FOUR MAIN GROUPS

- Type 1: Most common type.
  Painless slow growing anterior orbital mass .
  Cohesive lesion that moulds to adjacent structures.
  Little or no functional disability.
  Subconjunctival "salmon patch".
- Type 2: Fulminant orbital infiltration.
  Patients with lymphoproliferative or leukemic disorders.
  To be differentiated from infections and severe inflammations.
- Type 3: Secondary infiltration from bone.
  Burkitt's lymphoma, multiple myeloma.
  Presence of orbital masses with adjacent bony destruction.
  To be differentiated from metastatic carcinoma.
- Type 4: Neuro-ophthalmic complications of lymphoproliferative or leukemic disorders.

Ultrasonography is a good diagnostic tool and can also be used for performing an ultrasound guided fine needle aspiration biopsy to confirm the diagnosis.

ULTRASONOGRAPHY

- Homogenous, well defined, ovoid or elongated low reflective lesion, mostly in the superior orbit.
- Essentially extraconal.
- Tendency to mold to either the globe or orbital structures.
- No orbital bone involvement in type 1 lesions.
- Infiltrative lesions may be irregular, heterogenous and cause bony erosion.
- Can be bilateral.

NUGGETS

Using a standoff technique, one can follow the lesion from the anterior part, well into the orbit.

The lesion may not always be separable from the muscles or the lacrimal gland.

In any echolucent or very low reflective circumscribed lesion, rule out the presence of a localized highly reflective scolex of cysticercosis.

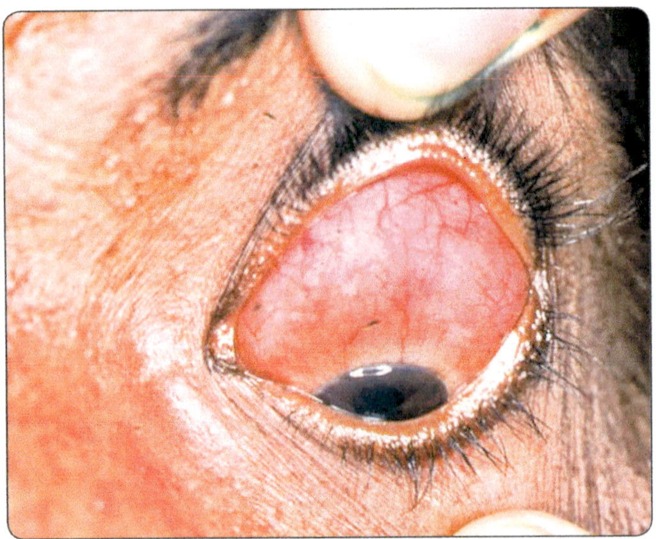

Figure 39.1A: External photograph of a patient with a salmon colored mass lesion in the superior subconjunctival space.

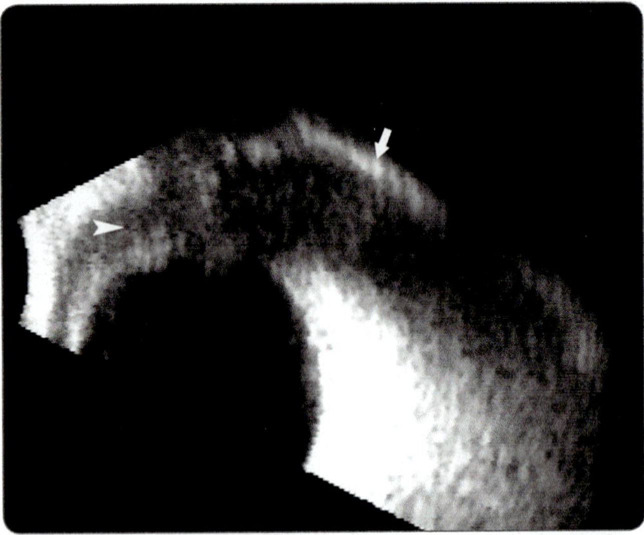

Figure 39.1B: Longitudinal B scan image using standoff showing a homogenous, well-defined, low reflective mass (arrowhead) extending posteriorly along the entire superior orbit (arrow = orbital roof).

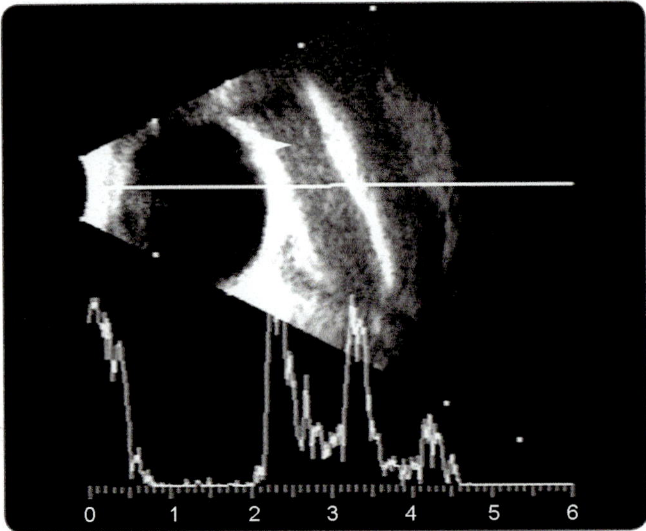

Figure 39.1C: Shows the same mass with an A scan vector confirming the low reflective nature. Also note that the mass is extraconal and molds to the orbital wall, features typical of a lymphoma.

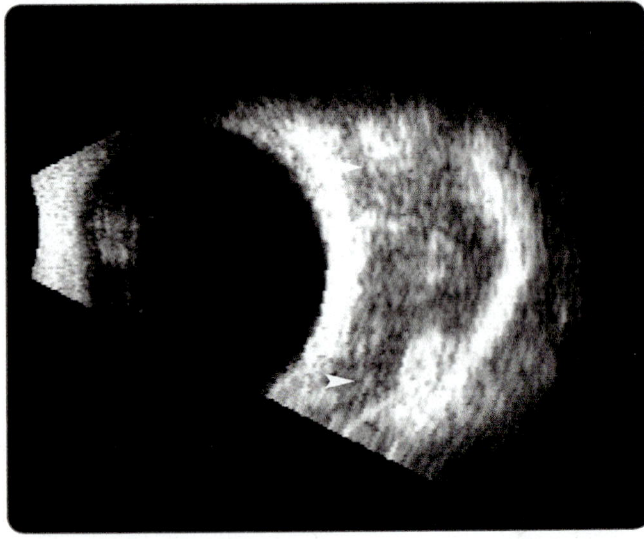

Figure 39.1D: Horizontal transverse view of the same mass (arrowhead) showing its lateral extent.

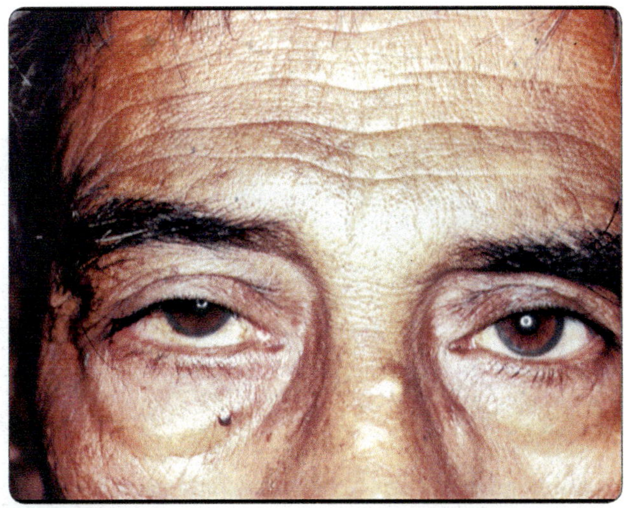

Figure 39.2A: Clinical photograph of a patient showing hypertropia and mild fullness of the right temporal area. There was restriction of abduction on the right side.

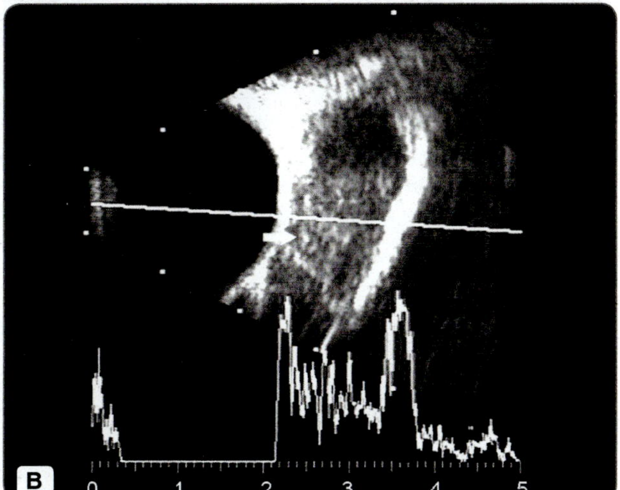

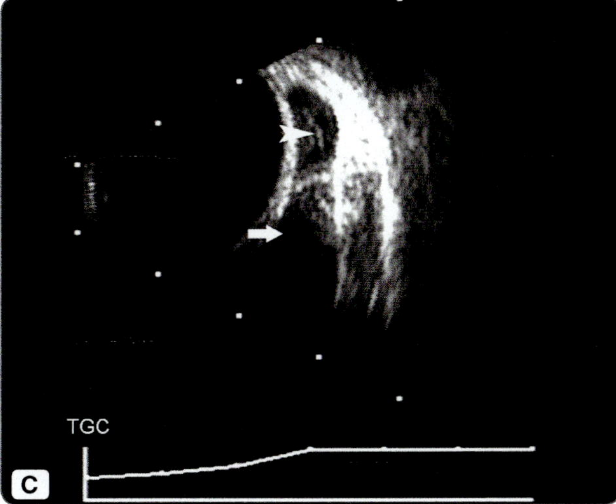

Figures 39.2B and C: Scan image showing a well-defined extraconal mass (arrow) in the inferior and lateral orbit, with lacrimal gland involvement (arrowhead). Lymphomas can sometimes show an irregular low to medium internal reflectivity as seen in this lesion. Lymphomas commonly involve the lacrimal gland as well and may not be easily distinguishable from the latter.

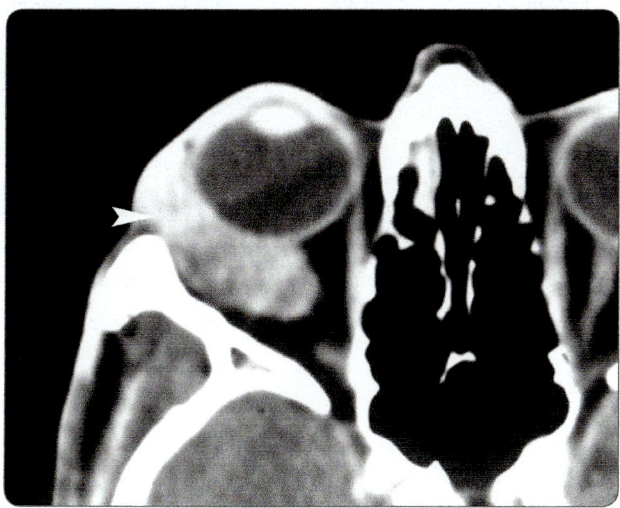

Figure 39.2D: CT scan of the orbit showing the homogenous mass (arrowhead) molding the globe and orbital wall.

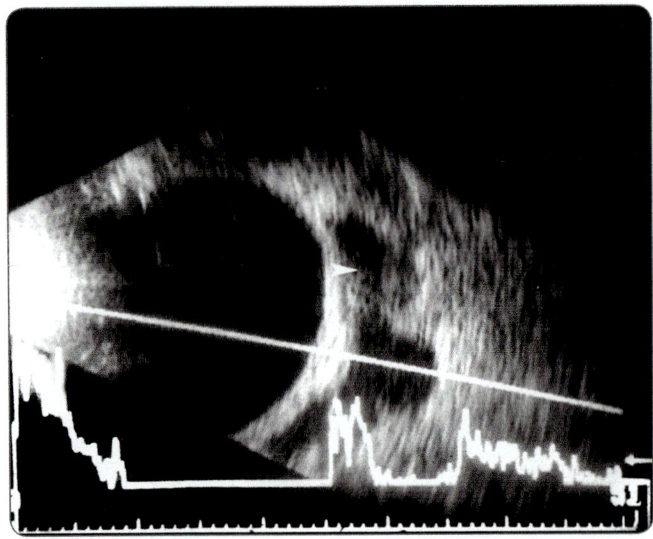

Figure 39.3A: B scan with vector A showing a very low reflective mass (arrowhead) molding to the posterior globe wall. It has an irregular posterior border.

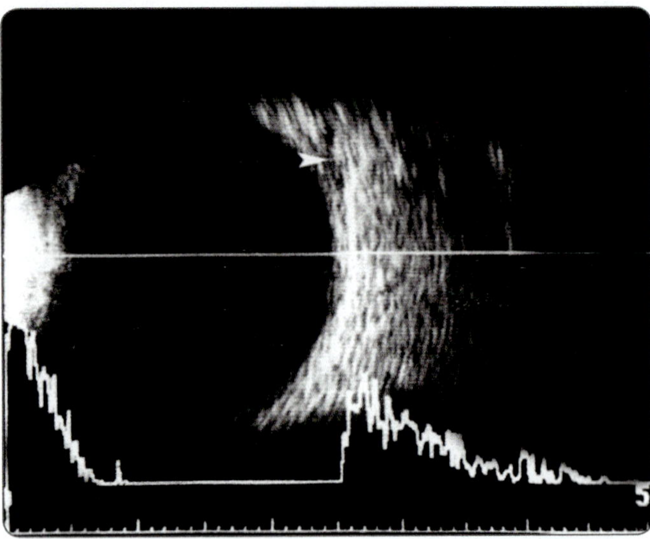

Figure 39.3B: B scan image postoperatively after the patient underwent orbitotomy showing a small residual area (arrowhead) adjacent to the globe wall.

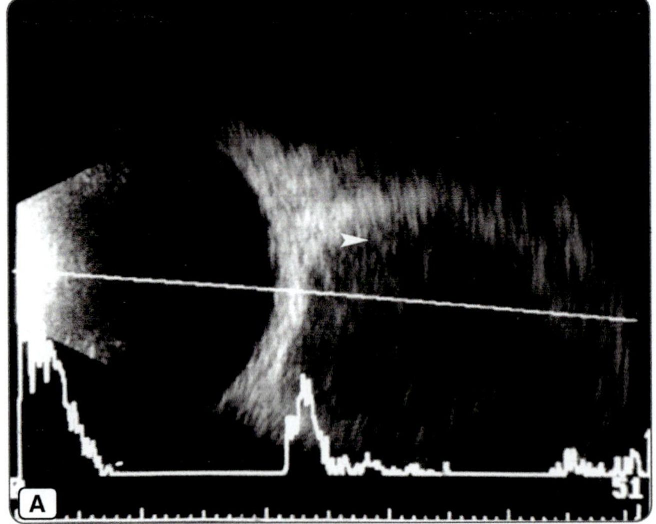

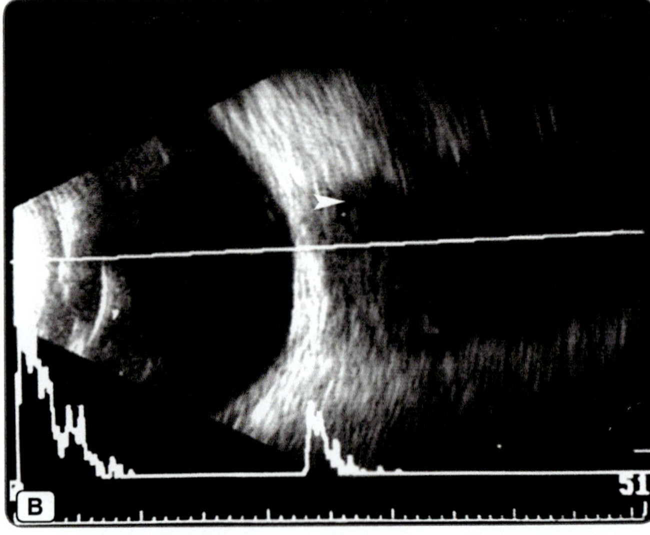

Figures 39.4A and B: B scan with vector A showing a low reflective homogenous lesion in the intraconal space (arrowhead). It appears to surround the optic nerve, which cannot be distinguished from it. HPE diagnosis was non-Hodgkin's lymphoma of the orbit, possibly secondary to a systemic lymphoma.

40 Lacrimal Gland Tumors

Common lesions that can occur in the lacrimal fossa region include:

- Pseudotumor
- Lymphoma
- Primary lacrimal gland epithelial tumors
- Cysts.

PLEOMORPHIC ADENOMA

CLINICAL FEATURES

- The most common benign tumor of the lacrimal gland.
- Usually develops from the orbital lobe and extends posteriorly. The posterior margin is arc-like.
- Can cause indentation of ocular coats, choroidal folds and bony excavation.
- Downward and nasal displacement of the globe.
- Well encapsulated.
- Malignant transformation can occur, particularly if the capsule has been damaged as a result of incomplete surgical excision.

ULTRASONOGRAPHY

- Well defined round to oval encapsulated lesion.
- Medium to high reflective regular internal structure.
- Moderate sound attenuation.
- May contain cystic cavities.
- Bony excavation of the adjacent orbital wall may be seen but there is no bone destruction.

ADENOID CYSTIC CARCINOMA

CLINICAL FEATURES

- Most common primary malignant lacrimal gland tumor.
- Highly infiltrative.
- Patient presents with pain due to infiltration of the orbital nerves.

ULTRASONOGRAPHY

- Infiltrative lesion (occasionally well circumscribed).
- Medium to high reflective irregular internal structure.
- Moderate to strong sound attenuation.
- Often contain cystic cavities
- Calcification may be seen.
- Bony destruction of adjacent orbital wall.

LYMPHOMAS AND PSEUDOTUMOR

CLINICAL FEATURES

- Cause diffuse expansion of the gland
- Firm in consistency
- Ten to seventeen percent are bilateral

ULTRASONOGRAPHY

- Usually irregular due to lack of a capsule.
- Low reflective.
- Low sound attenuation.
- Do not indent the globe but tend to mold around it.
- Do not cause changes in the adjacent bony wall.
- Changes due to inflammation in the adjacent extraocular muscles and orbital tissue can be seen in pseudotumor.

NUGGETS

Benign tumors can cause bony excavation due to their slow progression. The presence of bony destruction however, points to the malignant nature of the lesion.

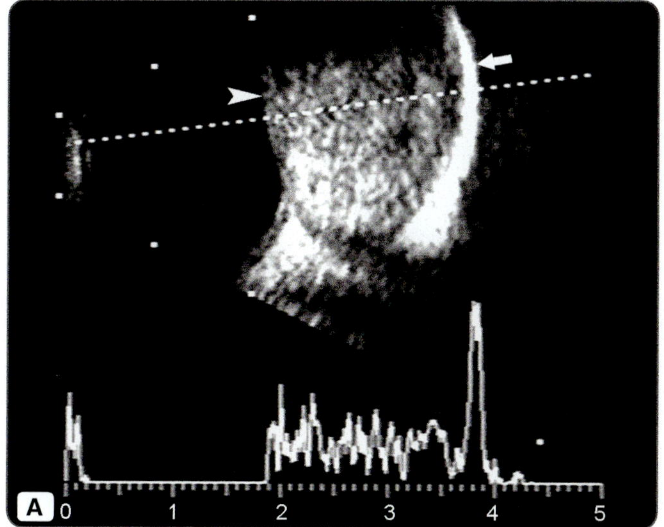

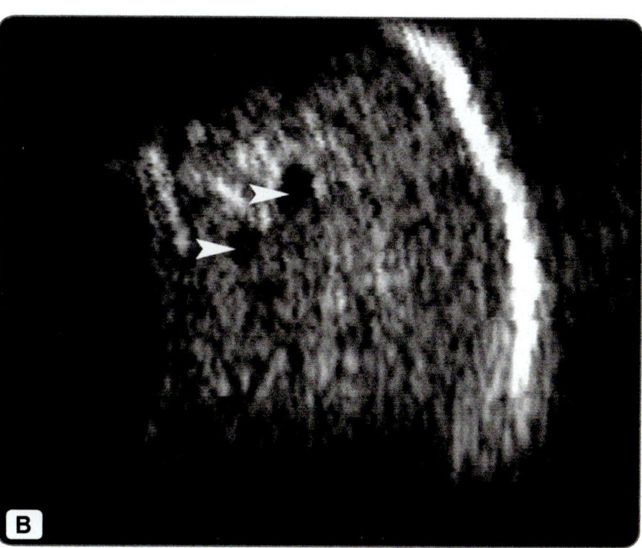

Figures 40.1A and B: B scan with vector A scan showing an oval, well-encapsulated orbital mass causing globe wall indentation (arrowhead) and orbital wall excavation (arrow). The internal structure is fairly regular, moderately reflective on the A scan. There are also a few cystic spaces within the mass. Figure B is a magnified view of the same mass showing the cystic spaces (arrowheads). The diagnosis was pleomorphic adenoma of the lacrimal gland.

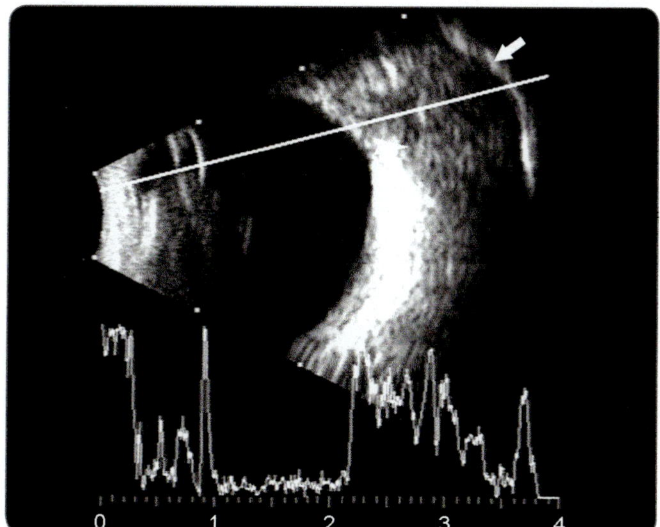

Figure 40.2: B scan with vector A showing a lacrimal tumor (arrowhead), causing both globe wall indentation and orbital wall excavation (arrow). The internal reflectivity is moderate to high with no cystic changes.

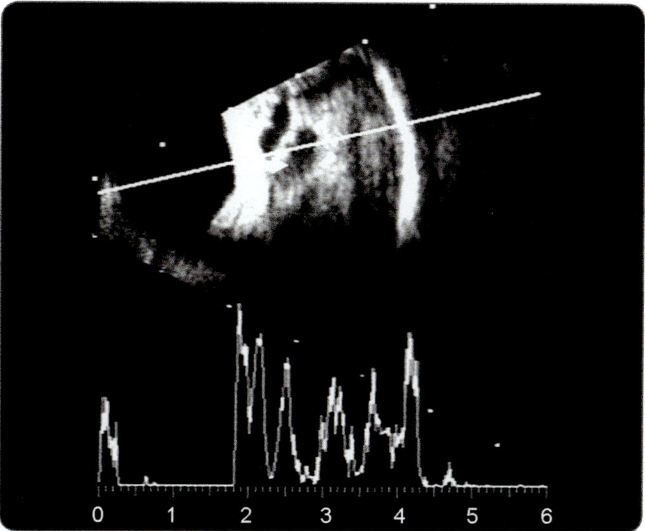

Figure 40.3: B scan with vector A scan showing a large mass lesion involving the lacrimal gland. Here the cystic spaces (arrow) are large and well defined.

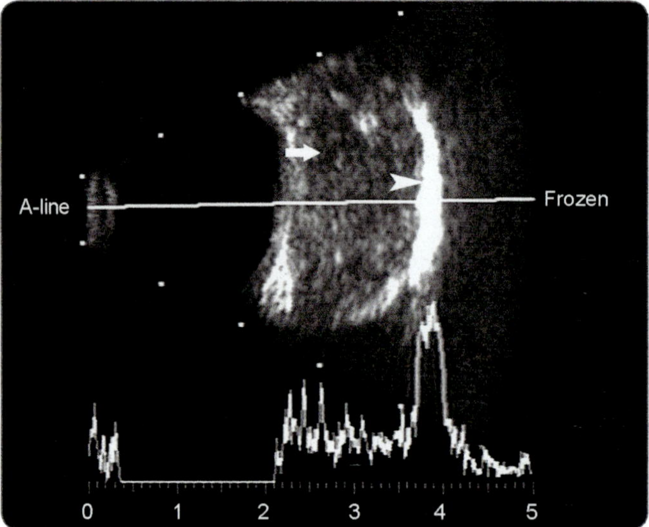

Figure 40.4A: B scan with vector A showing a mass in the lacrimal gland (arrow) causing minimal globe indentation and bony excavation (arrowhead). The internal reflectivity appears fairly regular. Few areas of high reflectivity are seen.

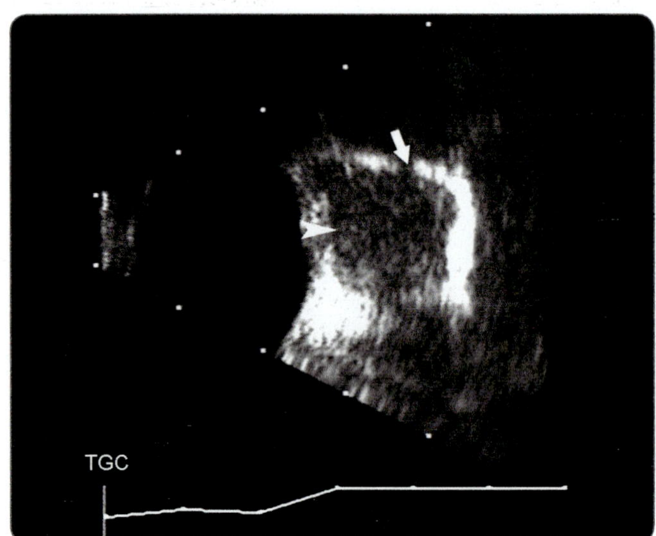

Figure 40.4B: B scan longitudinal view of the same lesion (arrowhead) showing irregular bony contour with bony destruction (arrow). The lower border of the mass is irregular and not well defined. This was a malignant lacrimal gland tumor, diagnosed on HPE to be a malignant transformation of a pleomorphic adenoma.

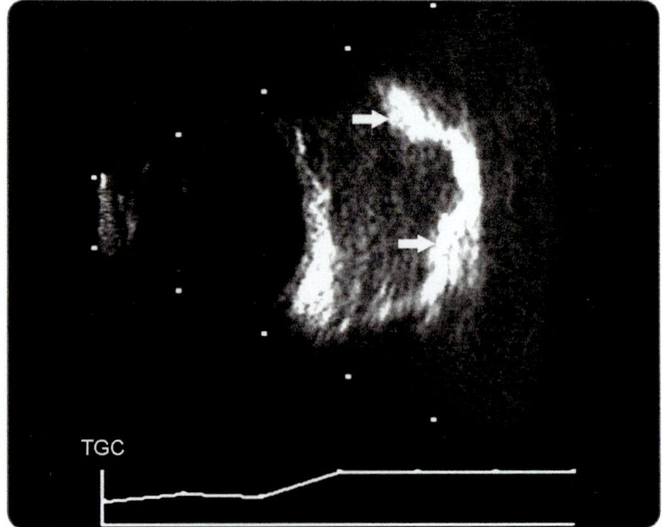

Figure 40.4C: This transverse B scan image shows the irregular contour of the mass as well as the irregular pattern of orbital wall changes (arrows).

41 Idiopathic Orbital Inflammation

CLINICAL FEATURES

- Also known as inflammatory pseudotumor of the orbit.
- Involves any or all orbital tissues, hence the clinical presentation can be varied.
- Associated with pain, proptosis, chemosis, visual loss and/or diplopia in varying proportions depending on the structures involved.
- Characterized by response to corticosteroids, but with a high incidence of recurrences.
- Most commonly unilateral.
- Myositis is the most common form of this disease.
- Ultrasound can help differentiate this from other mass lesions and also monitor response to therapy.

ULTRASONOGRAPHY

- Low reflective enlargement of a single or multiple extraocular muscles, which may appear irregular in shape. The low reflectivity is due to diffuse infiltration of the muscle fibers with inflammatory cells.
- Ill-defined orbital mass lesion which may be diffuse and involve adjacent structures.
- Associated scleritis or Tenon's widening adjacent to the involved muscle tendon.
- Widening of the perineural space may be seen.
- Absence of orbital bone contour alteration.
- Lacrimal gland enlargement may be seen.
- In chronic cases, the reflectivity may be high due to fibrotic and sclerotic changes.

NUGGETS

Extraocular muscle involvement in thyroid orbitopathy usually spares the tendon whereas myositis involves the entire extent.

Lymphomas are also low reflective but usually do not cause scleritis or adjacent muscle thickening.

Look for the presence of a scolex if there is thickening of the belly of one EOM.

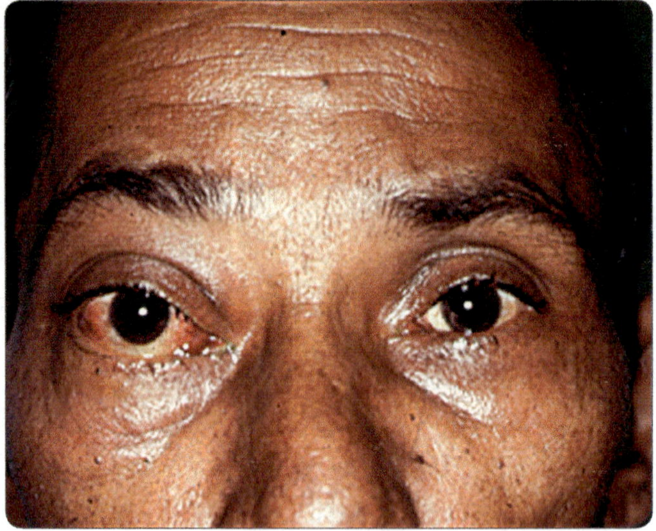

Figure 41.1A: External photograph of a patient with painful proptosis of the right eye due to idiopathic orbital inflammation.

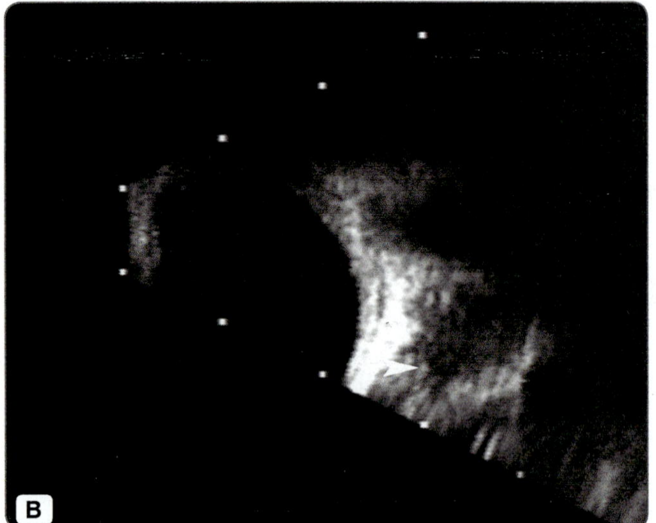

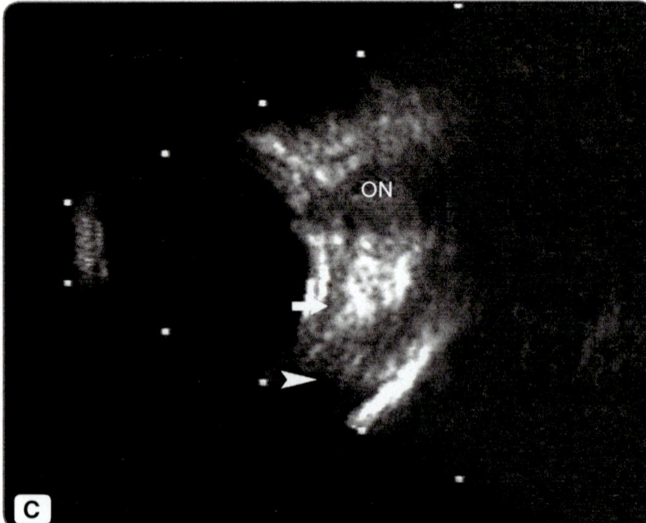

Figures 41.1B and C: B scan images showing low reflective thickening of the muscle along its entire extent (arrowhead). In addition there is widening of the Tenon's space (arrow) indicating an inflammatory etiology. The optic disc (ON) is also elevated.

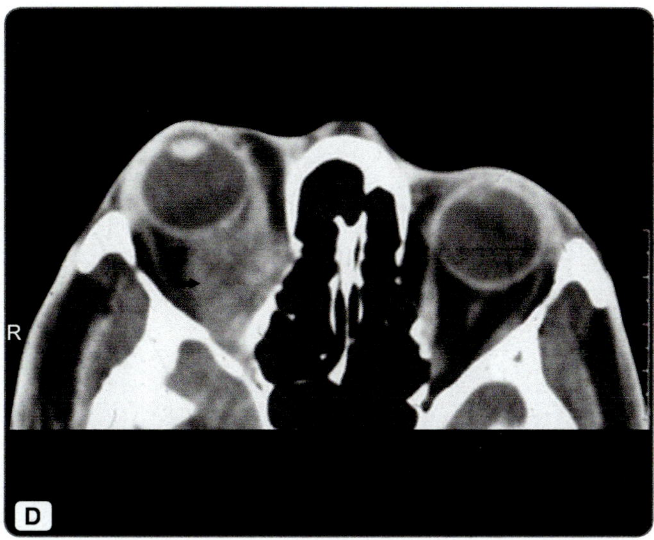

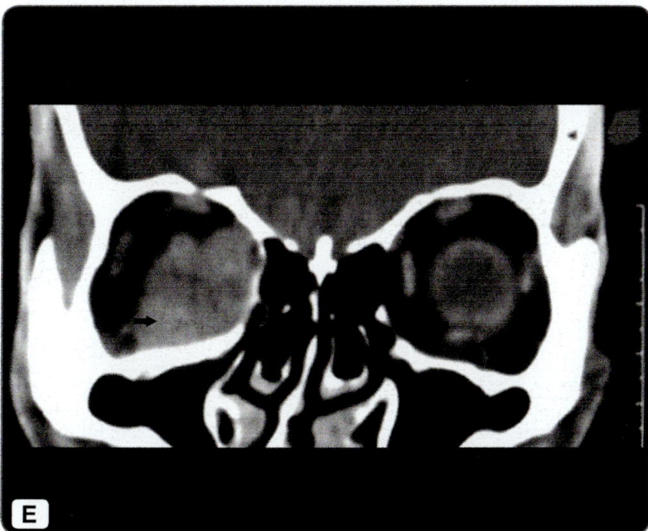

Figures 41.1D and E: Axial and coronal CT scan images of the same patient showing an irregular mass lesion in the inferomedial orbit (arrow), extending to the orbital apex. The diagnosis was orbital pseudotumor.

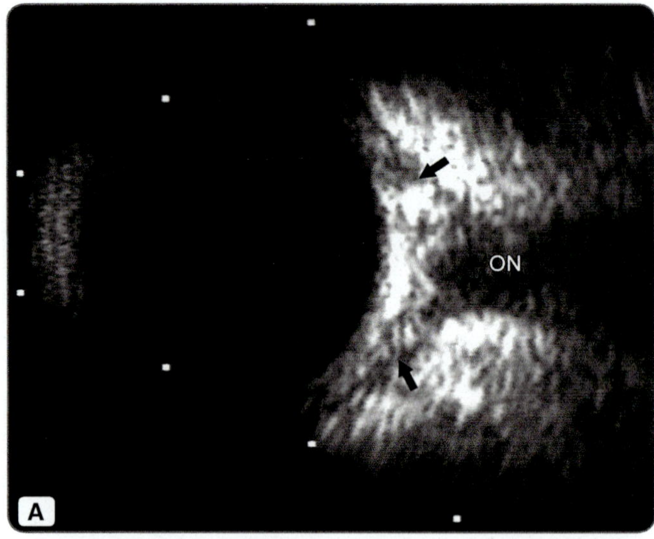

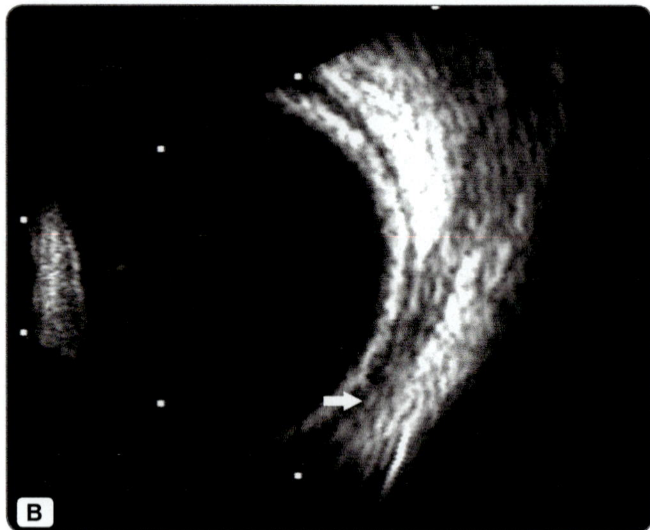

Figures 41.2A and B: B scan images showing irregular low reflective thickening of the Tenon's space (arrows), more obvious around the optic nerve (ON). Figure B shows thickening of the muscle belly adjacent to the Tenon's widening (arrow).

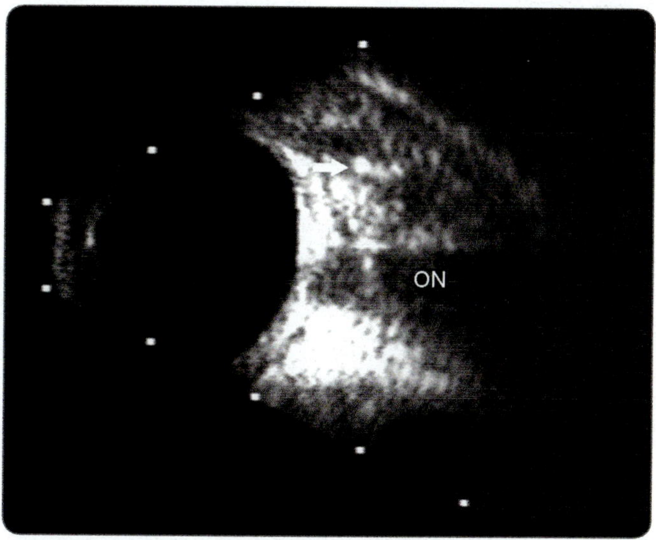

Figure 41.3: A more ill-defined lesion seen in the upper part of the echogram, irregular and low reflective, along the extent of the muscle (arrow). Tenon's widening is seen in this image as well.

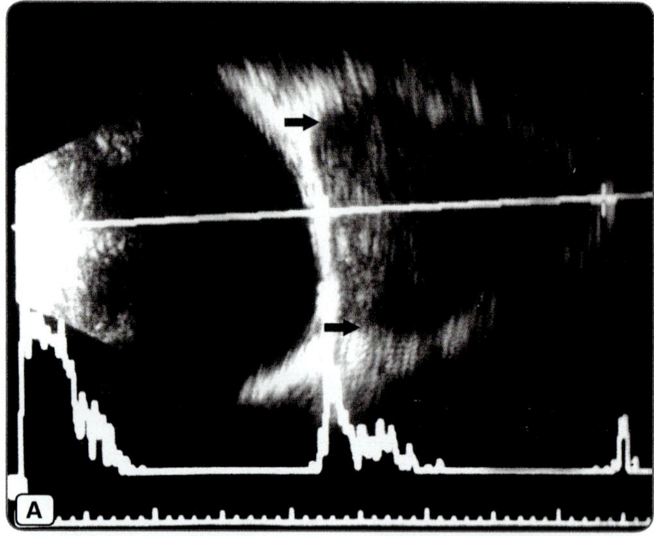

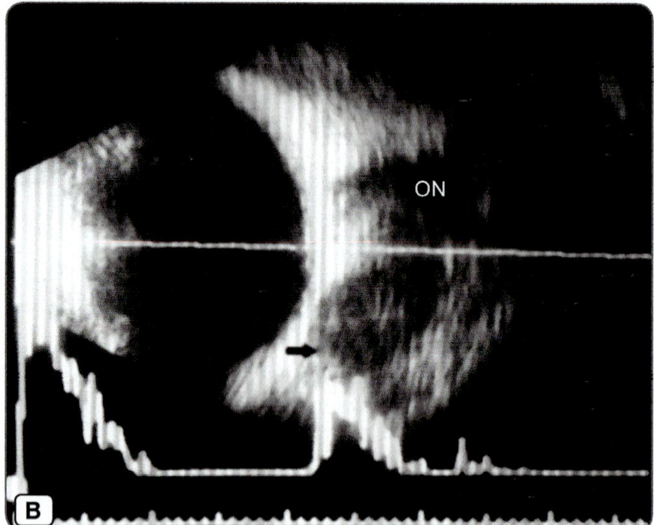

Figures 41.4A and B: A well-defined intraconal mass lesion surrounding the optic nerve (arrows). The lesion shows very low reflectivity on A scan. The second image shows the residual mass (arrow) nasal to the optic nerve, after orbitotomy. Histopathology was suggestive of a pseudotumor with fibrosis.

42 Orbital Abscess and Hematoma

CLINICAL FEATURES

- Can cause painful proptosis.
- Precipitating features like trauma or blood dyscrasias may be present in case of a hematoma.
- History of sinus infection or penetrating injury may be present in an orbital abscess.
- External features such as lid edema, chemosis and local rise of temperature may be present in both, but are more severe in case of an abscess. Associated systemic features such as fever and toxic signs may be present in an abscess.
- Ultrasound is indicated to diagnose the condition, follow-up for results of treatment and aid in fine needle aspiration of these lesions. Orbital foreign bodies need to be ruled out in case of trauma.
- CT scan may also be performed to rule out orbital fractures and other bony changes.

ULTRASONOGRAPHY

- Well-circumscribed lesion with low internal reflectivity.
- May be multiloculated or solitary.
- If subperiosteal in nature, the lesion may be well separated from the orbital soft tissues and communication with the adjacent paranasal sinuses may be demonstrable.
- In the case of an abscess, adjacent Tenon's widening or muscle thickening may be present. The T sign may be visible.

NUGGETS

Layering of echoes or a fluid level is more often seen in a blood filled cyst than an abscess.

A blood cyst is more likely to spontaneously decrease in size over a period of time.

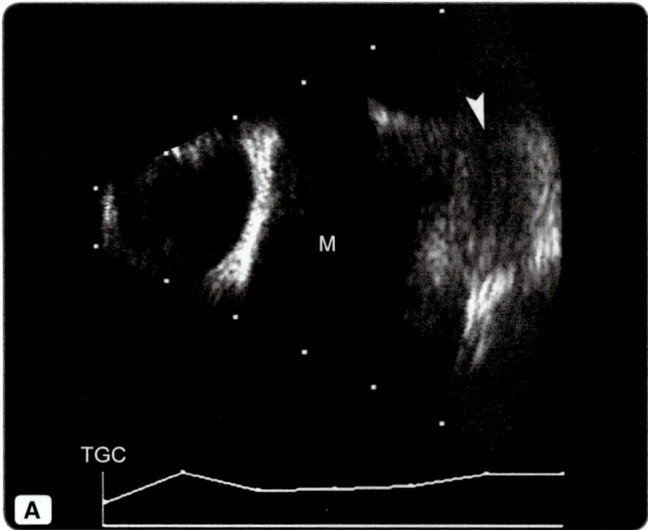

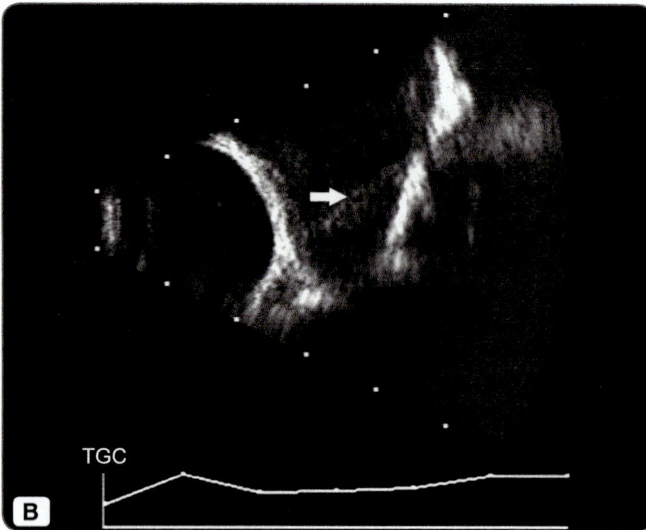

Figures 42.1A and B: B scan images of an elderly lady with progressive proptosis. There is a large orbital mass (M) with low reflectivity and causing erosion of the lateral orbital wall (arrowhead). Figure B shows the same mass lesion showing a fluid level (arrow), this suggests the presence of an abscess cavity or a blood filled cyst.

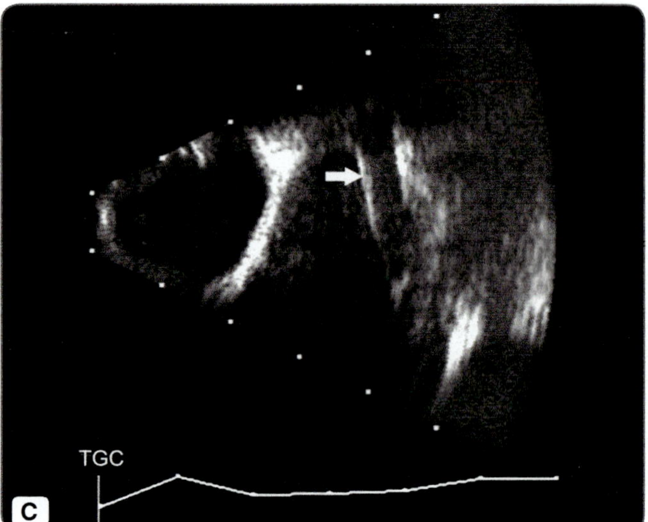

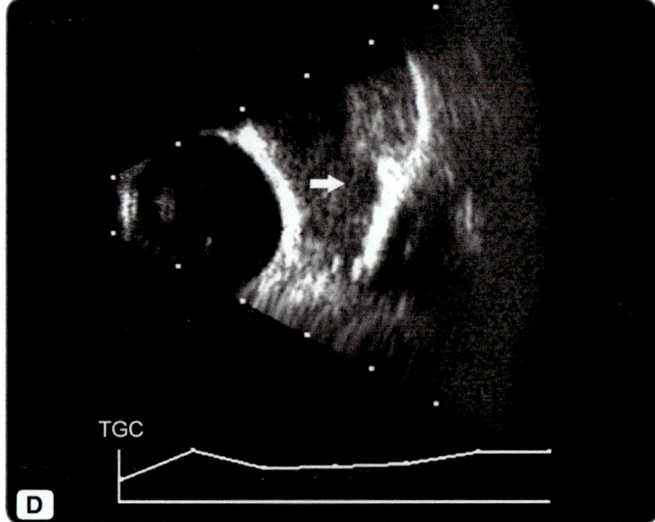

Figures 42.1C and D: The patient underwent an ultrasound guided fine needle aspiration procedure. The B scan image on the left shows the needle (arrow) within the mass. The aspirate appeared yellowish white in color, suggestive of purulent material. Smear showed septate fungi. The B scan image on the right after the procedure showing a reduction in size of the lesion along with disappearance of the fluid level. The echoes are more evenly distributed within the mass.

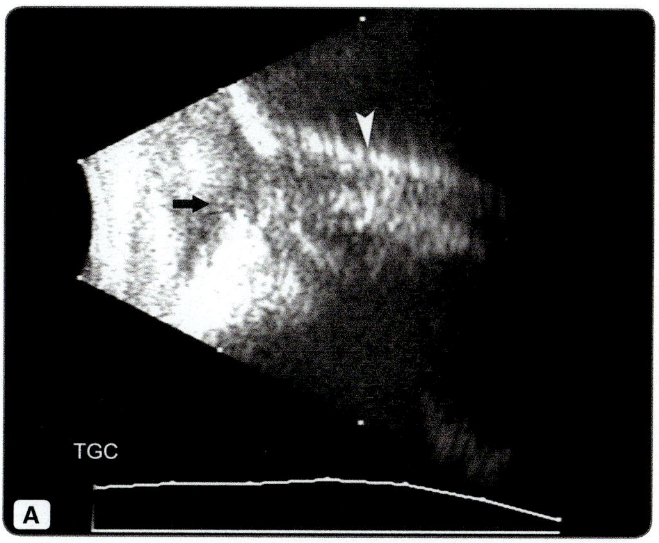

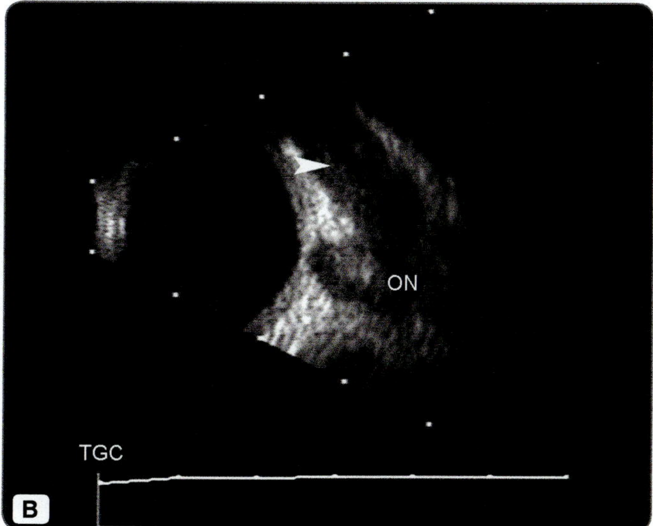

Figures 42.2A and B: B scan image of a patient with history of partial drainage of a superomedial anterior orbital mass. The aspirate yielded purulent material indicative of an abscess. This para axial scan shows a heterogenous preseptal mass lesion above the globe (arrow), which appears to have a posterior extension into the orbit along the orbital roof (arrowhead). The lower image is a transocular scan of the same patient showing the low reflective mass (arrowhead) extending along the medial rectus into the orbit.

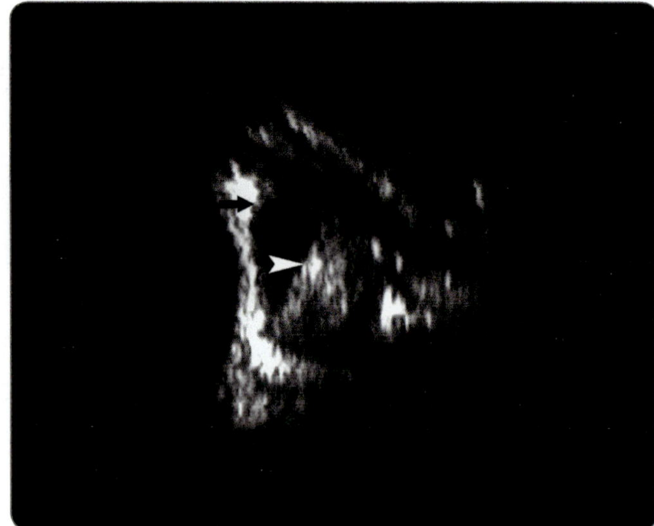

Figure 42.3: B scan image of a patient with a traumatic intraconal hematoma (arrow) of the orbit. The lesion is well circumscribed and shows a fluid level (arrowhead).

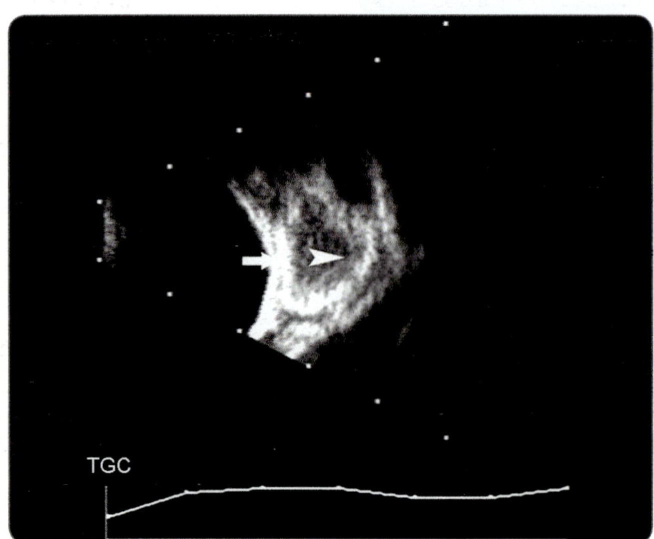

Figure 42.4: B scan image of a patient with a thick walled intraconal mass (arrow). This patient had painful proptosis and a suspected intracranial vascular malformation. The echoes within the cyst are low reflective, along with a fluid level (arrowhead). Aspiration of the cyst resulted in reduction of the mass. The cyst contents consisted of a mixture of blood and pus.

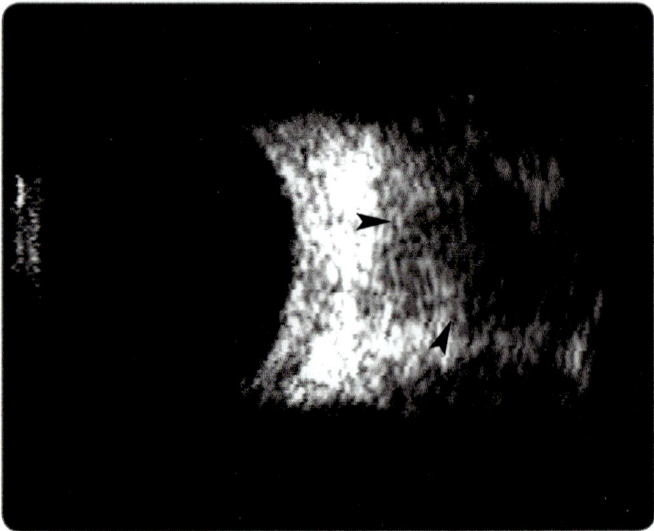

Figure 42.5: Transocular B scan of a patient with history of hemophilia and proptosis. Note the low reflective intraconal lesion (arrowheads), which appears well circumscribed and represents a hematoma.

43 Ultrasound-guided Fine Needle Aspiration Biopsy (FNAB)

INDICATIONS

- Suspected orbital metastasis from a distant or adjacent source
- Orbital abscess or hematoma
- Orbital mass in patients with systemic lymphoma

CONTRAINDICATIONS

- Tumors that are mainly in the posterior orbit or directly above or below the globe.
- Suspected inflammatory masses—the sample obtained may not represent the true composition of the lesion and hence may not contribute to the diagnosis.
- Well-encapsulated lesions—damage to the capsule during FNAB may interfere with complete removal later by orbitotomy, also there is the fear of spread of a potentially malignant mass.
- Lacrimal gland tumors especially pleomorphic adenoma where damage to the pseudocapsule can promote recurrences.
- Patients with bleeding disorders.

PROCEDURE

- The lesion is first evaluated on ultrasound
- 22 gauge needle mounted on a 5 cc syringe is used
- Infiltration of a local anesthetic is performed around the proposed site of needle puncture. In children it is performed under general anesthesia
- The area of the biopsy site is cleaned
- As the needle is introduced, the probe is used to scan longitudinally along the path to visualize the needle along its length
- Once the needle is inside the lesion, the required quantity of material is aspirated
- The needle is withdrawn along the same path, visualizing its exit on ultrasound.

COMPLICATIONS

- Globe perforation with the needle
- Orbital hemorrhage
- Damage to the optic nerve
- Seeding of the tumor along the needle path
- Ocular motility disturbances
- Ptosis

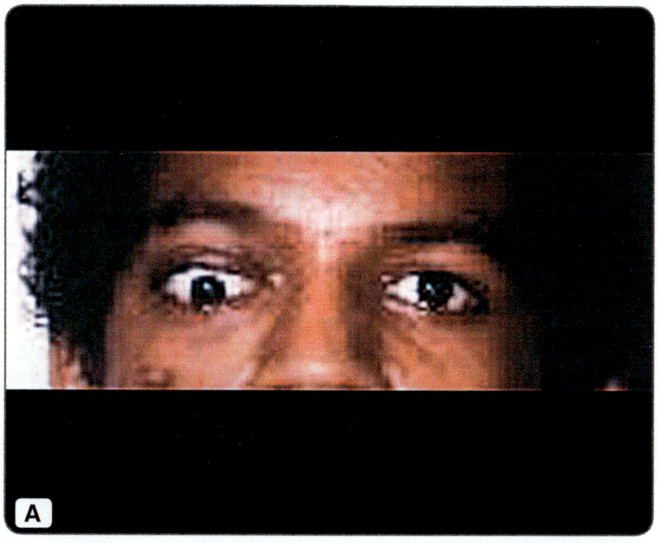

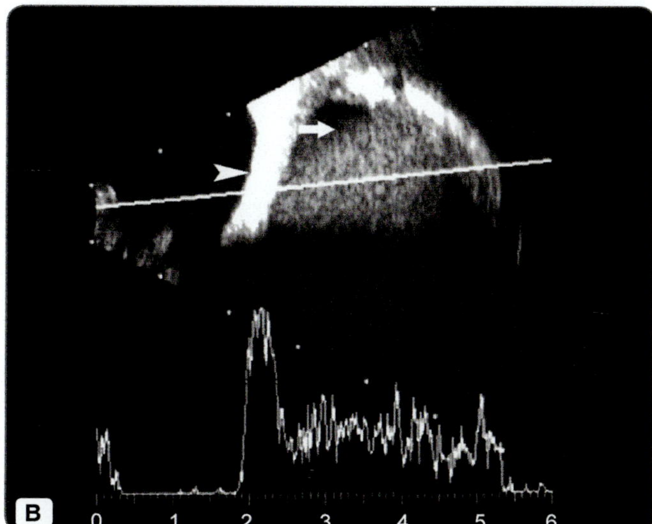

Figures 43.1A and B: Clinical photograph and B scan of a patient with proptosis and upper lid swelling. The B scan with vector A scan shows a large orbital mass with moderate to low reflective echoes. Note the globe indentation caused by the mass (arrowhead) and a small echolucent area at the superior aspect indicating a fluid level (arrow). This was a case of hematinic cyst following a road traffic accident.

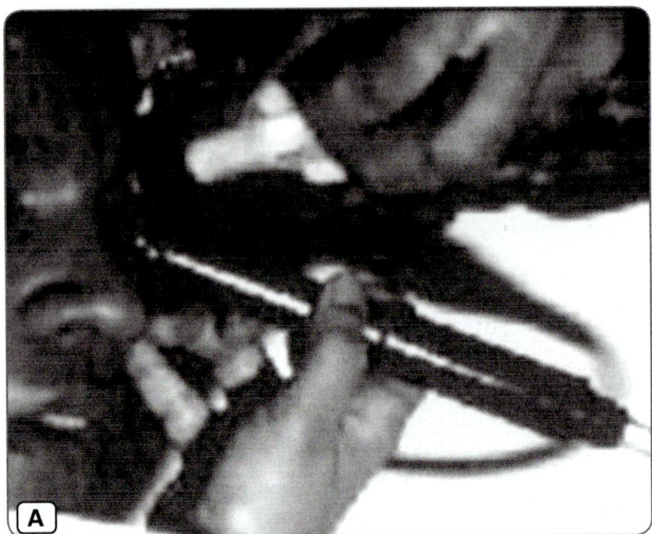

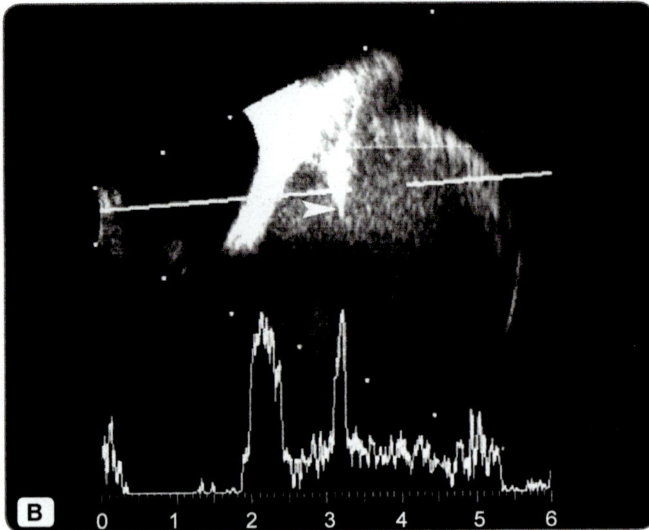

Figures 43.2A and B: Clinical photograph and B scan taken during ultrasound guided FNAB. Note the high reflective linear echo indicating the needle tip (arrowhead) within the lesion.

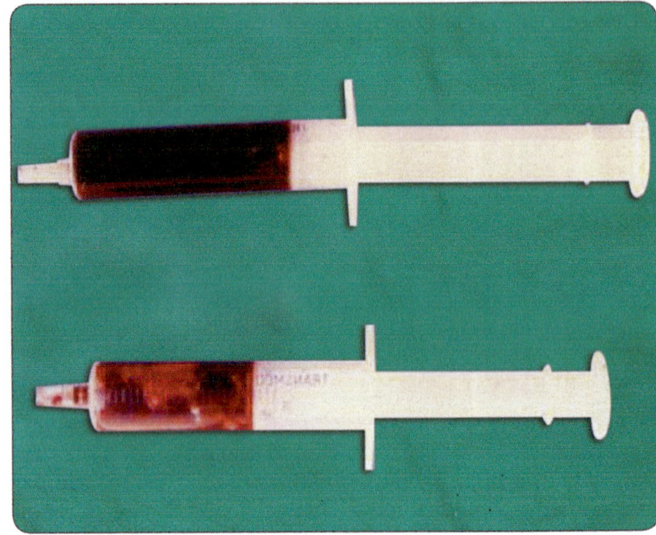

Figure 43.2C: 10 ml of blood was aspirated from the mass.

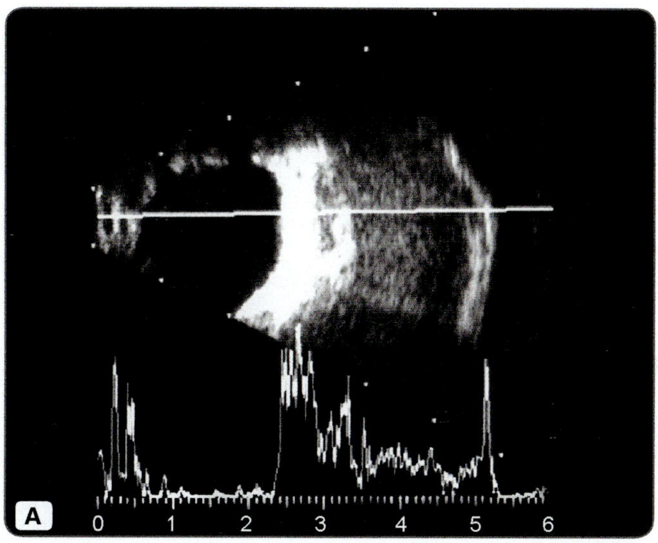

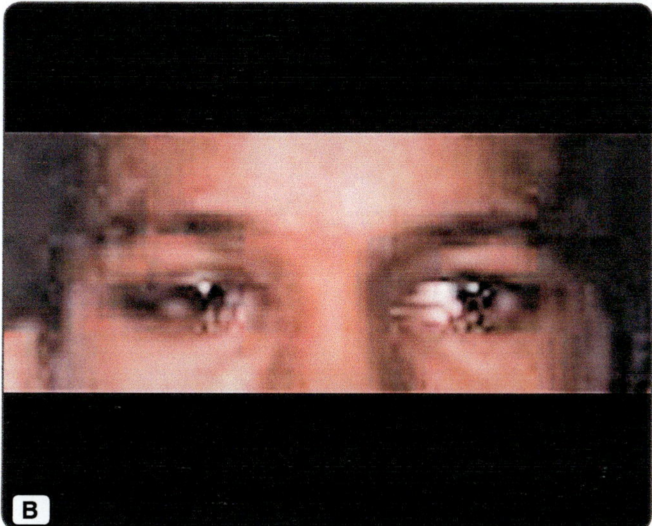

Figures 43.3A and B: At conclusion of the procedure note the reduction in the upper lid swelling on clinical photograph and a decrease in the size of the mass on B scan ultrasound. A diagnosis of hematinic cyst was confirmed.

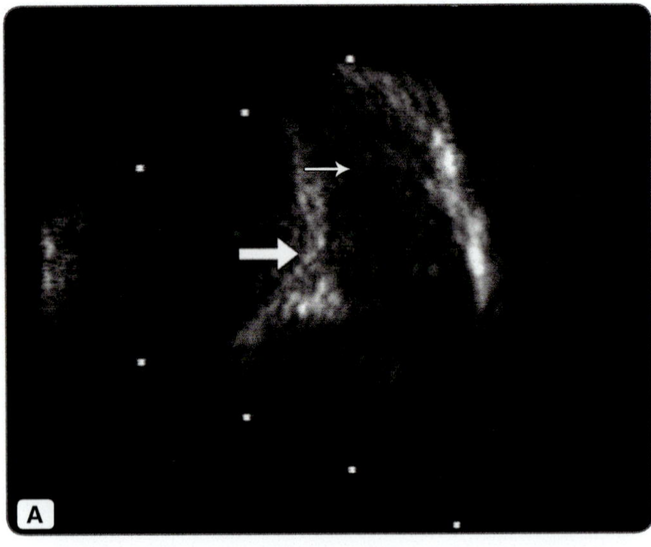

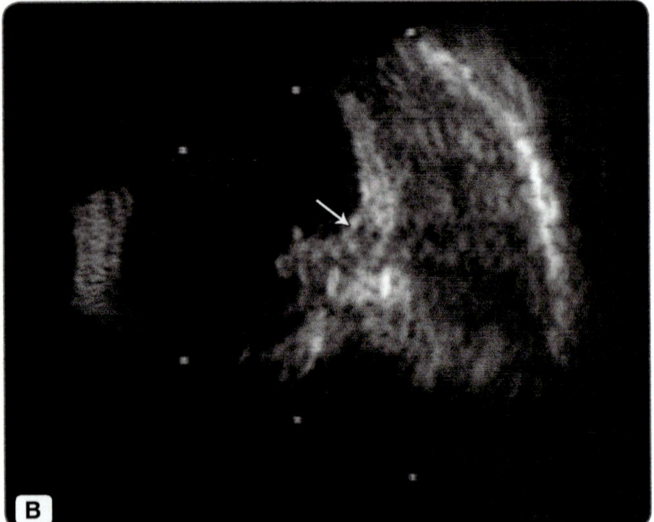

Figures 43.4A and B: 12-year-male child who underwent fine needle aspiration for an orbital mass and reported loss of vision after the procedure. The B scan images show a mass adjacent to the lateral rectus muscle (thin arrow) with low reflective echoes. Figure B shows intragel echoes converging on the globe wall adjacent to the mass lesion indicative of globe perforation (thin arrow) during attempted drainage of the abscess.

44 Orbital Schwannoma

CLINICAL FEATURES

- Also known as neurilemmoma
- May be isolated or can occur in association with neurofibromatosis
- Can be either intraconal or extraconal in location
- Causes gradual progression of proptosis and decreased vision.

ULTRASONOGRAPHY

- Oval, well-encapsulated lesions
- Regular structure with low internal reflectivity
- May have septae or cystic spaces.

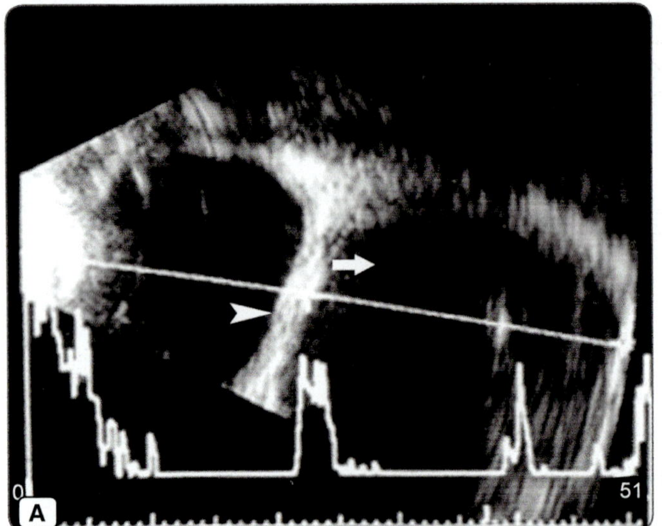

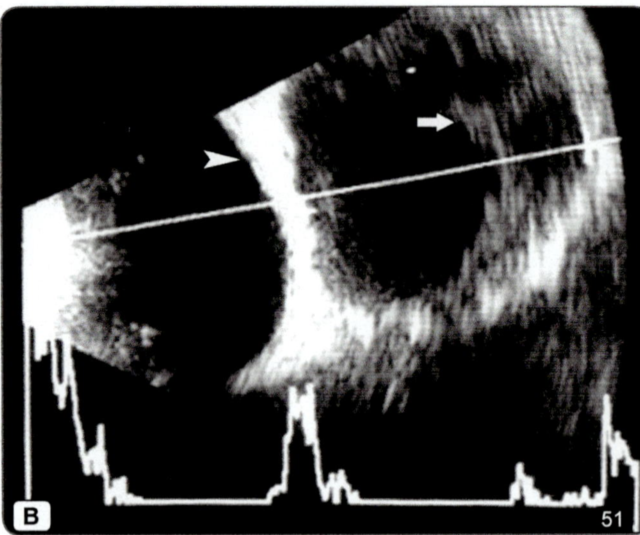

Figures 44.1A and B: Transocular scans of a patient with painless progressive proptosis. There is a large well-encapsulated mass lesion in the intraconal space (arrow), causing globe wall indentation (arrowhead). The internal structure shows large echolucent spaces suggestive of cystic changes. Orbitotomy was performed and HPE diagnosis was schwannoma.

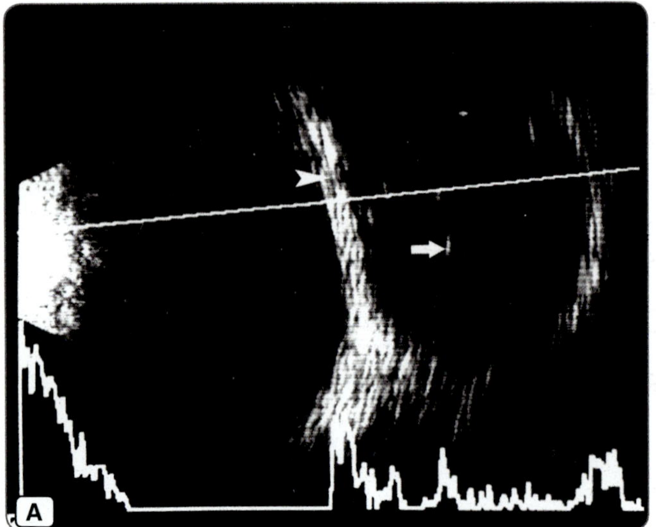

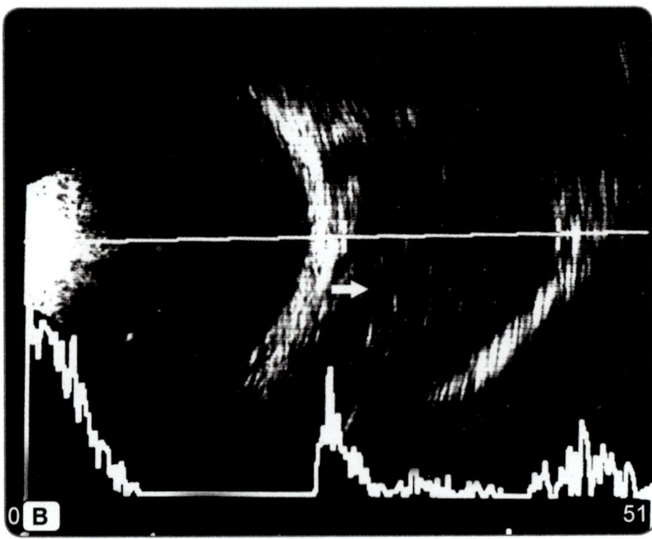

Figures 44.2A and B: Transocular scans of a large, well-encapsulated orbital mass with well-defined borders and a very low internal reflectivity (arrow). Few dot like moderately reflective echoes are seen within the mass, which is also seen to indent the optic nerve. Globe wall indentation is also seen (arrowhead). HPE of this mass showed features of a schwannoma.

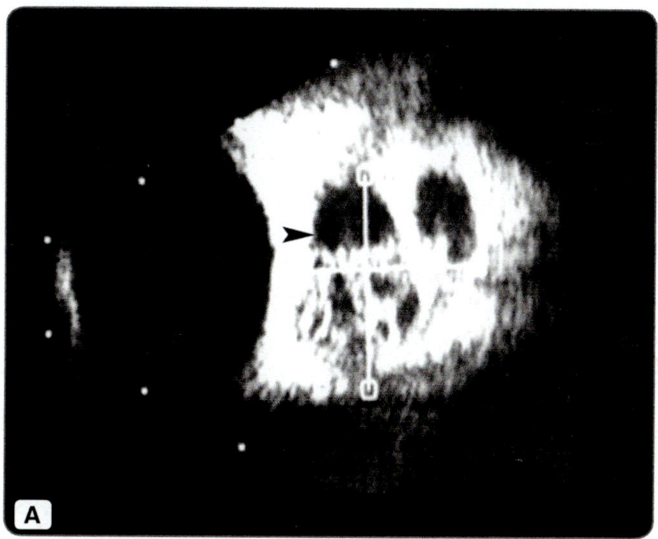

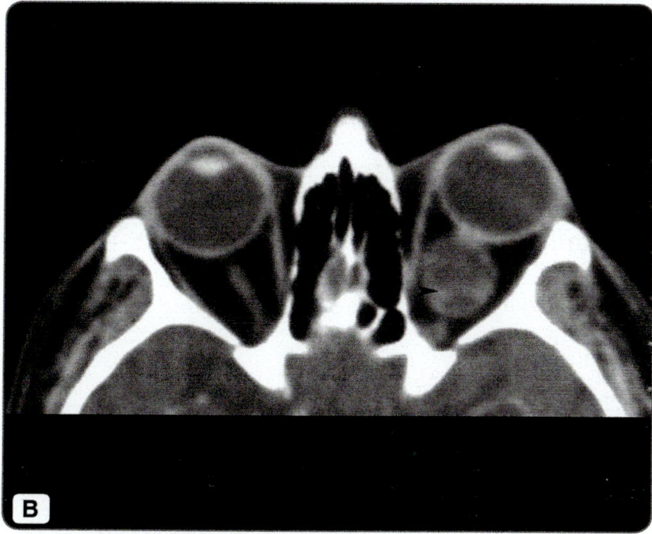

Figures 44.3A and B: B scan image showing a well-encapsulated intraconal mass with cystic spaces (arrowhead). CT scan shows the cystic spaces as well. HPE confirmed the presence of a cystic schwannoma.

45 Rhabdomyosarcoma

CLINICAL FEATURES

- Commonest primary malignant orbital tumor in children.
- Rapidly growing proptosis in a young child.
- May mimic an acute inflammatory condition.

ULTRASONOGRAPHY

- Well-circumscribed lesions.
- Tend to be unilateral and extraconal.
- Low to medium internal echoes.
- Adjacent bone may be intact or eroded.
- Internal vascularity may be demonstrated on the A scan.

NUGGETS

Rhabdomyosarcoma may appear clinically and echogenically like a pseudotumor. However, associated features like Tenon's widening, scleritis, and muscle thickening are absent.

Bony defects are more likely in rhabdomyosarcoma than pseudotumor.

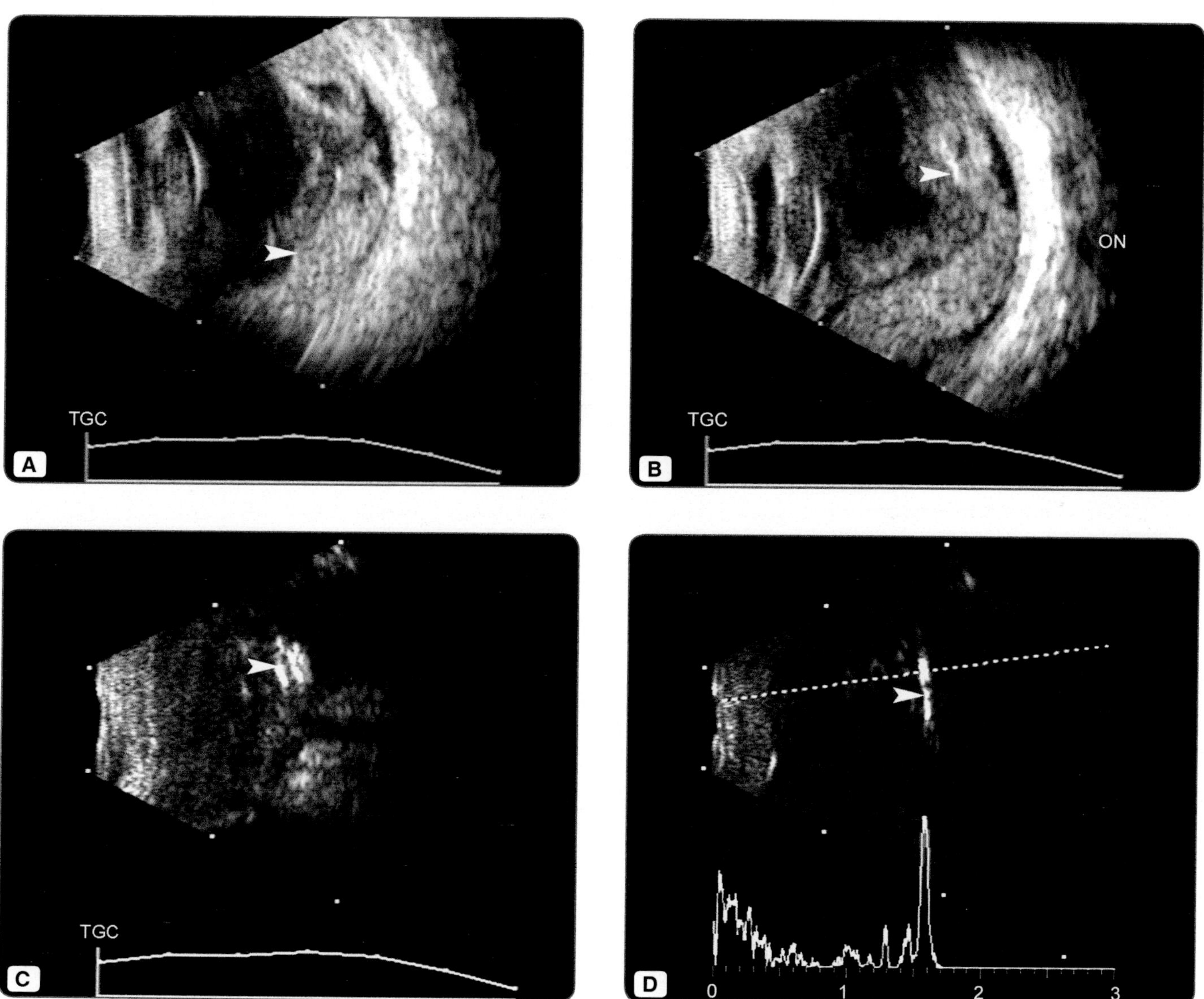

Figures 46.1A to D: B scan images of a young girl with bilateral retinoblastoma. The axial B scan shows a large exophytic mass (arrowhead). The eye was enucleated and HPE confirmed the diagnosis of retinoblastoma. B scan of the orbit six months after enucleation and chemotherapy. The patient presented with proptosis and an extruded prosthesis. The scan shows a calcific lesion (arrowhead) which was found to be an orbital recurrence and showed necrotic tumor cells on HPE. This is an example of local tumor recurrence.

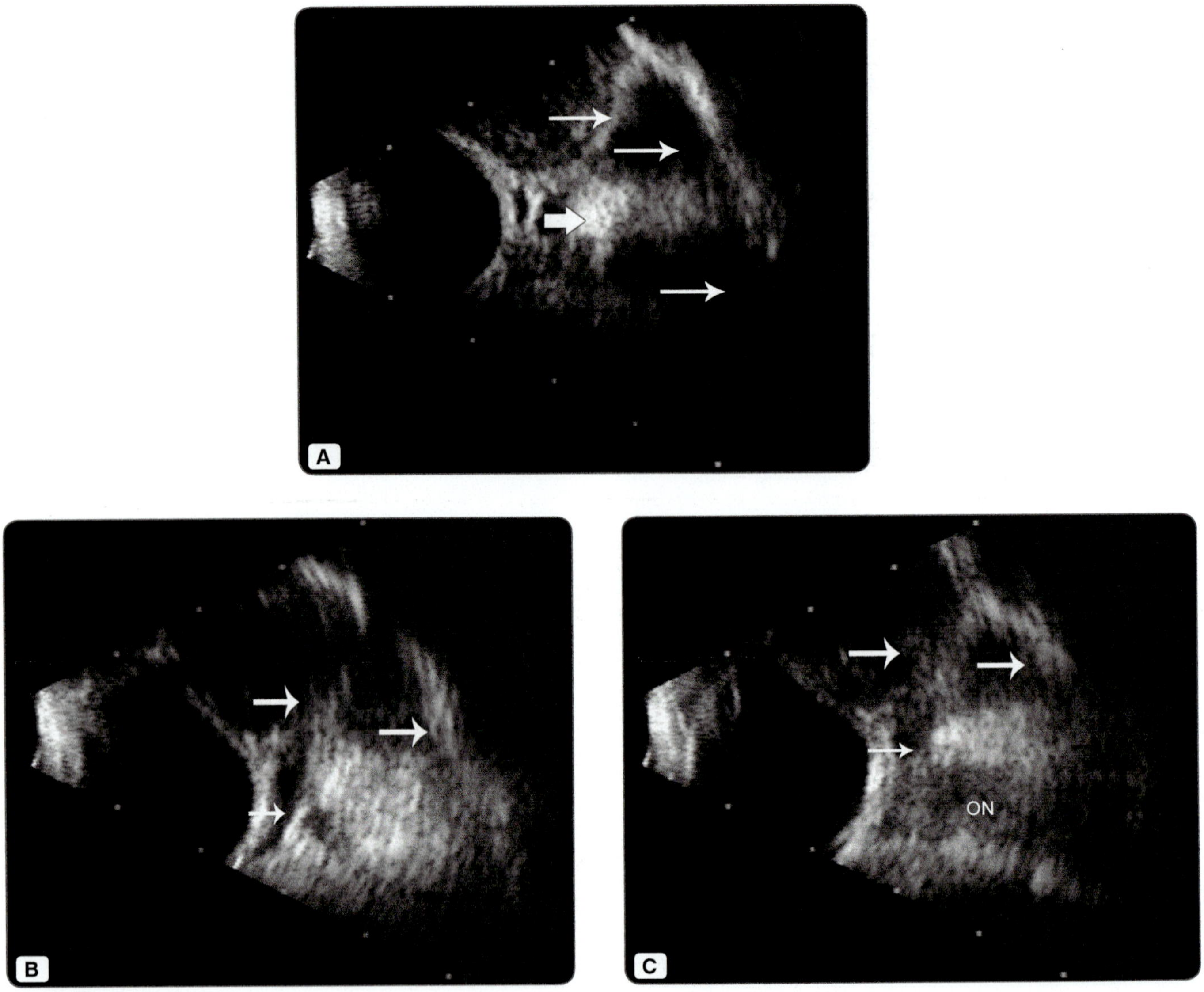

Figures 46.2A to C: Ultrasound B scan images of the left orbit of a 2-year-old child with progressive proptosis that increased on crying. Examination revealed the proptosis to be reducible with a palpable thrill. Ultrasound revealed a large ill-defined lesion in the superomedial orbit that consisted predominantly of areas of echolucency (arrows) with a few high reflective areas (broad arrow) and septae. The mass changed features when the child was crying (Fig. B). The optic nerve is not well seen (ON). MRI and Doppler imaging characterized this as a venolymphatic malformation extending into the paranasal sinuses as well as intracranially.

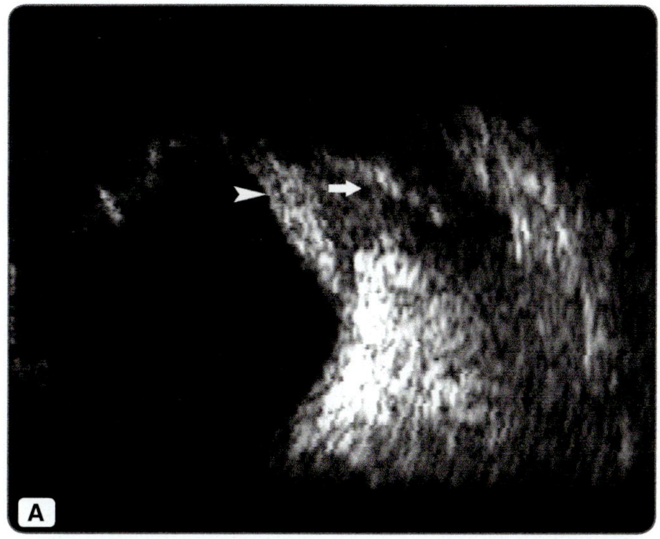

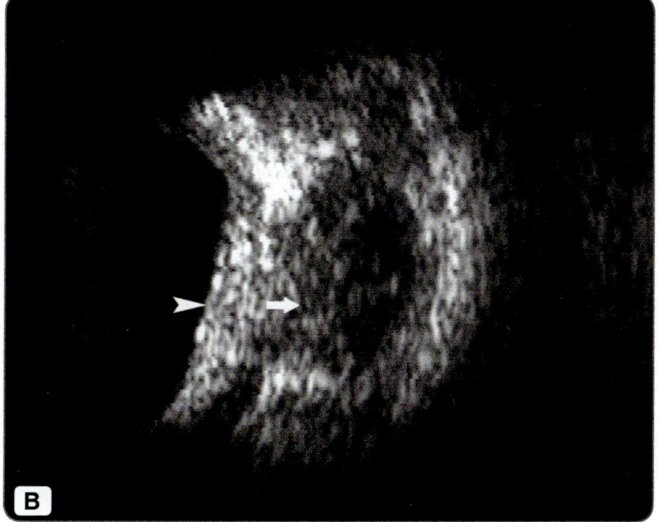

Figures 46.3A and B: Longitudinal and transverse transocular B scan ima ges of a middle-aged man with a conjunctival mass, diagnosed as squamous cell carcinoma. The orbital scan shows a low reflective mass lesion in the superior orbit (arrow) extending posteriorly from the conjunctiva, along the superior rectus muscle. The mass also involves the sclera and causes globe wall indentation (arrowhead). This is an example of contiguous tumor spread into the orbit.

Section 9

Optic Nerve Disorders

47 Optic Nerve Thickening

CLINICAL SITUATIONS

- Normal diameter of the retrobulbar optic nerve ranges from 2.2 to 3.3 mm with a mean value of 2.5 mm.
- Difference of more than 0.5 mm between the two nerves is of significance.
- Thickening may be due to widening of the parenchyma, perineural sheaths or increase in subarachnoid fluid.
- Though MRI and CT scans are more useful in imaging the optic nerve, an ultrasound may give useful initial information to the ophthalmologist.

ULTRASONOGRAPHY

- Lesions involving the parenchyma such as tumors and inflammations cause homogenous thickening of the nerve
- Lesions involving the sheaths such as nerve sheath meningiomas cause irregularly thickened nerves with heterogenous internal echoes
- Lesions causing increased subarachnoid fluid such as pseudotumor cerebri cause a low reflective widening of the subarachnoid space around the nerve—the 30 degree test may be positive. The 'doughnut sign' may be present in gross thickening.

NUGGETS

In case of a tumor near the apex, the only finding seen on ultrasound may be thickening of the proximal part of the nerve due to stasis of subarachnoid fluid.

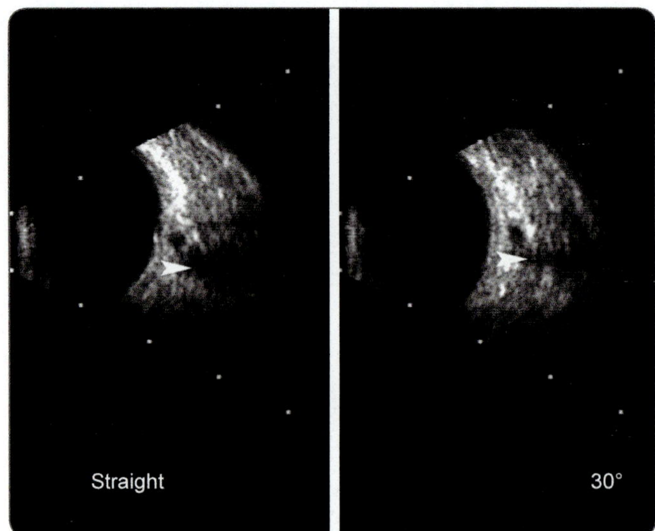

Figure 47.1A: Dual B scan image of the right optic nerve of a patient with bilateral papilloedema due to pseudotumor cerebri. The scan on the left shows the widened subarachnoid space due to fluid collection, in the primary position (arrowhead). The scan on the right shows the decrease in the thickness with the eye moved 30 degrees temporally—a positive thirty degree test.

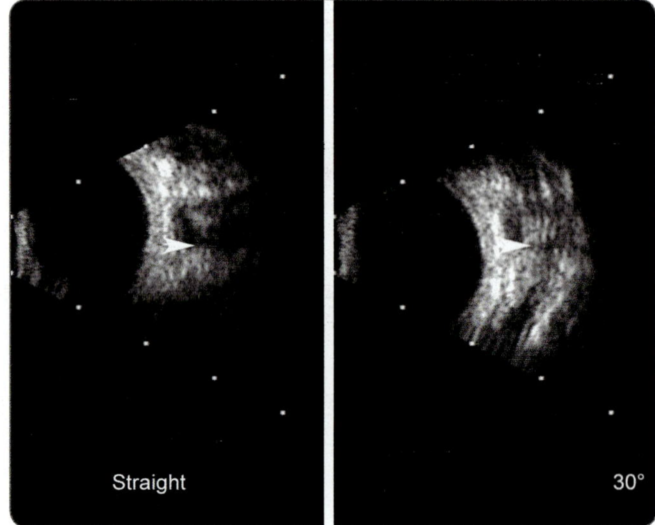

Figure 47.1B: Dual B scan images of the left optic nerve of the same patient, with similar findings.

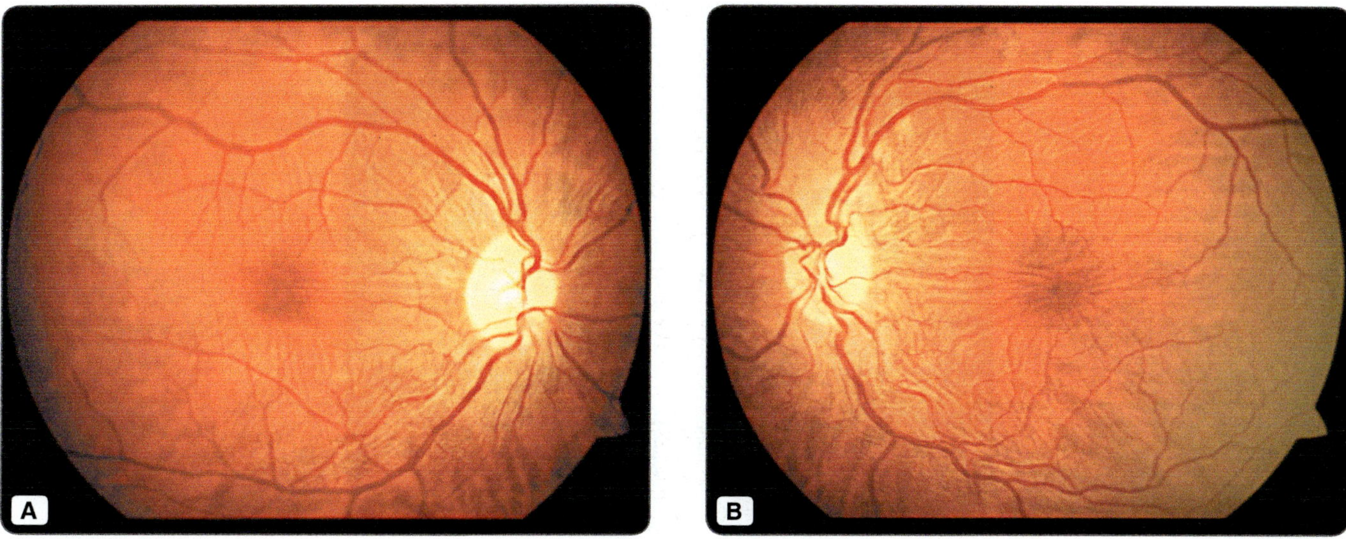

Figures 47.2A and B: Color fundus photographs of both eyes of a middle-aged male who presented with decreased vision in both eyes. The posterior pole shows evidence of internal limiting membrane striae. The vessels in the left eye appear tortuous.

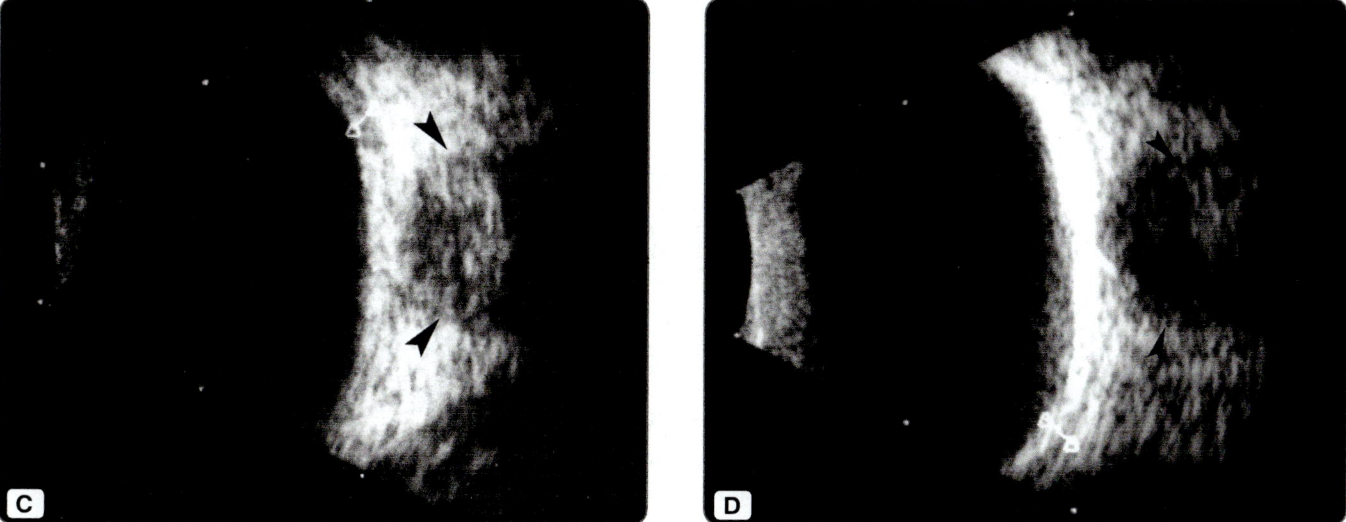

Figures 47.2C and D: B scan images of both eyes show evidence of globe wall flattening with choroidal thickening. Both optic nerves appear grossly widened (arrowheads). MRI confirmed the presence of bilateral optic nerve thickening. The patient responded to high dose systemic steroids.

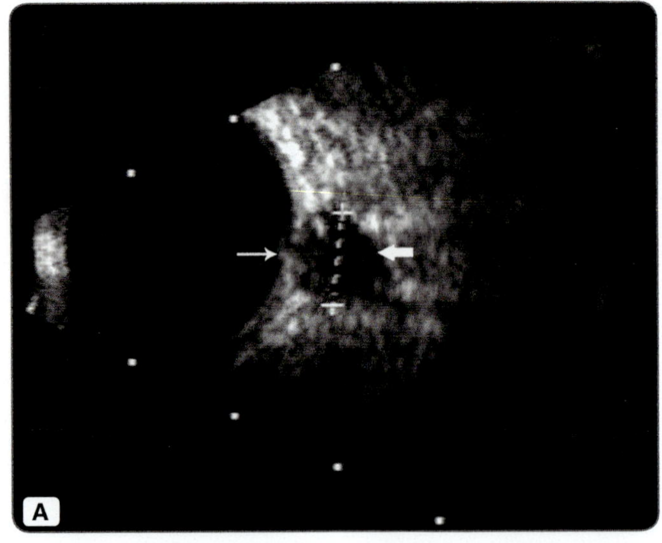

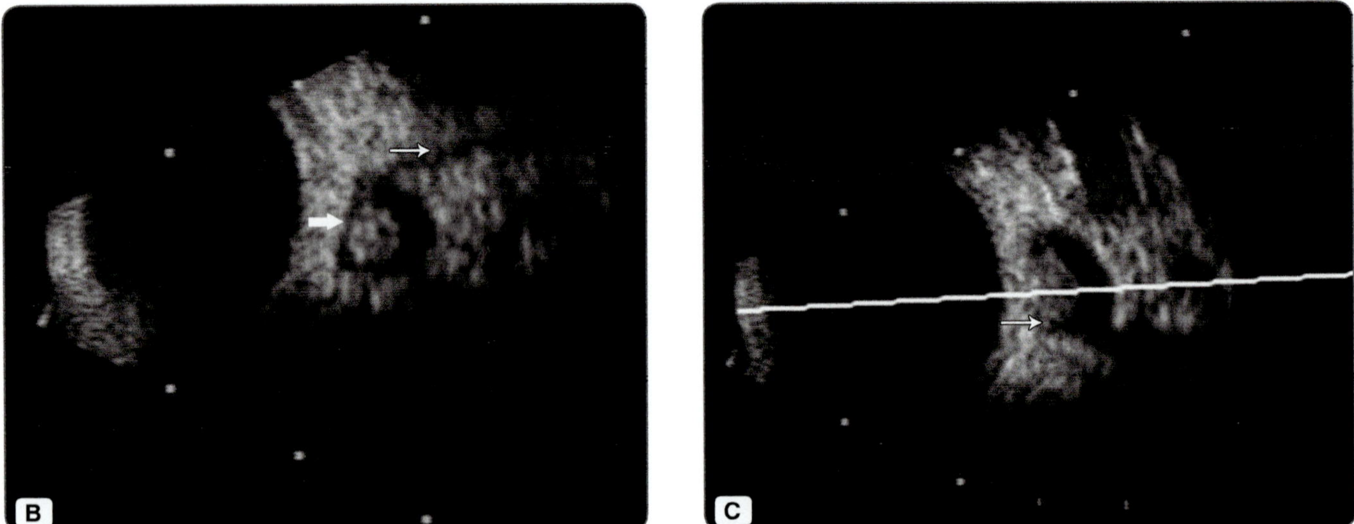

Figures 47.3A to C: Ultrasound images of a case of optic disc edema. Figure A shows the disc elevation (arrow) and widening of the optic nerve sheaths near the entry into the globe (fine arrow). Figure B shows the typical "doughnut" sign seen with concentric widening of the sheath. Figure C shows the decrease in the widening with abduction of the eye.

48 Tumors of the Optic Nerve

CLINICAL FEATURES

The two most primary common optic nerve tumors are optic nerve glioma and optic nerve meningioma.

Optic Nerve Glioma

- Optic nerve glioma is typically a tumor of childhood. If present in adults, it is more aggressive in nature.
- The symptoms are usually related to visual loss due to compression of the optic nerve. If restricted to the optic nerve, they cause unilateral loss of vision.
- Proptosis, diplopia and ptosis may occur.
- It may be associated with neurofibromatosis I. Optic atrophy in a child with no retinal or macular degeneration points to an optic nerve glioma, especially in neurofibromatosis.

Optic Nerve Sheath Meningioma

- Typically a tumor of adulthood, seen more frequently in middle-aged women. Meningiomas rarely occur in childhood, but if they do, they are usually intraorbital and more aggressive than those in adults
- The term optic nerve sheath meningioma (ONSM) does not indicate a definite site of origin. It may be either primary, which arises from the cap cells of the arachnoid surrounding the intraorbital or intracanalicular optic nerve, or secondary when it is an extension of an intracranial meningioma into the orbit
- The characteristic profile of a compressive optic neuropathy, such as that caused by ONSM, is usually painless, chronic progressive visual loss that may be accompanied by proptosis.

ULTRASONOGRAPHY

- MRI is the best method of optic nerve evaluation. However, ultrasonography may be the initial investigation performed in an ophthalmologist's clinic especially if the patient presents with proptosis
- Optic nerve gliomas present as smooth fusiform thickening of the optic nerve shadow. The reflectivity is homogenous and low. In long-standing cases, cystic areas may be seen
- Optic nerve sheath meningiomas also show thickening of the optic nerve shadow, but have an irregular structure, and may show areas of calcification.

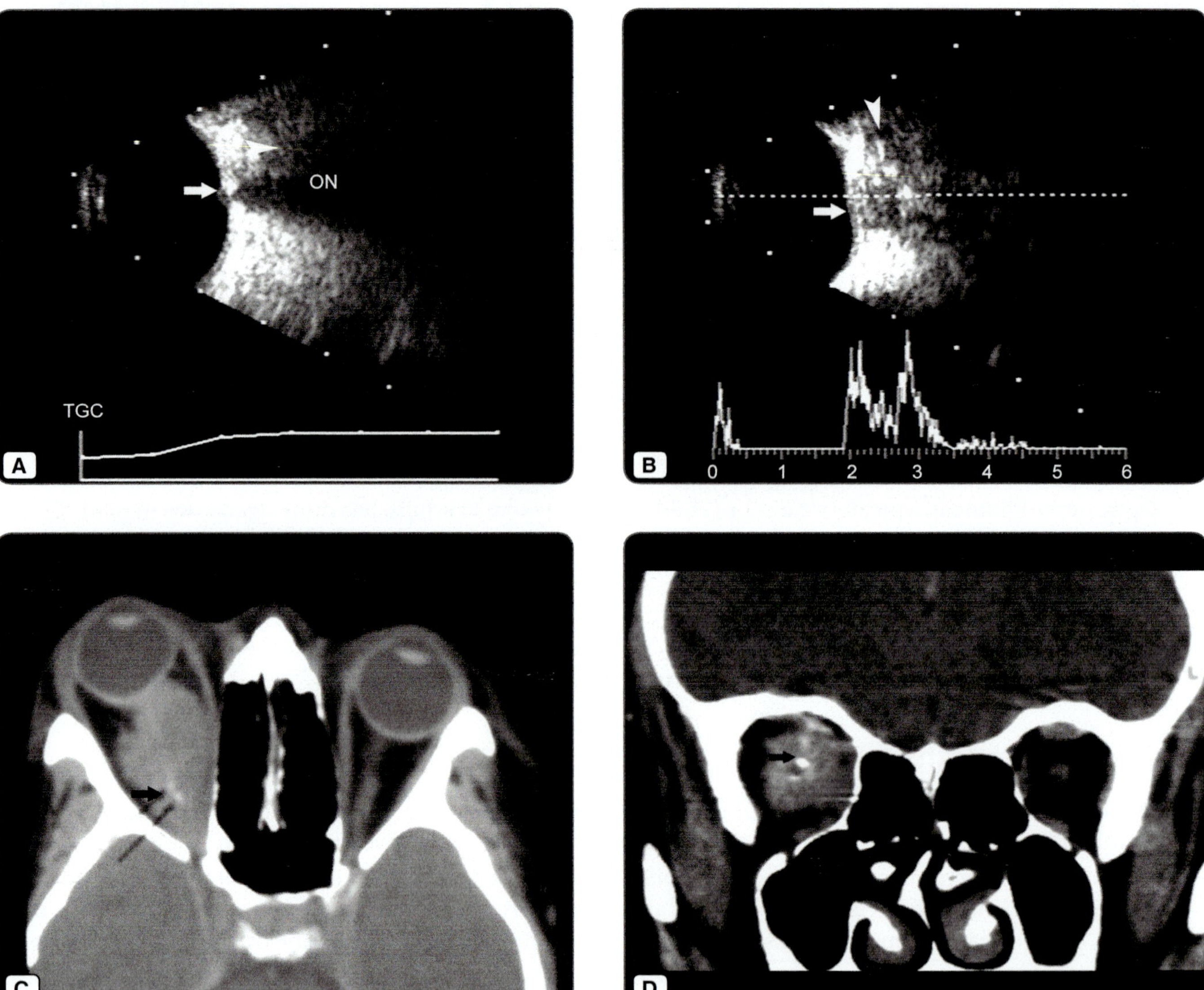

Figures 48.1A to D: B scan images of a young girl with decreased vision in the right eye, disc edema and choroidal folds. The disc elevation is seen (arrow) along with an irregular thickening of the superior aspect of the optic nerve (arrowhead). Figure B shows an irregular mass with heterogenous reflectivity (arrowhead) involving the optic nerve. Note the globe wall flattening (arrow) caused by the mass, along with a high reflective clump of echoes within the mass suggestive of calcification. Axial and coronal plain CT images showing a mass lesion involving the optic nerve sheath and extending till the orbital apex. There are specks of calcification along the nerve (arrow). The mass showed brilliant enhancement with contrast and was proven to be a case of optic nerve sheath meningioma.

NUGGETS

Suspect a tumor of the optic nerve if there is solid thickening of the nerve to double or more than the opposite normal side.

Lesions that are anterior can be picked up on ultrasound, but lesions near the apex may be suspected because of secondary changes such as increased fluid anteriorly.

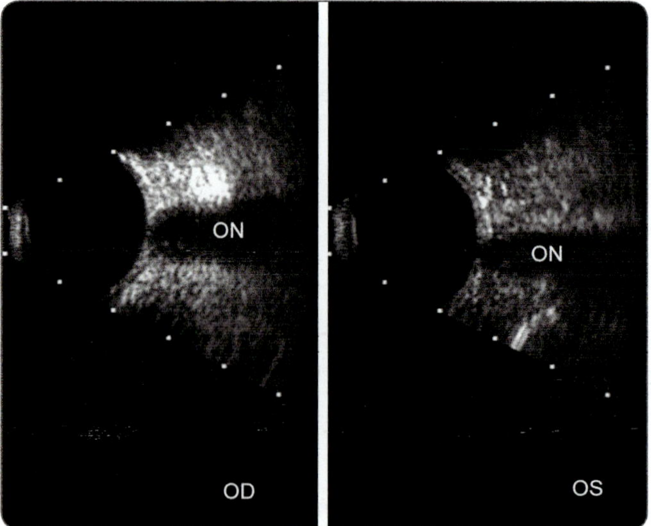

Figure 48.2: B scan images of the right and left eyes of a patient with disc edema of the right eye and a suspected optic nerve tumor. Note the subtle thickening of the right optic nerve (OD) compared to the left (OS). The MRI showed evidence of an optic nerve glioma near the orbital apex with thickening of the anterior part of the optic nerve. The dual B scan comparing the two optic nerves helps to diagnose the subtle thickening.

49 Optic Nerve Injury

CLINICAL SITUATIONS AND FEATURES

Direct Trauma to the Optic Nerve

- Penetrating wound of the orbit.
- Fracture of the orbital walls, optic canal or superior orbital fissure.
- Blunt injury causing contusion of the optic nerve with edema and/or hemorrhage.
- Avulsion of the optic nerve is suspected when there is no light perception and a picture of peripapillary hemorrhage and choroidal/scleral rupture near the optic disc. The vessels may appear tortuous, attenuated or appear to end abruptly at the avulsion. Arteriolar occlusion or segmentation of the blood column may be seen. If the media is clear, a hole or cavity in the region of the optic disc is seen where the disc has retracted into the dural sheath.
- Orbital surgery itself, due to hemorrhage, direct manipulation, tight postoperative dressings.
- Direct injury due to faulty needle positioning during retrobulbar anesthesia.

Indirect Injury Due to Orbitofacial or Closed Head Trauma

- Usually occurs where the nerve is tightly tethered to the walls of the optic canal.
- Hemorrhage or edema within the canal can compress the nerve.
- Shearing forces at both ends of the canal, where the brain and orbital contents are free to move but the intracanalicular part of the nerve is not.

ULTRASONOGRAPHY

- Not classically used to diagnose optic nerve injury as it is unable to image the nerve in its complete extent. The changes seen on ultrasound are not specific to any particular form of damage.
- The retrobulbar optic nerve shadow may be enlarged due to hemorrhage or edema.
- Thirty degree test may be positive.
- Low reflective areas within the orbit can indicate orbital hemorrhage.

- Optic nerve avulsion may be diagnosed by demonstrating scleral discontinuity near the exit of the nerve and clumps of vitreous echoes over the peripapillary region signifying hemorrhage. Tenon's space widening around the optic nerve insertion may also be seen. Once the acute phase has passed, the only feature may be an alteration in the direction or appearance of the nerve where it inserts into the globe.

NUGGETS

Ultrasonography is helpful but not specific in diagnosing optic nerve injury.

As orbital appearances are very variable it is helpful to compare with the opposite side before diagnosing any pathology.

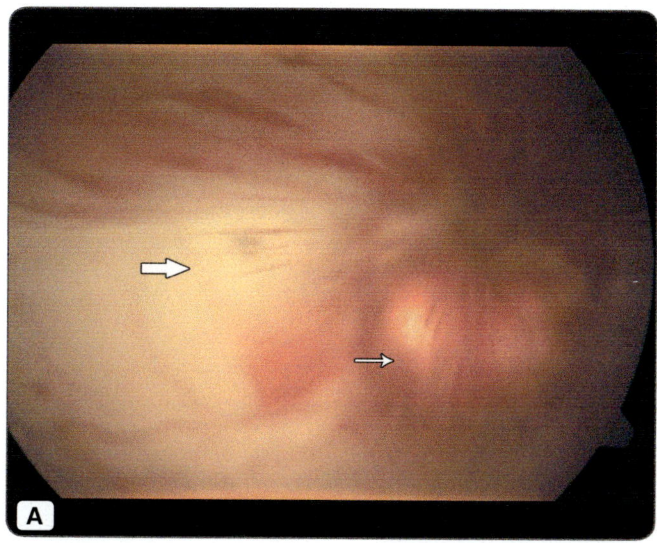

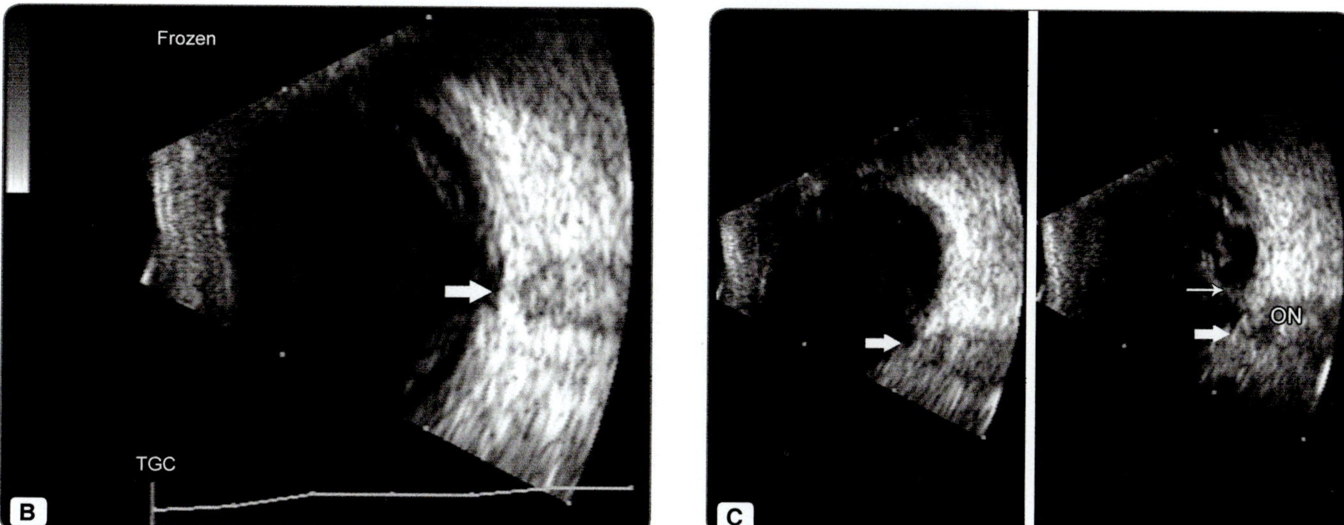

Figures 49.1A to C: 11-year-child presented with loss of light perception in after a road traffic accident. Right eye fundus showed vitreous hemorrhage tracking from the area of the optic disc. Whitening of the retina was noted (thick arrow). There was a large area of excavation (thin arrow) and bare sclera noted in the area of the disc. Ultrasound images show membrane echoes inserting into the margin of the area near the optic nerve (thin arrow in Figure C). There is an excavated area (arrow) seen at the expected point of entry of the nerve (ON). There is discontinuity between this point and the optic nerve signifying avulsion.

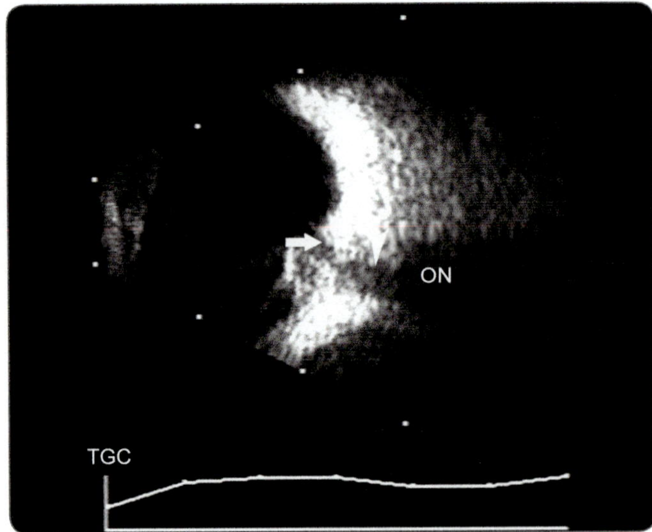

Figure 49.2: B scan ultrasound image of an eye with optic nerve avulsion showing a clump of moderate reflective echoes overlying the optic nerve head (arrow). The echoes are seen to radiate from within the optic nerve (ON). The optic nerve shadow also appears distorted (arrowhead).

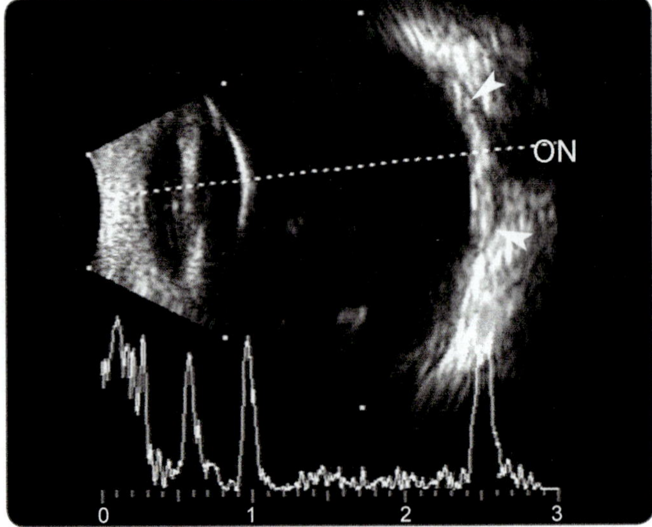

Figure 49.3: B scan image showing widening of the optic nerve shadow (ON) with an area of echolucency in the Tenon's space (arrowheads) around the optic nerve suggestive of optic nerve avulsion.

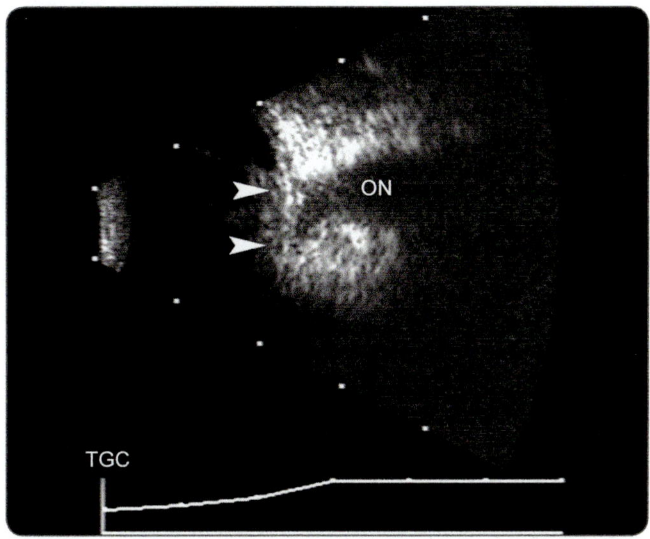

Figure 49.4: B scan image showing radiating echoes from the optic nerve head (arrows). The optic nerve (ON) insertion into the globe is also distorted.

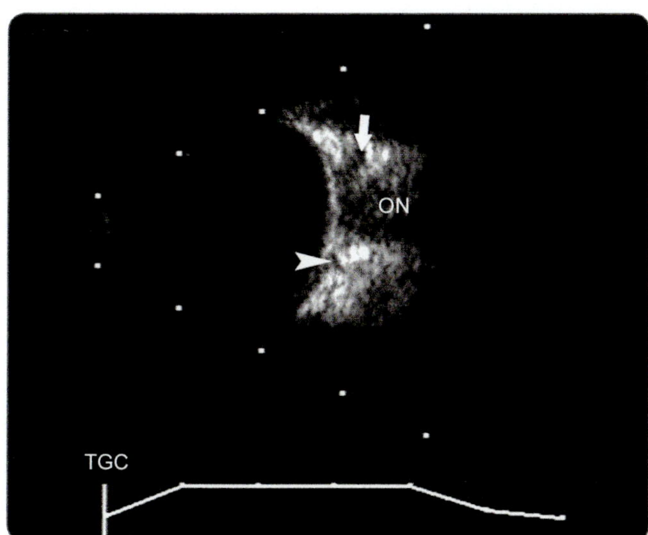

Figure 49.5: B scan image showing widening of the optic nerve shadow (ON). In addition, there is a sharp discontinuity within the coats (arrowhead) just adjacent to the optic nerve head. An area of echolucency continuous with and above the optic nerve shadow (arrow), signifying either hemorrhage or edema in the perineural area, is seen.

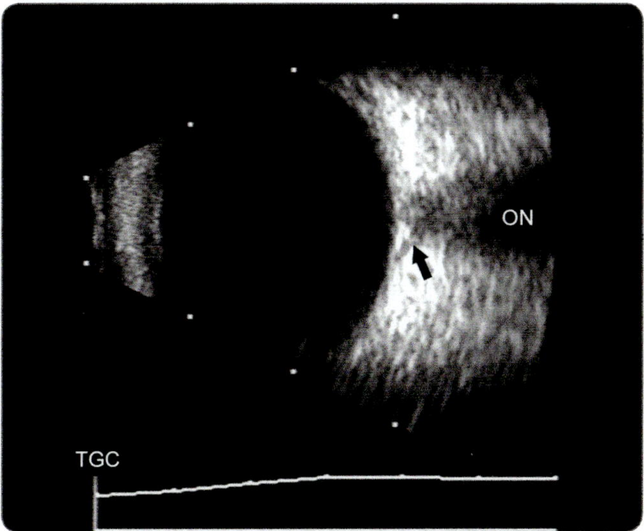

Figure 49.6: B scan image showing a localized area of low reflectivity (arrow) adjacent to the optic nerve head (ON) in a patient with traumatic optic neuropathy.

50 Optic Disc Abnormalities

OPTIC DISC DRUSEN

Clinical Features

- Causes disc swelling that is commonly misdiagnosed as papilloedema
- Usually bilateral
- Present from birth but usually buried and not clinically visible until later in life
- Ultrasound is indicated to confirm pseudopapilloedema.

Ultrasonography

- Seen as bilateral high reflective nodules within the optic nerve head
- Persist at very low gain when all other echoes disappear from the image.

OPTIC DISC CUPPING

Clinical Features

- May be physiological or due to advanced glaucoma
- Ultrasonography is of particular use in assessing eyes with corneal scars for penetrating keratoplasty and eyes with advanced cataract and raised intraocular pressure.

Ultrasonography

- Best imaged with a vertical transverse B scan view
- Different views may give an idea of the shape and size
- Seen as an excavation at the site of optic nerve entry into the globe.

NUGGETS

Reducing the gain in an eye with a high reflective lesion either overlying or within a swollen disc is essential to rule out drusen.

A minimum cup disc ratio of 0.5 is necessary to detect cupping on ultrasonography.

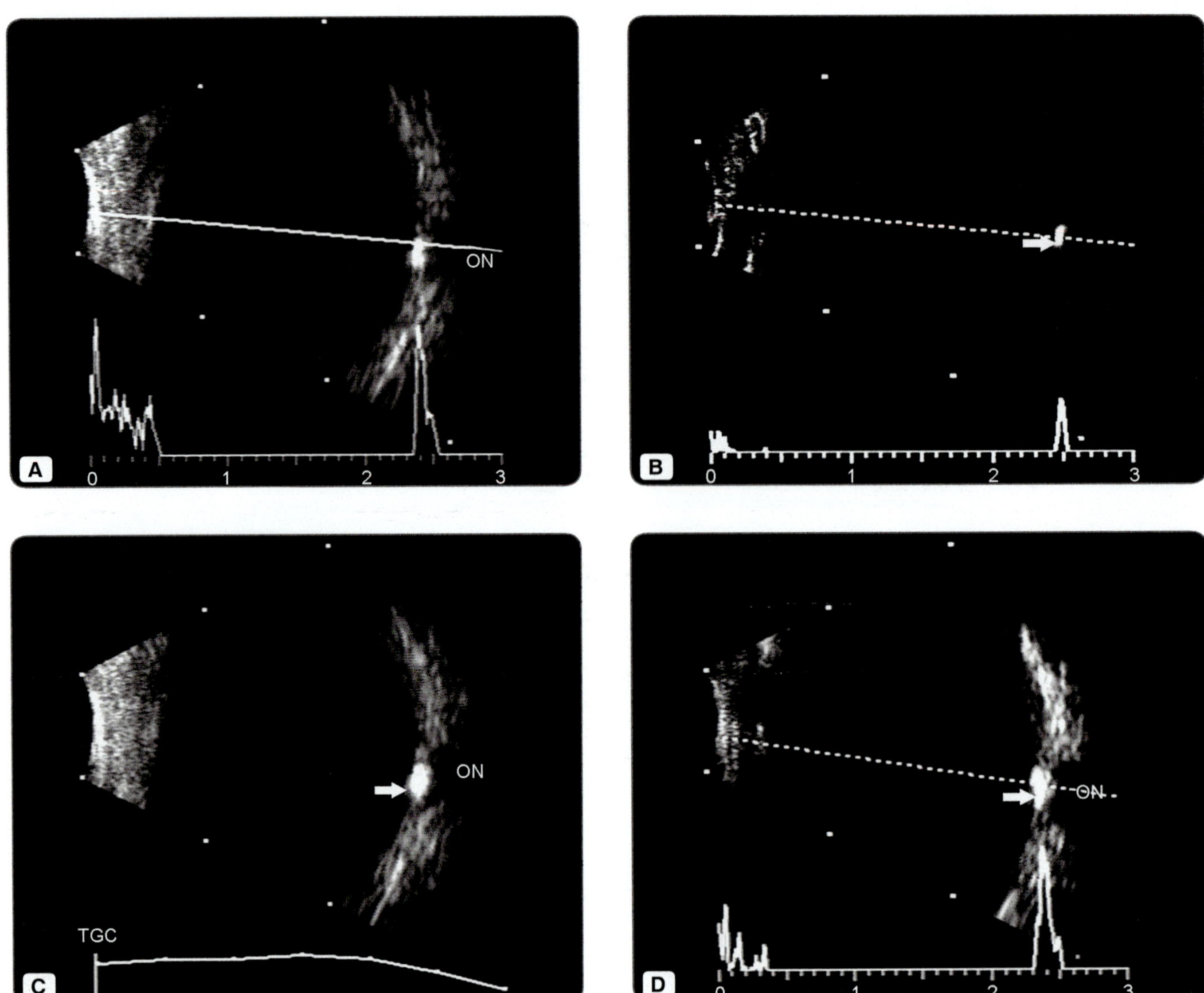

Figures 50.1A to D: B scan with vector A scans of a patient with bilateral disc swelling. Note the high reflective nodule within the optic nerve head (arrow) that persists at low gain. This is classical for optic disc drusen.

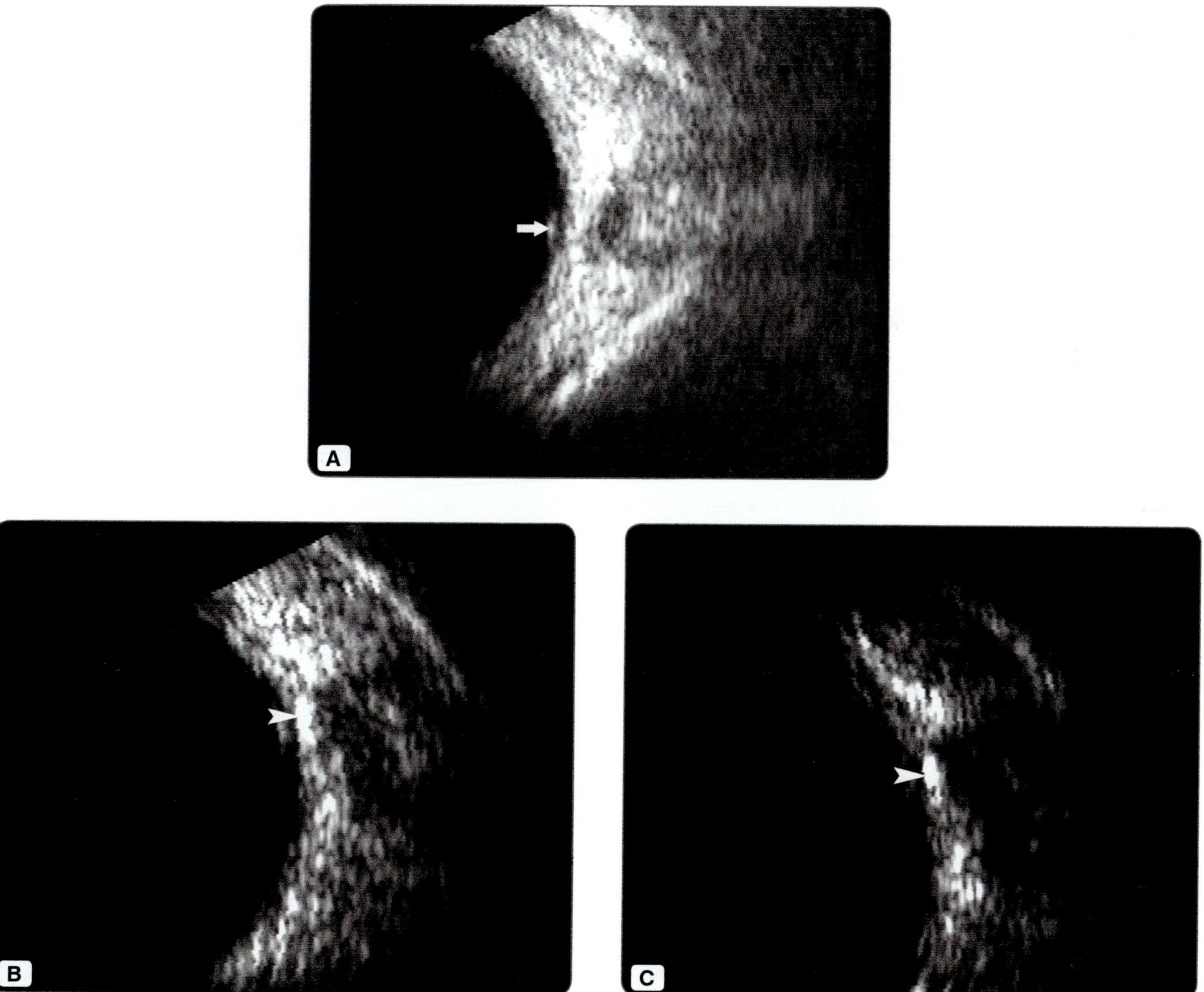

Figures 50.2A to C: B scan images of a patient with disc swelling. Note the elevated disc in Figure A (arrow). The rest of the image appears normal. Figures B and C, scanned at lower gain and with a high magnification shows a small high reflective nodule within the disc (arrowhead) that persists at lower gain, suggestive of disc drusen.

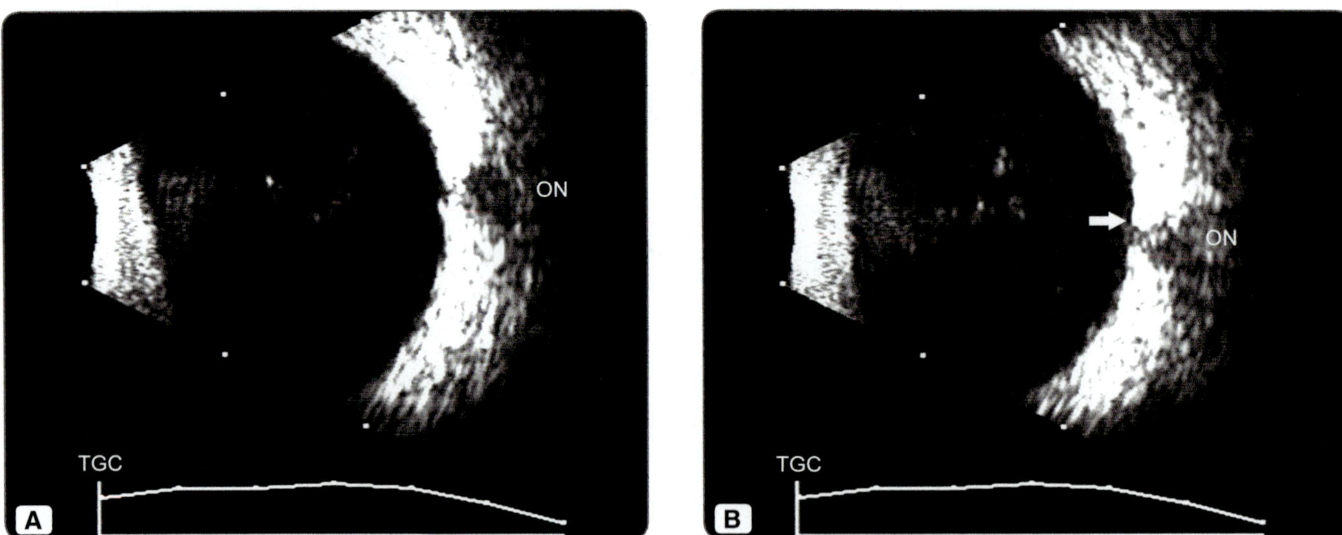

Figures 50.3A and B: B scan vertical and horizontal transverse views of an eye with optic disc cupping (arrow). Note the change in shape of the cup in both the views. ON= Optic nerve.

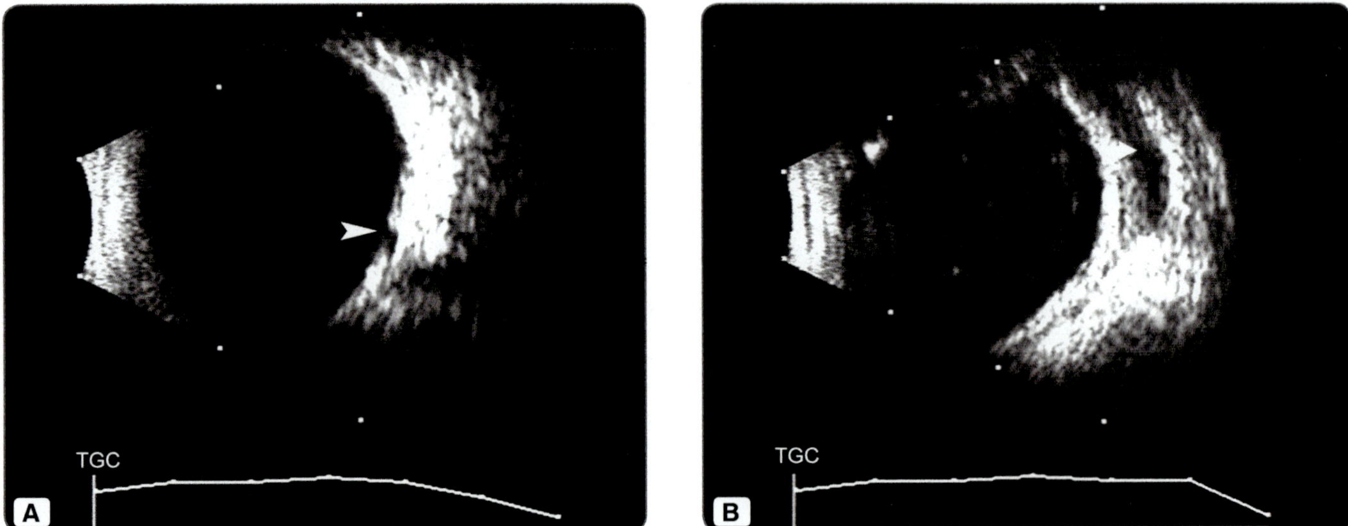

Figures 50.4A and B: B scan image showing significant optic disc cupping (arrowhead) in an eye with advanced glaucoma. Figure B is a transverse view showing an echolucent area external to the sclera (arrow) indicating the position of a glaucoma filtering device, in this case an Ahmed valve.

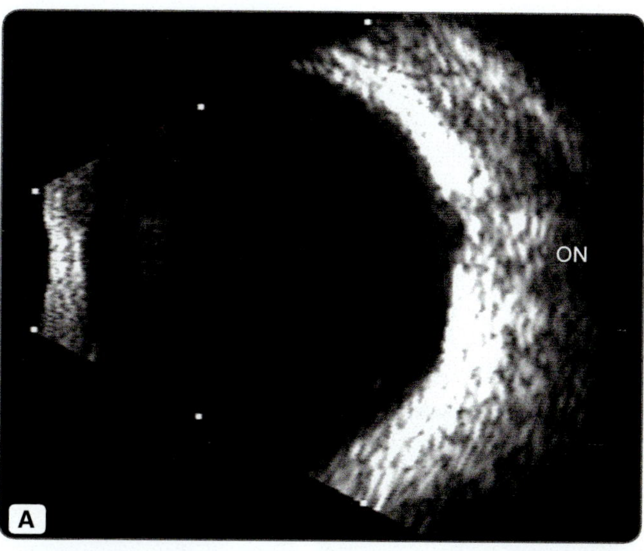

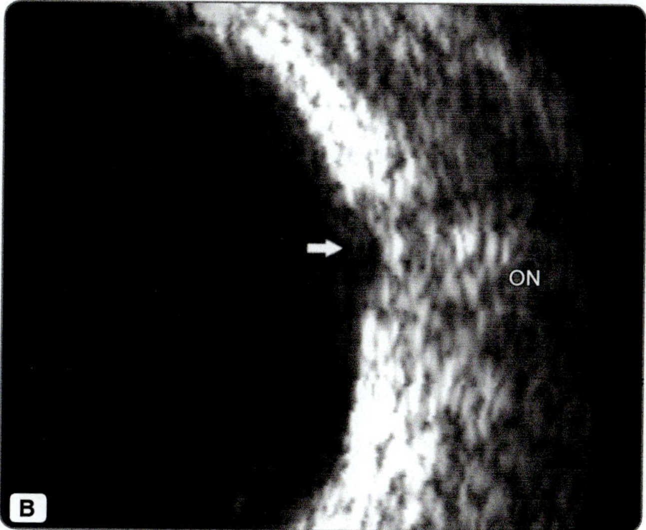

Figures 50.5A and B: B scan images showing advanced cupping (arrow) of the optic disc in a patient with phacomorphic glaucoma (ON= Optic nerve).

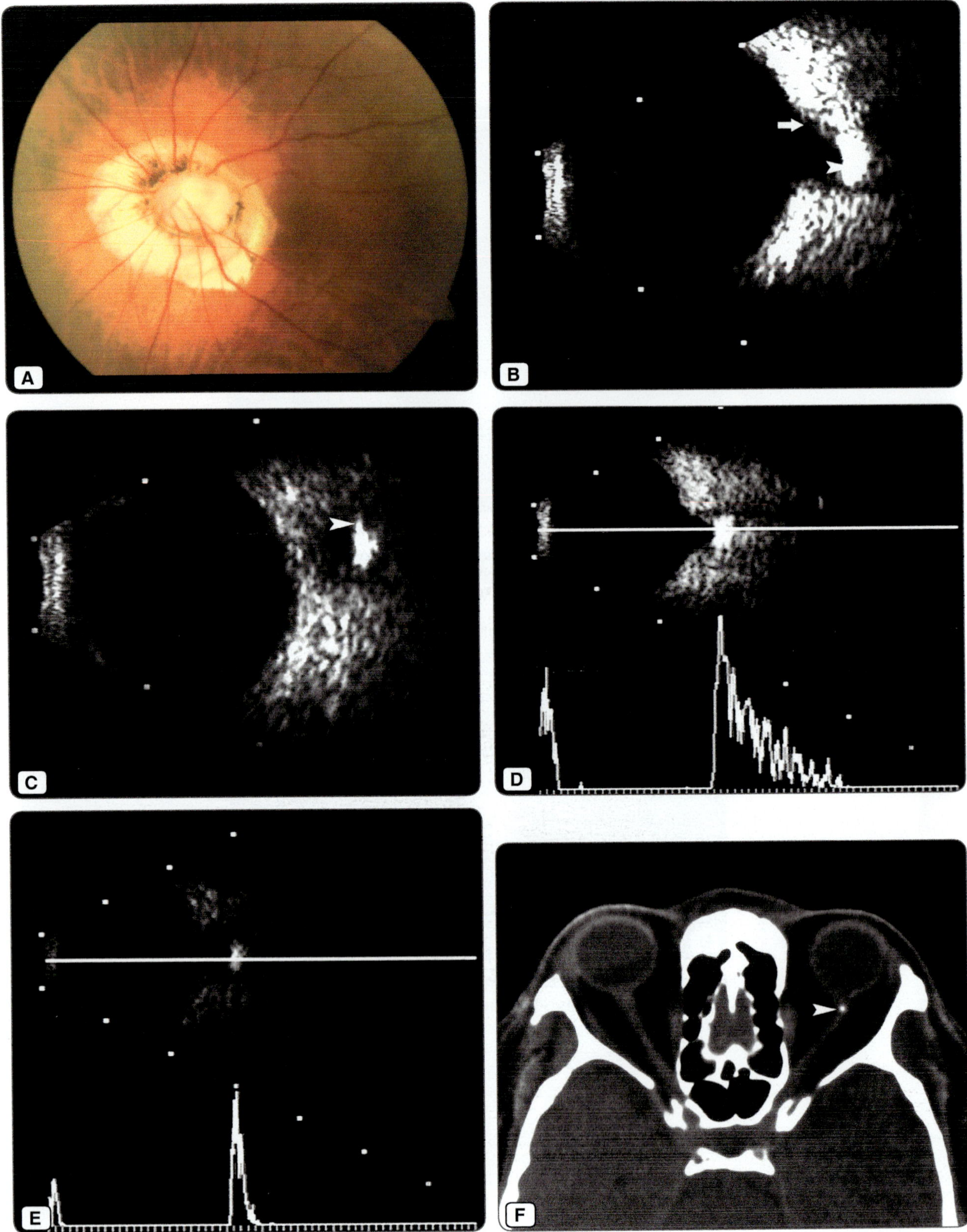

Figures 50.6A to F: A series of images showing a case of morning glory anomaly with optic disc drusen. Note the deep excavation of the optic disc (arrow) with an area of calcification at the base (arrowhead). This is seen to persist even at low gain and is confirmed on CT scan (F).

Section 10

Ultrasound Biomicroscopy

51 Ultrasound Biomicroscopy—An Introduction

The first practical ultrasound biomicroscopy (UBM) system for imaging of the eye was developed by Foster and Pavlin in the early 1990s.The first commercially available ultrasound biomicroscope, manufactured by Zeiss-Humphrey Instruments (San Leandro, CA, USA), was the result of this research. This initial instrument when commercially manufactured operated at a frequency of 50 MHz with a scan rate of 8 Hz, giving real-time imaging, with scans consisting of 256 vectors over a 5 × 5 mm field. The anterior segment upto the ciliary body and pars plana was imaged with this frequency and it proved to be a landmark achievement as far as anterior segment imaging was concerned. Areas previously inaccessible by traditional techniques such as the retroiridal space, ciliary processes, ciliary sulcus and ciliary body, the zonules and pars plana could be well visualized, though not often in a single frame. The piezoelectric element of conventional 10 MHz transducers is most often a ceramic material, lead zirconate (PZT). Use of PZT for frequencies above 15–20 MHz is impracticable because the brittle PZT crystal cannot be made thin enough to generate higher frequencies without cracking. Polyvinylidene fluoride (PVDF) is a piezopolymer that, unlike PZT, is highly flexible and readily available in thin sheets. A 9 mm thick PVDF membrane was initially used by Pavlin and Sherar to form the piezoelectric element of the 50 MHz probe. However, in newer systems the copolymer polyvinylidene fluoride trifluoroethylene (PVDF-TrFE) has largely replaced PVDF because of its greater sensitivity.

The advent of the 35 MHz UBM has further improved the extent of visualization by increasing the field of view both circumferentially and depth wise.

The comparison between properties of 10 MHz ultrasound and UBM is shown in Table 51.1.

IMAGE ACQUISITION TECHNIQUE

In the original model of the UBM, the probe was suspended from a gantry arm to minimize motion artifacts, and lateral distortion was minimized by a linear scan format. In the newer devices, the probe is small and light, and a sector scanning method is used. Scanning is performed with the patient in the supine position. Newer modifications for this include the sitting and prone positions. Before the advent of anterior segment OCT, a soft contact lens was used for scanning the anterior segment without disturbing a possible breach in continuity of the surface, though this resulted in loss of image quality. A plastic eyecup of the appropriate size is inserted between the lids, holding methylcellulose or normal saline coupling medium. For best signals, the transducer should be oriented so that the scanning beam strikes the target surface perpendicularly.

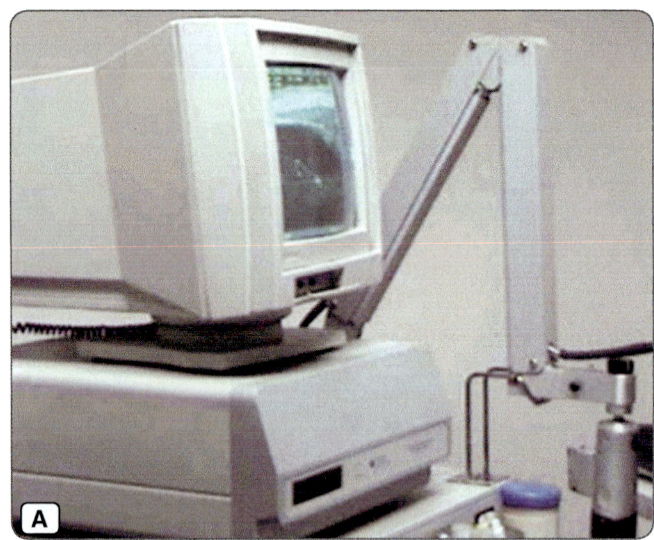

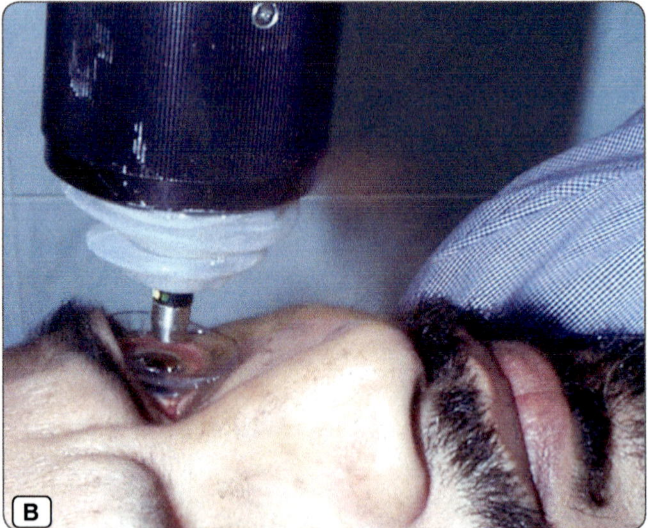

Figures 51.1A and B: 50 MHz UBM machine from Zeiss-Humphrey. The probe is seen immersed in the coupling solution, the lids kept apart with a PMMA shell.

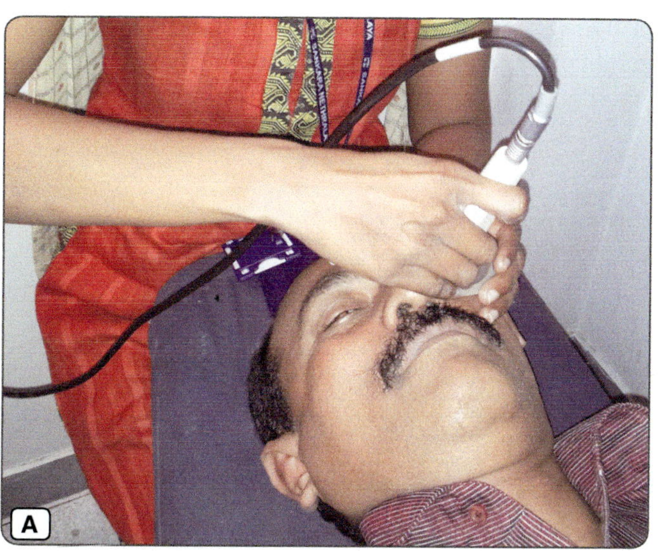

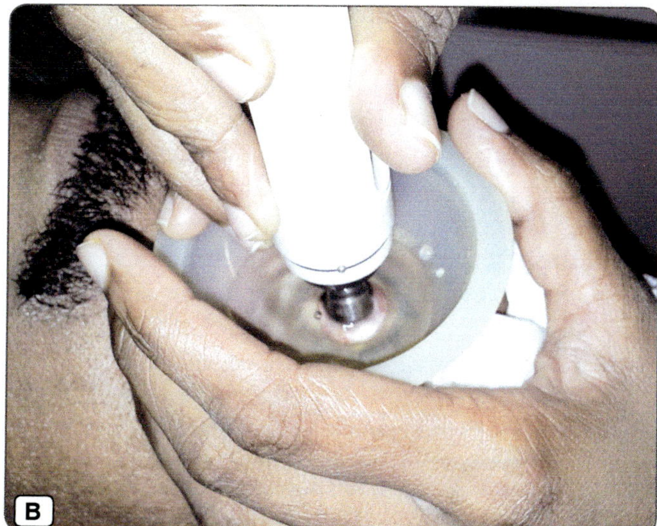

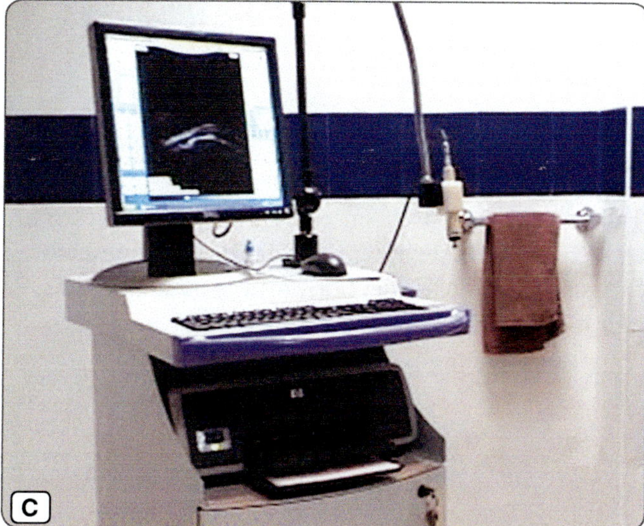

Figures 51.2A to C: The newer machines have a lighter probe in which the tip is uncovered, allowing for more flexibility.

Normal Structures as Seen on UBM

In the normal eye, the cornea, anterior chamber, posterior chamber, iris, ciliary body, and anterior lens surface can be recognized easily. The scleral spur is a constant landmark allowing one to interpret UBM images in terms of the morphologic status of the anterior chamber angle and is the key for analyzing angle pathology. The scleral spur is located where the trabecular meshwork meets the interface line between the sclera and ciliary body. The iris has a roughly planar configuration with slight anterior bowing, and the anterior chamber angle is normally wide and clear.

QUANTITATIVE UBM

Requirements

1. Good axial resolution and precision of measurements
2. Accuracy of measurements
3. Reproducibility of measurements

PARAMETERS OF MEASUREMENT

1. Angle opening distance (AOD)
2. Trabecular iris angle (TIA)
3. Trabecular-ciliary process distance (TCPD)
4. Iris thickness - 1,2,3 (ID1,2,3)
5. Iris-ciliary process distance (ICPD)
6. Iris-zonule distance (IZD)
7. Iris-lens contact distance (ILCD)
8. Iris-lens angle (ILA)
9. Iris concavity-convexity
10. Angle recess area (ARA)

APPLICATIONS

This technique has been extensively used in the understanding of mechanisms of various types of glaucoma as well as angle development. It has also been used to measure the extent of tumours of the anterior segment , measurements of ciliary body and corneal thickness and relative position of intraocular lenses, shape and position of the crystalline lens.

The subsequent chapters will demonstrate the usefulness of the UBM in various disease conditions.

Table 51.1: Comparative properties of typical 10 MHz ophthalmic B-scanner and UBM system

Characteristic	Conventional B-scanner	UBM
Frequency (MHz)	10	50
Aperture (mm)	10	6
Focal length (mm)	30	12
F-ratio	3	2
Axial resolution (μm)	150	30
Lateral resolution (μm)	450	60
Depth of field (mm)	9.6	0.85
Attenuation in water (dB/mm)	0.02	0.5

Source: Silverman, R. High resolution imaging of the eye. Clin Experiment Ophthalmol. 2009 January; 37(1):54-67

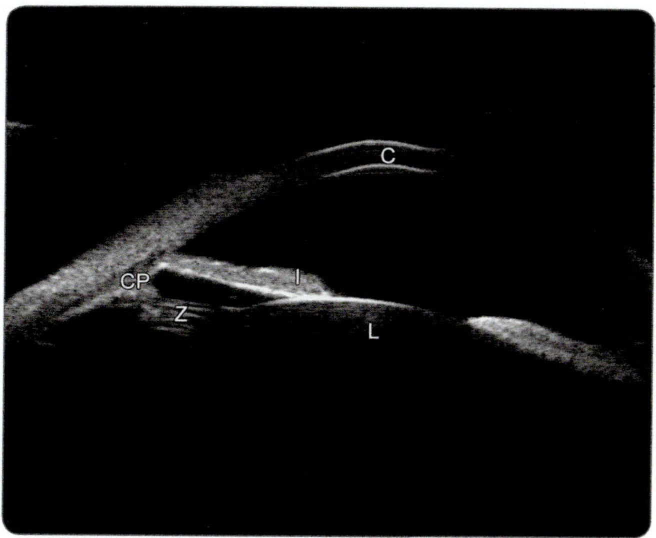

Figure 51.3A: UBM image of a normal eye showing the cornea (C), iris (I), ciliary processes (CP), zonules (Z) and anterior lens surface (L).

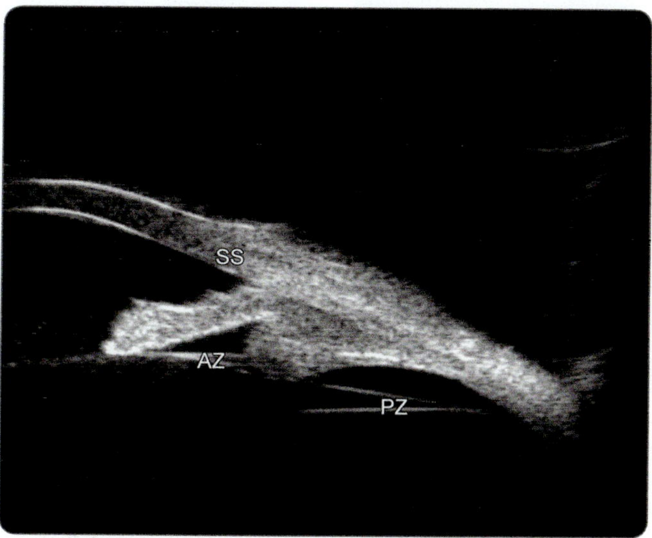

Figure 51.3B: Shows the zonules extending between the anterior surface of lens and ciliary processes (AZ), scleral spur (SS) and lens equator and pars plana (PZ).

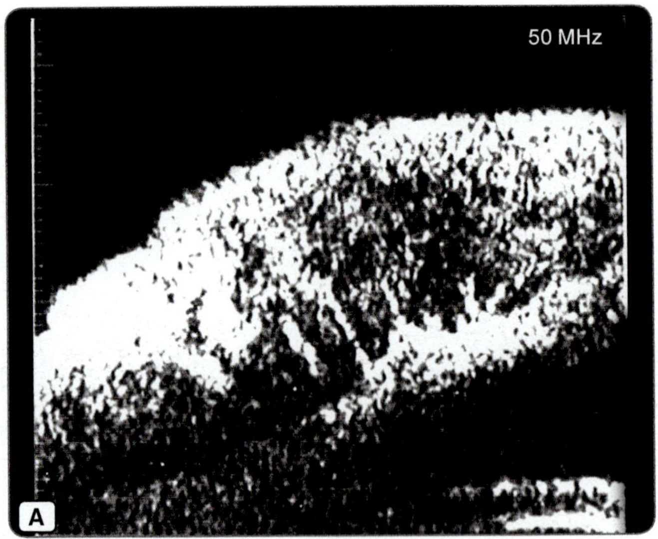

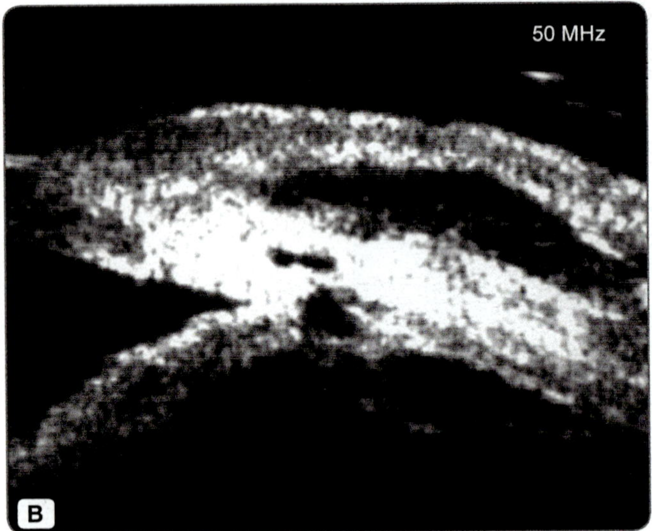

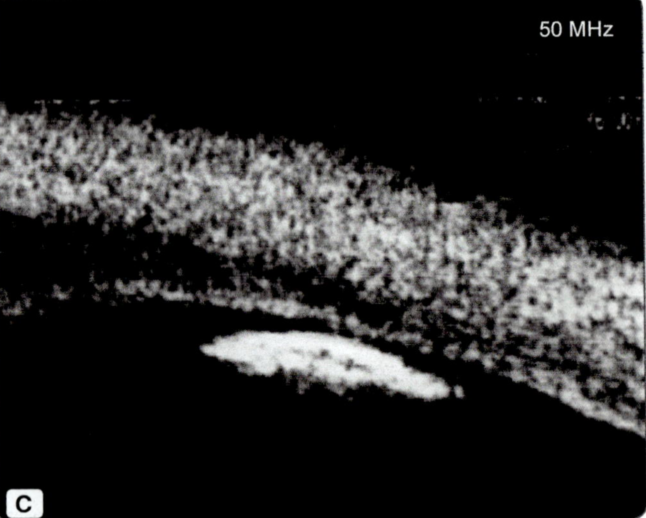

Figures 51.4A to C: 50 MHz UBM image of an eye with squamous cell carcinoma at the limbus. Note the detail visible in the image where the septae are clearly seen as also the absence of anterior chamber extension of the mass. The borders of the lesion are not well seen in this image. Figures B and C show excellent resolution of structures but limited field of view both in terms of depth and circumference. This frequency gives a much better interpretation of the internal structure of a lesion.

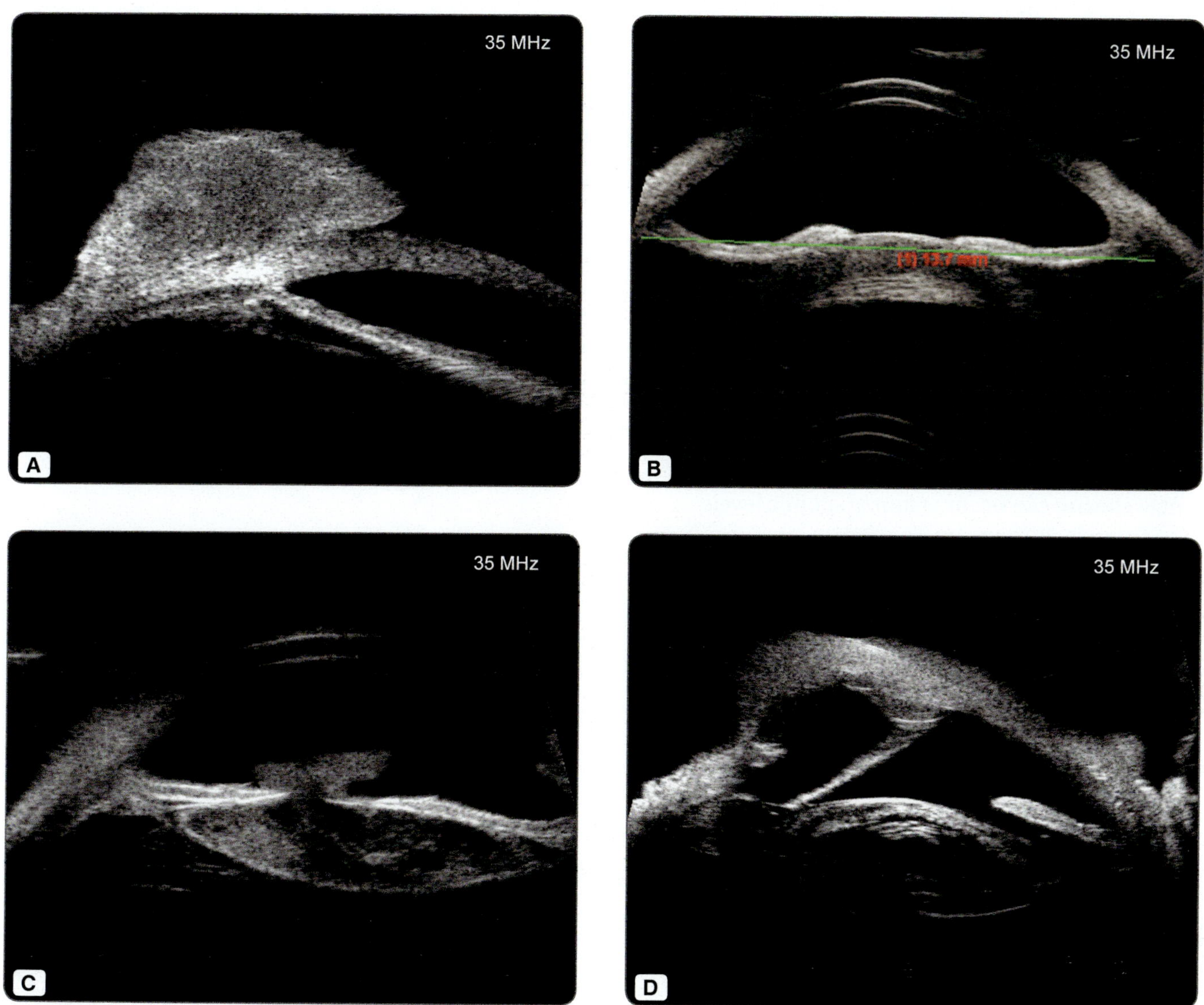

Figures 51.5A to D: 35 MHz UBM image of an eye with a limbal mass (A). Note the homogenous nature of the lesion, absence of deeper involvement, and most importantly the entire radial extent of the mass. Figures B to D show a significant increase in field of view—both in terms of ability to image limbus to limbus) as well as the integrity of the posterior capsule. This helps in better orientation and identification of the relationship between anterior segment structures.

52 Ultrasound Biomicroscopy in Glaucoma

The ability of the UBM to image structures of the eye that are involved in the pathogenesis of various types of glaucoma makes it an invaluable tool in investigation and management of glaucoma.

ANGLE CLOSURE DISEASE

Angle closure can occur at four anatomic levels;

1. Iris (Pupillary block)
2. Ciliary body (Plateau iris)
3. Lens (Phacomorphic glaucoma)
4. Anterior vitreous face (Malignant glaucoma).

Pupillary Block

- Shallow anterior chamber
- Narrow angle recess
- Forward bowing of iris
- Some eyes may have associated ciliary effusion.

Plateau Iris

- Primary angle closure without pupillary block
- Prominent peripheral roll of iris due to anteriorly directed ciliary processes
- Absence of ciliary sulcus
- Double hump sign on indentation UBM
- Will need laser iridotomy with/without iridoplasty
- Similar findings can occur with iridociliary cysts.

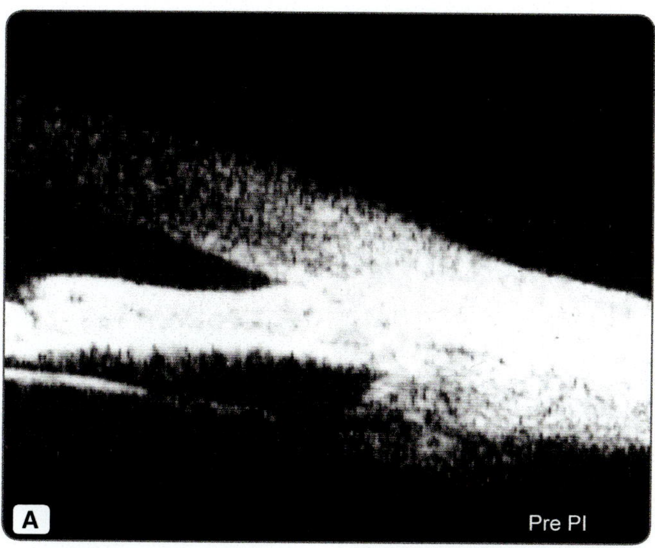

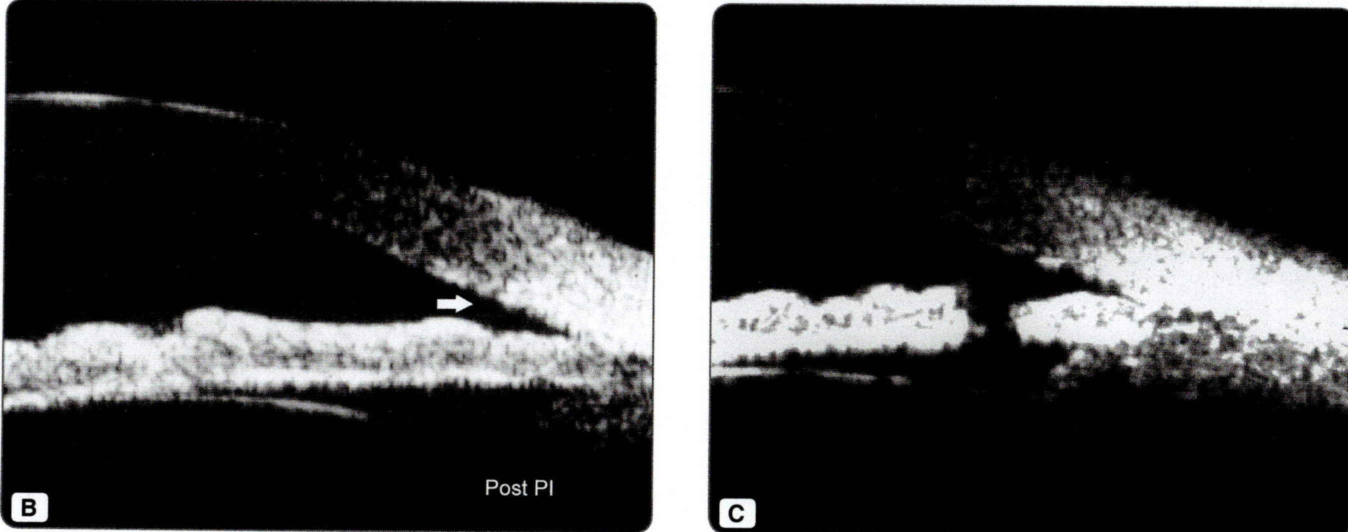

Figures 52.1A to C: (A) UBM image of an eye with closed angles. (B) UBM image of the same eye showing opening of the angle after peripheral iridotomy. (C) UBM image showing a full thickness patent iridotomy.

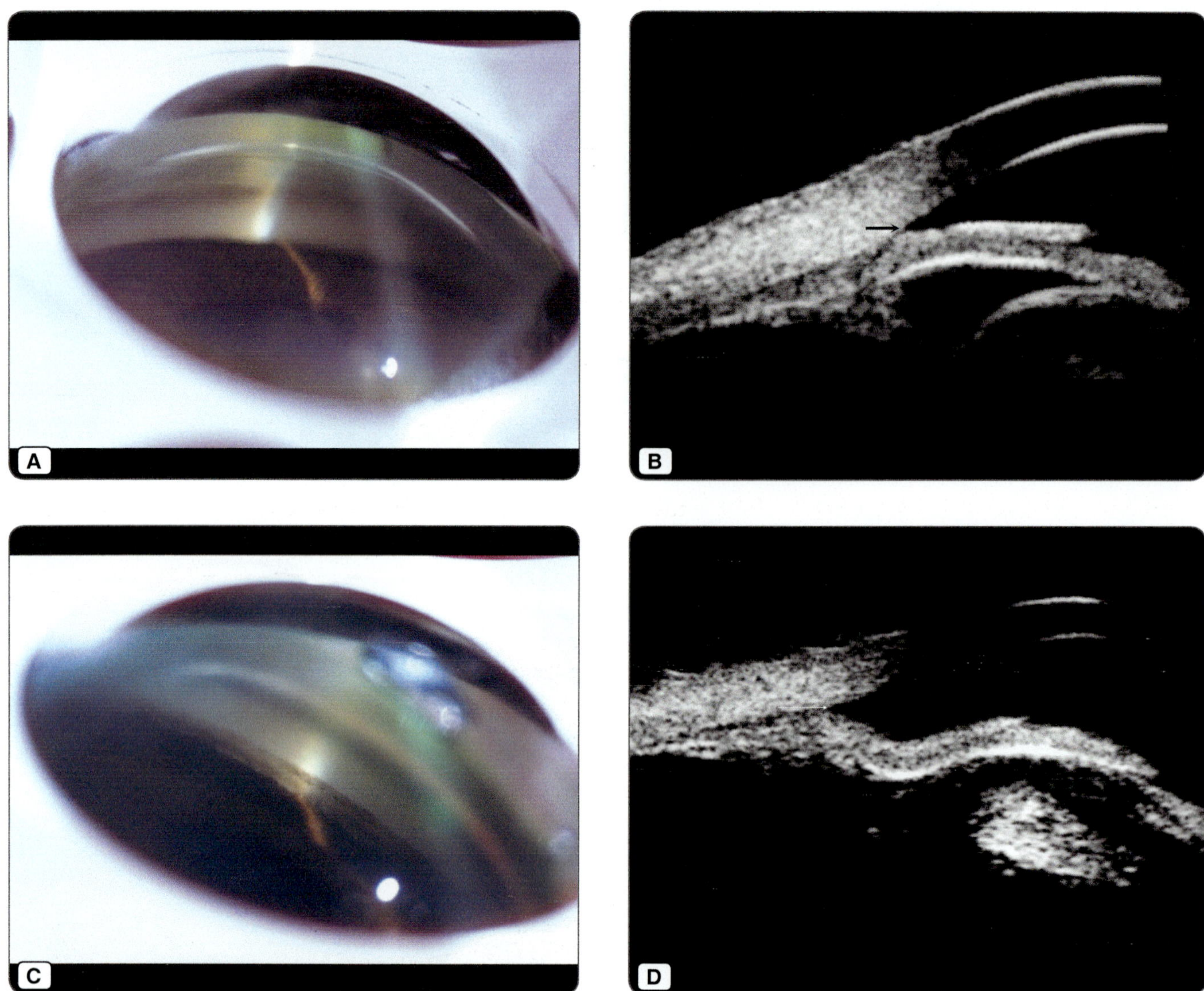

Figures 52.2A to D: (A) Gonioscopy image showing a closed angle with no structures visible. (B) UBM image of the same eye showing a convex iris and closed angle (arrow). (C) Indentation gonioscopy showing that the angle opens with compression. (D) Indentation UBM showing that the angle has now opened up.

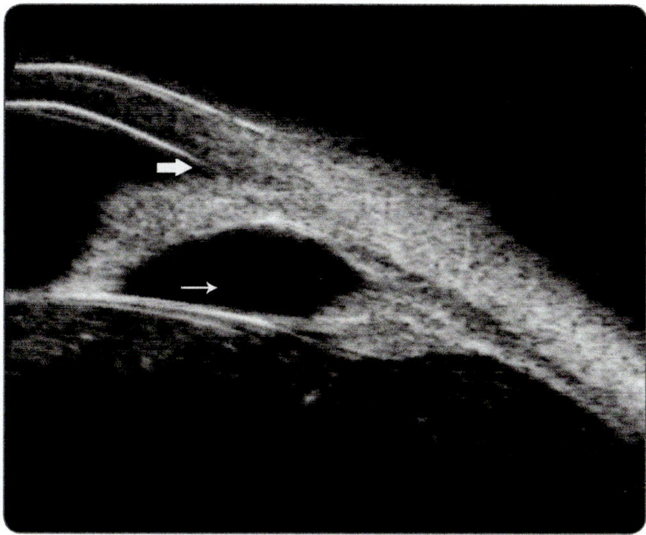

Figure 52.3: UBM image showing angle closure due to iris bombe (arrow) in an eye with history of uveitis. Note the deep posterior chamber (thin arrow).

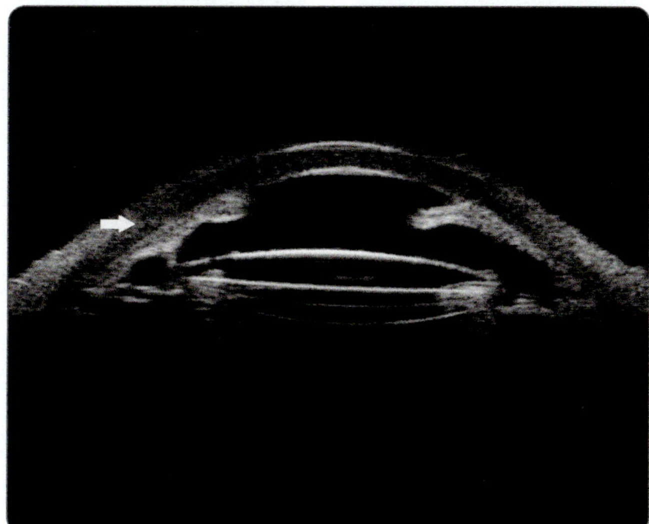

Figure 52.4: UBM image of a pseudophakic eye with closed angle (arrow) and uncontrolled glaucoma. The patient subsequently underwent diode laser cyclophotocoagulation.

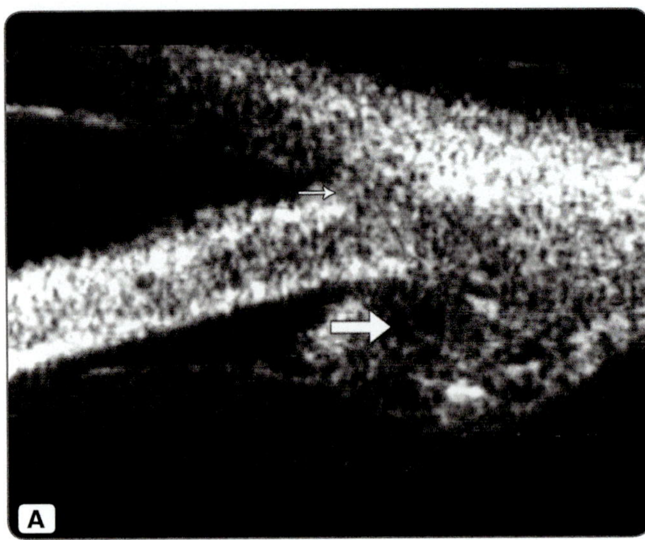

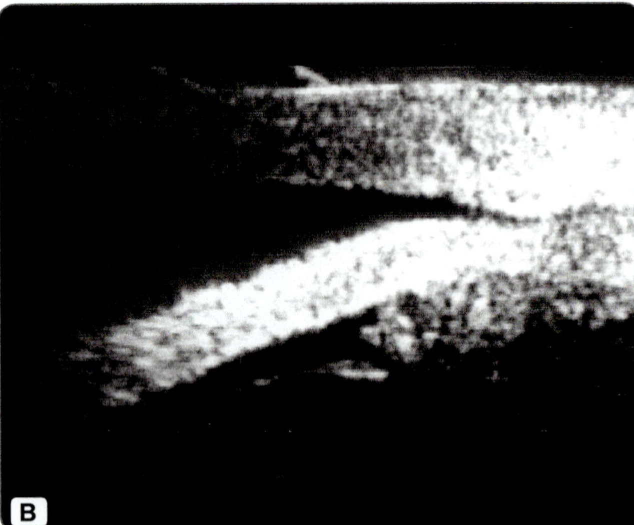

Figures 52.5A and B: (A) UBM of an eye with plateau iris. Note the peripheral roll of iris (thin arrow) caused by the bulky, anteriorly placed ciliary processes (broader arrow). (B) UBM image of the same eye following iridoplasty. Note the opening of the angle recess.

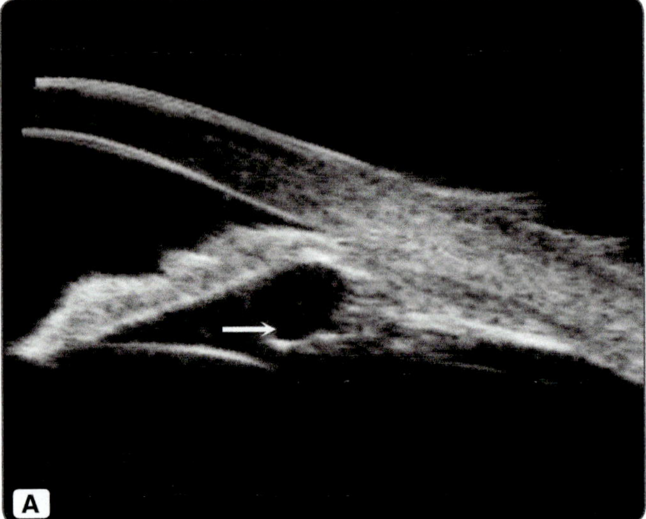

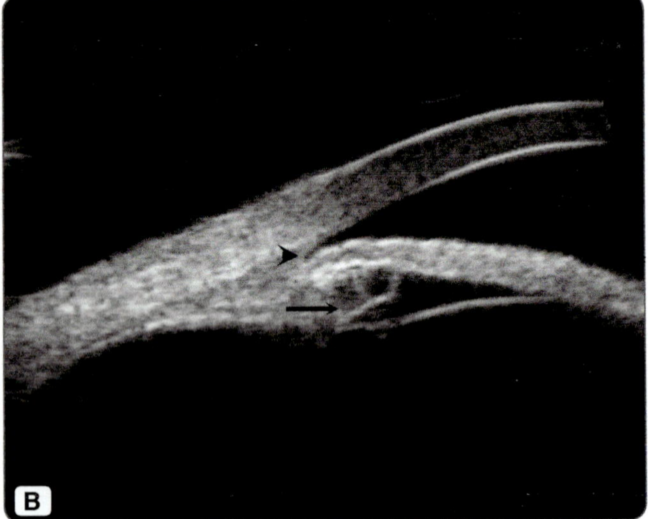

Figure 52.6A and B: UBM image of a solitary cyst of the ciliary process (Fig. A) and multiple cysts (Fig. B) causing a pseudo-plateau iris configuration.

SECONDARY ANGLE CLOSURE DUE TO DRUGS

- Acetazolamide, topiramate are known to cause ciliary effusion leading to secondary angle closure
- Stoppage of the drug leads to reversal of the changes and normalization of intraocular pressure.

MALIGNANT GLAUCOMA

- Also known as aqueous misdirection or ciliary block
- Can be an important cause of postoperative flat anterior chamber and a normal or raised intraocular pressure
- Shallow or flat anterior chamber with a closed angle
- Anterior rotation of ciliary processes
- Supraciliary effusion may or may not be present. The detection of supraciliary effusion on UBM is of significance as it indicates the need for aggressive medical management rather than immediate surgical intervention
- The presence of a deep posterior chamber indicates the presence of secondary pupillary block rather than ciliary block.

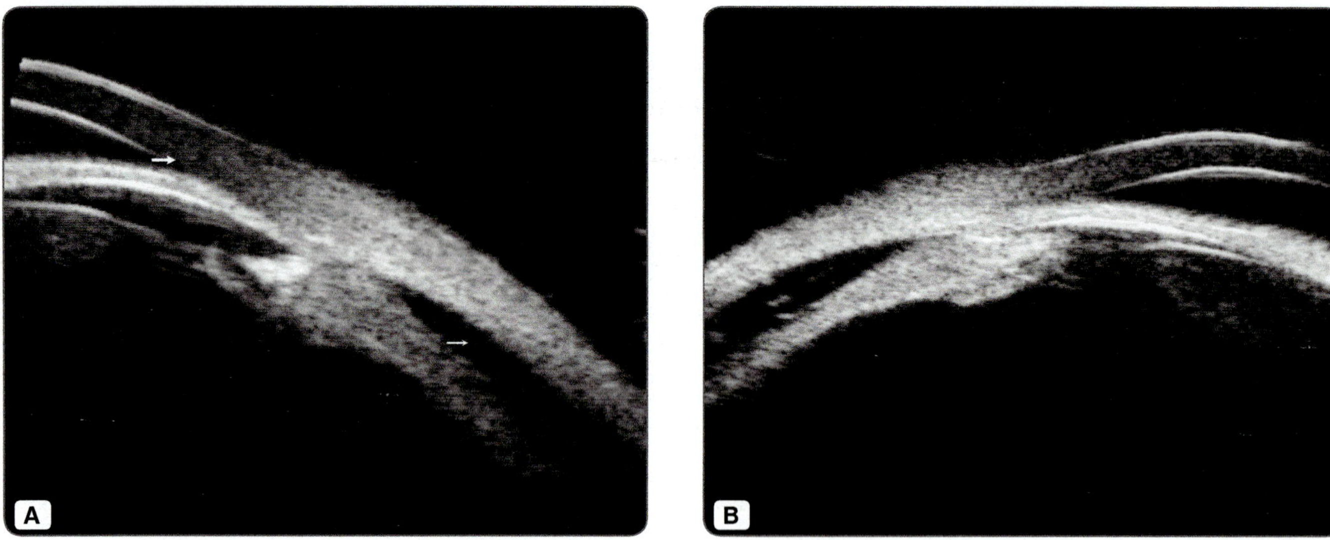

Figures 52.7A and B: UBM images of the right and left eyes of a patient with topiramate induced uveal effusion. Note the closed angle (wide arrow) and supraciliary effusion (thin arrow).

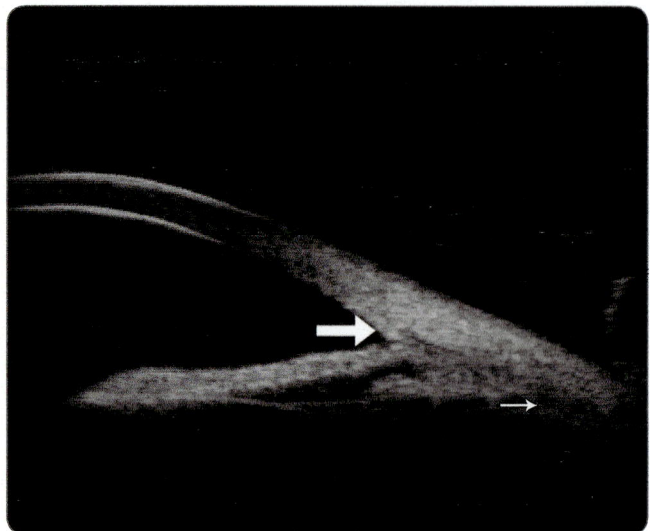

Figure 52.7C: UBM image of the same patient after successful treatment. Note the deepening of the anterior chamber (wide arrow) and absence of choroidal effusion (thin arrow).

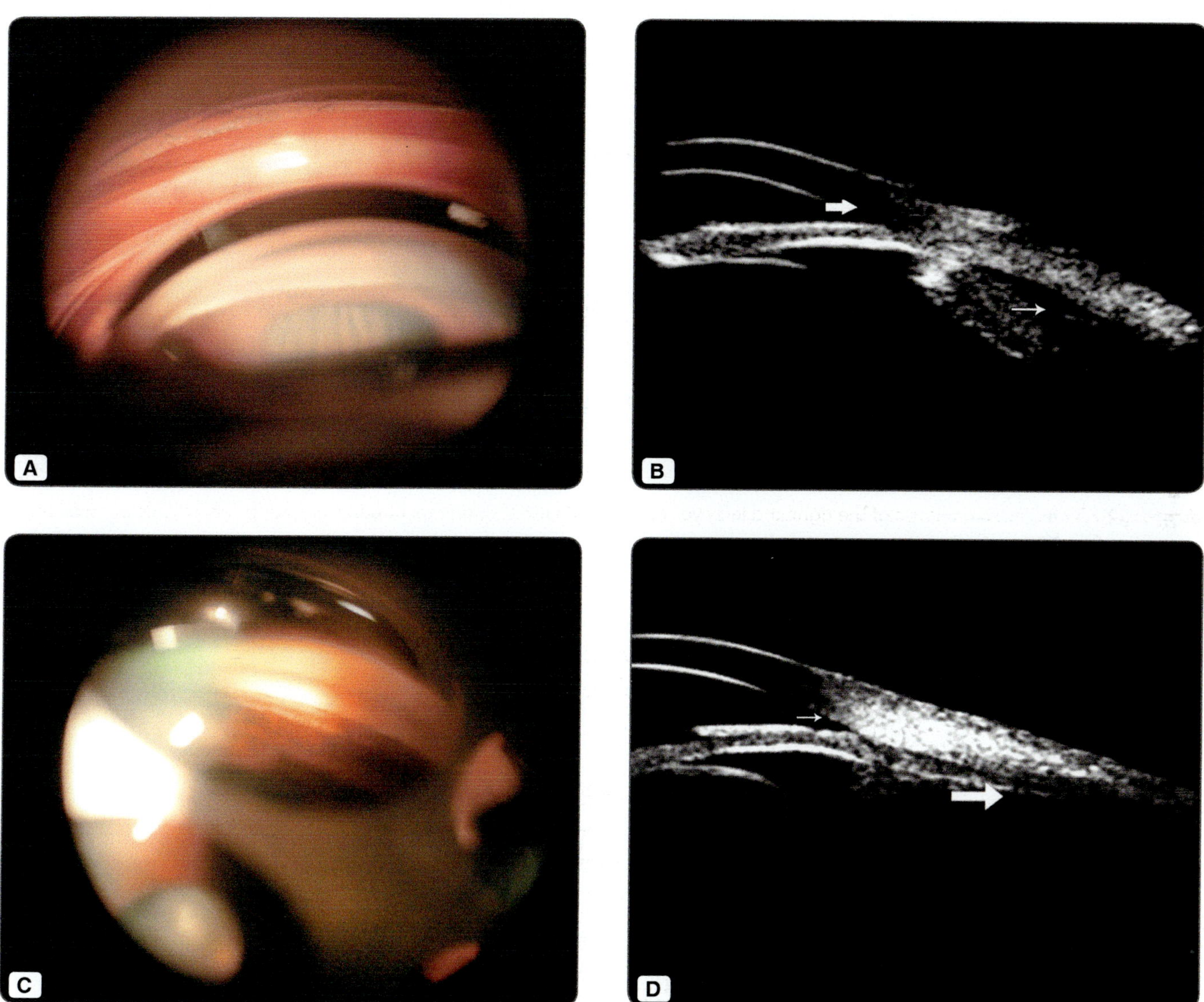

Figures 52.8A to D: (A) Gonioscopy image of an eye with a caroticocavernous fistula and angle closure due to uveal effusion. (B) UBM image of the same eye showing a closed angle (thin arrow) and suprachoroidal fluid (broad arrow). (C) Gonioscopy photograph showing opening of the angle after successful treatment. (D) UBM image of the same eye after successful treatment. Note the absence of suprachoroidal fluid (broad arrow) and the relative deepening of the anterior chamber (thin arrow).

OPEN-ANGLE GLAUCOMA

Pigment Dispersion Syndrome

- Deep anterior chamber with a concave iris leading to a reverse pupillary block
- Contact between the posterior surface of the iris and the anterior zonular fibers causing pigment dispersion can be seen
- The presence of iridozonular versus only iridolenticular contact is helpful in determining the need for intervention in the form of iridotomy.

Trauma

- UBM is especially helpful when there is a hyphema preventing accurate gonioscopy
- Detection of iridodialysis, angle recession and cyclodialysis clefts
- Associated lens and zonular damage can be identified along with foreign bodies in the angle
- UBM is useful to determine the cause and to plan surgical management in eyes with corneal opacification
- It helps to differentiate primary and secondary causes of angle closure.

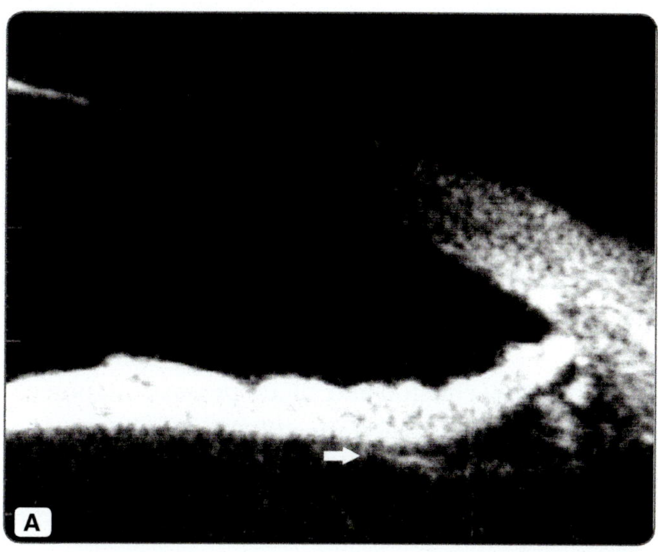

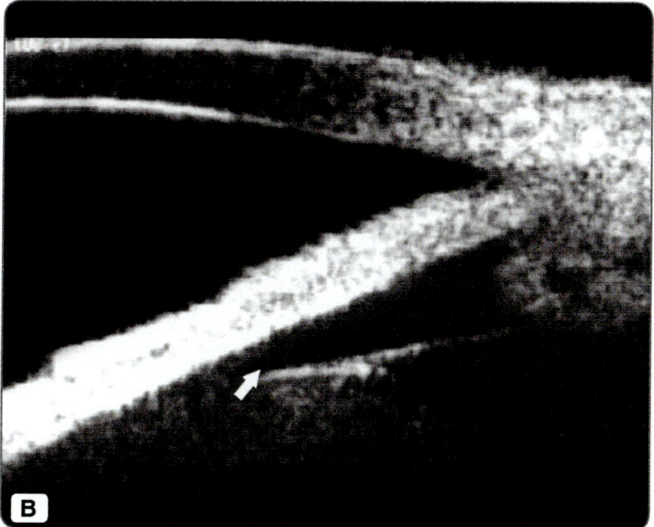

Figures 52.9A and B: (A) UBM of an eye with pigment dispersion syndrome. Note the deep anterior chamber, concave iris and iridozonular touch (arrow). (B) UBM of the same eye after iridotomy showing reversal of the iridozonular touch.

UBM IN ASSESSING EFFICACY OF THERAPY

Post Laser Iridotomy

- Assessing patency, effectivity and reasons for failure. The most important use of UBM post PI is the identification of anterior rotation of ciliary processes and absence of ciliary sulcus to identify plateau iris. The presence of cysts of the ciliary processes may be seen.

Post-glaucoma Surgery

- Stoma can be visualized and its patency verified
- Status of a filtering bleb–height, reflectivity within the bleb, patency of the stoma and connection to the bleb, apposition of scleral flap to sclera. A low reflective bleb with patent connection from the stoma to the bleb signifies a functioning bleb
- Associated features like suprachoroidal effusion and ciliary process rotation can be detected
- Intrascleral lakes of aqueous following non-penetrating filtering surgery can be visualized
- The patency of aqueous drainage tubes as well as the location can be determined
- Shrinkage and blunting of the ciliary processes after cyclophotocoagulation can be seen.

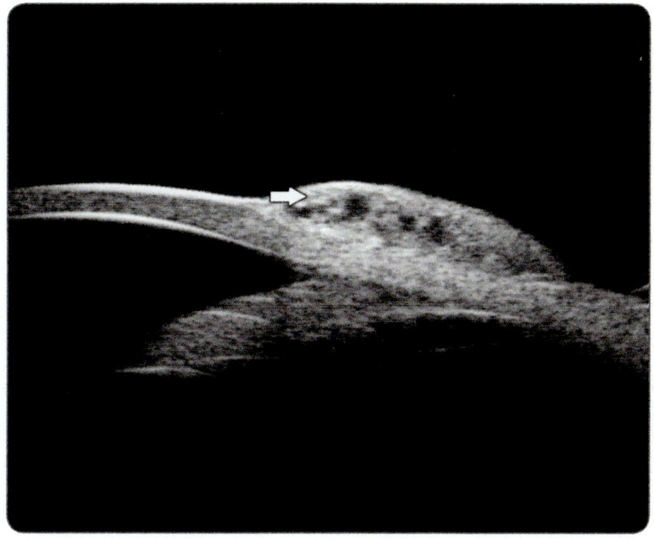

Figure 52.10: UBM image of an eye with a cystic bleb (arrow shows the multiple cysts).

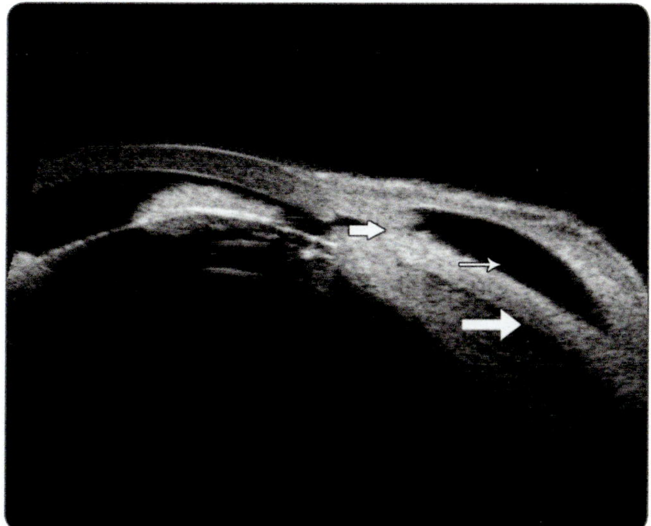

Figure 52.11: UBM image of an eye with a patent (arrow) trab stoma, large bleb (fine arrow) and a ciliochoroidal detachment (broad arrow). The patient underwent successful choroidal drainage.

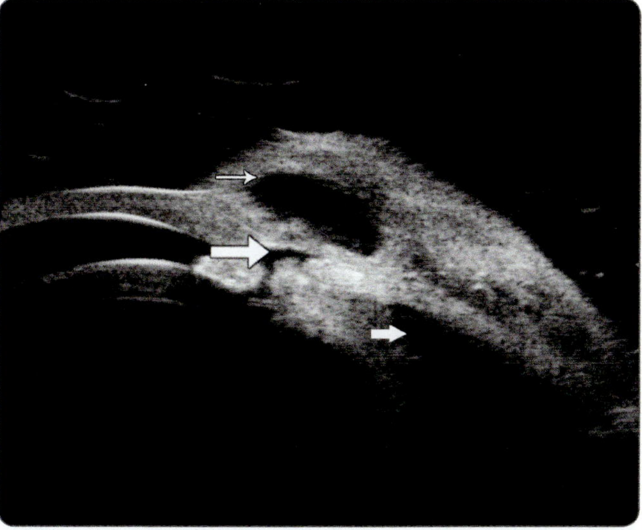

Figure 52.12: UBM image of an eye with shallow anterior chamber after trabeculectomy. Note the trabeculectomy stoma (thick arrow), thick walled bleb (fine arrow) and ciliochoroidal effusion (thin arrow).

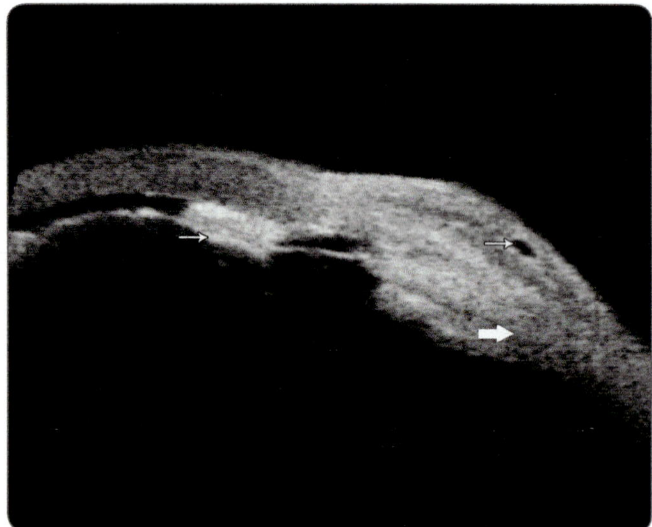

Figure 52.13: UBM image of an eye with post trabeculectomy malignant glaucoma. Note the flat anterior chamber (arrow) with anterior rotation of ciliary processes (thin arrow). The longer arrow points to a small fluid pocket at the site of the bleb.

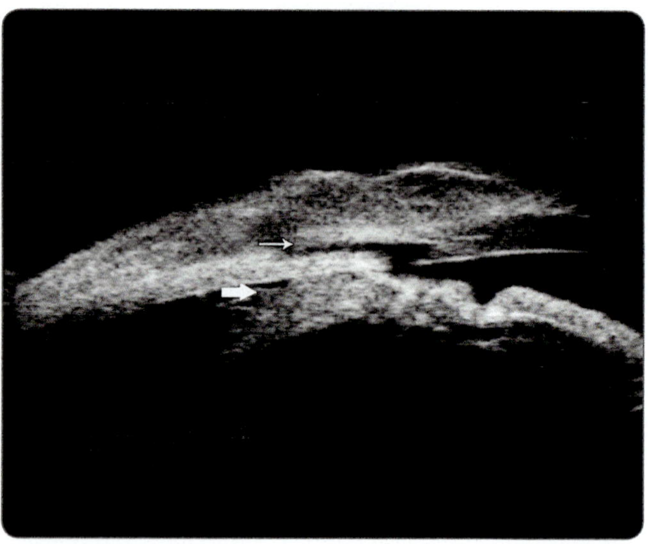

Figure 52.14: UBM image of an eye with a shallow anterior chamber and ciliochoroidal detachment after filtering surgery and autologous blood injection for a leaking bleb. The patient subsequently underwent a repeat injection.

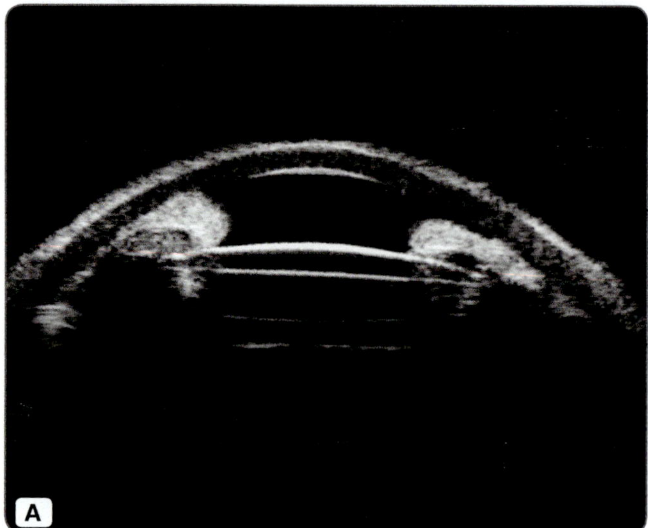

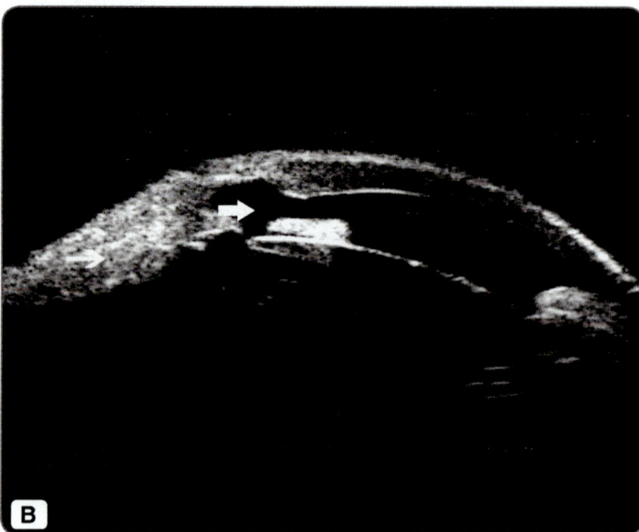

Figures 52.15A and B: (A) UBM images of a pseudophakic eye with malignant glaucoma after trabeculectomy with mitomycin C. Note the flat anterior chamber and absence of ciliochoroidal effusion. (B) Another image of the same eye showing the peripheral iridotomy (broad arrow), anterior rotation of ciliary processes (arrow) and absence of filtering bleb.

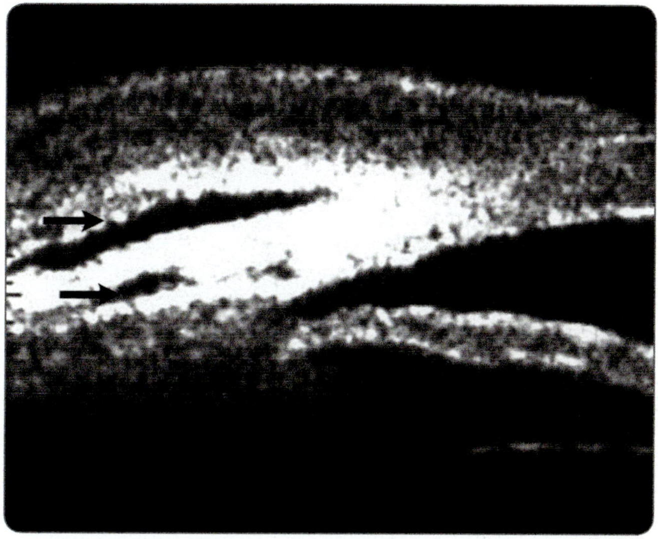

Figure 52.16: UBM of an eye after deep sclerectomy. Note the intrascleral aqueous lakes (arrows).

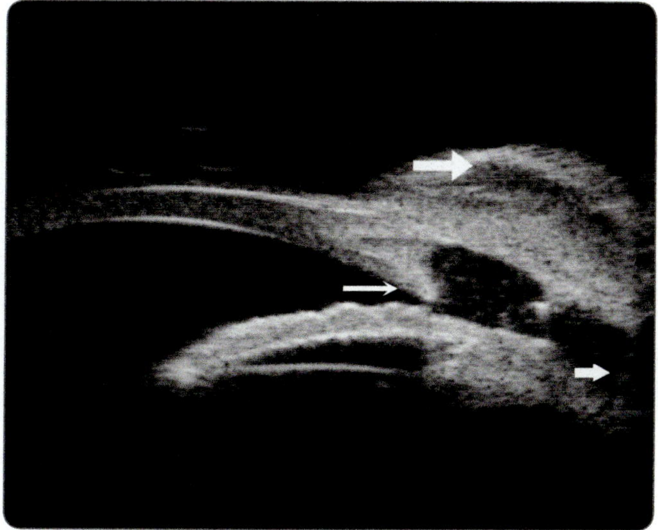

Figure 52.17: UBM image of an eye that has undergone deep sclerectomy. Note the intrascleral aqueous lake (arrow) as well as a bleb (broad arrow).

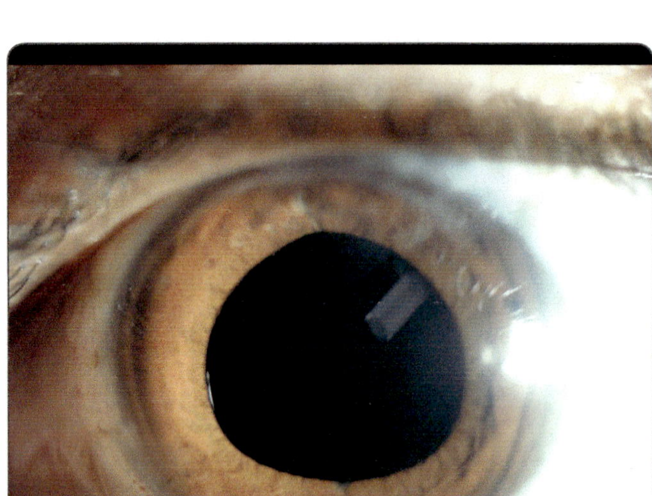

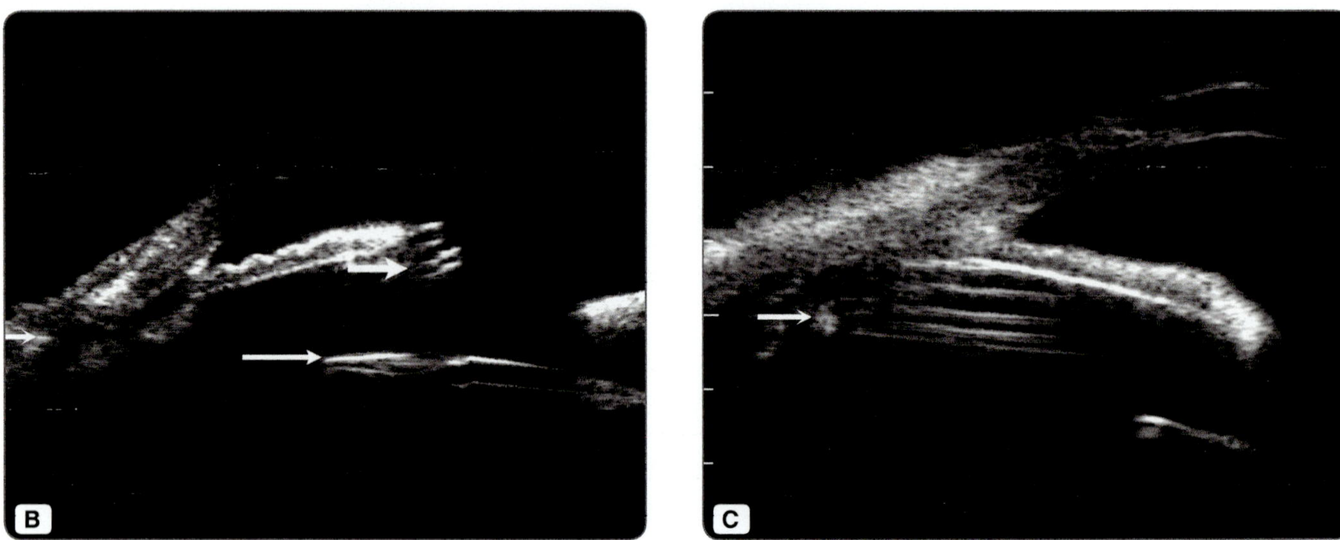

Figures 52.18A to C: An eye with scleral fixated IOL and a tube implant for angle recession glaucoma. (A) Slit lamp photograph showing a well-dilated pupil, the tube seen in the pupillary area and scleral fixated IOL behind it. (B) UBM and clinical pictures (thin arrow). UBM showing the scleral fixated IOL (thin arrow). Note the tube just behind the iris (arrow). The fine arrow shows the exit of the tube through the pars plana. (C) UBM image of the same eye showing the point of entry of the tube into the eye through the pars plana (arrow).

MODIFICATIONS IN TECHNIQUE

1. Indentation UBM - for relative pupillary block, PAS and plateau iris recognition.
2. UBM in sitting and prone positions - to study the relationship between various angle structures in these positions.
3. Quantitative UBM:
   - Pavlin and Foster have developed software for various measurements, using the scleral spur as a reference point (Table 52.1)
   - Measurements have to be performed in a standardized manner with standard room lighting and controlled accommodation.
   - Intraobserver agreement in this form of assessment is quite good; however, interobserver agreement is poor because of variation in placing the cursors for measurements
   - One of the limitations as far as measurement of the AOD and ACA is concerned is that the anterior surface of the iris shows a highly variable contour
   - Ishikawa et al. have come up with a software to measure the angle area instead; this is the area bounded by the anterior iris surface, the corneal endothelium, and a line perpendicular to the corneal endothelium drawn up to the anterior iris surface from a point on the corneal endothelium which is 750 millimicron from the scleral spur.

Table 52.1: Parameters used in quantitative UBM

Parameter (Abbreviation)	
Angle opening distance (AOD) 500/ 750	Distance between the trabecular meshwork and the iris at a point 500 μm or 750 μm anterior to the scleral spur
Trabecular iris angle (TIA)	Angle of the angle recess
Trabecular ciliary process distance (TCPD)	Distance between the trabecular meshwork and the ciliary process 500 μm anterior to the sceral spur
Iris thickness (ID-1)	Iris thickness 500 μm anterior to scleral spur
Iris thickness (ID-2)	Iris thickness 2 mm distance from iris root
Iris thickness (ID-3)	Iris thickness at pupillary edge
Iris-ciliary process distance (ICPD)	Distance between iris and ciliary body measured along the line of TCPD
Iris-zonule distance (IZD)	Distance between the iris and zonule along the line of TCPD
Iris-lens contact distance (ICLD)	Iris-lens contact distance
Iris-lens angle	Angle between iris and anterior surface of lens at pupillary margin

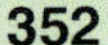

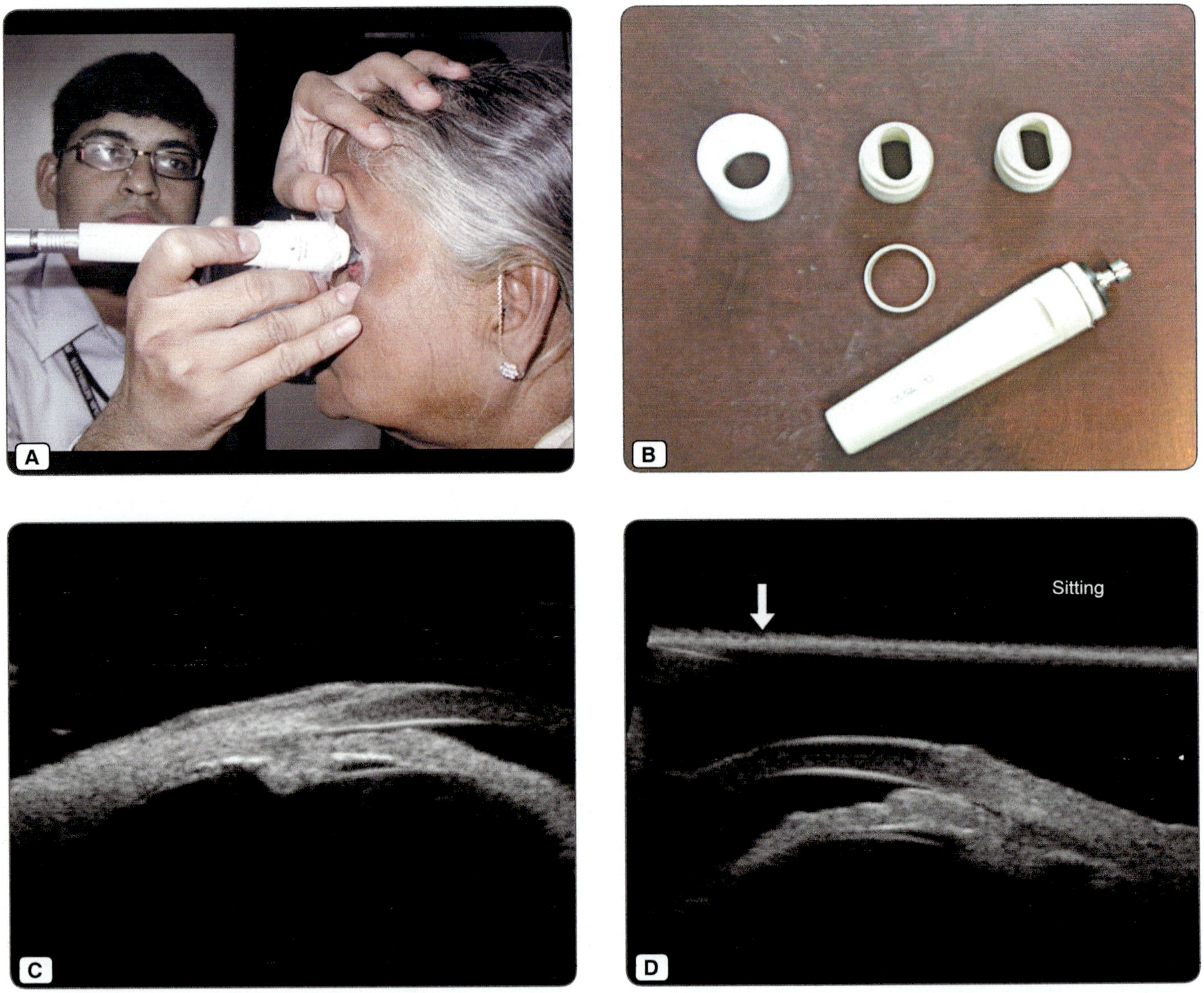

Figures 52.19A to D: Technique of performing UBM in the sitting position using special attachments to the transducers and a membrane over the attachment to avoid spillage of fluid. Figures C and D show the image obtained in supine and sitting positions showing good quality of images. Figure C without the membrane, and Figure D shows a linear high reflective structure indicative of the membrane.

53 Ultrasound Biomicroscopy in Anterior Segment Tumors

OBJECTIVES OF IMAGING MASS LESIONS WITH UBM

- To generate a differential diagnosis
- To identify the location of the tumor
- To measure the size of the lesion
- Follow-up.

UBM IN TUMORS INVOLVING THE ANTERIOR SEGMENT

- UBM gives an accurate estimate of tumor size, location and growth, tumor margins (both external and internal) which help in planning treatment and to also look for recurrence after treatment
- Tumor margin definition is important to plan iridocyclectomy and plaque brachytherapy
- Assessment of tumor features like internal reflectivity, hyper- or hypo-echoic patterns suggestive of vascular and cystic areas
- Superior to conventional 10 MHz B scan imaging in localization of ciliary body melanomas.
- **Superior to anterior segment OCT (AS-OCT) as the UBM** has fewer problems with posterior tumor shadowing and has a better image quality, better tumor visualization, better visualization of posterior margins and better resolution of iris and iridociliary tumors.
- UBM has a superior ability to penetrate large tumor, highly pigmented tumors and ciliary body tumors, however, the AS-OCT gives better resolution of anterior tumor surface and imaging of anterior segment anatomy.

Tumors Imaged on UBM

- Ocular surface tumors
- Iris tumors (pigmented and non-pigmented)
- Iridociliary cysts
- Iridociliary tumors
- Anterior margin of peripheral choroidal tumors.

OCULAR SURFACE TUMORS

Tumors arising from the squamous epithelium, melanocytes and lymphocytes of the conjunctiva.

Ocular Surface Squamous Neoplasia (OSSN)

- Intraepithelial and invasive squamous cell carcinoma of the conjunctiva and cornea
- Could be benign (squamous papilloma), precancerous (actinic keratosis), carcinoma *in situ* or invasive squamous carcinoma
- Xeroderma pigmentosa and HIV are associated with an increased incidence of OSSN
- Invasive carcinomas can spread intraocularly and metastasize both to regional lymph nodes and distant sites.

Melanocytic Tumors

- Classified into nevi (congenital or acquired), melanosis (congenital or acquired), indeterminate melanocytic proliferations, and malignant melanoma
- Could be benign (benign epithelial melanosis, nevi, ocular melanocytosis or nevus of Ota); premalignant (primary acquired melanosis) or malignant (conjunctival melanoma)
- Local recurrence of melanomas is common and the risk of regional and distant metastases is high.

Lymphoid Tumors

- Rare
- Characteristics similar to mucosa associated lymphoid tissue (MALT)
- May be indolent and localized
- Salmon patch/fish flesh appearance.

UBM in Surface Tumors

- Part of diagnosis and investigation along with photography, MRI and CT scans, pathologic examination and systemic evaluation
- Delineation of surface and borders
- Determination of surface and intralesional characteristics
- Determination of scleral and/or intraocular invasion
- Helps in preoperative planning.

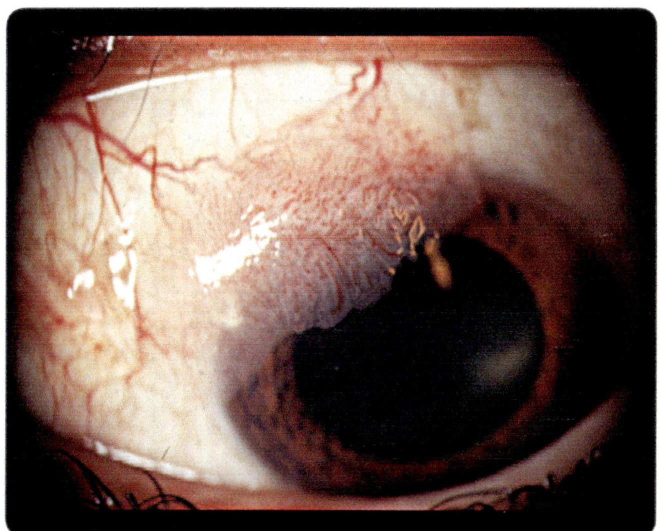

Figure 53.1A: Color photograph of the right eye of a patient showing a limbal mass overhanging the cornea, having multiple papillary projections.

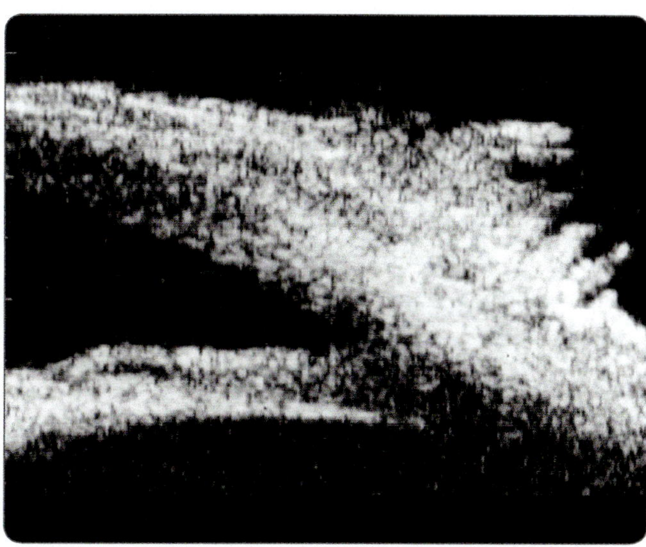

Figure 53.1B: 50 MHz UBM image of the same eye showing the finger-like projection of the mass and the lack of deeper involvement.

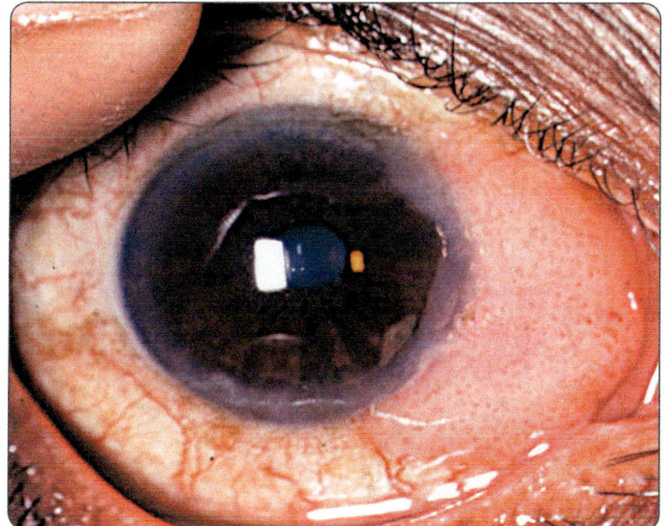

Figure 53.2A: Anterior segment photograph of the right eye of a patient showing a mass lesion involving the nasal bulbar conjunctiva and overhanging the limbus.

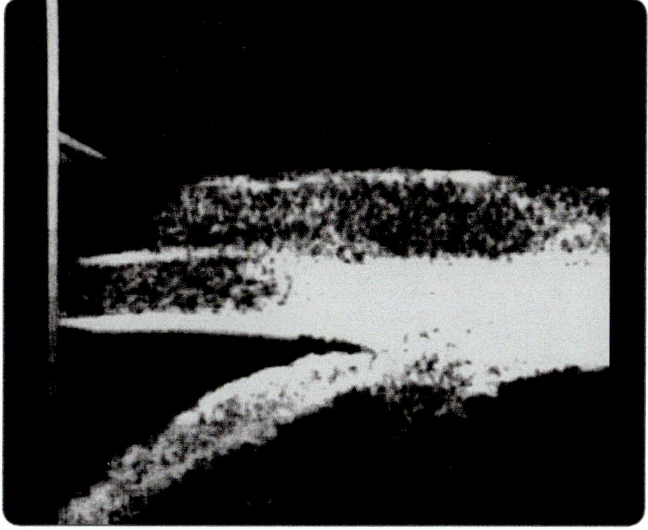

Figure 53.2B: 50 MHz UBM image of the same eye showing a homogenous mass involving only the conjunctiva, and overhanging the limbus without involving the cornea.

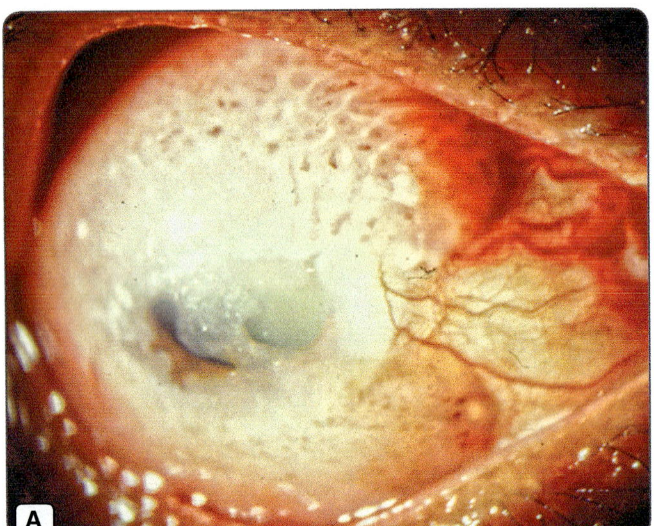

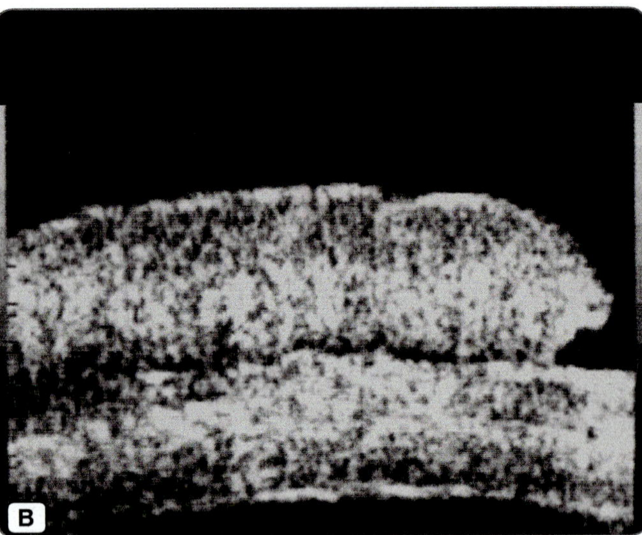

Figures 53.3A and B: Clinical photograph and 50 MHz UBM images of a large limbal mass showing apparent involvement of more than half the cornea. The UBM images show the mass lesion with a clear demarcataion between the mass and cornea indicating that the lesion overhangs but does not directly involve the cornea.

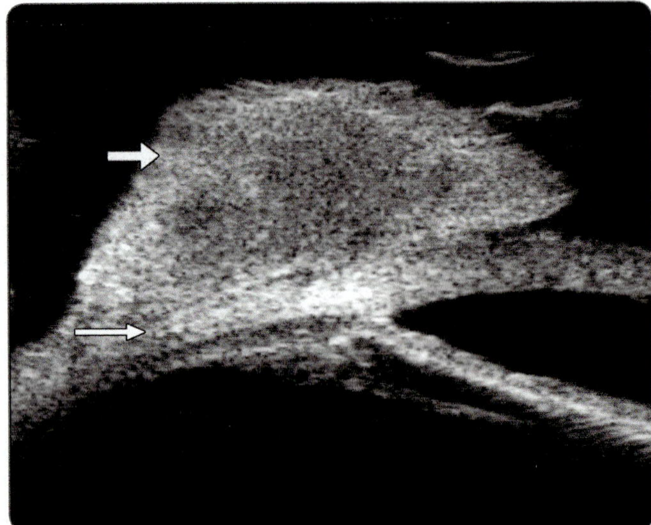

Figure 53.4: 35 MHz UBM image of a limbal surface tumor (broad arrow). Note the homogenous nature of the lesion and the clear demarcation (thin arrow) from the underlying episclera.

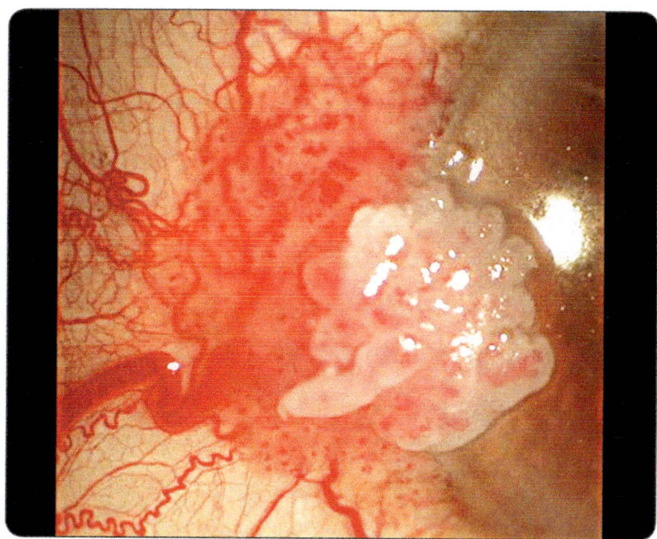

Figure 53.5A: Papillomatous limbal mass with a dilated feeder vessel.

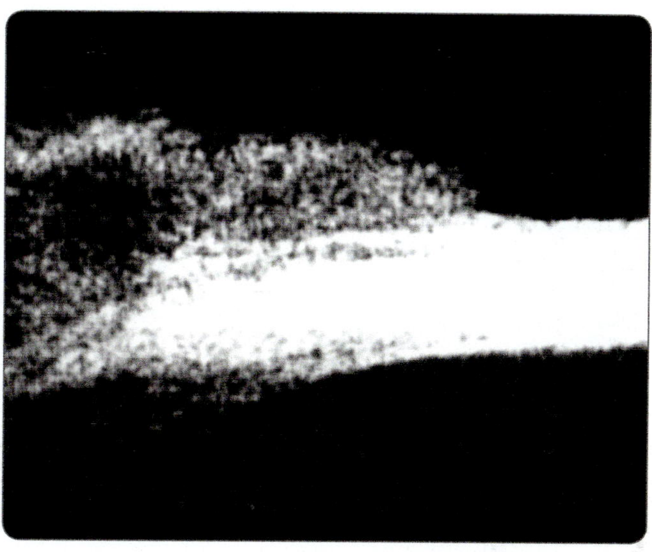

Figure 53.5B: 50 MHz UBM image of the same eye showing a conjunctival mass lesion. The feeder vessel is seen as an echolucent structure entering the mass.

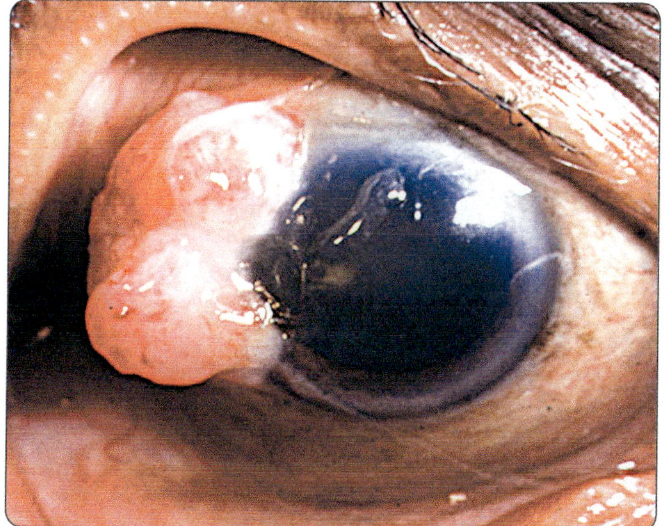

Figure 53.6A: A large mass lesion with irregular surface seen at the temporal limbus.

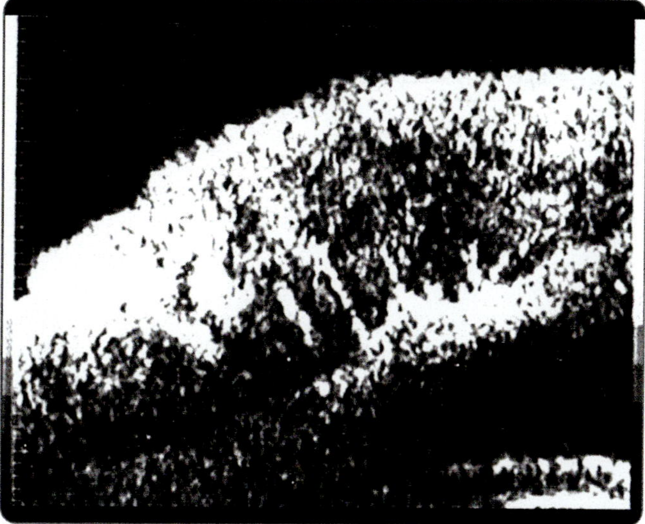

Figure 53.6B: 50 MHz UBM image of the same eye, shows a conjunctival mass lesion with septae, involving the superficial cornea and episcleral tissue. This proved to be a squamous cell carcinoma.

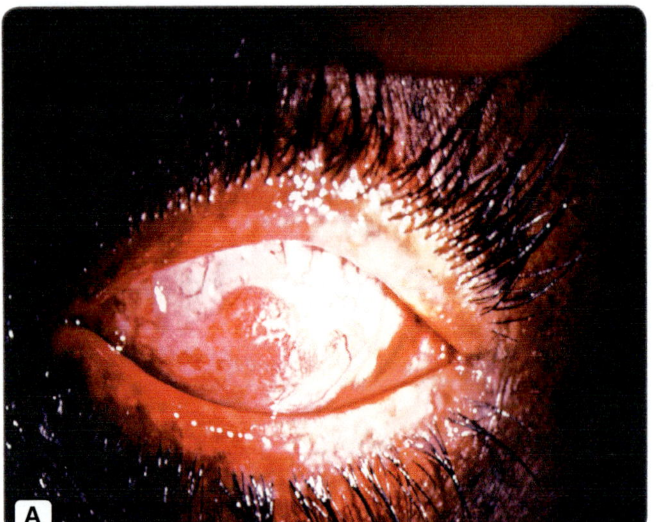

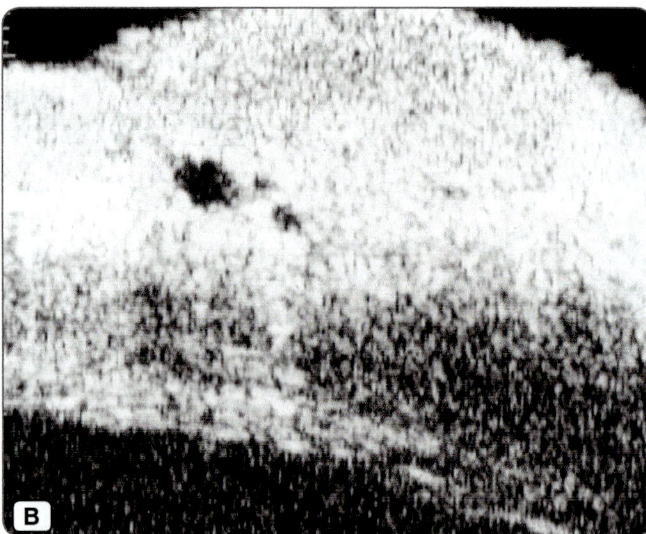

Figures 53.7A and B: Clinical photograph and 50 MHz UBM image of an eye with xeroderma pigmentosa and a large mass lesion concealing the anterior segment details. The UBM shows a high reflective conjunctival mass with areas of echolucency that could signify necrosis. Importantly, there is no clear demarcation between the surface mass and the deeper structures indicating its invasive nature.

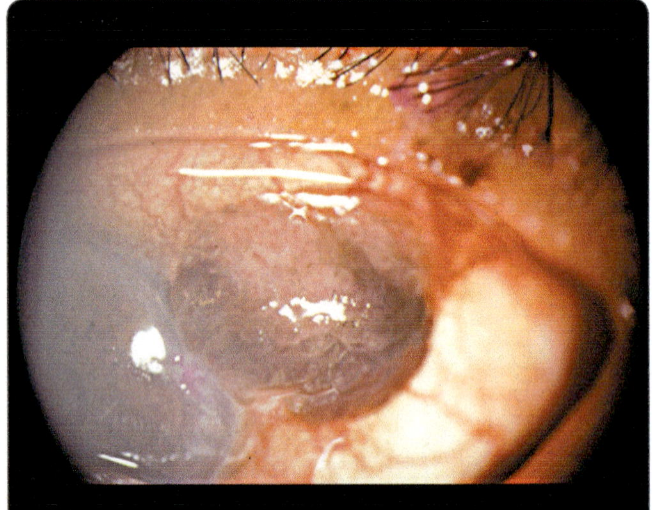

Figure 53.8A: A pigmented mass lesion seen at the superotemporal limbus.

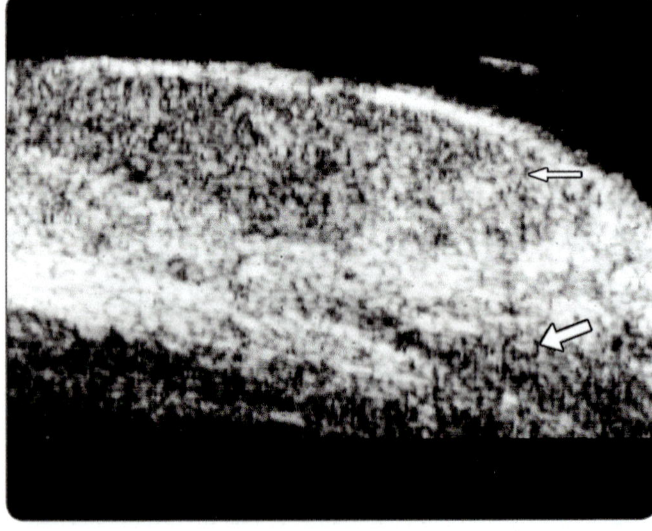

Figure 53.8B: 50 MHz UBM image of the same eye showing a homogamous well encapsulated mass that is probably involving the episcleral layer.

IRIS LESIONS

Primary Neuroepithelial Cyst

- May be bilateral or multiloculated
- Highly reflective, smooth cyst wall
- Anechoic center with no solid component.

Implantation Cyst

- Diffuse/dense internal echoes
- The site of origin of the cyst, e.g. limbal or corneal wound, may be demonstrated.

Iris Nevus

- Solid plaque-like lesion on the anterior iris surface and/or stroma
- Heterogeneous internal reflectivity
- Posterior iris surface flat or smoothly concave
- Minor degrees of pupil distortion
- Minimal or no growth tendency on serial biometry.

Iris Melanoma

- Solid irregular iris mass
- Variable internal reflectivity
- Distortion of surrounding structures
- Irregularity or convex bowing of posterior iris plane
- Enlargement on serial biometry
- Surface plaque is hyporeflective if cells are packed (spindle cell type) and hyper-reflective if cells are loosely packed (epithelioid cell type)
- Internal vascularity—UBM detects internal vascularity reliably in 93% of cases. Large vessels are seen as hyper reflective areas with hypoechoic spaces whereas small vessels are seen as hyper reflective areas
- Delineates tumor and ciliary body interface more reliably than clinical examination and helps in planning treatment. This also helps to prognosticate as ciliary body involvement is associated with a poor prognosis
- Detects disruption of posterior surface of iris pigment epithelium which is a sign of posterior tumor extension
- Detects extra scleral extension
- Involvement of iris root is a risk factor for metastasis.

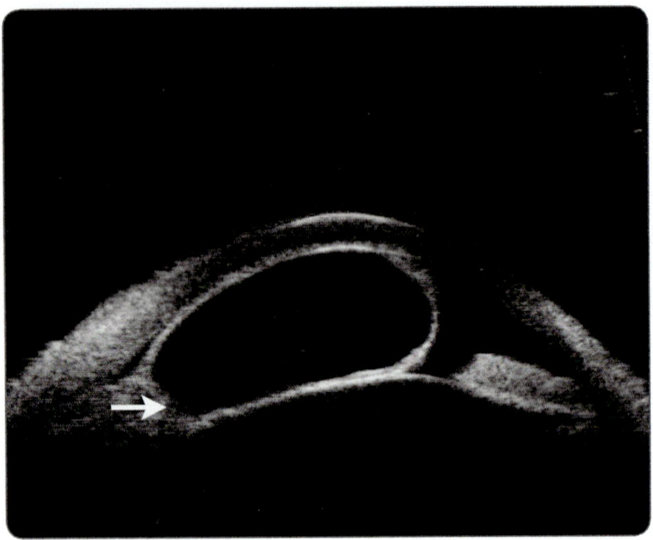

Figure 53.9: UBM image of a large iris cyst occupying more than half the anterior chamber. Note the absence of posterior extension.

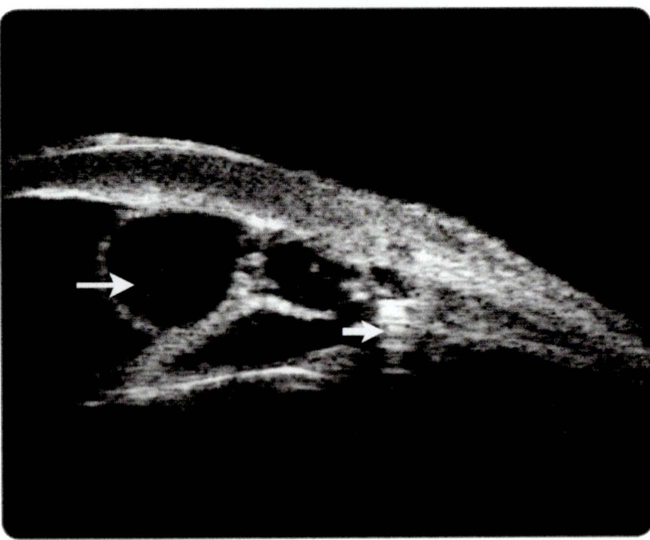

Figure 53.10: UBM image showing multiple implantation cysts (thin arrow) in a pseudophakic eye having a poorly healed section. The IOL haptics are seen in the sulcus (broad arrow).

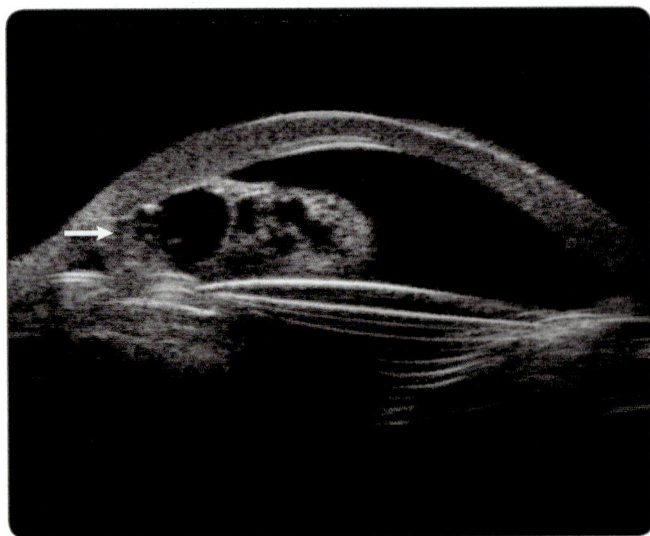

Figure 53.11: 35 MHz UBM image of a cystic iris mass lesion in a pseudophakic eye. The arrow shows the origin of the mass corresponding to the cataract surgery wound.

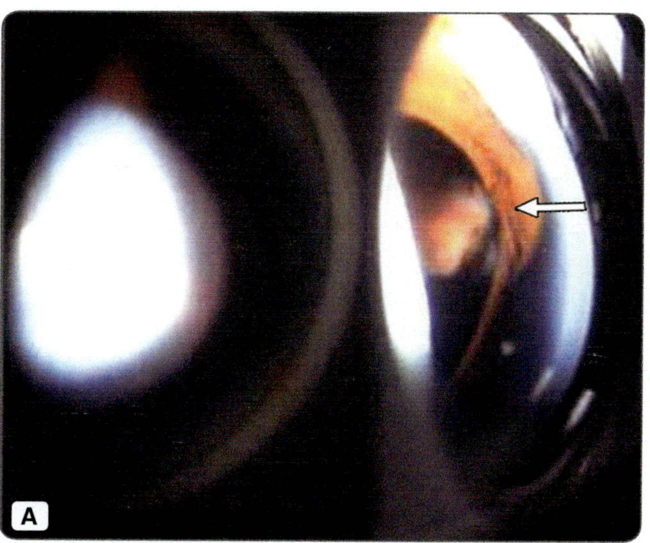

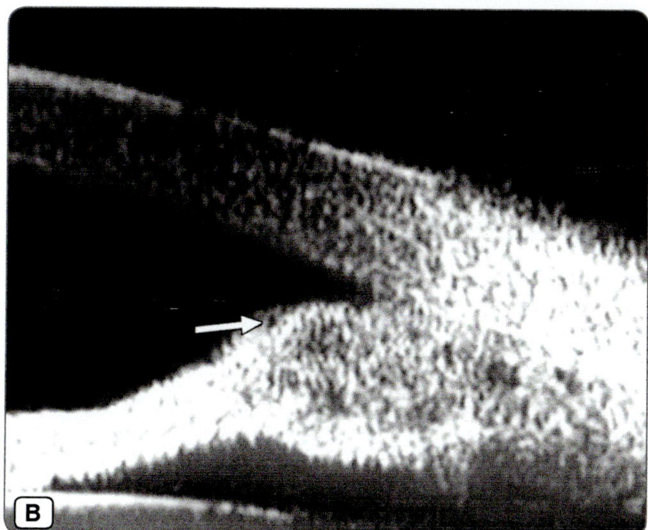

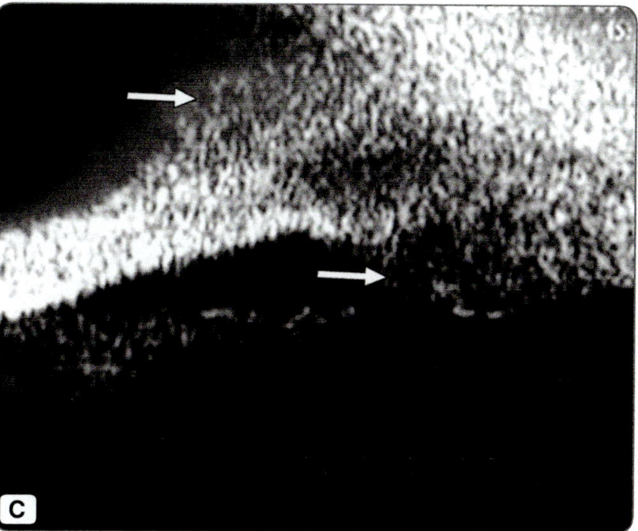

Figures 53.12A to C: Clinical photographs and UBM image (50 MHz) of an eye with an iris tumor. The feature of iris bowing seen on the clinical photograph is due to tumor infiltration of the iris stroma which displaces the surfaces. The presence of acoustically empty or cystic spaces is suggestive of tumor vascularity. Loss of the normal high reflectivity of the angle is suggestive of iris root involvement (arrow). Ciliary body involvement is also seen in this image (lower arrow in Figure C).

CILIARY BODY LESIONS

Ciliary Body Melanoma

- Oval shaped mass centered on the ciliary body
- Usually solid, cavitation may occur
- Low to medium internal reflectivity
- Invasion of adjacent tissues may be evident.

Diffuse Melanoma

- Diffuse melanoma of ciliary body with >180 degree involvement is called ring melanoma
- Must be suspected in eyes with unilateral refractory glaucoma with iris hyperchromia
- Associated with visual field loss, hyphema, RD and extraocular extension
- High-risk of extrascleral extension and metastasis
- Transillumination is not adequate in non-pigmented tumors
- All ciliary body tumors must be followed circumferentially to assess the extent
- UBM detects abnormal ciliary body architecture and reflectivity.

Melanocytoma

- Benign if seen to be long standing without any growth
- UBM shows a ciliary body mass with low internal reflectivity
- Low internal reflectivity is a feature of cohesiveness of cells
- Lack of internal vascularity (feature against melanoma).

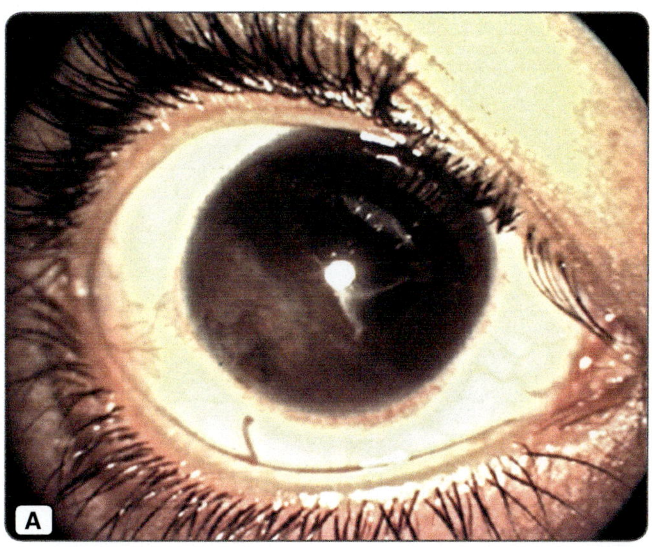

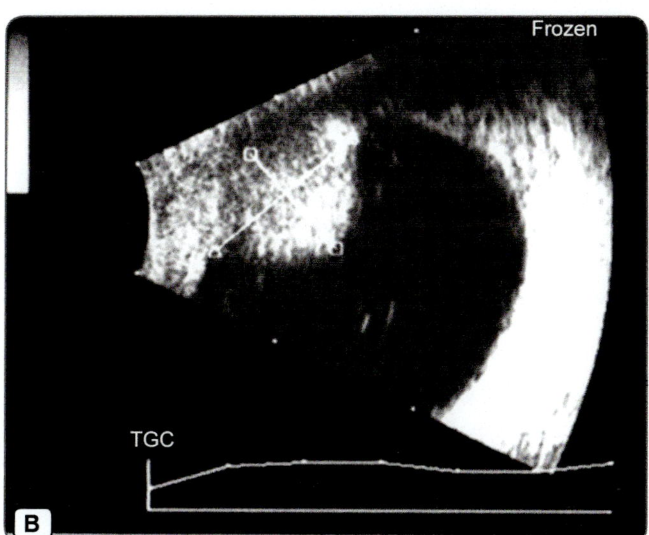

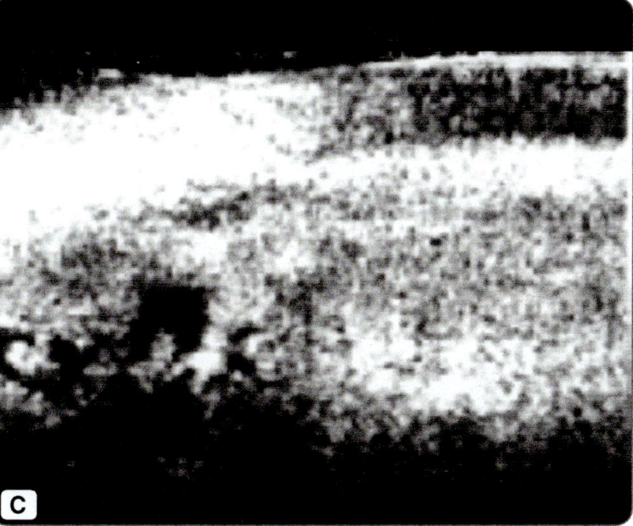

Figures 53.13A to C

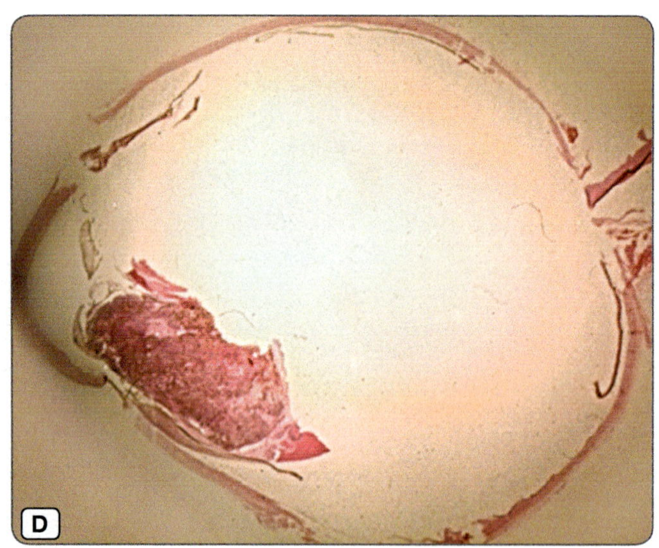

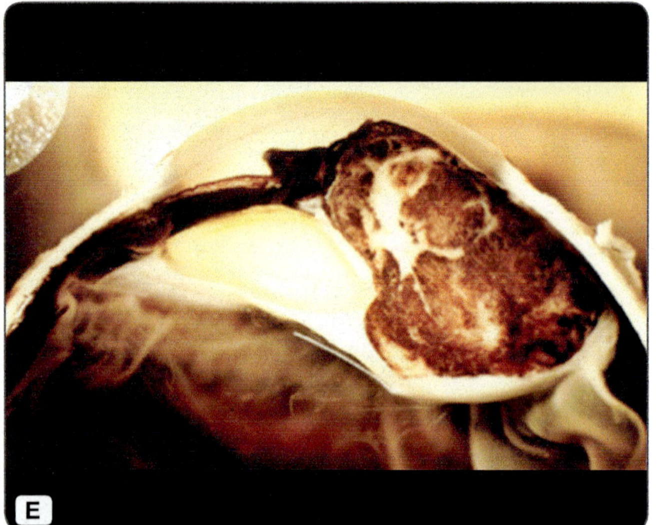

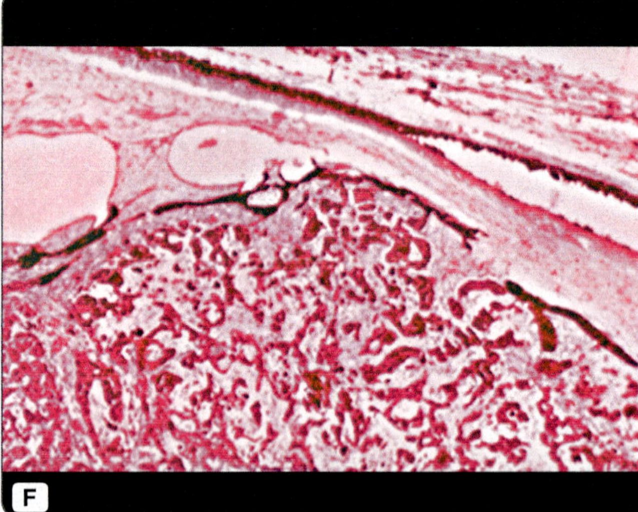

Figures 53.13A to F: Clinical photograph, ultrasound, UBM and HPE images of an eye with a vascularized ciliary body mass extending into the angle of the anterior chamber. The ultrasound B scan shows a high reflective mass in the ciliary body region. UBM shows the mass lesion which extends from the ciliary body into the anterior chamber. The mass is high reflective with a few echolucent spaces. The gross images of the eye after enucleation show the location of mass and HPE image shows the cell pattern to be that of a medulloepithelioma.

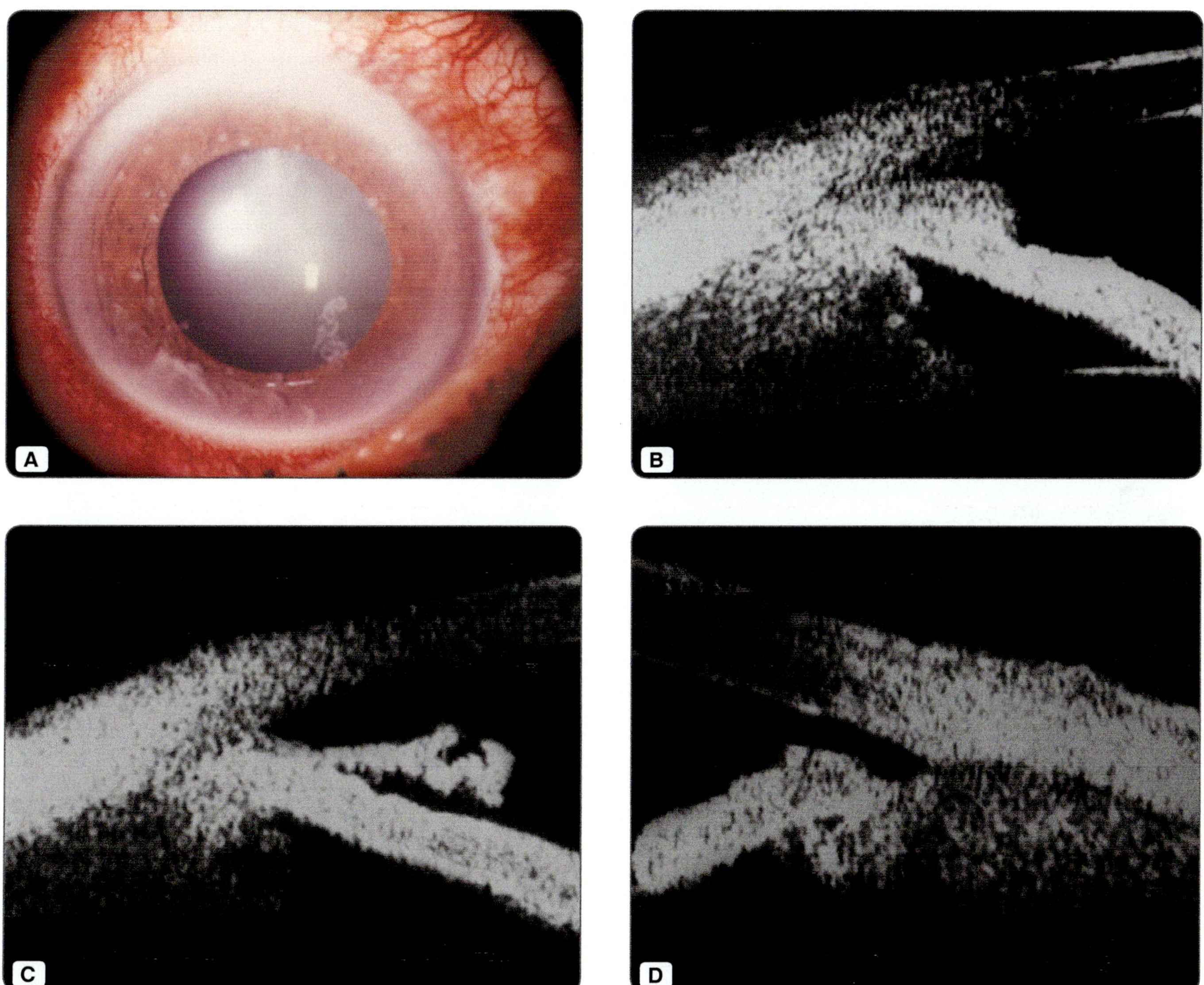

Figures 53.14A to D: Clinical photograph and UBM images of an eye with secondaries from breast carcinoma. The clinical picture shows iris nodules and white deposits in the anterior chamber. The UBM images show the thickening of the ciliary body and iris which is low reflective. The anterior chamber deposits are seen as highly reflective irregular echoes on the iris surface.

ANTERIOR EXTENSION OF POSTERIOR LESIONS

Anterior Choroidal Melanoma

- Ciliary body/iris extension of a peripheral choroidal melanoma can be appreciated by UBM
- Invasion usually appears as tissue of reduced reflectivity compared to the surrounding ciliary body/iris.

Retinoblastoma

- UBM is found to be a crucial tool in the intraocular staging of disease of children with advanced retinoblastoma
- Provides sensitive and reproducible visualization of the anterior retina, ciliary body region, and anterior segment, thereby optimizing patient management of cases with severe retinoblastoma
- Involvement of the anterior retina and ciliary body region with the tumor is associated with a poor prognosis. Failure to detect anterior tumors early can compromise the chances of saving the eye and increase the risk of extraocular disease
- Determination of the mechanism of glaucoma in these eyes.
  1. Angle closure and pupillary block
  2. Neovascular glaucoma
  3. Tumor obstruction of the iridocorneal angle.

Follow-up

- Most small tumors show little growth over extended periods
- Long-term follow-up is needed to look for growth in height, lateral extension and need for surgery
- Important to look for lateral growth to avoid overlooking early diffuse or ring tumor formation
- Growth documentation is the most important point to distinguish iris nevi from melanoma. Here the growth may be seen on the undersurface of lesion which makes it difficult to appreciate clinically.

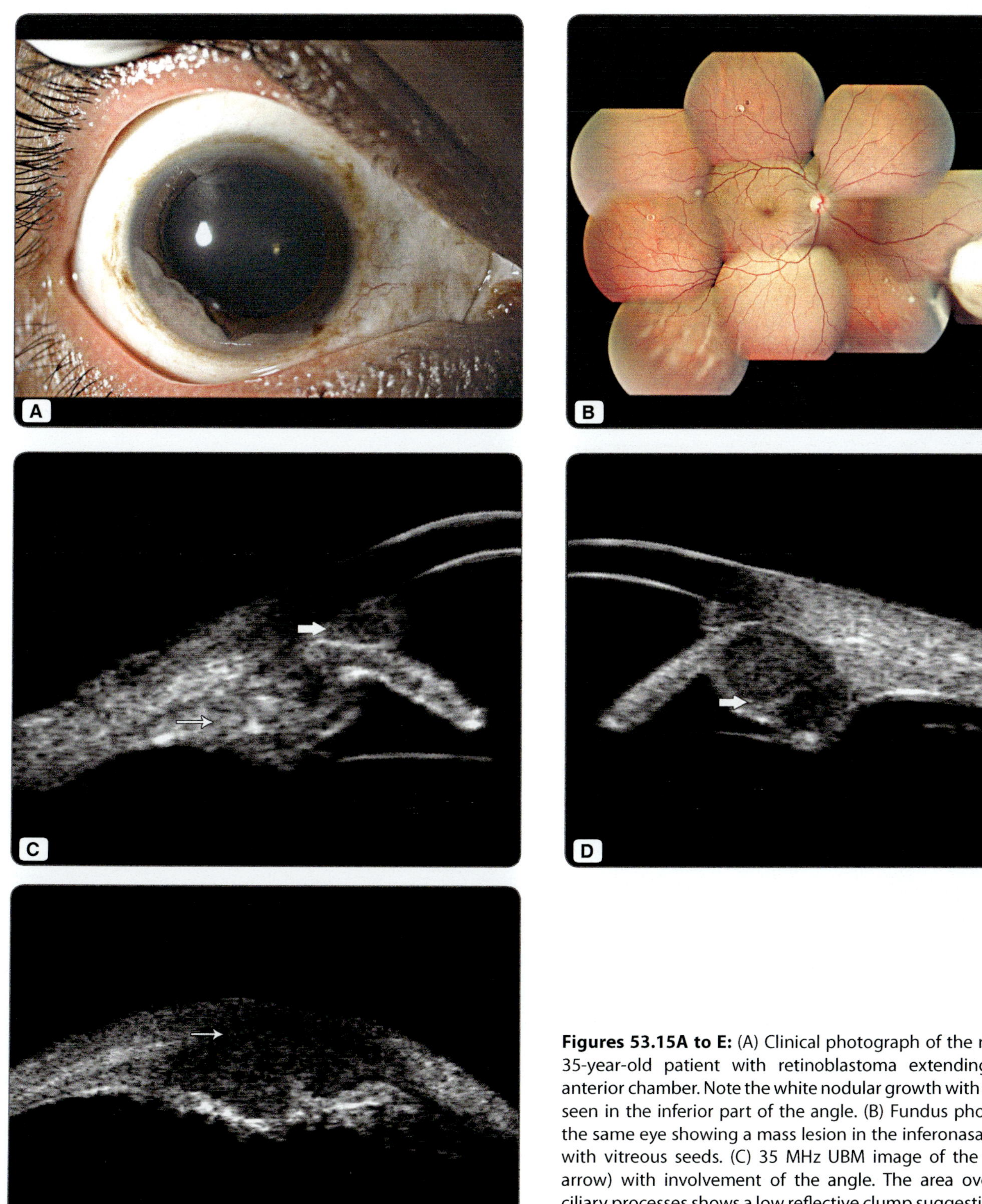

Figures 53.15A to E: (A) Clinical photograph of the right eye of 35-year-old patient with retinoblastoma extending into the anterior chamber. Note the white nodular growth with vascularity, seen in the inferior part of the angle. (B) Fundus photograph of the same eye showing a mass lesion in the inferonasal periphery with vitreous seeds. (C) 35 MHz UBM image of the mass (thin arrow) with involvement of the angle. The area overlying the ciliary processes shows a low reflective clump suggesting vitreous seeds. (D) 35 MHz image of a well circumscribed ciliary body mass (arrow) with angle involvement. Note the clear demarcation from the position part of the ciliary body. (E) Circumferential view of the same mass lesion showing the invasion through the angle (arrow).

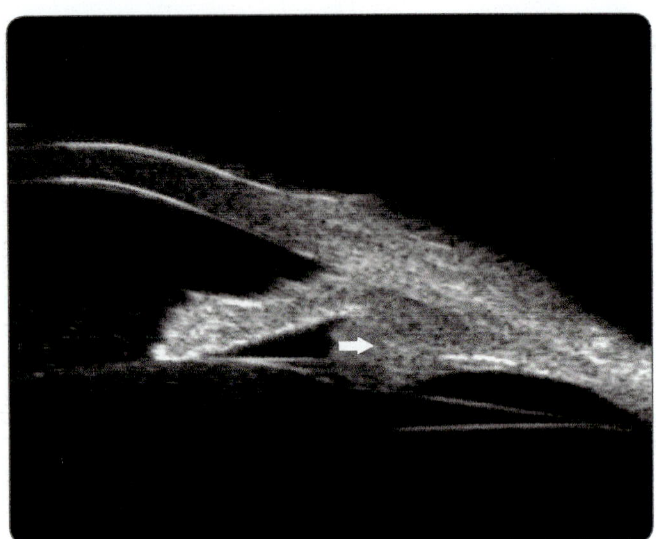

Figure 53.16A: 35 MHz UBM image of a small ciliary body mass (arrow). Note the absence of angle and peripheral choroidal involvement. The dot-like echoes in the anterior chamber are possibly cells.

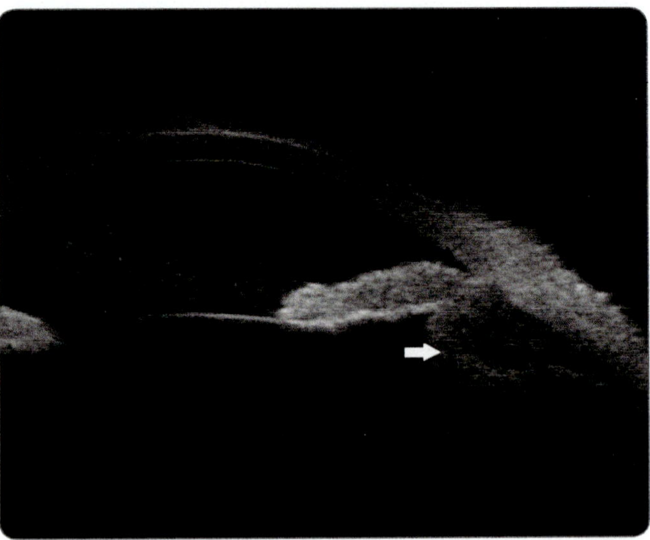

Figure 53.16B: 35 Mz image of an eye with anterior chamber cells. Note the low reflective ciliary body mass (arrow) pushing up the peripheral iris.

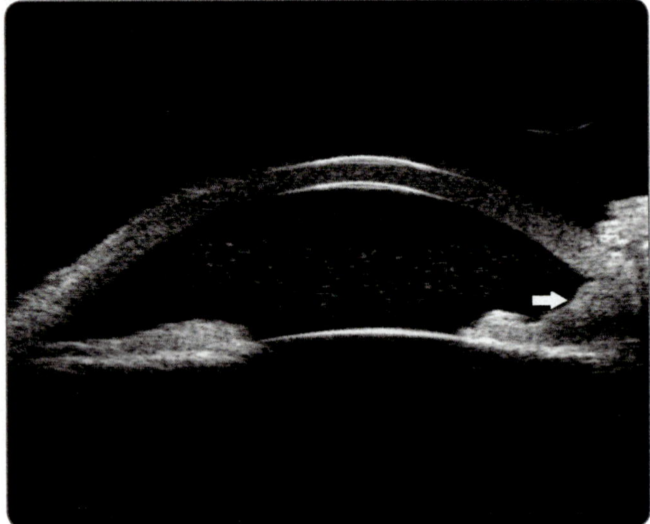

Figure 53.16C: 35 MHz image of the same eye in a different area showing that the mass lesion involves the iris root (arrow) and extends into the anterior chamber.

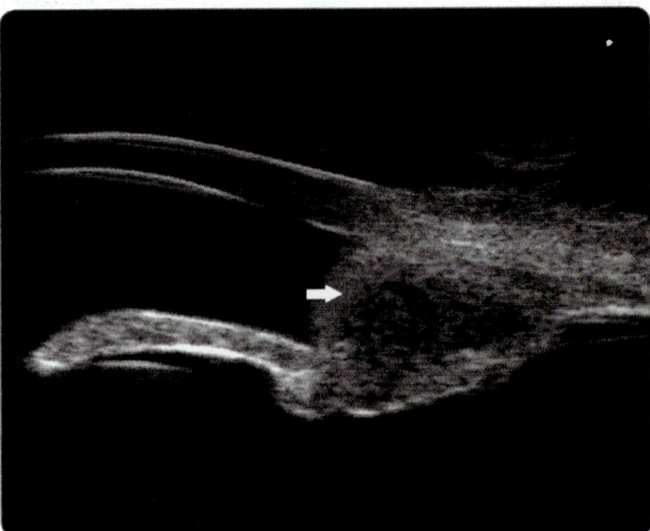

Figure 53.17: 35 MHz UBM image of a homogenous mass lesion involving the iris root and extending into the anterior chamber.

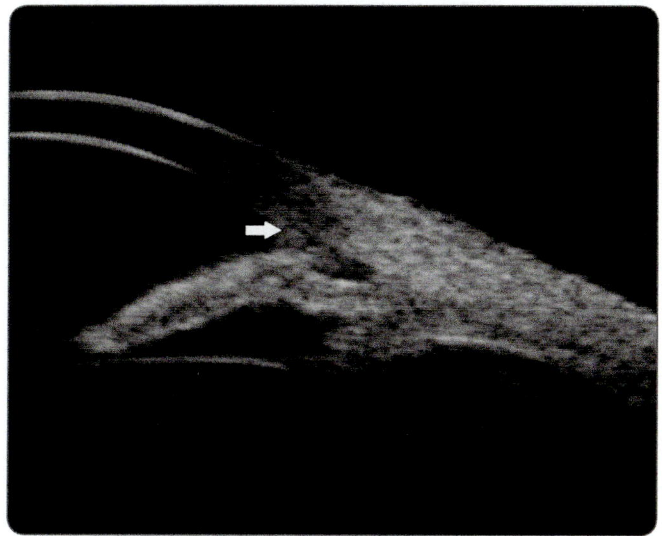

Figure 53.18: A small area (arrow) of involvement of the angle is seen in this 35 MHz image of an eye with a mass lesion involving the iris root.

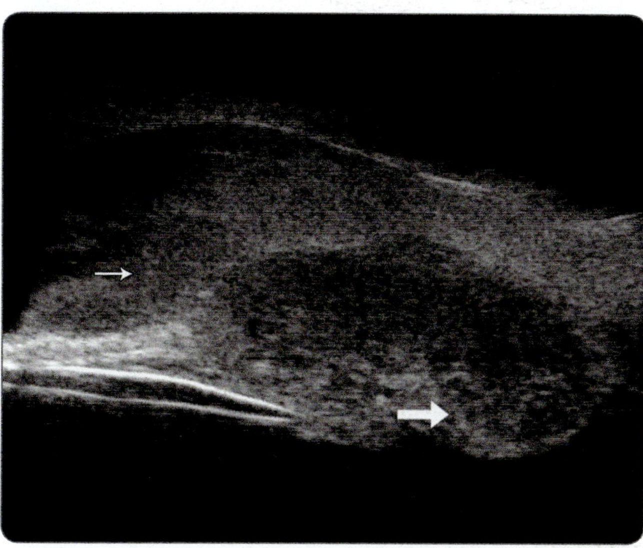

Figure 53.19A: 35 MHz image of a ciliary body mass lesion extending into the anterior chamber through the iris root (thin arrow).

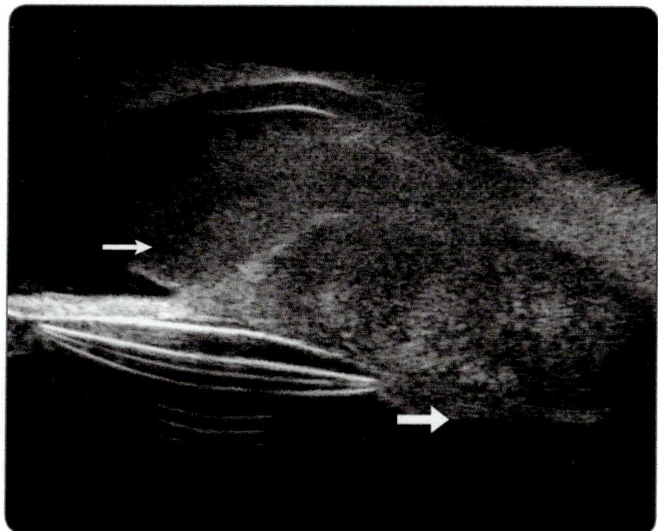

Figure 53.19B: 35 MHz UBM image of a pseudophakic eye showing a heterogeneous mass lesion involving the iris and ciliary body. The broad arrow shows that the mass extends beyond the ciliary body.

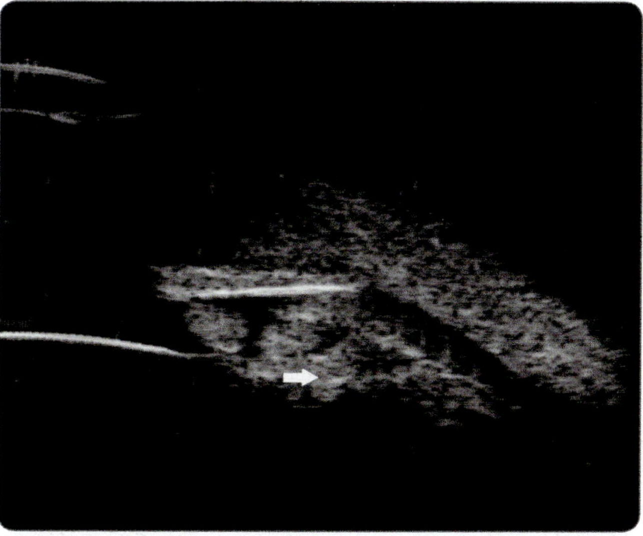

Figure 53.20: 35 MHz UBM image of a diffuse circumferential retino blastoma. The high reflective mass (arrow) is seen to extend under the iris and also involve the angle.

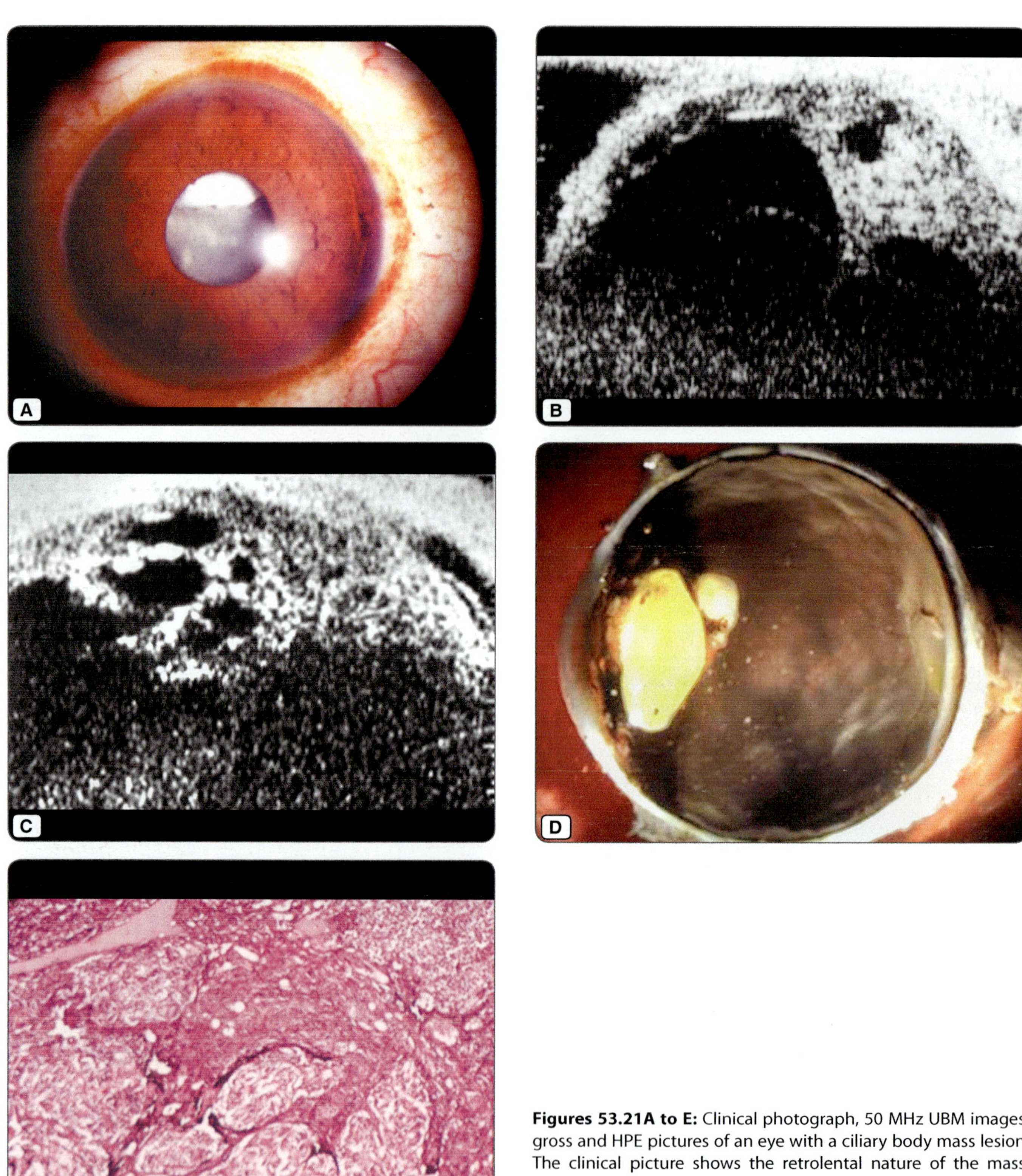

Figures 53.21A to E: Clinical photograph, 50 MHz UBM images, gross and HPE pictures of an eye with a ciliary body mass lesion. The clinical picture shows the retrolental nature of the mass. The UBM images show that the mass involves the ciliary body and consists of large cystic spaces. The gross photograph after enucleation shows the retrolental mass and HPE confirmed it to be an adenoma of the ciliary body.

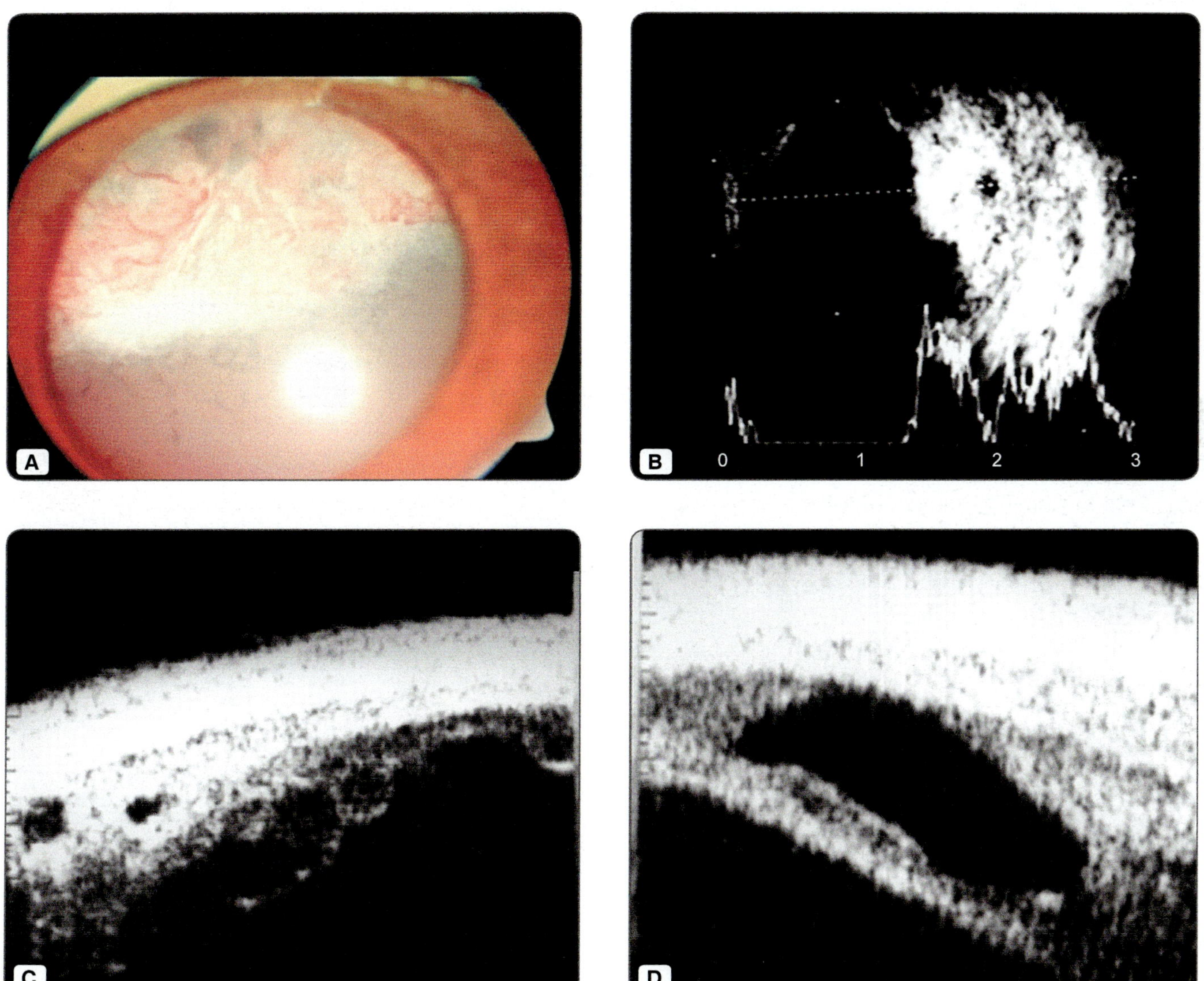

Figures 53.22A to D: Clinical photograph, ultrasound and UBM images of an eye with a mass lesion seen retrolentally with overlying fibrovascular tisuue. Ultrasound and UMB show the high reflective ciliary body mass with echolucent cystic spaces and overlying high reflective membranes , suggestive of a medulloepithelioma.

54 Ultrasound Biomicroscopy in Uveitis

INDICATIONS

- Intermediate uveitis with small pupil and/or complicated cataract
- Hypotony
- IOL induced uveitis
- Vogt Koyanagi Harada's disease
- Parasitic uveitis.

INTERMEDIATE UVEITIS

Clinical Features

- Intermediate uveitis is a type of uveitis in which there is accumulation of inflammatory material in the posterior ciliary body, pars plana and peripheral retina.
- Presence of snow banking and snow balls over the pars plana region is the clinical hallmark of the disease, in association with retrolental cells, cystoid macular edema and disc leak on FFA.
- Chronic cystoid macular edema (CME) is the commonest cause of visual loss.
- Presence of pars plana membranes and/or exudates in one or all quadrants along with ciliary body edema is a sign of active pars planitis which requires treatment. Presence of only pars plana membranes on UBM does not indicate activity.
- Investigations to rule out other causes of intermediate uveitis like tuberculosis, sarcoidosis, caterpillar hair induced uveitis should be done.
- Treatment is with oral and periocular steroids, and immunosuppressives in resistant cases.
- Surgical intervention, e.g. cataract surgery is not advised in the presence of active pars planitis.

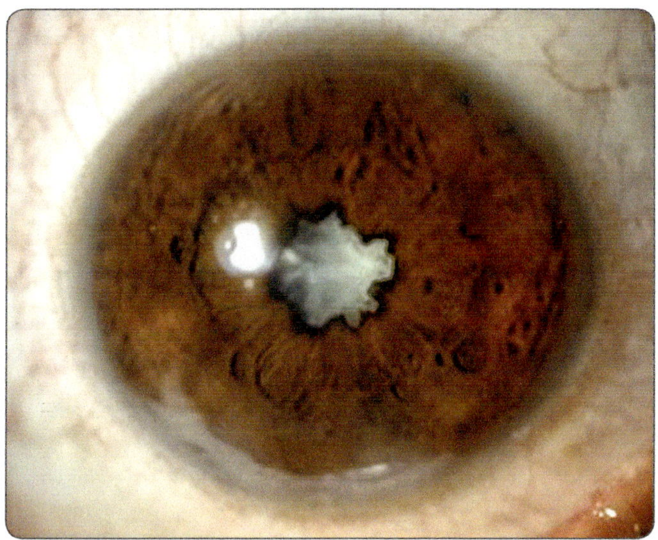

Figure 54.1A: Color photograph of an eye with posterior synechiae and complicated cataract.

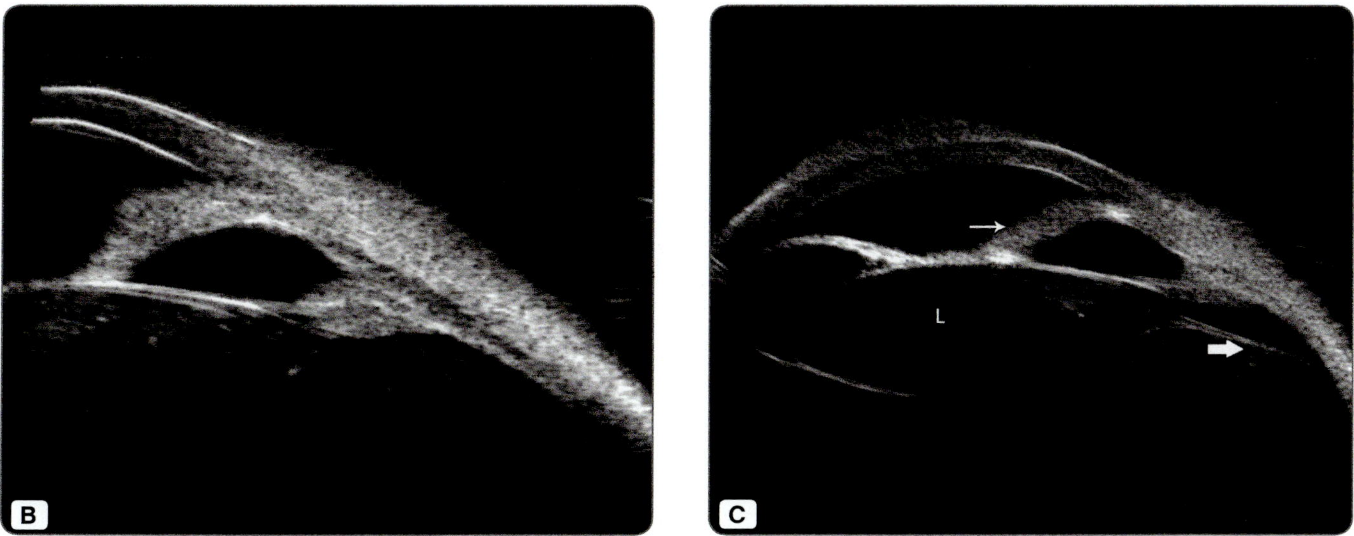

Figures 54.1B and C: UBM images of an eye with anterior uveitis, posterior synechiae and an iris bombe configuration. Note the absence of ciliary body edema and effusion.

UBM in Intermediate Uveitis

- Useful in cases of intermediate uveitis where the view of pars plana is precluded due to presence of complicated cataract and/or small pupil
- UBM in active intermediate uveitis shows a low reflective mass over the pars plana and ciliary body region suggestive of exudates along with low reflective ciliary body thickening suggestive of ciliary body edema
- UBM in inactive disease shows high reflective pars plana membranes all around or in few quadrants with or without traction on ciliary body and peripheral retina
- Demonstration of cilia in eyes with caterpillar hair induced uveitis.

HYPOTONY

Hypotony in uveitic eyes can occur in the following situations:

- Ciliary body atrophy: Normal ciliary processes are high reflective finger-like processes from ciliary body. Reduction in number and blunting of ciliary processes are seen in ciliary body atrophy. Significance→decrease/absence of aqueous secretion
- Supraciliary effusion/Choroidal effusion: Presence of echolucent space above ciliary body or choroid suggestive of effusion. Significance→needs aggressive medical management
- Traction on ciliary body: Thick pars plana membranes pull the ciliary body causing ciliary body detachment and hypotony. Significance→relief of traction in the presence of healthy ciliary processes may reverse hypotony.

IOL INDUCED UVEITIS

Clinical Features

- Recurrent episodes of inflammation post cataract surgery in a uveitic or non-uveitic eye
- A combination of uveitis, glaucoma and hypema can occur due to frequent chafing of the iris and ciliary body by the IOL haptics.

UBM Features

- UBM helps in locating the position of haptics below the iris, retained lens matter within the capsular bag, and associated features of preexisting uveitis like pars plana membranes which may explain the etiology of recurrent inflammation
- The relationship of the IOL haptic to the iris and angle structures can be ascertained
- The haptic may be in the bag or ciliary sulcus. In-the-bag haptics are seen medial to ciliary processes in close relation to irregularly reflective membranes formed by the zonules and capsule. Haptics not in the bag are imaged peripherally in the region of the ciliary sulcus
- Residual lens matter may be seen within the capsular bag
- Associated findings may include ciliary body edema, peripheral anterior synechiae and cyclitic membranes.

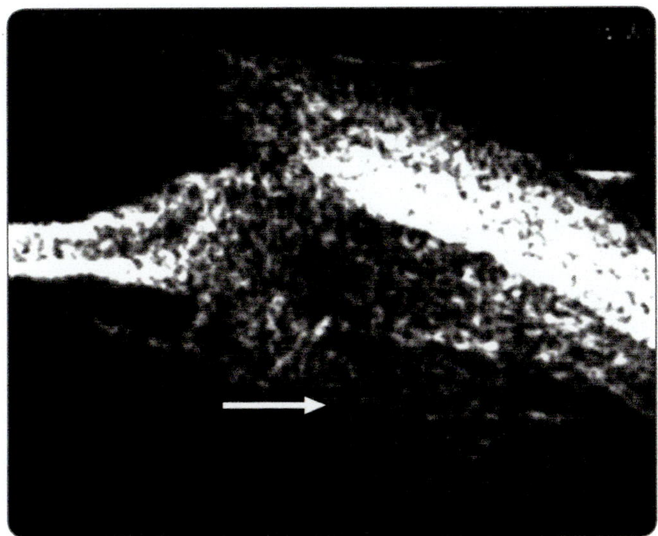

Figure 54.2: 50 MHz UBM image of an eye with active intermediate uveitis. The arrow marks a low reflective mass of echoes over the ciliary body suggestive of exudates.

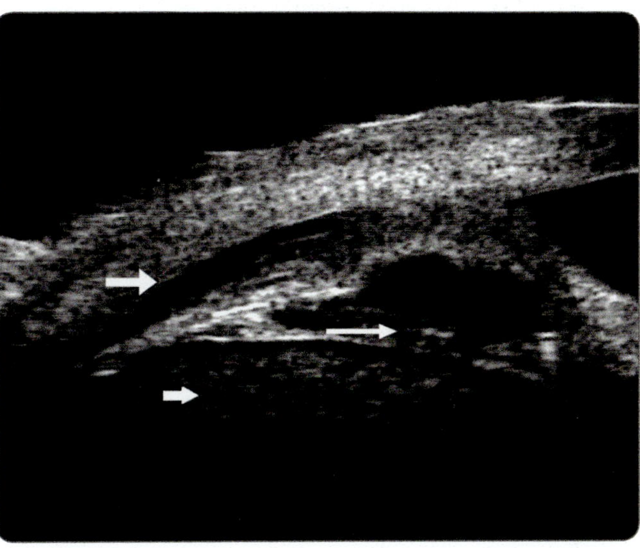

Figure 54.3: UBM showing ciliary body effusion (broad arrow) and vitreous cells (arrow). The membranes extending across the anterior hyaloid are seen (long arrow).

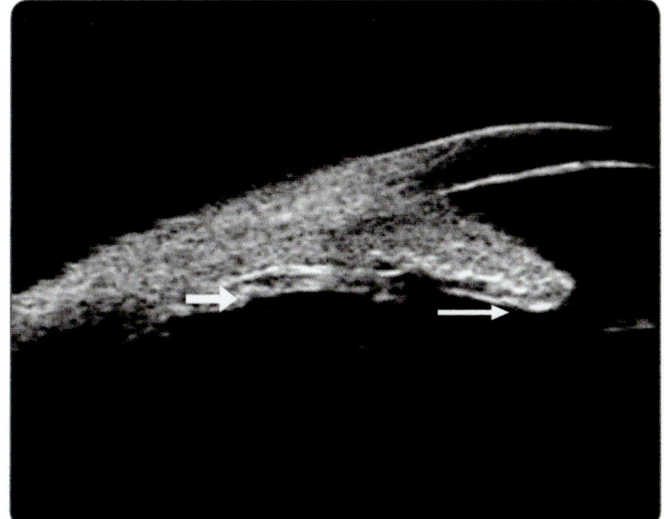

Figure 54.4: 35 MHz image of an eye with chronic hypotony showing a high reflective membrane covering the posterior surface of the iris (thin arrows) and extending to the ciliary body and peripheral retina (thick arrows). The ciliary processes are not seen.

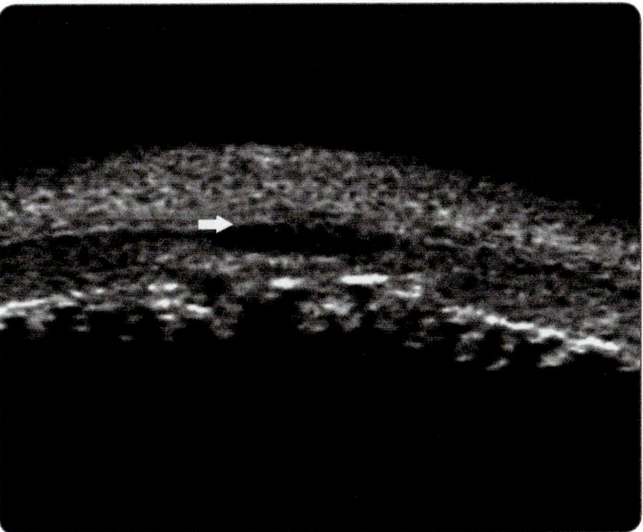

Figure 54.5: Circumferential view of supraciliary fluid (arrow) in an eye with uveitis.

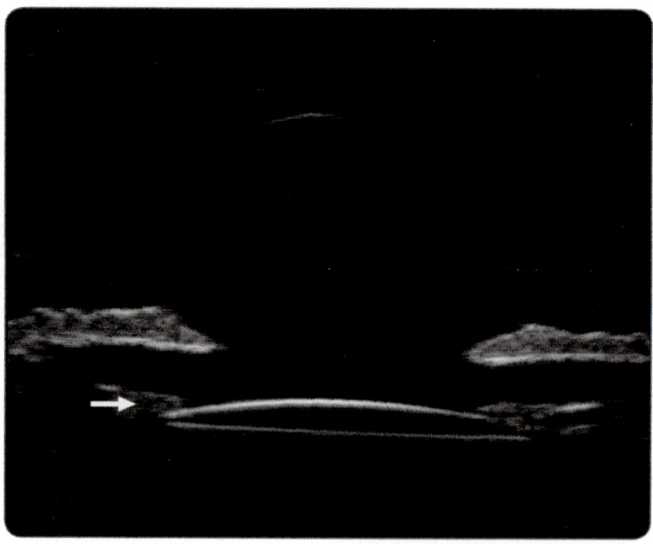

Figure 54.6: 35 MHz UBM image showing a well centered, in-the-bag IOL (Arrow showing the haptic optic junction in the bag).

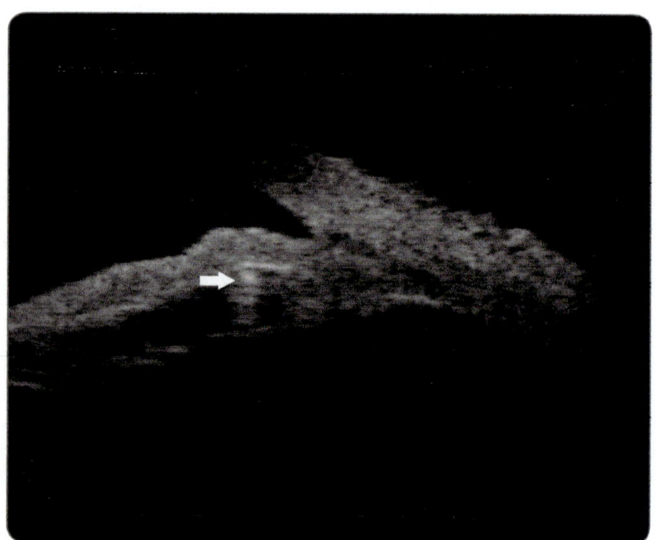

Figure 54.7: 35 MHz UBM image of an eye with recurrent postoperative inflammation. Note the IOL haptic (arrow) rubbing on the undersurface of the iris.

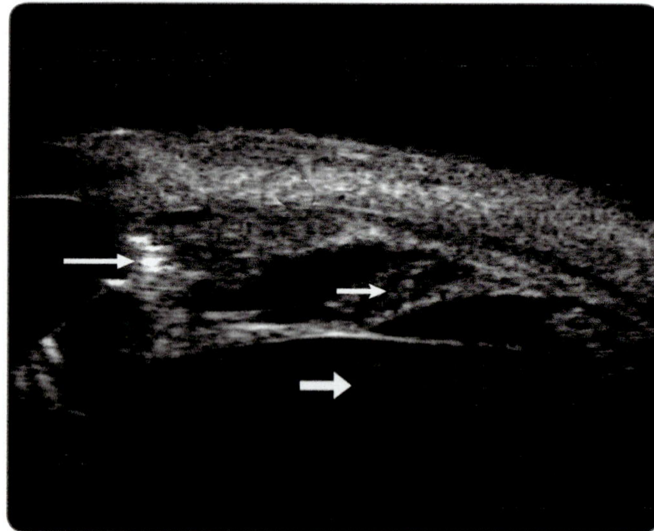

Figure 54.8: Vitreous and pars plana membranes with traction (arrows) in a pseudophakic eye with chronic uveitis. The IOL haptics are seen (long arrow).

ANTERIOR SCLERITIS

Clinical Features

- Inflammatory disease of anterior sclera
- Can be idiopathic, infective or secondary to collagen vascular disease
- Can be diffuse, nodular or necrotizing
- Treatment is with topical and oral NSAIDs, topical and systemic steroids. Immunosuppressives are used in scleritis associated with collagen vascular disorders.

UBM

- Episcleritis: Thickened episcleral tissue without involvement of the sclera
- Diffuse scleritis: Mottled internal reflectivity with areas of lower reflectivity scattered throughout the involved region. The diffuse mottling represents scleral infiltration with inflammatory cells and edema of collagen bundles
- Nodular scleritis: Thickened episclera with localized nodule of lower reflectivity than the surrounding sclera
- Necrotizing scleritis: Scleral thinning.

VKH DISEASE

- In acute stage, patient may present with angle closure glaucoma
- UBM in the acute stage shows anterior rotation of the ciliary body, supraciliary effusion and angle closure.

PARASITIC UVEITIS

- Intraocular parasites can cause intractable uveitis that is difficult to diagnose.
- UBM may be able to identify the parasite in the pars plana and ciliary body region.
- In toxocariasis, a peripheral granuloma with traction on the ciliary processes and peripheral retina, may be seen.

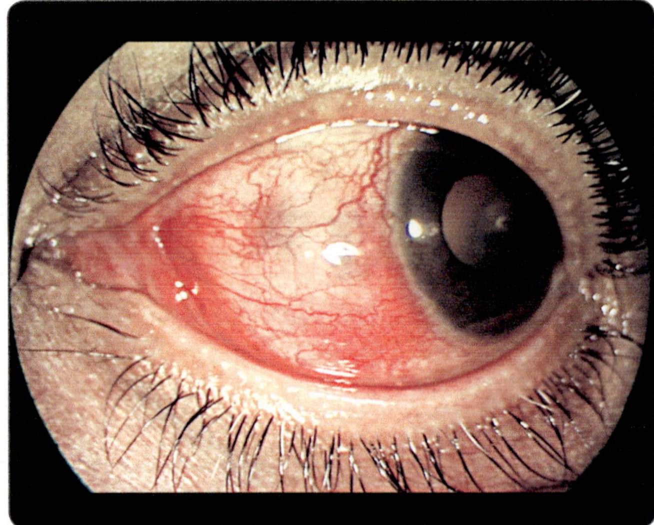

Figure 54.9A: External photograph of an eye with nodular anterior scleritis.

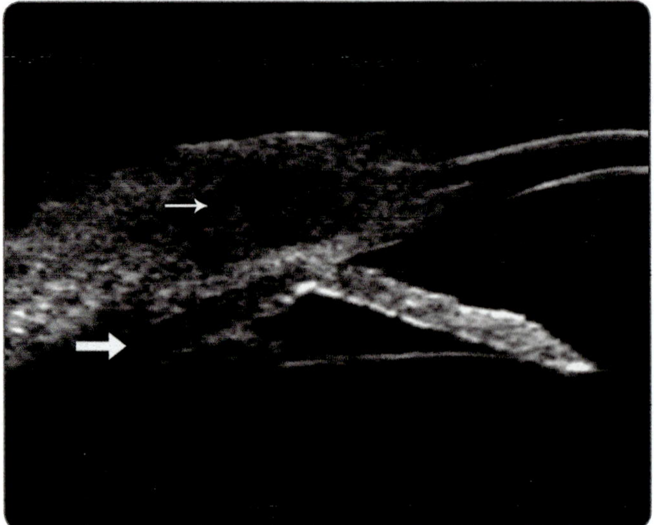

Figure 54.9B: UBM image of an eye with anterior scleritis. Note the low reflective thickening at the limbus (thin arrow). The underlying ciliary body also shows low reflective areas suggestive of edema.

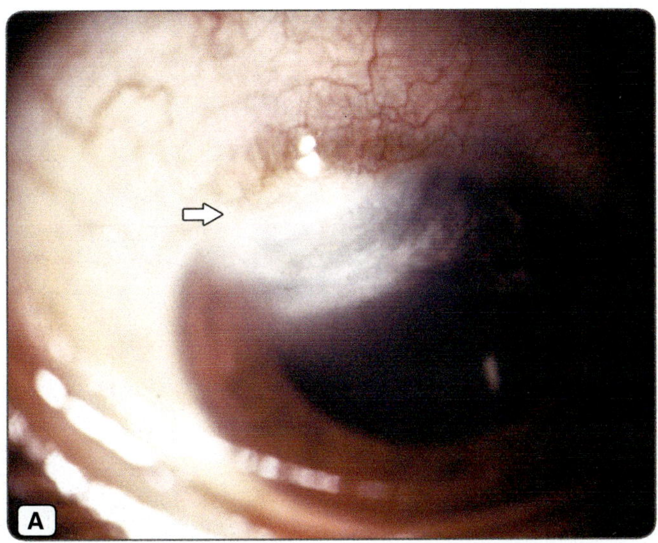

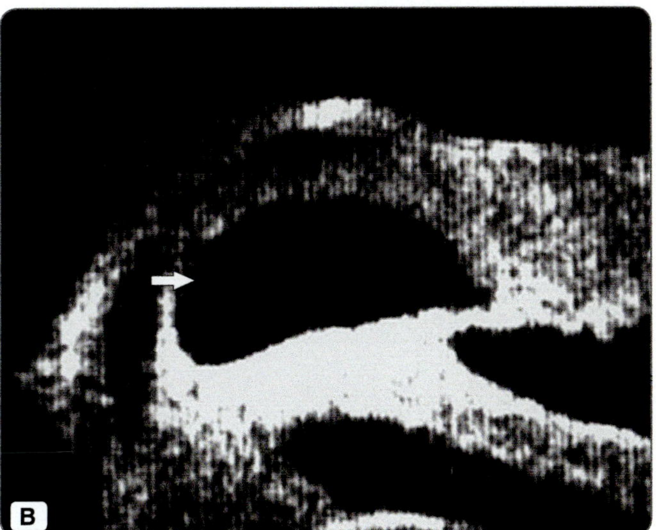

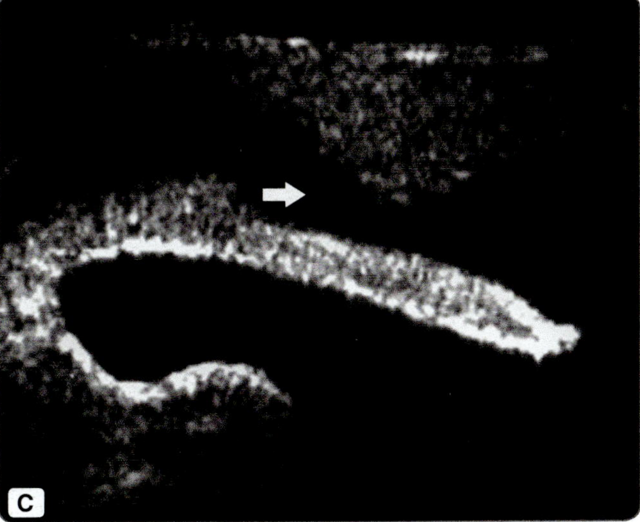

Figures 54.10A to C: Clinical photograph and UBM images of an eye with chronic sclerouveitis and a spontaneous bleb. Note the bleb at 12 o' clock position. The 50 MHz image shows a large echolucent space within the bleb. The third image shows the communication with the anterior chamber (arrow).

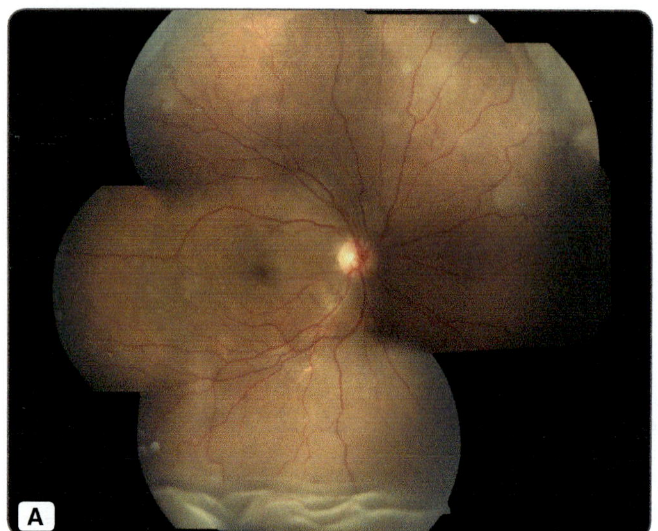

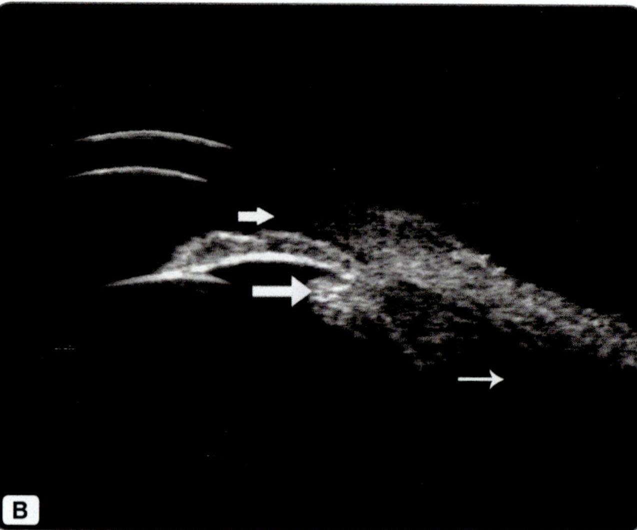

Figures 54.11A and B: Clinical photograph and UBM image of a middle aged female who presented with angle closure secondary to VKH syndrome. Note the exudative RD and peripheral choroidal detachment. The photograph was taken after the episode subsided and the pupil could be dilated. UBM shows the closed angle (arrow) due to ciliochoroidal effusion (long arrow) and anterior rotation of ciliary processes (broad arrow).

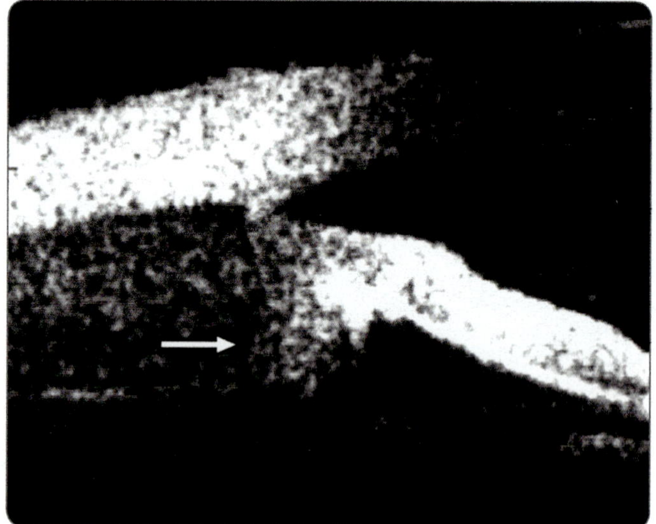

Figure 54.12A: 50 MHz UBM image of an eye with VKH showing the swollen ciliary processes.

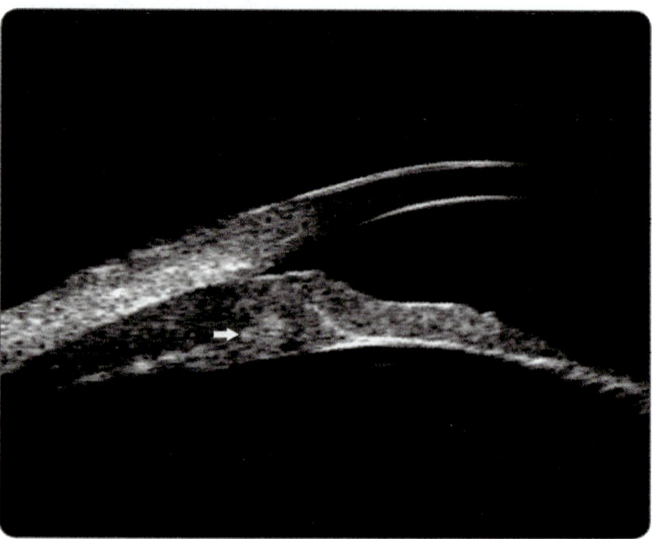

Figure 54.12B: 35 MHz UBM image of a patient with VKH syndrome showing the ciliary body edema.

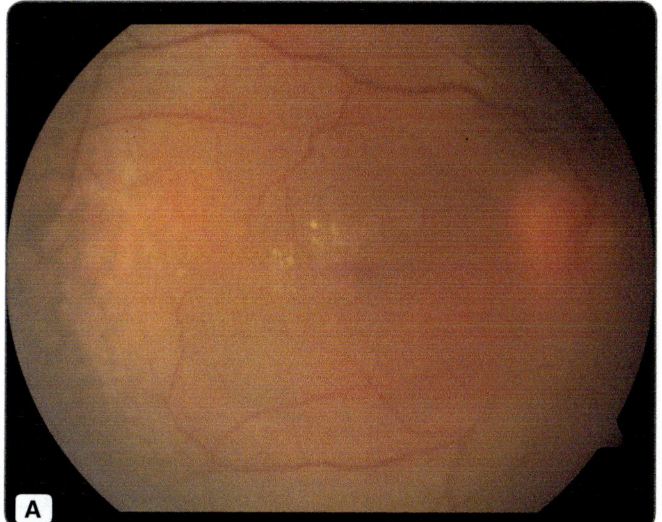

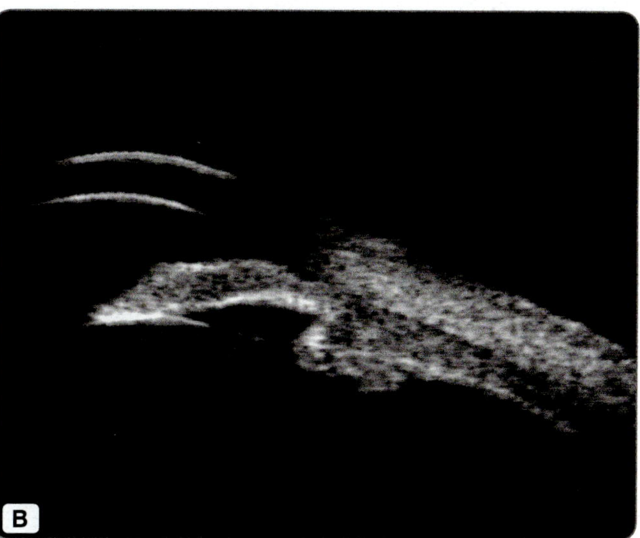

Figures 54.13A and B: Fundus photo and UBM image of a patient with VKH and angle closure. Note the hazy fundal view due to inflammation. The UBM shows the narrow angle and ciliary body edema.

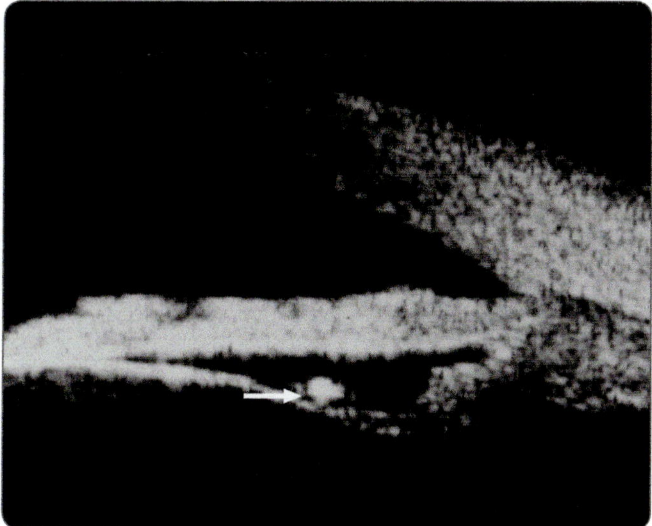

Figure 54.14: 50 MHz UBM image of an eye with recalcitrant uveitis showing a high reflective structure in the retro iridal space which proved to be a caterpillar hair.

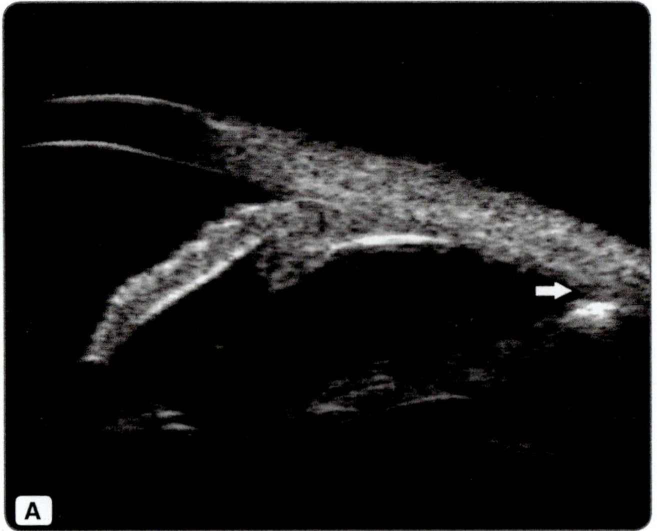

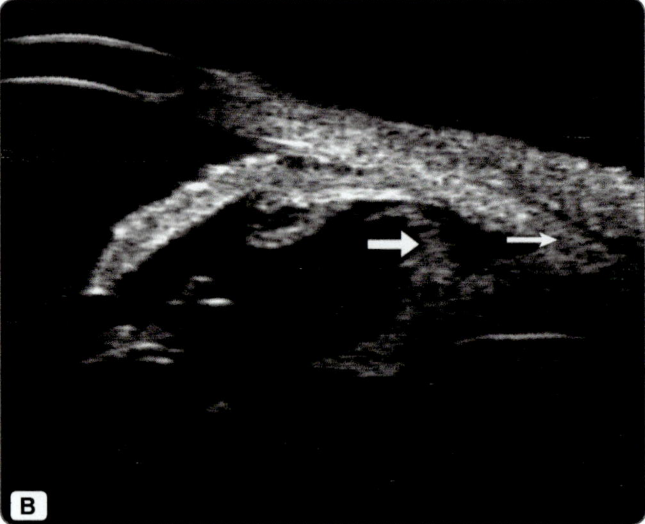

Figure 54.15A and B: 35 MHz UBM image of a young boy with suspected toxocara granuloma. Note the high reflective clump of echoes (arrow) on the peripheral retina and vitreous membranes extending from it. Figure B shows peripheral vitreous membranes (broad arrow) extending from the pars plana, causing ciliary effusion (thin arrow).

55 Ultrasound Biomicroscopy in Vitreoretinal Conditions

The ability of the UBM to image the ciliary sulcus, pars plana and peripheral retina permits evaluation of the diseases affecting these regions: traumatic zonular dehiscence, IOFB, cyclitic membrane, ROP, peripheral extent of ciliochoroidal masses, iris cysts, and fibrovascular proliferation in vitrectomized eyes or rarely, after permanent keratoprosthesis (modified osteo-odonto or Boston keratoprosthesis).
A better evaluation assists in surgical planning and thereby better outcome.

Preoperatively

- Eyes with history of trauma, in particular penetrating trauma to image retinal incarceration or anterior loop traction or IOFB
- Eyes with history of chronic uveitis to document cyclitic membrane over the ciliary body region causing hypotony, peripheral toxocara granuloma or rarely, caterpillar setae
- Aphakic eyes that have undergone penetrating keratoplasty or permanent keratoprosthesis to assess how far anteriorly the detached retina is pulled.

Postoperatively

- To study various healing patterns at the sclerotomy sites after vitreous surgery
- To identify fibrovascular ingrowth at the sclerotomy sites after vitrectomy accounting for rebleed

Significance

- To identify the possible cause of unexplained hypotony after vitreous surgery, such as sclerotomy gape, ciliary effusion, or traction
- To detect retained lens matter or IOFB in the angle particularly in eyes with persistent inflammation or rarely, iridolenticular abscess.
- Increase risk of bleeding in eyes with FVP or AHFVP. During reoperation meticulous dissection is needed to remove or cauterize these fibrovascular nails besides using adjunct steps such as additional laser, anti-VEGF drugs or silicone oil tamponade.

SPECIFIC CONDITIONS OF THE PERIPHERAL RETINA AND PARS PLANA

Retinoschisis

- Seen as a thin hyperreflective layer with an associated cavity.
- Schisis detachment is noted as a thicker more hyperreflective membrane underneath.
- May be associated with peripheral cystoid changes.
- X-linked retinoschisis may have multiple cystic cavities with bridging membranes.

Retinal Detachment

- Bilayered echogenic membrane.
- UBM helps in assessment of retinal detachment and its association vis-a-vis the ora serrata. In a case of retinal detachment, UBM demonstrates the retinal attachment at ora. In a case of dialysis, the retina is disinserted from the ora.

Associated Features which Can be Noted Include

- Pars plana epithelial tear due to trauma
- Intraretinal cyst suggestive of chronicity
- Operculum suggestive of relieved traction.
- Some other features like meridional fold, vitreoretinal tufts and par plana cysts may also be imaged.

Choroidal Hemorrhage

Irregular hyperreflective lesion extending into pars plana.

Serous Choroidal Effusion

Echolucent and is generally restricted to the suprachoroidal space.

Pars Planitis

- Thickened pars plana with overlying homogenous and moderately hyperreflective areas of snow banking.
- Secondary changes such as ciliary body traction, detachment, ciliary process atrophy can be seen.
- Detection of these changes can help in proper planning if surgery is required for complications of uveitis such as complicated cataract with chronic hypotony.
- As the pars plana is not fully developed and fibrous tissue is located close to the ciliary process, UBM is useful to identify the area anterior to the ciliary process for selecting the site of instrument entry. Particularly this is important in eyes where the anterior retinal loops are prominent and entry into the eye may result in dialysis formation.
- The anterior surgical space located between the retina and lens is not readily visible on indirect ophthalmoscopy because of the presence of retrolental membrane. The presence and configuration of the anterior surgical space decides whether a smaller gauge vitrectomy or an associated lensectomy needs to be planned.
- Disadvantage, is that the procedure would necessitate general anesthesia and may not be practical as a routine preoperative evaluation tool.

UBM TO ASSESS THE SCLEROTOMY SITES POSTOPERATIVELY

Patterns of UBM morphology at sclerotomy sites include:

- ***Well healed***: Sclerotomy site not well identified
- ***Gape***: Echolucency/very low reflective echo bridging the sclerotomy
- ***Plaque like*** area of moderate/high reflectivity at the sclerotomy with low reflective radiating strand into vitreous cavity but discontinuous from the vitreous
- ***Vitreous incarceration***: Moderate to high reflective membranous echoes extending from and continuous from the peripheral vitreous gel into the sclerotomy site
- ***Fibrovascular proliferation (FVP)*** at sclerotomy: High reflective stalk of echoes at sclerotomy with high reflective radiations extending both circumferentially and radially
- ***Anterior hyaloidal fibrovascular proliferation (AHFVP)***: High reflective membrane echoes which may or may not originate at the sclerotomy but extend all along the anterior hyaloid causing traction on the ciliary body and the peripheral retina.
  - Chances of rebleeding are higher in eyes with presence of FVP at sclerotomy sites/AHFVP
  - Presence of AHFVP necessitates extensive resurgery with membrane peeling, removal of fibrovascular proliferation and cauterization of the stump, additional laser with or without endotamponade.
- ***UBM*** has been used to study sclerotomy healing in eyes after small gauge sutureless vitrectomy. Complete closure without bleb formation is seen as early as day 1 in 20 gauge and 23 gauge 2-step sclerotomies. However, complete disappearance of the tunnel can take up to 30 days after MIVS.

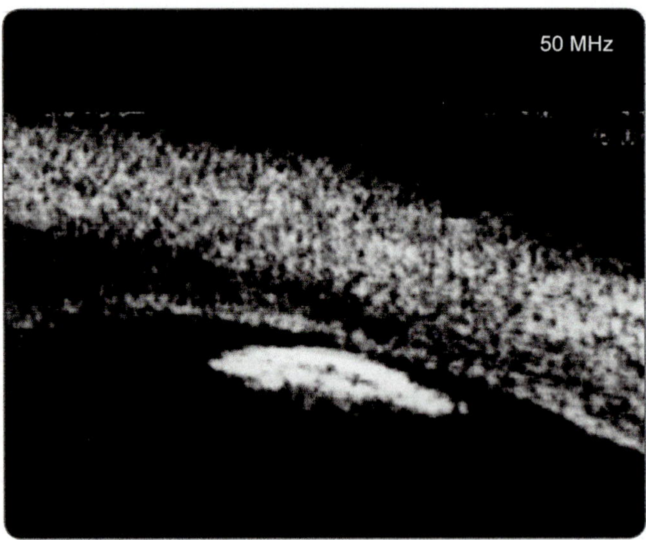

Figure 55.1: 50 MHz UBM image of an eye with a foreign body in the pars plana region.

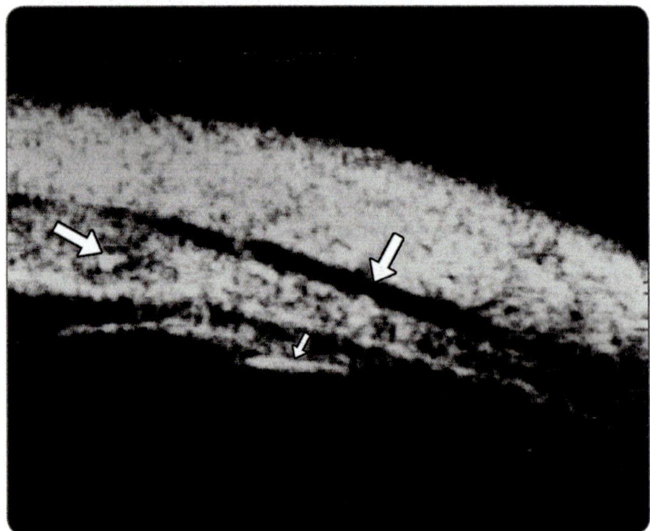

Figure 55.2: 50 MHz UBM image of an eye with severe uveitis due to intraocular caterpillar setae. The cilia are seen on the pars plana and embedded in the ciliary body. Ciliary effusion is also noted (arrow). The UBM localization of the cilia guided in their surgical removal.

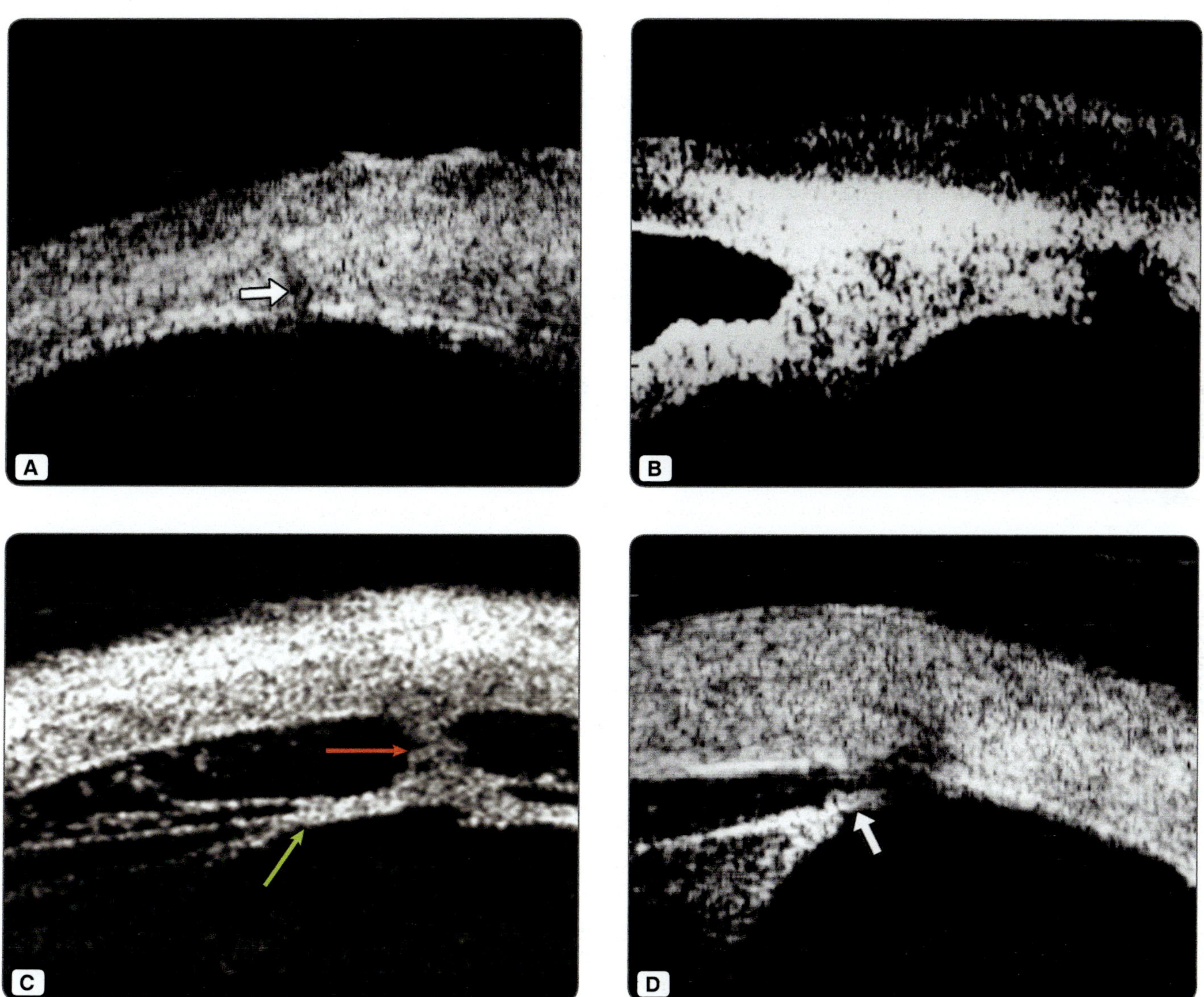

Figures 55.3A to D: 50 MHz UBM images showing healing patterns at the sclerotomies after 20, a vitrectomy for diabetic retinopathy. (A) well healed (B) gape (C) fibrovascular proliferation (D) vitreous incarceration.

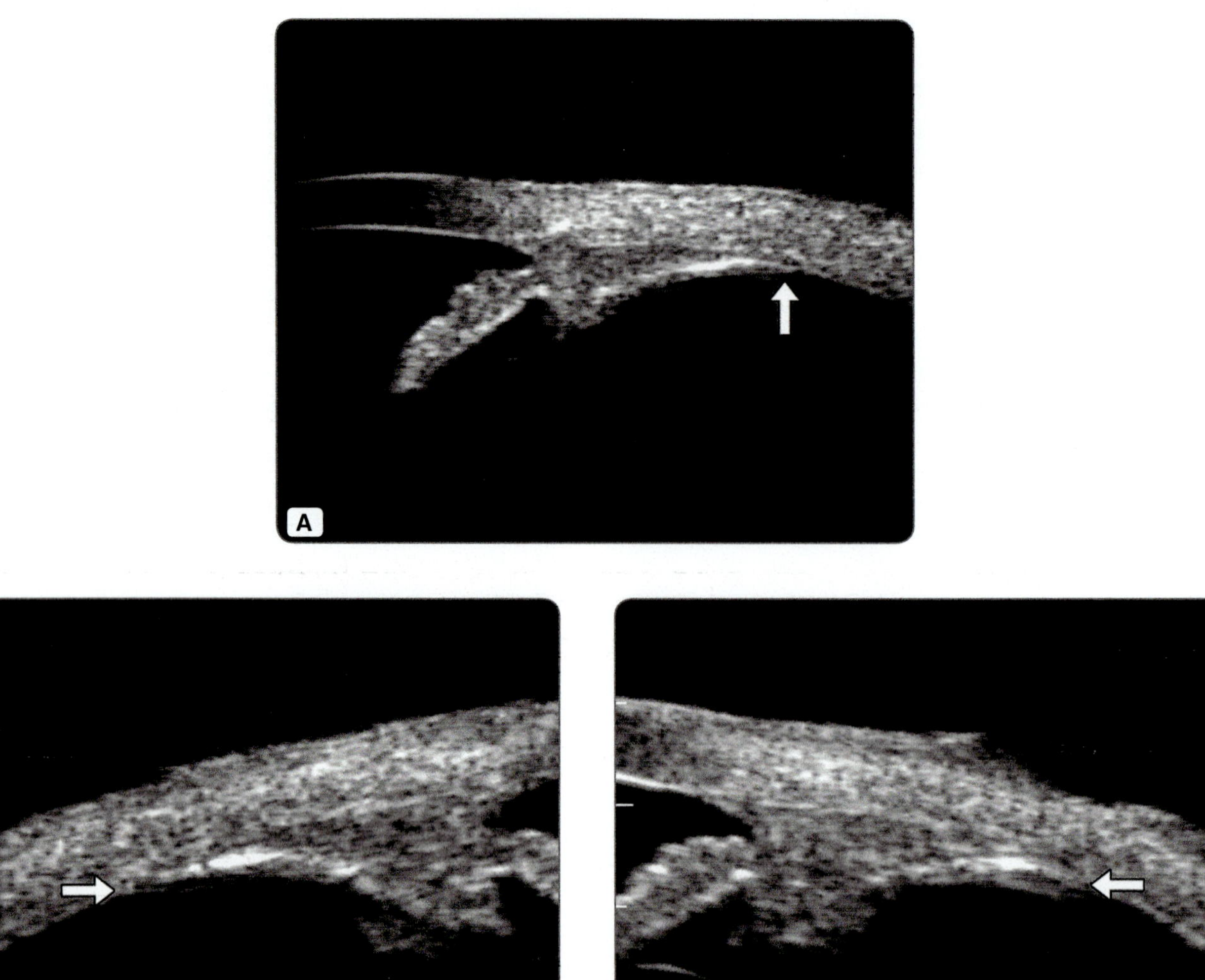

Figures 55.4A to C: UBM images of an eye that underwent 23 gauge pars plana vitrectomy 5 months earlier. Note the well-healed sclerotomies (arrow). A small irregularity at the inner lip marks the site of the sclerotomy. A vitreous strand is seen at the inner lip (B and C).

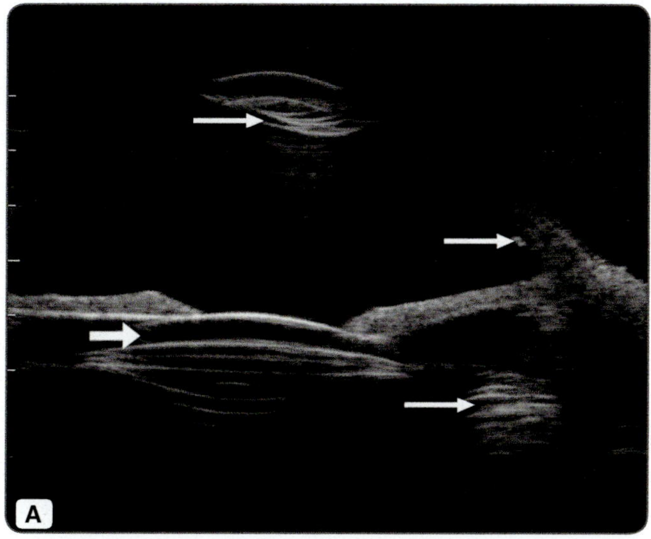

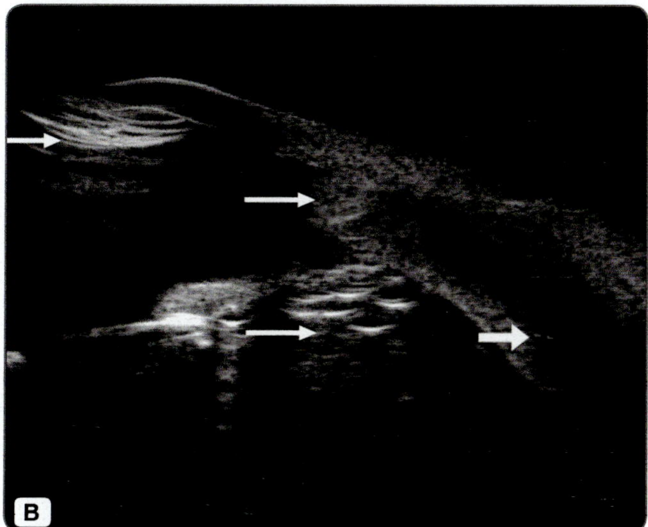

Figures 55.5A and B: UBM images of a pseudophakic eye that developed hypotony after removal of silicone oil. The arrows show the reverberations caused by residual emulsified oil droplets on the corneal endothelium, angle, between the zonules and in the sulcus. The IOL is depicted with a broad arrow (A). Figure B shows ciliary effusion (broad arrow) responsible for the hypotony.

56 Ultrasound Biomicroscopy in Trauma and Lens disorders

Clinical Evaluation

Clinical evaluation is difficult after trauma due to:

- Trauma related media opacities
- Hypotony
- Distorted anatomy.

Role of UBM (Table 56.1)

- Evaluation of zonular integrity
- Detection of foreign body
- Evaluation of hypotony
- Detection of angle structures (angle recession, cyclodialysis cleft, ciliary body status)
- Assessment of lens dislocation.

Table 56.1: UBM in trauma

Closed globe injury	Open globe injury
Zonular deficiency	Incarceration of iris tissue in wound
Lens dislocation	Peripheral anterior synechiae (PAS)
Angle recession	Angle abnormalities
Iridodialysis	Disruption of lens capsule
	Zonular deficiency
	Intraocular foreign body

Foreign Body

- Clinical detection of ocular foreign bodies after trauma can be hindered by their small size, haziness of the optical media, poor patient cooperation or hidden location.
- UBM helps in detection and accurate localization of anterior chamber foreign bodies till the pars plana and peripheral retina. Detects small, nonmetallic and anteriorly located foreign bodies which can be missed by CT scan
- IOFBs are noted as high reflective structures with posterior shadowing. Glass pieces are noted to have posterior reverberations
- The location of foreign body with respect to sclera is better compared to CT and conventional ultrasound.
- Detects associated structural damage to lens, zonules and pars plana.

Angle Recession

- Common finding following blunt ocular trauma
- Can lead to hyphema in the early stages and angle recession glaucoma later
- The ciliary body face is torn at the iris insertion, resulting in a wide-angle appearance

Cyclodialysis

- UBM is a safe, accurate and noninvasive diagnostic tool in the diagnosis of cyclodialysis clefts and is of particular use when other conventional methods of diagnosis are difficult, e.g. extreme hypotony, total hyphema
- Occasionally, partial closure of the anterior part of the cleft renders gonioscopy inconclusive. UBM can image the open posterior part of the cleft
- Typical finding is a disinsertion of the ciliary body from the scleral spur with a direct communication between the anterior chamber and suprachoroidal space
- UBM delineation of the cleft aids the precise identification and treatment thereby facilitating procedures for cleft closure and normalization of the IOP.

Post-traumatic Myopia

- Caused by shallowing of anterior chamber due to forward shifting of ciliary body, iris and lens or thickening of lens
- Due to ciliary body edema and annular ciliochoroidal effusion
- All the above features can be reliably detected by UBM.

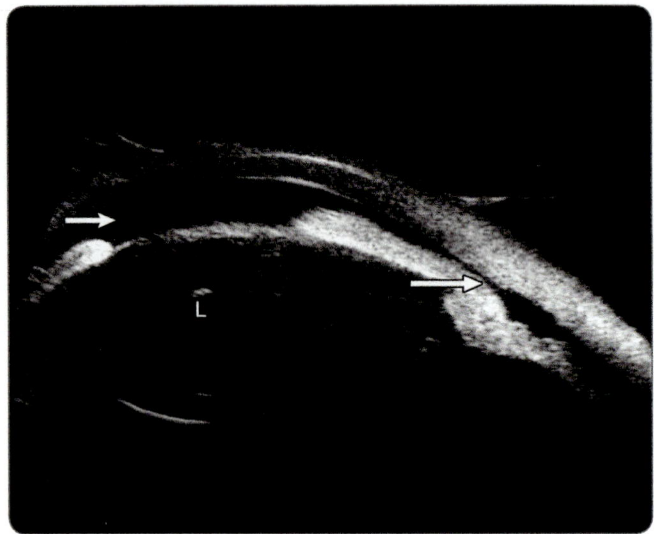

Figure 56.1A: 35 MHz UBM image of an eye with blunt trauma. Note the anterior displacement of the lens along with a cyclodialysis cleft and suprachoroidal effusion.

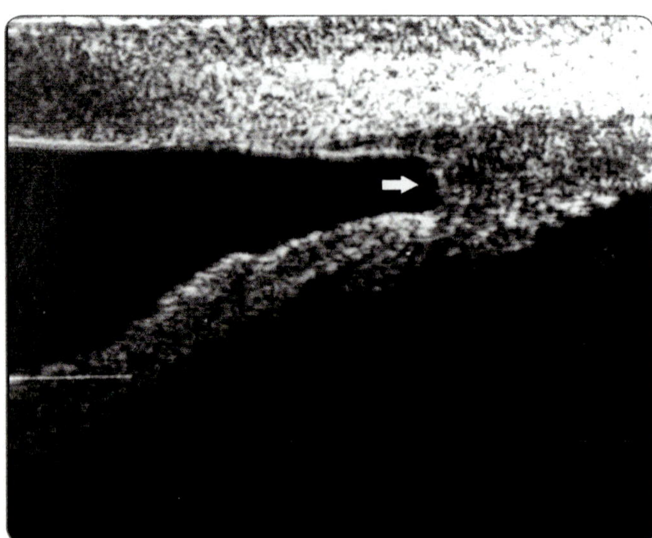

Figure 56.1B: UBM of an eye with angle recession post trauma. Note the deep anterior chamber and the tear at the base (arrow).

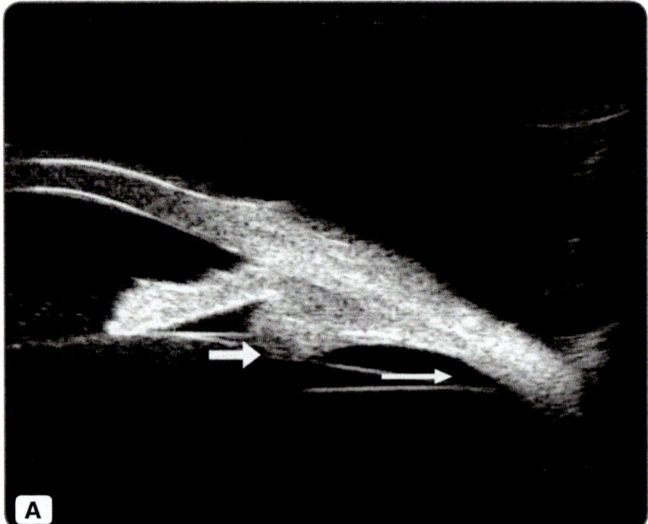

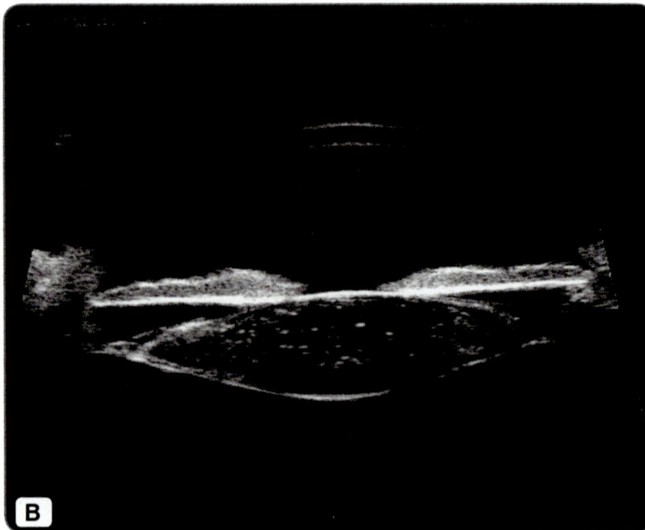

Figures 56.2A and B: UBM images showing the normal appearance of zonules and the lens equator.

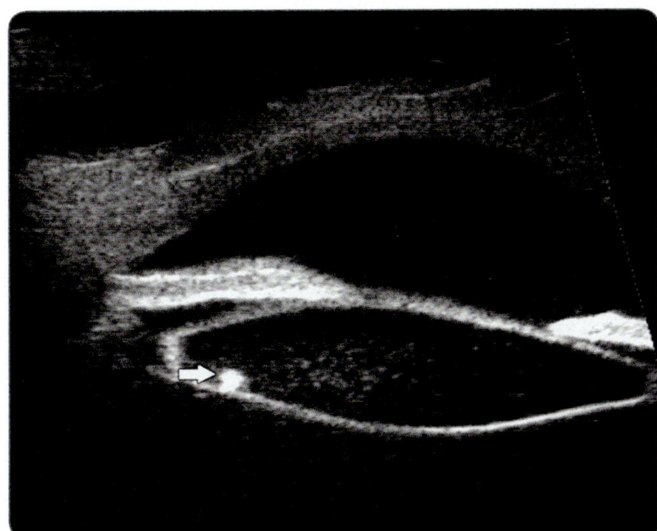

Figure 56.3: 35 MHz UBM image of an intralenticular foreign body (arrow) seen as a clump of high reflectivity within the lens. Note the intact posterior capsule. The dot echoes around the foreign body are suggestive of cataractous changes.

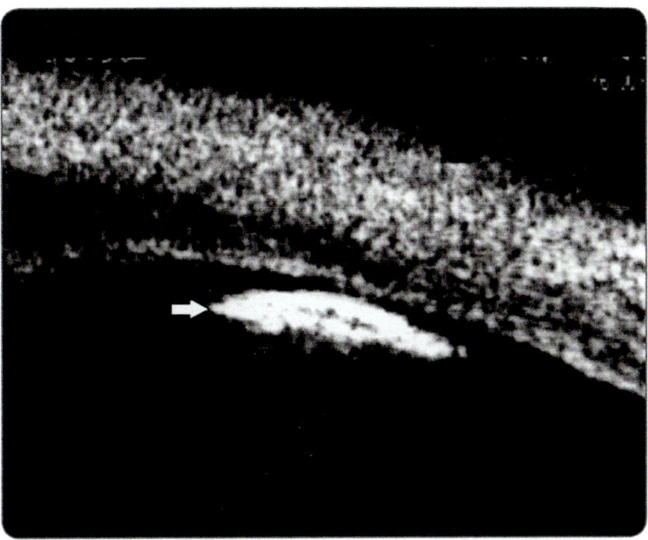

Figure 56.4: 50 MHz UBM of an eye with siderosis many years after penetrating injury. Previous investigations for IOFB proved inconclusive. UBM shows the foreign body as an area of high reflectivity over the pars plana (arrow).

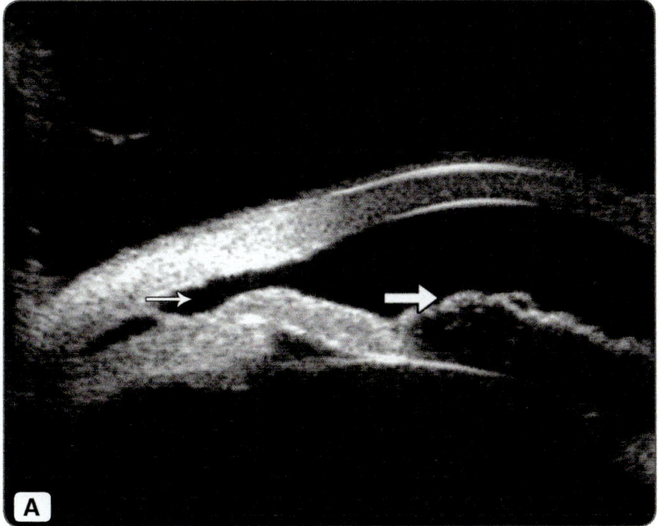

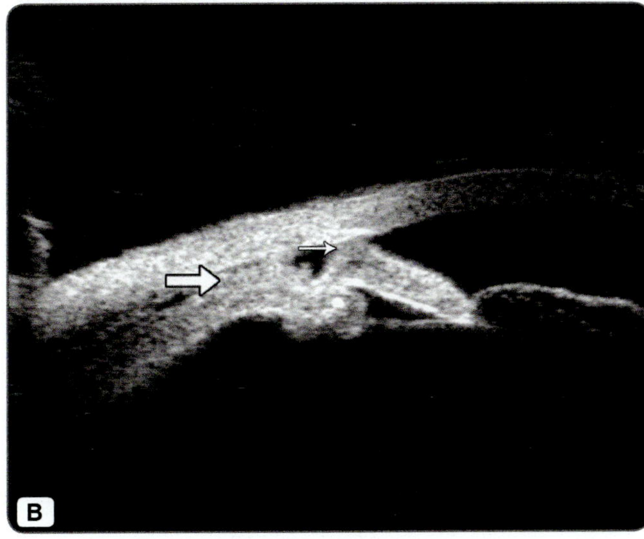

Figures 56.5A and B: 35 MHz UBM images of an eye with extreme hypotony following blunt trauma. The broad arrow points to vitreous prolapse into the anterior chamber through an area of zonular dialysis. The thin arrow shows the disinsertion of the ciliary body from the scleral spur giving rise to a communication between the anterior chamber and suprachoroidal space. There is a small residual membrane indicating choroidal tissue bridging the suprachoroidal space. Figure B shows an area where there is temporary closure of the anterior part of the cyclodialysis cleft (thin arrow) but the posterior part remains open with a slit like communication to the suprachoroidal space (broad arrow).

UBM in Disorders of the Crystalline Lens

- Both closed and open globe injury as well as certain congenital conditions, may result in damage to the crystalline lens
- This could be in the form of change in zonular tension, loss of zonules, or change in relative size of the lens to the sulcus
- Requires alteration of the surgical plan when cataract surgery is planned both in terms of type of surgery to be planned, type of lens that can be placed and haptic placement
- The normal lens equator changes to a rounded shape when there is loss of or laxity of zonules in that quadrant
- Occasionally, there is laxity of zonules all 360 degrees in which case the entire lens may take on a small, globular appearance
- In the presence of a normal or shallow anterior chamber, it may be possible to image a posterior capsular dehiscence or posterior lenticonus.

Post-cataract Surgery IOL Malpositions

- UBM is able to detect tilt, decentration and exact location of haptics in relation to the normal anatomic landmarks and possibly ascertain the cause of the symptoms
- Optic and haptic locations can be assessed accurately by looking for a strong echo at their interface plane. The most peripheral portion of the haptic defines its position in the capsular bag, ciliary sulcus, or a dislocated point
- This ability to image the IOL helps in determining whether structural changes induced by the IOL are responsible for postoperative complications such as poor quality of vision, recurrent inflammation, hyphema and glaucoma.

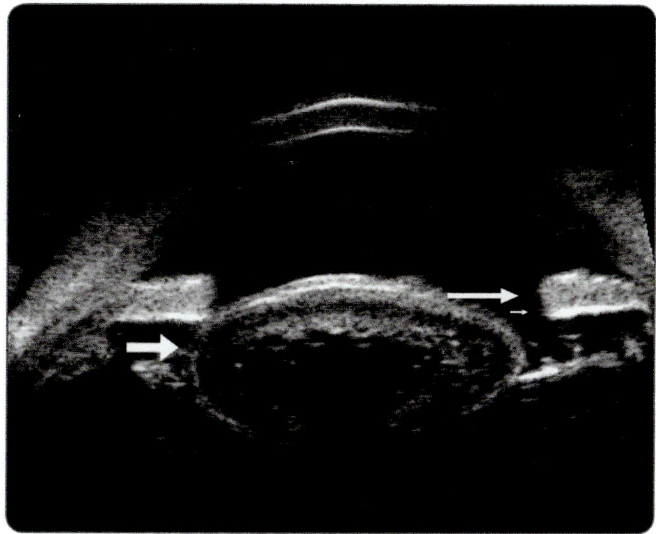

Figure 56.6: UBM images of an eye with subluxated lens following blunt trauma. Note the loss of contact of the lens with the iris. The lens equator has a variable contour with altered appearance of the zonule indicating damage to the zonular apparatus.

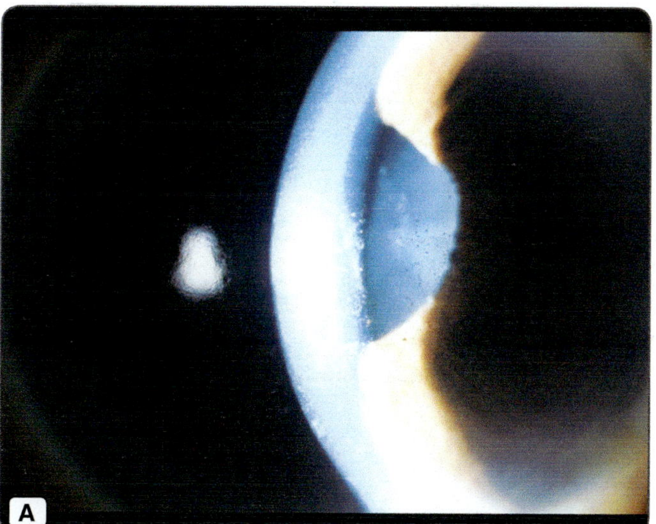

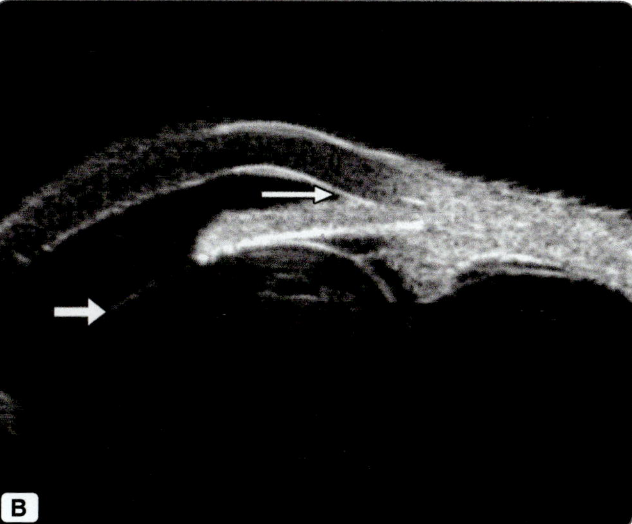

Figures 56.7A and B: Clinical photograph and UBM image of anteriorly subluxated lens in pseudoexfoliation syndrome. This occurs due to weakening of the zonular apparatus and can give rise to angle closure glaucoma.

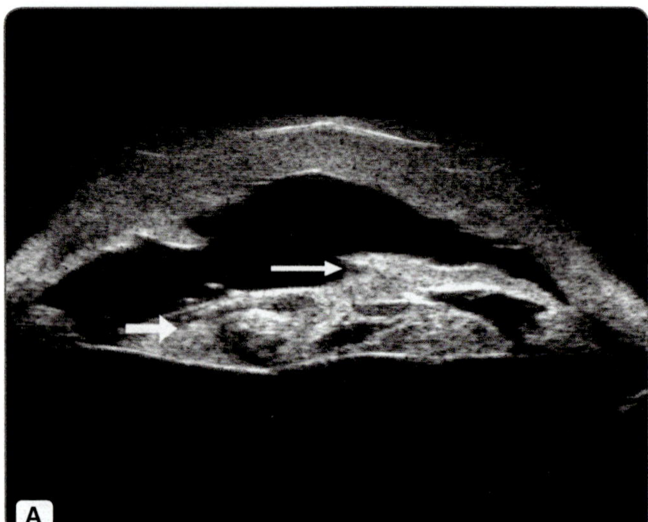

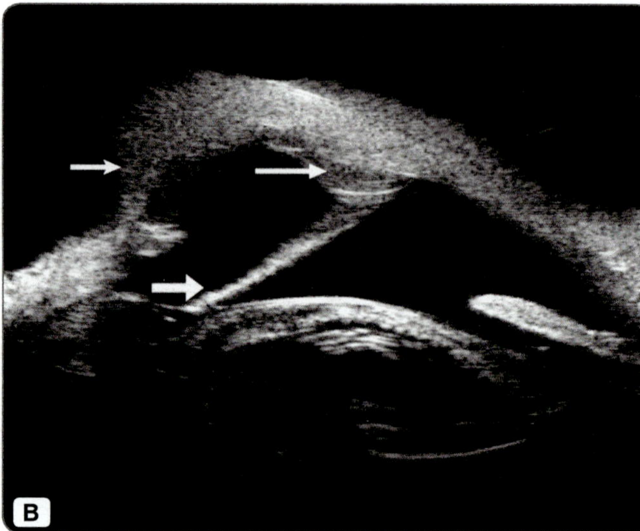

Figures 56.8A and B: UBM images of two eyes with long standing trauma and corneal changes with cataract. The corneal surfaced echoes are irregular indicative of opacification. (A) Shows a membranous cataract (broad arrow) with posterior synechia (thin arrow). (B) Shows a fibrotic band extending from the corneal wound (thin arrow) to the area of the zonules (thick arrow). A second band is seen corresponding to iris adhesion to the cornea (fine arrow).

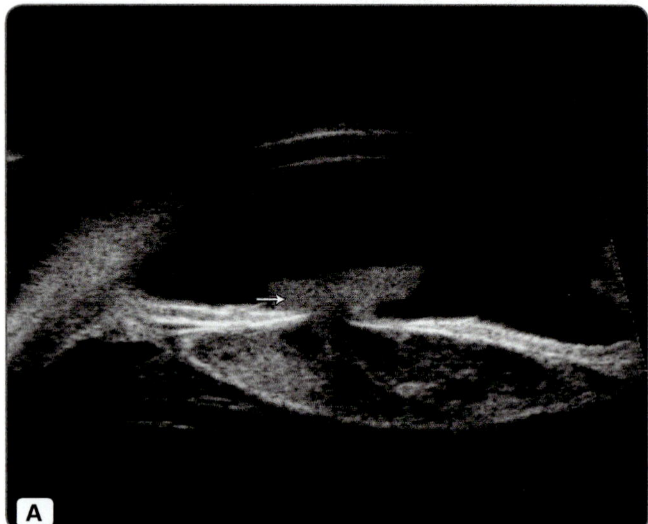

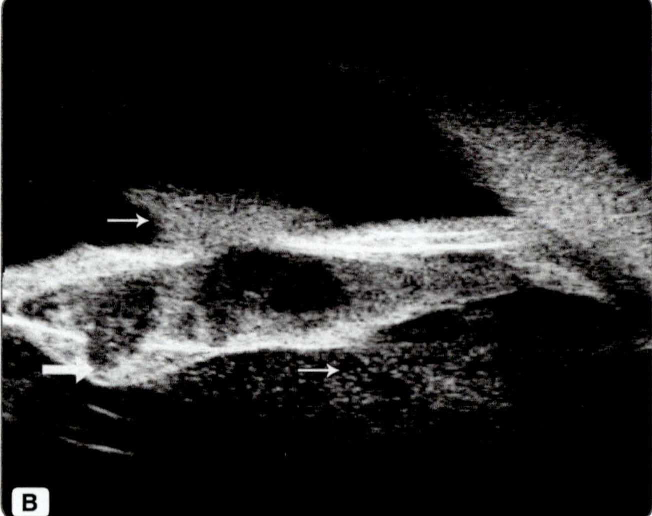

Figures 56.9A and B: UBM images of an eye with penetrating injury and traumatic cataract. The anterior (thin arrow) and posterior capsules (broad arrow) show loss of integrity with prolapse of lens matter into the anterior chamber and anterior vitreous. The fine arrow marks the associated inflammatory reaction seen as dot echoes.

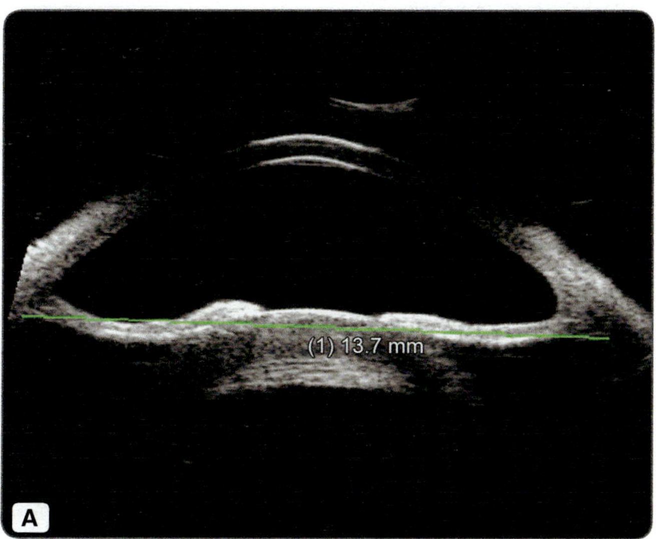

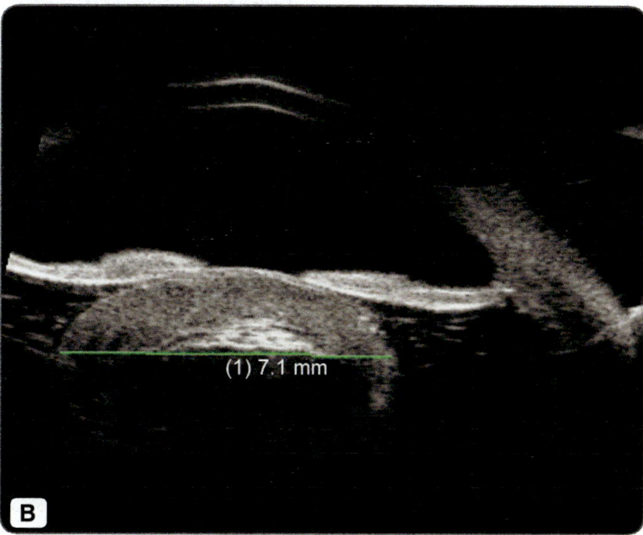

Figures 56.10A and B: UBM images of an eye with phacodonesis and cataract. Note the small globular appearing lens with a diameter of 7.1 mm and the sulcus to sulcus diameter of 13.7 mm. The increased length of zonules is clearly seen.

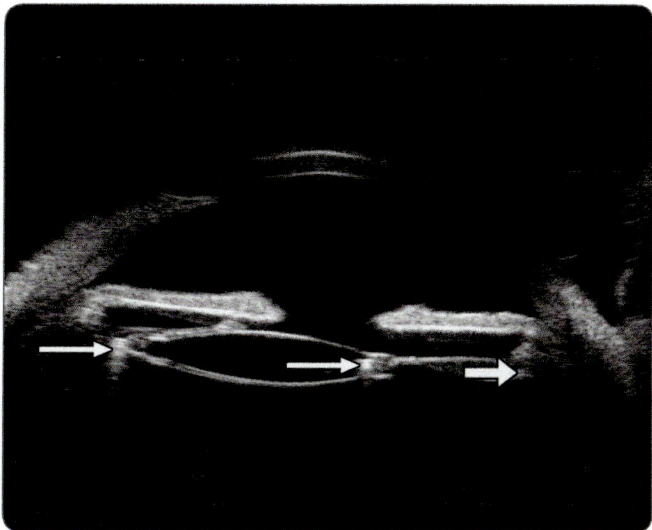

Figure 56.11: UBM image of an eye with a decentered posterior chamber IOL. Note the thin arrows marking the haptic-optic junction. The equatorial part of the capsular bag is marked with a broad arrow. The tilt of the IOL is evident from the difference in vertical distance from the posterior iris surface to the anterior surface of the IOL.

Bibliography

SECTION 1

1. Byrne SF, Green RL. Ultrasound of the eye and orbit. 2nd ed. Mosby, Inc. St. Louis. 2002.
2. Coleman DJ, Lizzi FL, Jack RL. Ultrasonography of the eye and orbit. Lea & Febiger, Philadelphia, 1977.
3. Curry III TS, Dowdey E, Murry Jr RE. Christensen's Physics of diagnostic radiology. Fourth ed. Lea & Febiger, 1990.
4. Ossoinig KC. Standardized echography: Basic principles, clinical applications and results. Int Ophthalmol Clin. 1979; 19(4):127.
5. Pavlin CJ, Foster FS. Ultrasound Biomicroscopy of the eye. Springer-Verlag, New York. 1995.
6. Scott IU, Smiddy WE, Feuer WJ, Ehlies FJ. The impact of echography on evaluation and management of posterior segment disorders. Am J Ophthalmol. 2004 Jan;137(1):24-29.
7. Silverman RH, Vinarsky E, Woods SM, Lizzi FL, Coleman DJ. The effect of transducer bandwidth on ultrasonic image characteristics. Retina. 1995;15(1):37-42.

SECTION 2

1. Allison KL, Price J, Odin LJ. Asteroid hyalosis and axial length measurement using automated biometry. Cataract Refract Surg. 1991 Mar;17(2):181-86.
2. Byrne SF, Green RL. Ultrasound of the eye and orbit. 2nd ed. Mosby, Inc. St. Louis. 2002.
3. Capeans C, Santos L, Tourino R, Otero JL, Gomez-Ulla F, Sanchez-Salorio M. Ocular echography in the prognosis of vitreous haemorrhage in type II diabetes mellitus. Int Ophthalmol. 1997-98;21(5):269-75.
4. Chu TG, Lopez PF, Cano MR, Freeman WR, Lean JS, Liggett PE, Thomas EL, Green RL. Posterior vitreoschisis. An echographic finding in proliferative diabetic retinopathy. Ophthalmology. 1996 Feb;103(2):315-22.
5. Fledelius HC, Fuchs HJ, Jensen PK, Scherfig E. Uveal effusion and ultrasonic imaging: a clinical series. Acta Ophthalmol Scand. 2002 Apr;80(2):202-10.
6. Genovesi-Ebert F, Rizzo S, Chiellini S, Di Bartolo E, Marabotti A, Nardi M. Reliability of standardized echography before vitreoretinal surgery for proliferative diabetic retinopathy. Ophthalmologica. 1998;212 Suppl 1:91-92.
7. Genovesi-Ebert F, Rizzo S, Chiellini S, Di Bartolo E, Marabotti A, Nardi M. Echographic study of the vitreoretinal interface in giant retinal tears. Ophthalmologica. 1998;212 Suppl 1:89-90.
8. Kelley LM, Walker JP, Wing GL, Raskauskas PA, Schepens CL. Ultrasound-guided cryotherapy for retinal tears in patients with vitreous hemorrhage. Ophthalmic Surg Lasers. 1997 Jul;28(7):565-69.
9. Miller DM, Benz MS, Murray TG, Dubovy SR. Intraretinal calcification and osseus metaplasia in Coats disease. Arch, Ophthalmol. 2004 Nov; (11):1710-12.
10. Nischal KK, James JN, McAllister J. The use of dynamic ultrasound B-scan to detect retinal tears in spontaneous vitreous haemorrhage. Eye. 1995;9 (Pt4):502-06.
11. Rabinowitz R, Yagev R, Shoham A, Lifshitz T. Comparison between clinical and ultrasound findings in patients with vitreous hemorrhage. Eye. 2004 Mar;18(3):253-56.

12. Rochels R, Hackelbusch R. Echographic findings in choroidal detachment. Klin Monatsbl Augenheilkd. 1983 Jan;182(1):54-56.
13. Scott IU, Flynn HW Jr, Hughes JR. Echographic evaluation of a patient with diabetes and dense vitreous hemorrhage: an avulsed retinal vessel may mimic a tractional retinal detachment. Am J Ophthalmol. 2001 Apr;131(4):515-16.
14. Wang F, Wang H, Zhuang J, Xu Q. Diagnostic value of B scan in exudative age related macular degeneration.Yan Ke Xue Bao. 1999 Dec; 15(4):233-35.
15. Wing GL, Schepens CL, Trempe CL, Weiter JJ. Serous choroidal detachment and the thickened-choroid sign detected by ultrasonography. Am J Ophthalmol. 1982 Oct;94(4):499-505.
16. Wong SC, Sampath R. Erroneous automated refraction in a case of asteroid hyalosis. J Cataract Refract Surg. 2002 Sep;28(9):1707-08.

SECTION 3

1. Byrne SF, Green RL. Ultrasound of the eye and orbit. 2nd ed. Mosby, Inc. St. Louis. 2002.
2. Kuhn F, Dante JP. Ocular Trauma, Principles and Practice. Thieme, NY, 2002.
3. Loewenstein A, McKinnon S, DiBernardo C. Echographic diagnosis of scleral fold in hypotony. Am J Ophthalmol. 1997 Aug;124(2):260-61.
4. Prakash G, Venkatesh P, Garg S. Clinical Case Notes. Unusual cause for non-detection of retained metallic foreign body on ocular ultrasonography. Clin Experiment Ophthalmol. 2005 Jun;33(3):333-34.
5. Rubsamen PE, Cousins SW, Winward KE, Byrne SF. Diagnostic ultrasound and pars plana vitrectomy in penetrating ocular trauma. Ophthalmology. 1994 May;101(5):809-14.
6. Zhang Y, Zhang J, Shi S. Determination of posterior lens capsule status in traumatic cataract with B-ultrasonography. Zhonghua Yan Ke Za Zhi. 1998 Jul;22:34(4):298-99.

SECTION 4

1. Benson WE, Shields JA, Tasman W, Crandall AS. Posterior scleritis. A cause of diagnostic confusion. Arch Ophthalmol. 1979 Aug;97(8):1482-86.
2. Biswas J et al. Posterior scleritis – Clinical profile and imaging characteristics. IJO 1998 Dec. 46(4):195-202.
3. Dacey MP, Vlencia M, Lee MR, et al. Echographic findings in infective endophthalmitis. Arch Ophthalmol. 1994; 112:1325.
4. Forster DJ, Cano MR, Green RL, Rao NA. Echographic features of VKH syndrome. Arch Ophthalmol. 1990 Oct; 108(10):1421-26.
5. Gulliani BP, Dadeya S, Malik KP, Jain DC. Bilateral cysticercosis of the optic nerve. J Neuro-ophthalmol. 2001 Sep;21(3):217-18.
6. Huang J, Wang Z, Zou L, Lin X, Luo Y, Yuan Z. Diagnostic ultrasound and pars plana vitrectomy in endophthalmitis. Yan Ke Xue Bao. 2004 Sep; 20(3):149-54.
7. Mc Cluskey PJ, et al. Posterior scleritis – Clinical features, systemic association and outcome in a large series of patients. Oph. 1999 Dec. 106(12):2380-86.

SECTION 5

1. Anteby II, Pe'er J. Need for confirmation of positioning of ruthenium plaques by postoperative B-scan ultrasonography. Ophthalmic Surg Lasers. 1996 Dec;27(12):1024-29.

2. Arevalo JF, Shields CL, Shields JA. Giant nodular posterior scleritis simulating choroidal melanoma and birdshot retinochoroidopathy. Ophthalmic Surg Lasers Imaging. 2003 Sep-Oct;34(5):403-05.
3. Augsburger JJ, Coats TD, Lauritzen K. Localized suprachoroidal hematomas. Ophthalmoscopic features, fluorescein angiography, and clinical course. Arch Ophthalmol. 1990 Jul;108(7):968-72.
4. Aylward WL, Byrne SF, Hughes JR, Hodapp EA. Dislocated lens nuclei simulating choroidal melanomas. Arch Ophthalmol. 1989 Oct;107(10):1463-64.
5. Balasubramanya R, Pushker N, Bajaj MS, Ghose S, Kashyap S, Rani A. Atypical presentations of retinoblastoma. J Pediatr Ophthalmol Strabismus. 2004 Jan-Feb;41(1):18-24.
6. Basta LL, Israel CW, Gourley RD, Acers TE. Which pathologic characteristics influence echographic patterns of retinoblastoma? Ann Ophthalmol. 1981 May;13(5):585-88.
7. Biswas J, Ahuja VK, Shanmugam MP, et al. Malignant melanoma of the choroid presenting as orbital cellulites. Report of two cases and review of literature. Orbit. 1999; 18:123.
8. Biswas J, Mani B, Shanmugam MP, Patwardhan D, Kumar KS, Badrinath SS. Retinoblastoma in adults. Report of three cases and review of the literature. Surv Ophthalmol. 2000 Mar-Apr;44(5):409-14.
9. Biswas J, Raghavendra R, Ratra V, Krishnakumar S, Gopal L, Shanmugam MP. Diffuse malignant melanoma of the choroid simulating metastatic tumour in the choroid. Indian J Ophthalmol. 2000 Jun;48(2):137-40.
10. Byrne SF, Green RL. Ultrasound of the eye and orbit. 2nd ed. Mosby, Inc. St. Louis. 2002.
11. Cham MC, Pavlin CJ. Ultrasound detection of posterior scleral bowing in young patients with choroidal melanoma. Can J Ophthalmol. 2000 Aug;35(5):263-66.
12. Collaborative Ocular Melanoma Study Group. Comparison of clinical, echographic, and histopathological measurements from eyes with medium-sized choroidal melanoma in the collaborative ocular melanoma study: COMS report no. 21. Arch Ophthalmol. 2003 Aug;121(8):1163-71.
13. Fuller DG, Snyder WB, Hutton WL, Vaiser A. Ultrasonographic features of choroidal malignant melanomas. Arch Ophthalmol. 1979 Aug;97(8):1465-72.
14. Gass JDM. Stereoscopic atlas of macular diseases—diagnosis and treatment. Vol 1, 4th edn. St Louis, Mosby, 1997.
15. Harbour JW, Murray TG, Byrne SF, Hughes JR, Gendron EK, Ehlies FJ, Markoe AM. Intraoperative echographic localization of iodine 125 episcleral radioactive plaques for posterior uveal melanoma. Retina. 1996;16(2):129-34.
16. Kaiserman I, Anteby I, Blumenthal E L, Kliers I, Pe'er J. Changes in ultrasound findings in posterior uveal melanoma after ruthenium 106 brachytherapy. Ophthalmology. 2002 Jun; 109(6): 1137-41.
17. Kielar RA. Choroidal melanoma appearing as vitreous hemorrhage. Ann Ophthalmol. 1982 May;14(5):461-64.
18. Kiratli H. Persistent intraschisis hemorrhage simulating choroidal melanoma. Jpn J Ophthalmol. 2002 Mar-Apr;46(2):222-25.
19. Lin DT, Munk PL, Maberley AL, Cooperberg PL, Rootman J. Ultrasonography of pathologically proved choroidal melanoma with a high-resolution small-parts scanner. Can J Ophthalmol. 1987 Apr;22(3):161-64.
20. Nemeth J, Szabo A, Vegh M. Unusual echographic form of retinoblastoma. Acta Ophthalmol Suppl. 1992;(204):107-09.
21. Pearce IA, Smith PA, Damato BE. Pseudocystic ultrasound appearance of choroidal melanoma. Br J Ophthalmol. 1997;81:513.
22. Read RW, Green RL, Rao NA. Metastatic adenocarcinoma with rupture through the Bruch membrane simulating a choroidal melanoma. Am J Ophthalmol. 2001 Dec;132(6):943-45.
23. Rochels R, Nover A. Small choroidal melanoma with diffuse orbital involvement detected and differentiated with standardized echography—with special reference to the reliability of sonography in predicting scleral tumoral infiltration. Ophthalmologica. 1986;192(1):39-45.
24. Seitz B, Jonas JB. Solitary retinal astrocytoma with "acoustic shadowing". Klin Monatsbl Augenheilkd. 1995 Mar;206(3):188-89.

25. Shields CL, Shields JA, Augsburger JJ. Choroidal osteoma. Surv Ophthalmol. 1988; 33:17-27.
26. Shields CL, Shields JA, Eagle RC Jr, Cangemi F. Progressive enlargement of acquired retinal astrocytoma in 2 cases. Ophthalmology. 2004 Feb;111(2):363-68.
27. Shields JA, Shields CL. Intraocular tumors: a text and atlas. WB Saunders Company 1992.
28. Shields JA, Stephens RF, Eagle RC Jr, Shields CL, De Potter P. Progressive enlargement of a circumscribed choroidal hemangioma. A clinicopathologic correlation. Arch Ophthalmol. 1992 Sep;110(9):1276-78.
29. Sneed SR, Byrne SF, Mieler WF, Nicholson DH, Olsen K, Hughes JR. Choroidal detachment associated with malignant choroidal tumors. Ophthalmology. 1991 Jun;98(6):963-70.
30. Sobottka B, Kreissig I. Ultrasonography of metastases and melanomas of the choroid. Curr Opin Ophthalmol. 1999 Jun;10(3):164-67.
31. Spraul CW, Kim D, Fineberg E, Grossniklaus HE. Mushroom-shaped choroidal hemangioma. Am J Ophthalmol. 1996 Sep; 122(3): 434-36.
32. Thijssen JM, Verbeek AM, Romijn RL, de Wolf-Rouendaal D, Oosterhuis JA. Echographic differentiation of intraocular melanomas by computer analysis. Acta Ophthalmol Suppl. 1992;(204):26-34.
33. van Gool CA, Thijssen JM, Verbeek AM. B-mode echography of choroidal melanoma; echographic and histological aspects of choroidal excavation. Int Ophthalmol. 1991 Sep;15(5):327-34.
34. Verbeek AM, Koutentakis P, Deutman AF. Circumscribed choroidal hemangioma diagnosed by ultrasonography. A retrospective analysis of 40 cases. Int Ophthalmol.1995; 19(3):185-89.
35. Verbeek AM, Thijssen JM, Cuypers MH, Brink H, Deutman AF. Echographic classification of intraocular tumors. A 15 year retrospective analysis. Acta Ophthalmol (Copenh). 1994 Aug; 72(4):416-22.
36. Verma N, Ghose S, Chandrasekhar G. Ultrasonic evaluation of retinoblastoma. Jpn J Ophthalmol. 1984;28(3):223-29.
37. Ward SD, Byrne BJ, Kincaid MC, Mann ES. Ultrasonographic evidence of a mushroom-shaped choroidal metastasis. Am J Ophthalmol. 2000 Nov;130(5):681-82.
38. Yap EY, Robertson DM, Buettner H. Scleritis as an initial manifestation of choroidal malignant melanoma. Ophthalmology. 1992 Nov;99(11):1693-97.
39. Yeo JH, Jakobiec FA, Iwamoto T, Brown R, Harrison W. Metastatic carcinoma masquerading as scleritis. Ophthalmology. 1983 Feb; 90(2):184-94.

SECTION 6

1. Byrne SF, Green RL. Ultrasound of the eye and orbit. 2nd ed. Mosby, Inc. St. Louis. 2002.
2. de Juan E Jr, Shields S, Machemer R. The role of ultrasound in the management of retinopathy of prematurity. Ophthalmology. 1988 Jul;95(7):884-88.
3. Fisher YL. Microphthalmos with communicating orbital cyst – ultrasonic diagnosis. Ophthalmology. 1978;85:1208.
4. Pulido JS, Byrne SF, Clarkson JG, Di Bernardo CL, Howe CA. Evaluation of eyes with advanced stages of retinopathy of prematurity using standardized echography. Ophthalmology. 1991 Jul;98(7):1099-1104.

SECTION 7

1. Bhavsar AR, Fong DS, Kerman B, Yoshizumi MO. Intraorbital air simulating an intraocular foreign body. Am J Ophthalmol. 1997 Jun;123(6):835-37.
2. Clemens S, Kroll P. Echographic findings following intravitreous silicone injections. Klin Monatsbl Augenheilkd. 1984 Jul; 185(1):17-21.

3. Fledelius HC, Scherfig E. The acoustic lighthouse effect. An ultrasonic response met in eyes after vitreoretinal surgery with silicone oil. Acta Ophthalmol Scand. 2000 Feb;78(1):89-92.
4. Krasnik V, Strmen P, Furdova A, Hasa J. Ultrasonic diagnosis of retinal detachment after internal tamponade with silicone oil. Cesk Slov Oftalmol. 1998;54(5):305-09.
5. Kumar A, Sharma N, Singh R. Prone position ultrasonography in silicone filled eyes. Acta Ophthalmol Scand. 1998 Aug; 76(4):496-98.
6. Kumar N, Zeldovich A, Chang A. Scleral buckle intrusion. Clin Experiment Ophthalmol. 2004 Apr; 32(2):228-29.
7. Murray DC, Durrani OM, Good P, Benson MT, Kirkby GR. Biometry of the silicone oil filled eye: II. Eye. 2002 Nov; 16(6):727-30.
8. Murray DC, Potamitis T, Good P, Kirkby GR, Benson MT. Biometry of the silicone oil filled eye. Eye. 1999 Jun, 319-24.
9. Stone RD, Irvine AR, Santos E. An ultrasonographic study of the persistence of buckle height three years after segmental sponge explants. Am J Ophthalmol. 1977 Oct; 84(4):508-13.
10. Whitacre MM. B scan ultrasonography of eyes containing intravitreal gas. Am J Ophthalmol. 1991 Sep 15; 112(3):272-77.

SECTION 8

1. Balchunas WR, Quencer RM, Byrne SF. Lacrimal gland and fossa masses: evaluation by computed tomography and A-mode echography. Radiology. 1983 Dec;149(3):751-58.
2. Boonman ZF, De Keizer RJ, Graniewski-Wijnands HS, Watson PG. Orbital myositis in scleritis. Br J Ophthalmol. 2003 Jan;87(1):38-42.
3. Brooks SE, Pillai JJ, Bains H. Orbital cellulitis due to occult orbital lymphangioma. South Med J. 2001 May;94(5):532-35.
4. Bullock JD, Goldberg SH, Connelly PJ. Orbital varix thrombosis. Ophthalmology. 1990 Feb;97(2):251-56.
5. Buys R, Abramson DH, Kitchin FD, Gottlieb F, Epstein M. Simultaneous ocular and orbital involvement from metastatic bronchogenic carcinoma. Ann Ophthalmol. 1982 Dec;14(12):1165-67, 1170-71.
6. Byrne BM, van Heuven WA, Lawton AW. Echographic characteristics of benign orbital schwannomas (neurilemomas). Am J Ophthalmol 1988 Aug 15;106(2):194-8.
7. Byrne SF, Glaser JS. Orbital tissue differentiation with standardized echography. Ophthalmology. 1983 Sep;90(9):1071-90.
8. Byrne SF, Green RL. Ultrasound of the eye and orbit. 2nd ed. Mosby, Inc. St. Louis. 2002.
9. Cappaert WE, Kiprov RV, Frank KE. Sector B-scan ultrasonographic 'hemangiomalike' pattern. Arch Ophthalmol 1983 Jan;101(1):74-77.
10. Char DH, Norman D. The use of computed tomography and ultrasonography in the evaluation of orbital masses. Surv Ophthalmol. 1982 Jul-Aug;27(1):49-63.
11. Cockerham GC, Jakobiec FA. Lymphoproliferative disorders of the ocular adnexa. Int Ophthalmol Clin. 1997;37:39-59.
12. Coleman DJ, Jack RL, Franzen LA. B-scan ultrasonography of orbital lymphangiomas. Br J Ophthalmol. 1973 Mar;57(3):193-98.
13. Coleman DJ, Jack RL, Franzen LA. High resolution B-scan ultrasonography of the orbit. II. Hemangiomas of the orbit. Arch Ophthalmol. 1972 Oct;88(4):368-74.
14. Coleman DJ, Jack RL, Franzen LA. High resolution B-scan ultrasonography of the orbit. III. Lymphomas of the orbit. Arch Ophthalmol. 1972 Oct;88(4):375-79.
15. Coleman DJ, Jack RL, Franzen LA. High resolution B-scan ultrasonography of the orbit. IV. Neurogenic tumors of the orbit. Arch Ophthalmol. 1972 Oct;88(4):380-84.

16. Coleman DJ, Lizzi FL, Jack RL. Ultrasonography of the eye and orbit. Lea & Febiger, Philadelphia, 1977.
17. Coleman DJ. Reliability of ocular and orbital diagnosis with B-scan ultrasound. II. Orbital diagnosis. Am J Ophthalmol. 1972 Oct;74(4):704-18.
18. Coupland SE, Hummel M, Stein H. Ocular adnexal lymphomas: Five case presentations and a review of the literature. Surv Ophthalmol. 2002;47:470-90.
19. Dadd M, Hughes H, Kossoff G. Ultrasonic examination of orbital vasculature. J Clin Ultrasound. 1978 Feb;6(1):36-40.
20. Davis KR, Hesselink JR, Dallow RL, Grove AS Jr. CT and ultrasound in the diagnosis of cavernous hemangioma and lymphangioma of the orbit. J Comput Tomogr. 1980 Jun;4(2):98-104.
21. Dick AD, Nangia V, Atta H. Standardised echography in the differential diagnosis of extraocular muscle enlargement. Eye. 1992;6(Pt 6):610-7.
22. Divine RD, Anderson RL. Metastatic small cell carcinoma masquerading as orbital myositis. Ophthalmic Surg. 1982 Jun;13(6):483-87.
23. Dyer J, Atkinson L. Cavernous haemangioma of the orbit. Aust NZJ Surg. 1985 Jun; 55(3):269-73.
24. Friberg TR, Grove AS Jr. Choroidal folds and refractive errors associated with orbital tumors. An analysis. Arch Ophthalmol. 1983 Apr;101(4):598-603.
25. Fujitani A, Hayasaka S. Concurrent acute angle-closure glaucoma, choroidal detachment and exudative retinal detachment in a patient with spontaneous carotid cavernous fistula. Ophthalmologica. 1995;209(4):220-22.
26. Harr DL, Quencer RM, Abrams GW. Computed tomography and ultrasound in the evaluation of orbital infection and pseudotumor. Radiology. 1982 Feb;142(2):395-401.
27. Harris GJ, Sakol PJ, Bonavolonta G, De Conciliis C. An analysis of thirty cases of orbital lymphangioma. Pathophysiologic considerations and management recommendations. Ophthalmology. 1990 Dec;97(12):1583-92.
28. Hasenfratz G, Riedel KG, Markl A, Stefani FH. Echographic findings in metastization in an extraocular muscle Klin Monatsbl Augenheilkd 1987 Sep;191(3):229-33.
29. Hasenfratz G. Orbital tumours—the importance of standardized echography. Acta Ophthalmol Suppl. 1992;(204): 82-86.
30. Jorgensen JS. An unusual case: episcleral and orbital varicose veins. Klin Monatsbl Augenheilkd. 1987 Aug;191(2): 146-48.
31. Kenney AH, Hafner JN. Ultrasonic evidence of inflammatory thickening and fluid collection within the retrobulbar fascia: the T sign. Ann Ophthalmol. 1977 Dec;9(12):1557-63.
32. Li KC, Poon PY, Hinton P, Willinsky R, Pavlin CJ, Hurwitz JJ, Buncic JR, Henkelman RM. MR imaging of orbital tumors with CT and ultrasound correlations. J Comput Assist Tomogr. 1984 Dec;8(6):1039-47.
33. Mazzeo V, Galli G, Signori D, Perri P. Spontaneous choroidal detachment and 'red-eyed shunt syndrome': two clinical entities with the same cause? Int Ophthalmol. 1985 Sep;8(3):129-38.
34. Menon SV, Shome D, Mahesh L, Subramanian N, Krishnakumar S, Biswas J, Noronha OV. Thrombosed orbital varix — a correlation between imaging studies and histopathology. Orbit. 2004 Mar;23(1):13-18.
35. Nasr AM, Huaman AM. Anterior orbital varix presenting as a lacrimal sac mucocele. Ophthal Plast Reconstr Surg. 1998 May;14(3):193-97.
36. Neudorfer M, Kessler A, Anteby I, Goldenberg D, Barak A. Co-existence of intraocular and orbital lymphoma. Acta Ophthalmol Scand. 2004 Dec;82(6):754-61.
37. Neudorfer M, Leibovitch I, Stolovitch C, Dray JP, Hermush V, Nagar H, Kessler A. Intraorbital and periorbital tumors in children—value of ultrasound and color Doppler imaging in the differential diagnosis. Am J Ophthalmol. 2004 Jun;137(6):1065-72.
38. O'Mahony D, O'Neill E. Recurrent proptotic diplopia due to congestive expansion of cavernous haemangioma with relapsing right-sided cardiac failure. Postgrad Med J. 1999 Oct;75(888):607-09.

39. Ossoinig KC. Standardized echography: Basic principles, clinical applications and results. Int Ophthalmol Clin. 1979; 19(4):127.
40. Parentin F, Borzaghini L, Perissutti P. The role of ultrasonography in the diagnosis of orbital lymphangiomas. Ophthalmologica. 2001 May-Jun;215(3):238-40.
41. Perri P, Brienza D, Mazzeo V, Ravalli L, Lubrano L, Police G, Pastena B, Rossi A. Orbital metastases: echographic findings our experience. Ophthalmologica. 1998;212 Suppl 1:82-74.
42. Rastogi A, Jain S. Fine needle aspiration biopsy in orbital lesions. Orbit. 2001 Mar;20(1):11-23.
43. Rootman J. Diseases of the orbit. JB Lippincott Co, Philadelphia. 1988.
44. Sharara N, Holden J, Wojno WH. Ocular adnexal lymphoid proliferations: clinical, histologic, flow cytometric, and molecular analysis of forty-three cases. Ophthalmology. 2003;110:1245-54.
45. Siatkowski RM, Capo H, Byrne SF, Gendron EK, Flynn JT, Munoz M, Feuer WJ. Clinical and echographic findings in idiopathic orbital myositis. Am J Ophthalmol. 1994 Sep 15;118(3):343-50.
46. Sklar EL, Quencer RM, Byrne SF, Sklar VE. Correlative study of the computed tomographic, ultrasonographic, and pathological characteristics of cavernous versus capillary hemangiomas of the orbit. J Clin Neuro-ophthalmol. 1986 Mar;6(1):14-21.
47. Slavin ML, Glaser JS. Idiopathic orbital myositis: report of six cases. Arch Ophthalmol. 1982 Aug;100(8):1261-65.
48. Spoor TC, Kennerdell JS, Dekker A, Johnson BL, Rehkopf P. Orbital fine needle aspiration biopsy with B-scan guidance. Am J Ophthalmol. 1980 Feb; 89(2):274-77.
49. Tychsen L, Tse DT, Ossoinig K, Anderson RL. Trochleitis with superior oblique myositis. Ophthalmology. 1984 Sep; 91(9):1075-79.
50. Wan WL, Cano MR, Green RL. Orbital myositis involving the oblique muscles. An echographic study. Ophthalmology. 1988 Nov;95(11):1522-8.
51. Xiao LH, Lu XZ, Wei H. Diagnosis by ultrasonography and CT scan in orbital vascular tumors and malformations. Zhonghua Yan Ke Za Zhi. 2004 Jun;40(6):364-67.
52. Yan J, Wu Z, Li Y. The differentiation of idiopathic inflammatory pseudotumor from lymphoid tumors of orbit: analysis of 319 cases. Orbit. 2004 Dec;23(4):245-54.

SECTION 9

1. Atta HR. Imaging of the optic nerve with standardised echography. Eye. 1988;2 (Pt 4):358-66.
2. Boldt HC, Byrne SF, DiBernardo C. Echographic evaluation of optic disc drusen. J Clin Neuroophthalmol. 1991 Jun;11(2):85-91.
3. Foster BS, March GA, Lucarelli MJ, Samiy N, Lessell S. Optic nerve avulsion. Arch Ophthalmol. 1997 Aug;115(8):1070.
4. Gans MS, Byrne SF, Glaser JS. Standardized A-scan echography in optic nerve disease. Arch Ophthalmol. 1987 Sep;105(9):1232-36
5. Haritoglou C, Herzum H, Ehrt O, Ossoinig KC, Kampik A. Echographic differential diagnosis of optic nerve widening. Ophthalmologe. 2002 Jul;99(7):559-65.
6. Kenney AH, Hafner JN. Ultrasonic evidence of inflammatory thickening and fluid collection within the retrobulbar fascia: the T sign. Ann Ophthalmol. 1977 Dec;9(12):1557-63.
7. Kheterpal S, Good PA, Beale DJ, Kritzinger EE. Imaging of optic disc drusen: a comparative study. Eye 1995;9 (Pt 1): 67-69.
8. Kurz-Levin MM, Landau K. A comparison of imaging techniques for diagnosing drusen of the optic nerve head. Arch Ophthalmol. 1999 Aug;117(8):1045-49.

9. McNicholas MM, Power WJ, Griffin JF. Sonography in optic disk drusen: imaging findings and role in diagnosis when funduscopic findings are normal. AJR Am J Roentgenol. 1994 Jan;162(1):161-63.
10. Neroev VV, Karlova IZ, Zaitseva OV, Kruzhkova GV, Boiko AN. Role of ultrasonic B-scanning in differential diagnosis and prognosis of the course of optic neuritis. Vestn Oftalmol. 2001 Nov-Dec;117(6):25-29.
11. Pierro L, Guarisco L, Zaganelli E, Freschi M, Brancato R. Capillary and cavernous hemangioma of the optic disc. Echographic and histological findings. Acta Ophthalmol Suppl. 1992;(204):102-06.
12. Sawhney R, Kochhar S, Gupta R, Jain R, Sood S. Traumatic optic nerve avulsion: role of ultrasonography. Eye. 2003 Jul;17(5):667-70.

SECTION 10

1. Azad R, Mannan R, et al. "Role of ultrasound biomicroscopy in management of eyes with stage 5 retinopathy of prematurity." Ophthalmic Surg Lasers Imaging. 2010;41(2):196-200.
2. Berinstein DM, Gentile RC, Sidoti PA, et al. Ultrasound biomicroscopy in anterior segment trauma. Ophthalmic Surg Lasers. 1997;28;201-7.
3. Bhende M, Agraharam SG, et al. "Ultrasound biomicroscopy of sclerotomy sites after pars plana vitrectomy for diabetic vitreous hemorrhage." Ophthalmology. 2000;107(9):1729-36.
4. Bhende M, Biswas J, et al. "Ultrasound biomicroscopy in the diagnosis and management of intraocular gnathostomiasis." Am J Ophthalmol. 2005;140(1):140-2.
5. Bhende M, Biswas J, et al. "Ultrasound biomicroscopy in the diagnosis and management of pars planitis caused by caterpillar hairs." Am J Ophthalmol. 2000;130(1):125-6.
6. Bhende M, Lekha T, Vijaya L, Gopal L, Sharma T, Parikh S. Ultrasound Biomiscroscopy in the diagnosis and management of cyclodialysis clefts. Indian J Ophthalmol 1999;47:19-23.
7. Bianciotto C, Shields CL, Guzman JM, et al. Assessment of anterior segment tumors with ultrasound biomicroscopy versus anterior segment optical coherence tomography in 200 Cases. Ophthalmology. 2011.
8. Braich PS, Chang JS, Albini TA, Schefler AC. Irido-lenticular abscess as the initial sign of Candida albicans endogenous endophthalmitis. Ophthalmic Surg Lasers Imaging. 2011 Dec 8;42 Online:e107-9. doi: 10.3928/15428877-20111201-01. PubMed PMID: 22150597.
9. Brancato R, Carassa RG. Value of ultrasound biomicroscopy for ciliodestructive procedures; Curr opin Ophthalmol. 1996;7(2);87-92.
10. Brent MH, Pavlin CJ, et al. "Ultrasound biomicroscopy in the screening of retinopathy of prematurity." Am J Ophthalmol. 2002;133(2): 284-5.
11. Conway RM, Chew T, Golchet P, Desai K, Lin S, O'Brien J. Ultrasound biomicroscopy: role in diagnosis and management in 130 consecutive patients evaluated for anterior segment tumours. Br J Ophthalmol. 2005;89:950-5.
12. Dada T, Gadia M, Sharma A, et al. Ultrasound Biomicroscopy in glaucoma; Surv Ophthalmol. 2011;56:433-450.
13. Deramo VA, Shah GK, Baumal CR, et al. Ultrasound biomicroscopy as a tool for detecting and localizing occult foreign bodies after ocular trauma. Ophthalmology 1999;106:301-5.
14. Endo S, Ishida N, Yamaguchi T. Tear in the trabecular meshwork caused by an airsoft gun. Am J Ophthalmol 2001;131: 656-7.
15. Finger PT, Tran HV, Turbin RE, Perry HD, Abramson DH, Chin K, et al. High-frequency ultrasonic evaluation of conjunctival intraepithelial neoplasia and squamous cell carcinoma. Arch Ophthalmol. 2003;121(2):168-72.
16. Gentile RC, Berinstein DM, et al. "High-resolution ultrasound biomicroscopy of the pars plana and peripheral retina." Ophthalmology 1998;105(3):478-84.

17. Giuliari GP, McGowan HD, Pavlin CJ, Heathcote JG, Simpson ER. Ultrasound biomicroscopic imaging of iris melanoma: a clinicopathologic study. Am J Ophthalmol. 2011;151:579-85 e1.

18. Guha S, Bhende M, Baskaran M, Sharma T. Role of ultrasound biomicroscopy (UBM) in the detection and localisation of anterior segment foreign bodies. Ann Acad Med Singapore 2006;35:536-45.

19. Gupta P, Gupta A, Gupta V, Singh R. Successful outcome of pars plana vitreous surgery in chronic hypotony due to uveitis. Retina. 2009 May;29(5):638-43. PubMed PMID: 19262435.

20. Gutfleisch M, Dietzel M, Heimes B, Spital G, Pauleikhoff D, Lommatzsch A. Ultrasound biomicroscopic findings of conventional and sutureless sclerotomy sites after 20-, 23-, and 25-G pars plana vitrectomy. Eye (Lond). 2010 Jul;24(7):1268-72. Epub, 2009 Dec 11. PubMed PMID: 20010792.

21. Hwang JM, Ahn K, Kim C, Park KA, Kee C. Ultrasonic biomicroscopic evaluation of cyclodialysis before and after direct cyclopexy. Arch Ophthalmol 2008;126:1222-5.

22. Ikeda N, Ikeda T, Nagata M, Mimura O. Pathogenesis of transient high myopia after blunt eye trauma. Ophthalmology 2002;109:501-7.

23. Ishikawa H, Liebmann J, Ritch R. Quantitative assessment of the anterior segment using ultrasound biomicroscopy. Curr Opin Ophthalmol. 200;11:133-9.

24. Kazakova D, Roters S, Schnyder RS, Ultrasound biomicroscopy images: long-term results after deep sclerectomy with collagen implant. Grarefes Arch Clin Exp Ophthalmol. 2002:240(11):918-23.

25. McWhae JA, Crichton AC, Rinke M. Ultrasound biomicroscopy for the assessment of zonules after ocular trauma. Ophthalmology 2003;110:1340-3.

26. Mohamed MD, Gupta M, Parsons A, Rennie IG. Ultrasound biomicroscopy in the management of melanocytoma of the ciliary body with extrascleral extension. Br J Ophthalmol. 2005;89:14-6.

27. Noble J, Qazi FA, Lakosha HK, et al. Extrascleral extension in association with ciliochoroidal melanoma: ultrasound biomicroscopy with histopathological correlation. Can J Ophthalmol. 2005;40:616-8.

28. Othman IS. Ocular surface tumors. Oman J Ophthalmol. 2009;2(1)3-14.

29. Ozdal MP, Mansour M, Deschenes J. Ultrasound biomicroscopic evaluation of the traumatized eyes. Eye (Lond) 2003;17:467-72.

30. Pavlin CJ, Foster FS. Ultrasound biomicroscopy of the eye. New York; Springer, 1995.

31. Pavlin CJ, Harasiewicz H, Eng P, et al. Clinical uses of ultrasound biomicroscopy. Ophthalmology. 1991;98:287-95.

32. Pavlin CJ, Vasquez LM, Lee R, Simpson ER, Ahmed, II. Anterior segment optical coherence tomography and ultrasound biomicroscopy in the imaging of anterior segment tumors. Am J Ophthalmol. 2009;147:214-9 e2.

33. Potash SD, Tello C, Liebmann J, et al. Ultrasound biomicroscopy in pigment dispersion syndrome. Ophthalmology. 1994;101;332-9.

34. Shields JA, Shields CL, Mercado G, Gunduz K, Eagle RC, Jr. Adenoma of the iris pigment epithelium: a report of 20 cases: the 1998 Pan-American Lecture. Arch Ophthalmol. 1999;117:736-41.

35. Sihota R, Kumar S, Gupta V, et al. Early predictors of traumatic glaucoma after closed globe injury: trabecular pigmentation, widened angle recess, and higher baseline intraocular pressure. Arch Ophthalmol 2008;126:921-6.

36. Silverman RH. High-resolution ultrasound imaging of the eye—a review. Clin Experiment Ophthalmol 2009;37:54-67.

37. Tello C, Liebmann J, Potash SD, et al. Measurement of ultrasound biomicroscopy images; intraobserver and interobserver reliability; Invest Ophthalmol Vis Sci. 1994;35;3549-52.

38. Tello C, Tran HV, Liebermann J, Ritch R. Angle closure; classification, concepts, and the role of ultrasound biomicroscopy in diagnosis and management. Seminars in Ophthalmology. 2002;17:69-78.

39. Vasquez LM, Pavlin CJ, McGowan H, Yucel Y, Simpson ER. Ring melanoma of the ciliary body: clinical and ultrasound biomicroscopic characteristics. Can J Ophthalmol 2008;43:229-33.

40. Weisbrod DJ, Pavlin CJ, Emara K, Mandell MA, McWhae J, Simpson ER. Small ciliary body tumors: ultrasound biomicroscopic assessment and follow-up of 42 patients. Am J Ophthalmol. 2006;141:622-8.
41. Weisbrod DJ, Pavlin CJ, Xu W, Simpson ER. Long-term follow-up of 42 patients with small ciliary body tumors with ultrasound biomicroscopy. Am J Ophthalmol. 2010;149:616-22.
42. You C, Wu X, Ying L, Xie L. Ultrasound biomicroscopy imaging of sclerotomy in children with cataract undergoing 25-gauge sutureless pars plana anterior vitrectomy. Eur J Ophthalmol. 2010 Nov-Dec;20(6):1053-8. PubMed PMID: 20491045.
43. Zhang Y, Wu Q, Zhang M, et al. Evaluating subconjunctival bleb function after trabeculectomy using slit-lamp optical coherence tomography and ultrasound biomicroscopy.Chin Med J (Engl). 2008;121(14):1274-9.

Index

Page numbers followed by *f* refer to figure and *t* refer to table, respectively.

D

E

F

G

H

I

L

M

Q

R

S

T

U

V

W

Z